Obstetrics and Gynaecology

Murdoch G. Elder
Imperial College School of Medicine, UK

Obstetrics and Gynaecology

Clinical and Basic Science Aspects

ICP
Imperial College Press

Published by

Imperial College Press
57 Shelton Street
Covent Garden
London WC2H 9HE

Distributed by

World Scientific Publishing Co. Pte. Ltd.
P O Box 128, Farrer Road, Singapore 912805
USA office: Suite 1B, 1060 Main Street, River Edge, NJ 07661
UK office: 57 Shelton Street, Covent Garden, London WC2H 9HE

British Library Cataloguing-in-Publication Data
A catalogue record for this book is available from the British Library.

OBSTETRICS AND GYNAECOLOGY: CLINICAL AND BASIC SCIENCE ASPECTS

ISBN 1-86094-276-8
ISBN 1-86094-279-2 (pbk)

Printed in Singapore by Mainland Press

Preface

Why another undergraduate book in Obstetrics and Gynaecology? The older books have started from the basis of didactic teaching of clinical management while their editors have tried to keep pace with the changes in the specialty. There is no emphasis on the underlying biochemistry and pathogenesis of the various clinical conditions. Rather, it is a concentration on clinical diagnosis and management.

Medicine in general has changed rapidly and this will continue for the foreseeable future. Obstetrics and Gynaecology has been at the forefront of these developments. Some examples are a trend away from gynaecological surgery towards other forms of management; continuing development of sub-specialties of fetal-maternal medicine, reproductive medicine, and gynaecological oncology; women with serious medical disorders can now have children when in the past this was impossible or very dangerous. These changes are driven by the need and ability to understand at least some of the basic science behind the clinical problems. It is important that medical students ask questions as to what is going on at a molecular, cellular, and tissue level and to then understand what can or can't be done and why. This book starts from this premise and attempts to give the reader a broader and more scientific perspective than most of the current undergraduate books.

It contains more information than the standard undergraduate needs to pass his exam in O & G but hopefully it will begin to enthuse some students towards a specialty that is increasingly diverse and at the forefront of so many aspects of human biology. It will also be invaluable to junior doctors in the specialty who will find it especially useful for postgraduate studies such as the MRCOG. This book will be a very valuable addition between the basic undergraduate textbooks and the very large and very comprehensive postgraduate books and as such is recommended to the junior specialist in training.

Contributors

M M Afnan FRCOG
Consultant Obstetrician and Gynaecologist
Director of the Assisted Conception Unit
Birmingham Women's Hospital
Metchley Park Road
Edgbaston, Birmingham B15 2TG

Katy Clifford MA MD MRCOG
Consultant in Obstetrics and Gynaecology
St Mary's Hospital
London W2 1PG

C Kotzias MRCOG
Specialist Registrar in Obstetrics and Gynaecology
Lister Hospital
Stevenage
Herts SG1 4AB

Michael Darling FRCOG
Consultant Obstetrician and Gynaecologist
Rotunda Hospital
Dublin

D Keith Edmonds FRCOG FRANZCOG
Consultant Obstetrician and Gynaecologist
Queen Charlotte's and Chelsea Hospital
Du Cane Road
London W12 0HS

M G Elder DSc MD FRCS FRCOG
Emeritus Professor of Obstetrics and Gynaecology
Easter Calzeat
Broughton
Biggar
ML12 6HQ

H El-Refaey MD MRCOG
Senior Lecturer and Consultant in Obstetrics and Gynaecology
Imperial College School of Medicine
Chelsea and Westminster Hospitals
369 Fulham Road
London SW10 9NH

Jacqueline Feld MSc BA CQSW
Infertility Counsellor
IVF Unit
Hammersmith Hospital
Du Cane Road
London W12 0HS

David Harding PhD MRCP
Lecturer in Neonatal Medicine
University of Bristol Medical School
St Michael's Hospital
Bristol BS2 8EG

D F Hawkins DSc FRCOG FACOG
Emeritus Professor of Obstetric Therapeutics
University of London
Blundell Lodge
Blundell Lane
Cobham
Surrey

Jenny Higham MD MRCOG MFFP
Senior Lecturer in Obstetrics and Gynaecology
Imperial College School of Medicine
St Mary's Campus
Norfolk Place
London W2

Pam Johnson MD MRCGP MRCOG
Senior Lecturer and Honorary Consultant Obstetrician
Imperial College School of Medicine
Queen Charlotte's and Chelsea Hospital
Du Cane Road
London W12 0HS

R Khan BSc MBBS
Research Fellow
Imperial College School of Medicine
Chelsea and Westminster Hospital
369 Fulham Road
London SW10 9NH

Lennox Kane BA MD FRCOG
Consultant Gynaecologist at St Albans and Hemel Hempstead Hospitals
St Albans City Hospital
Waverley Road
St Albans
Herts AL3 5PN

R J Lilford PhD FRCOG FRCP MFPHM
Director of Research and Development
NHS Executive
West Midlands Regional Office
142 Hagley Road
Birmingham B16 9PA

K B Lim MRCOG
Consultant Obstetrician and Gynaecologist
Southend Hospital
Southend
Essex

Naomi Low-Beer MBBS
Clinical Research Fellow
Imperial College School of Medicine
St Mary's Hospital and Chelsea and Westminster Hospital
London

Angus McIndoe PhD FRCS MRCOG
Consultant in Gynaecological Oncology
Hammersmith Hospitals Trust
Du Cane Road
London W12 0HS

Norman A McWhinney BA FRCS(Ed) FRCOG
Consultant Obstetrician and Gynaecologist
St Helier Hospital
Carlshalton

R A Margara MD
Reader in Fertility Studies
Imperial College School of Medicine
Hammersmith Campus
Du Cane Road
London W12 0NN

B Ola FWACS MRCOG
Assisted Conception Unit
Birmingham Women's Hospital
Metchley Park Road
Edgbaston, Birmingham B15 2TG

Leslie Regan MD FRCOG
Professor of Obstetrics and Gynaecology
Imperial College School of Medicine
St Mary's Campus
Norfolk Place
London W2 1PG

Gill Rose MD MRCOG
Consultant Gynaecologist
Queen Charlotte's and Chelsea Hospital
Du Cane Road
London W12 0HS

J Richard Smith MD MRCOG
Consultant and Honorary Senior Lecturer in Obstetrics and Gynaecology
Imperial College School of Medicine
Chelsea and Westminster Hospital
369 Fulham Road
London SW10 9NH

W S Soutter MD MSc FRCOG
Reader in Gynaecological Oncology
Imperial College School of Medicine
Hammersmith Campus
Du Cane Road
London W12 0NN

P J Steer BSc MD FRCOG
Professor of Obstetrics and Gynaecology
Imperial College School of Medicine
Chelsea and Westminster Hospital
369 Fulham Road
London SW10 9NH

G H Trew MRCOG
Consultant in Reproductive Medicine
and Surgery
Hammersmith Hospital
Honorary Senior Lecturer
Imperial College School of Medicine
Du Cane Road
London W12 0HS

Beverley Webb FRCS(Eng) FRCOG
Consultant Obstetrician and Gynaecologist
The Lister Hospital
Stevenage
Herts SG1 4AB

Andrew Whitelaw MA MD MRCP FRCPCH
Professor of Neonatal Medicine
University of Bristol
Southmead Hospital
Bristol BS10 5NB

Gordon Williams MS FRCS FRCS(Ed)
Consultant Urological Surgeon
Hammersmith Hospital
Du Cane Road
London W12 0HS

Contents

1

Approach to the Patient

Patients approach a doctor in the hope of a cure for their ills. Diagnosis is the first stage of the process, and is both a science and an art. The science is the reasoning which promotes the correct conclusions based on the facts assimilated from a good history and clinical examination, including the assessment of both positive and negative findings. The art is the skilful collection of these facts, and is learned and mastered only with much practice. All diagnoses are based on the three firm foundations of history, physical signs and the results of necessary investigations. The first two of these will be considered in more detail.

THE HISTORY

History taking is of paramount importance. The ability to obtain a good history is partly based on instruction, partly initiative and partly acquired by experience.

It is essential to hear the woman's story in order to learn the exact nature of her complaints. Each individual symptom should be dealt with in detail; the date and mode of onset, subsequent progression, exacerbating and relieving factors, previous treatment, etc. The symptom of pain must always be carefully considered and its site, nature, severity, duration, frequency, periodicity, radiation and relation to menses, micturition, defaecation and fetal movements, should all be recorded. She should not be allowed to leapfrog from one symptom to another before a complete account of each individual symptom has been rendered. Leading questions should be kept to a minimum, but may be necessary to elucidate the full story in a logical pattern. Direct questions may yield important information quickly, but should not suggest an answer. Once the voluntary history is complete, direct questioning is used for the assessment of the remaining systems and the student should be familiar with the essential questions for each system.

Having dealt with the general aspects of history taking which are applicable to any specialty, the woman with gynaecological symptoms will now be specifically considered.

History of the Gynaecological Patient

Many women of differing age, social class and culture find it difficult to discuss gynaecological and sexual matters. The doctor must adopt a tactful, understanding and unhurried approach to gain the full confidence of the patient. It is often best to obtain general information first such as age, marital status, number of children, obstetric, family and social history, to allow the woman time to settle. She should then be encouraged to tell the story in her own words with gentle guidance to encourage the taciturn and direct the garrulous. As with all clinical documentation, the details should be recorded in a clear, precise and legible manner.

Presenting complaint(s)

Often there are two or more symptoms and these should be enumerated to allow the doctor a clear picture in his/her mind of the facts which must subsequently be recorded in more detail. It is useful to note how long the symptoms have been present and record them in the woman's own words: (1) heavy periods for

6 months; (2) vaginal discharge for 3 years; (3) heavy feeling down below for 5 years. It is often of value to note which symptom is the most troublesome.

History of presenting complaints. Each symptom enumerated above should now be dealt with in detail and interrelated to each other and/or bodily functions where appropriate, e.g. pelvic pain and menstruation; uterovaginal prolapse and urinary symptoms. The features of any pain should be recorded as previously outlined.

Remaining gynaecological history

The following points should also be elicited as they will cast further light on the presenting symptoms or will bring out other possible problems:

1. Date of onset of last menstrual period, if not already noted.
2. Duration of menstruation.
3. Amount of blood loss — this may be recorded in terms of heavy, average or light, or by the amount of protection required.
4. The presence or absence of clots in the menstrual loss.
5. Length and regularity of menstrual cycle.
6. Age of menarche.
7. Age of menopause.
8. Dysmenorrhoea (pelvic pain associated with menstruation) — premenstrual, menstrual or both; site of the discomfort; severity; radiation; associated nausea; previous treatment.
9. Breast discomfort associated with menstruation.
10. Intermenstrual bleeding.
11. Postcoital bleeding.
12. Dyspareunia (pain on intercourse) — superficial (i.e. discomfort at the introitus or vaginal walls) or deep (i.e. pelvic pain experienced on full penetration of the penis).
13. Vaginal discharge — timing in relation to menstrual cycle; duration; character; amount; odour; irritation.
14. Pruritus — vulvul irritation or itch.
15. Climacteric symptoms — hot flushes; dry vagina; irritability; insomnia; etc.
16. Contraception.
17. Urinary symptoms — frequency; dysuria; incontinence — stress or urge; nocturia; haematuria.
18. Bowel function — frequency; consistency and colour of stool; straining, pain on defaecation; blood or mucus per rectum.

PHYSICAL EXAMINATION

The thought of a physical examination is likely to cause anxiety due to embarrassment and the fear of discomfort or pain. This is especially true for pelvic examination which is always performed last. The obstetrician/gynaecologist should approach the examination of the woman in a reassuring and gentle manner, remembering that she is not simply a carrier of pelvic organs but an entire human entity. An assessment of her general physical condition is required to provide valuable information as a background to her local pelvic condition. It is often of value to explain what is being done at each stage of the examination and to give a warning of anything which might be unexpected, such as pressure of the examining hand on the abdomen, the temperature of the bell of the stethoscope, vaginal speculum, etc.

An attendant nurse is essential during the examination. She can reassure the woman and, by allaying her fears, help her to relax. The nurse can also verify the correctness of the examination should the need ever arise in a medico-legal inquiry.

Ideally, the woman should be shown into an examination room. If this is not possible, she is left with the nurse to prepare for examination, which includes removal of all her clothes, although for antenatal appointments, this in unnecessary. A gown allowing easy access for examination should be available or she should be placed supine on a couch with two sheets covering her, one across the upper half of her body and the other across the lower half. This allows exposure of the part of the body to be examined, yet maintains a degree of modesty.

The order of examination will vary from one doctor to another, and the student should decide for him/herself which system to adopt and adhere to it thereafter. An orderly, logical approach will avoid missing important signs. On the other hand, the methods for elucidating clinical signs have stood the test of time and the student should be attentive in learning the correct methods from his/her seniors. Inspection, touching, palpation and hearing are the cornerstones of physical examination. Leonardo's motto was *Sapere vedere* — learn to see things. As the woman walks into the examination room, an impression of height, weight, gait and body posture (kyphosis, lordosis) can be gained.

Examination of Head and Neck

The woman's facies, e.g. pallid, florid, cyanotic, is noted and the mucous membranes checked for the presence of anaemia. The eyes are observed for any suggestion of exophthalmos and any change in colour of the sclera. Any loss of normal texture, brittleness or excessive dryness of the hair should also be recorded. Lymphadenopathy is always important and the glands of the supraclavicular region, anterior and posterior triangles of the neck are examined. The thyroid gland is gently examined for asymmetry, enlargement or other irregularities, remembering that a slight, diffuse enlargement may occur in pregnancy. The tongue, tonsils and teeth require inspection, the latter being particularly important in pregnancy as any caries present will almost certainly worsen as pregnancy advances.

Examination of the Breasts

Breast examination is important in both obstetric and gynaecological examinations and should never be omitted. The breasts are first inspected with the patient sitting upright, her arms by her side. Their size, shape and position of the nipples are compared. Prominent veins, retracted nipples, discharge from the nipples and prominent Montgomery's tubercles in the primary areola are noted. The woman is then asked to raise her arms above her head and the features outlined above are again checked. Any indentation or bulge in the contour of the breast or retraction of a nipple may indicate underlying pathology. The axillae are next examined, but this is only satisfactorily achieved if the pectoral muscles are relaxed. The woman should rest her forearm on the examiner's arm while the axilla is carefully palpated. She is then placed supine and the breast gently palpated with the flat portion of the fingers. This should be done systematically, starting with the upper inner quadrant and finishing with the upper outer quadrant. Finally, the nipple should be palpated and gently squeezed to release any secretion which might be present.

Examination of the Abdomen

In order to examine the abdomen properly, both the woman and the examiner must adopt the correct position. The former should be placed supine, as flat as is tolerable, with her arms at her sides. The examiner should be seated or on one knee, so that even pressure may be applied with the flat of the hand. The abdomen should be examined in sequence and is best divided into nine imaginary portions (Fig. 1.1). The sequence for the examination is inspection, palpation, percussion and auscultation.

Inspection allows assessment of the condition of the abdominal wall, and size and contour of the abdomen. Previous surgical wounds are noted as are any motile phenomena, such as movement with respiration, visible peristalsis or pulsation.

Palpation is performed gently, noting the presence of superficial or deep tenderness and any rigidity of the abdominal wall. If pain is a presenting symptom, palpation should commence in the diagonally opposite region, so that the area of pain is palpated last. The viscera should be checked for enlargement of

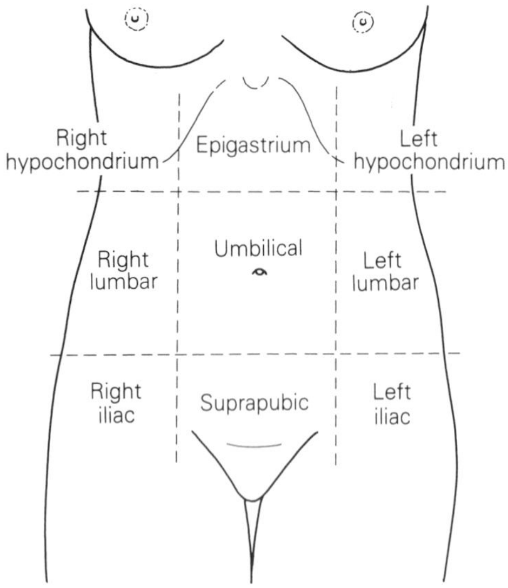

Fig. 1.1 *The regions of the abdomen.*

liver, spleen and kidneys, and abnormal masses are noted, specifically those arising from the pelvic viscera — bladder, uterus, ovaries. Site, size, shape, contour, consistency and mobility are recorded. Hernial orifices should be checked routinely.

Percussion may add confirmatory information in the case of enlarged viscera and tumours and is the only technique in most patients for establishing the presence of ascites.

Auscultation is used to confirm the presence and nature of bowel sounds.

It should be emphasised that abdominal examination is an essential part of the gynaecological examination and should never be omitted. Occasionally, a tumour arising from a pelvic viscus is only palpable per abdomen and it is not unknown for uterovaginal prolapse to be caused by the raised intra-abdominal pressure of ascites or an ovarian cyst.

The foregoing is of necessity a superficial and incomplete account of the general medical examination of a patient. However, the obstetrician/gynaecologist must be capable of performing such an examination correctly. Coexisting conditions will affect his/her patient throughout pregnancy or influence the anaesthetic and postoperative risks of the woman requiring surgery for a gynaecological complaint. No one can be an expert at everything, but a proper examination allows for appropriate referral for advice. Examination of the respiratory, cardiovascular and nervous systems have been omitted and reference should be made to a textbook of medicine. The importance of neurological examination must never be forgotten. The woman presenting to the gynaecological clinic with urinary incontinence and is found to have saddle anaesthesia is most unlikely to have a gynaecological cause for her complaint.

The Pelvic Examination

As previously mentioned, the pelvic examination must be approached by the examiner in a reassuring and gentle manner in order to allow the woman to relax as much as possible. Adequate palpation of the pelvic viscera is extremely difficult, if not impossible, when the abdominal and pelvic musculature is contracted.

There are several positions which can be employed for the pelvic examination and each has its adherents for many and differing reasons. Only the two most commonly used will be described here.

The full dorsal position. This is the most commonly used position. The woman is placed supine with the hips flexed and abducted as fully as possible, the knees flexed and the ankles or soles of feet in apposition. The woman will feel much less exposed if the lower abdomen and upper thighs are covered with a sheet. This is the best position for inspection of the vulva, visualisation of the cervix with a bivalve speculum and for bimanual palpation of the uterus, fallopian tubes and ovaries. It is of less value than the lateral position for inspection of the vagina and assessing uterovaginal prolapse.

Modified Sim's or left lateral position. The woman is placed on her left side and near the edge of the examining couch. The left leg is kept straight, extended at the knee, while the right hip and knee are fully flexed so that the leg is over the abdomen. It is valuable if the nurse can help support the right leg at the knee and also gently retract the right buttock upwards. The anus, perineum and posterior vulva can be inspected and, using a Sim's speculum, the vagina is easily visualised. This is the best position for assessing uterovaginal prolapse. Bimanual examination is possible, but not as satisfactory as with the woman in the dorsal position.

Inspection of vulva and perineum

Adequate lighting must be available for this part of the examination. Points to note are local hair growth; the state of the skin — erythema, excoriation, rashes; ulceration; tumours; development of external genitalia — hypotrophic or hypertrophic labia, clitoral hypertrophy; presence of excessive vaginal discharge; presence of haemorrhoids; and any previous vaginal delivery. The woman is asked to strain down to detect any evidence of uterovaginal prolapse.

Speculum examination

Speculum examination is required to allow inspection of the vaginal tissues and cervix, and to assess any degree of uterovaginal prolapse. The woman should be told what is happening at each stage of the examination. The index finger and thumb of the left hand are used to gently separate the labia minora to expose the vestibule. The speculum, which should be at body temperature and slightly lubricated, is gently inserted in an oblique position and in a cephalad and posterior direction with a gentle rotating action to bring it to lie in the transverse axis of the vagina. A speculum should not be inserted with its blade(s) in the axis of the vulval cleft as pressure on the urethra and clitoral region is painful. The blades of a bivalve speculum should only be opened when the instrument is fully inserted. The woman can be told as the examiner gently opens the blades of the speculum that she might experience a little pressure. The cervix is usually easily visualised. If a cervical smear is required, it should be taken at this stage. Opinions differ as to whether the speculum should be lubricated when a smear is required, but it is our opinion that a little lubrication never causes problems in obtaining an adequate cervical sample and enhances patient comfort and continuing co-operation.

The cervix is inspected for size, colour, contour, evidence of previous damage, eversion, infection, polyps and discharge form the canal. The finding of an irregular, injected, granular-looking cervix requires further diagnosis by cytology and possibly colposcopy.

The speculum is then withdrawn slowly and the vaginal walls inspected as they come into view. Colour, erythema, petechiae, ulcerations and adherent discharge are noted. If the woman has been examined in the dorsal position, an impression of the degree of any uterovaginal prolapse may be formed if she is asked to bear down as the speculum is removed. If prolapse is present, the woman may then be examined in the modified Sim's position using a Sim's speculum and the degree of prolapse assessed more accurately.

If vaginal infection is suspected, swabs for culture are obtained from the posterior vaginal fornix and the endocervical canal during the speculum examination. A urethral swab is also sometimes of value and should be taken once the speculum has been removed.

Bimanual vaginal examination

It should be stressed that this part of the examination requires two hands, each assuming equal importance. Most gynaecologists use their right hand for the vaginal examination and the left as the abdominal counterpart. After the labia minora have been parted using the left hand, one finger of the lubricated right hand is introduced, passing upwards and backwards. As previously mentioned, pressure on the posterior vaginal wall and rectum is much less uncomfortable than pressure on the urethra and anterior vagina wall. Once the woman has started to relax the muscles around

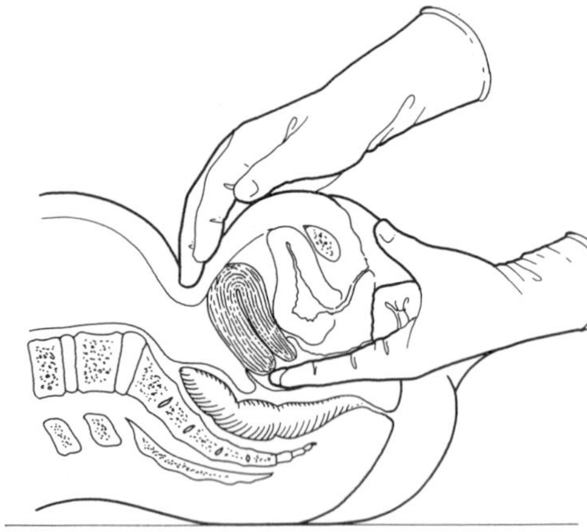

Fig. 1.2 *Bimanual examination, step 1. Two fingers are gently inserted into the vagina. The consistency and symmetry of the cervix are noted. The uterus is then elevated towards the abdominal wall to enable the size of the uterus to be ascertained. (Modified from A.S. Duncan, 1955. In* British Gynaecological Practice, *1st edn., A. Bourne, ed. Philadelphia: Davis.)*

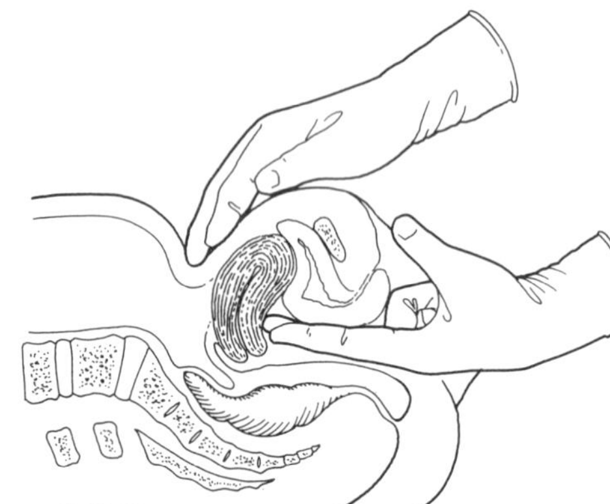

Fig. 1.3 *Bimanual examination, step 2. The vaginal fingers are moved into the anterior fornix and the body of the uterus is palpated. Size, contour, consistency and mobility are noted.*

the vagina, and it is clear that vaginal capacity is adequate, a second finger may be gently introduced. Slight pressure exerted by the abdominal hand brings the pelvic viscera into easier reach of the vaginal fingers.

The cervix is palpated for size, consistency, contour, lateral lacerations and mobility. It should be moved in both anteroposterior and lateral directions to ascertain that such movement causes no discomfort (Fig. 1.2). If there

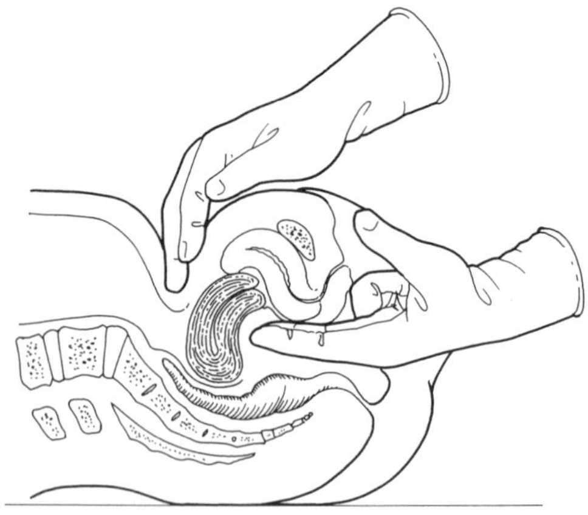

Fig. 1.4 *Bimanual examination, step 3. If the tips of the vaginal and abdominal fingers meet when performing step 2, it can be concluded that the uterus is retroverted or, less commonly, axial. The vaginal fingers are then moved to the posterior fornix. Contour, symmetry, consistency and mobility of the corpus uteri are assessed.*

is sharp pelvic pain related to cervical movement, this is called excitation pain.

The uterus must then be palpated between the hand on the abdomen and the fingers in the vagina. The vaginal fingers should move the cervix backwards to rotate the fundus of the uterus downwards and forwards. The abdominal hand is placed just below the umbilicus and gradually moved lower until the fundus is caught against the fingers in the anterior fornix (Fig. 1.3). If the uterus remains impalpable, then it is in a retroverted position and may be felt by the vaginal fingers when placed in the posterior fornix (Fig. 1.4). The uterine size, shape, contour, regularity, consistency and mobility are noted, along with any tenderness.

The abdominal hand is now moved to the left iliac fossa and the vaginal fingers to the left lateral fornix (Fig. 1.5). This allows palpation of the left adnexa. Features such as thickening, tenderness, ovarian outline, mobility, and the presence of a mass should be noted. The procedure is then repeated on the right side. It should be noted that normal fallopian tubes are rarely, if ever, palpable and often normal ovaries are not felt.

Bimanual examination should impose no significant discomfort. If a painful lesion is

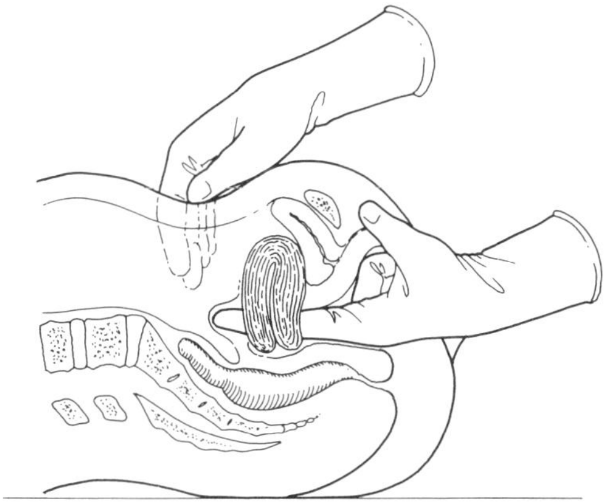

Fig. 1.5 *Bimanual examination, step 4. The vaginal fingers are moved to one of the lateral fornices and the abdominal fingers are moved towards the ipsilateral iliac fossa. The two are then approximated as closely as possible and the intervening tube and ovary palpated.*

encountered, extreme gentleness is required and the woman must never feel that she has been needlessly hurt by the examination.

Rectal examination

Rectal examination may replace vaginal examination in children or in adults who are *virgo intacta.* It can prove a useful adjunct to vaginal examination especially in the assessment of the uterosacral ligaments, pouch of Douglas and outer portions of the broad ligaments. Occasionally, a combined rectovaginal examination, with the index finger in the vagina and the middle finger in the rectum, is of value for assessing lesions of the rectovaginal septum or bowel.

COMMUNICATION

When the examination is complete, the woman dresses and there should then follow an explanation, in terms that can be understood, of the findings, the diagnosis and its implications and any investigations or treatment that are required. It is well known that much of what a doctor tells a patient is immediately forgotten and some points may require reiteration. She should then be encouraged to ask questions and these should be answered patiently, honestly and clearly. There will be times when the news is not good and such situations will be briefly considered further with both patient and doctor in mind.

The Approach to Difficult Situations

Situations arise in every practitioner's lifetime when events will be difficult for both doctor and patient to discuss. Obstetric and gynaecological practice is no exception. What should be done when an ultrasound examination reveals an abnormal fetus? How should we deal with the parents whose baby has died in the first few days of life or has survived with a congenital anomaly or has suffered cerebral damage? Should we tell the truth to the woman with gynaecological malignancy? Views on these subjects vary greatly among all those concerned with patient care and among patients themselves. Only a brief consideration is possible here, but may provide an introduction for further thought.

The ability of the doctor to provide comfort while imparting bad news will, to a large extent, depend on the doctor's own reactions and feelings. The art of communication with the dying patient remains a difficult and uncertain area, often inducing insecurity and anxiety, and may lead to doing nothing in such a situation. Such feelings may be enhanced by a fear of being blamed by the patient as the cause of her illness, rather than acceptance as the healer, soother or comforter. A patient's reaction to bad news if often difficult to predict, and the need for knowledge of how to deal with the consequences of the news we break to an individual enshrines a universal criterion of all medical practice. Fear of expressing emotion may also prove restricting, as all our clinical training is directed to encourage a calm approach, even in emergencies, and stifle any emotional response invoked by the situation or the individual patient. It is necessary to learn to show sincere sympathy. Junior doctors commonly express the fear of incomplete knowledge, and not knowing all the answers is a real handicap when facing difficult situations. All confidence can be totally undermined. While ignorance should not be condoned, it is worth remembering that often the patient realises that the answers to his/her questions are unknown, or even does not want the answers, but simply needs someone to listen. The skill of talking to patients about difficult matters is an acquired talent. Those who do it often and do it well, should be encouraged to teach the rest of us. Guidance as to how to relate to parents suffering bereavement due to loss of pregnancy or a child is given in Chapter 16.

The aim in all these situations is broadly to provide the best possible degree of health for the woman in mind and body. This requires patience and commitment by all those involved and perhaps reflects the vocational element of 'medical' practice.

FURTHER READING

Jenkins D. (1986). *Listening to the Gynaecological Patient's Problems.* London: Springer-Verlag.

Buckman R. (1992). *How to Break Bad News: A Guide for Health-Care Professionals.* London: Papermac.

2

The Reproductive Organs: Structure and Function

EMBRYOLOGY

Ovary

Primitive germ cells are first apparent in the endoderm of the yolk sac from where they migrate to the gut and through the mesentery to the genital ridge on the medial aspect of the mesonephros. The primitive gonad consists of the thickened coelomic epithelium of the genital ridge, the underlying mesoderm and the germ cells (oogonia). By 5–6 weeks, the epithelium has grown inwards as a series of gonadal cords. Further development of these cords obliterates the mesenchymal elements. The epithelial elements and oogonia proliferate vigorously up to 14 weeks; the predominance of cortical tissue distinguishes the early ovary from the testis. From this stage, stromal cells develop from the mesenchyme in the hilum and spread peripherally. When the process is complete, the primary oocytes are surrounded by a ring of epithelial granulosa cells embedded in the stroma. The identity of the gonad is apparent by 7 weeks in the testis and a little later in the ovary.

During the process of formation of the primary oocytes, the germ cells enter the diplotene stage of the prophase of the first meiotic division. They remain in this stage until ovulation occurs, which may be decades later. The number of germ cells reaches a maximum of 7 million in each ovary at 15–20 weeks, falling to 2 million at birth and 400, 000 by puberty.

The early ovary is attached to the inguinal fold and uterus by a fibromuscular band, the gubernaculum, along which it is drawn to its definitive site. The cranial part of the gubernaculum becomes the ovarian ligament and the caudal part becomes the round ligament. The lower end of the gubernaculum is associated with a peritoneal projection, the processus vaginalis, which may persist in the labia majora as the canal of Nuck.

Uterus and Fallopian Tubes

The paramesonephric (müllerian) duct develops on the lateral aspect of the mesonephros at 5–6 weeks and extends caudally to reach the urogenital sinus at 9 weeks (müllerian tubercle). At 8 weeks, both the müllerian and wolffian ducts are present and sex differentiation begins. In the female, the wolffian ducts degenerate due to a lack of testosterone. The lower portions of the müllerian ducts fuse to form the uterus and cervix, while the upper portions remain separate as the fallopian tubes. In the male, the müllerian system degenerates under the influence of a glycoprotein inhibitory factor from the Sertoli cells of the testis, the müllerian inhibitory factor, which is locally active. Remnants of the wolffian duct system may be evident as cysts in the vagina (Gartner's duct) or the broad ligament (paraovarian cysts).

Vagina

Paired sinovaginal bulbs on the posterior aspect of the urogenital sinus fuse with the lower end of the müllerian ducts to form the vaginal plate. This consists of solid epithelium which grows rapidly and then becomes canalised at 16–18 weeks.

External Genitalia

The primitive cloaca becomes divided by a transverse septum which fuses with the cloacal membrane at 7 weeks. The anterior part is the urogenital sinus and on the external surface there is a conical projection, the genital tubercle. Proliferation of the mesoderm leads to the formation of the genital folds medially and the genital swellings laterally. At this point, male and female development is identical.

Normal female development does not depend on gonadal hormones. Instead, it is a "neuter" state, which occurs in the absence of the testis. The testis has three endocrine effects: (1) secretion of müllerian inhibitory factor; (2) secretion of testosterone which directly promotes wolffian development; and (3) conversion of testosterone to dihydrotestosterone by 5-α-reductase which promotes male development of the external genitalia.

ANATOMY

A simplified diagram of the female reproductive organs is shown in Fig. 2.1

Vulva

The vulva comprises the mons pubis, the labia majora and minora and the clitoris, and overlaps with the vaginal vestibule (Fig. 2.2). Before puberty, the mons pubis is flat, the labia majora are small and the vaginal orifice is virtually occluded by the hymen. At puberty, the fatty pad of the mons pubis develops, labia majora and minora enlarge considerably, the vaginal orifice becomes bigger and the hymen provides a partial barrier to the vagina. Pubic hair grows, with the upper margin being the upper edge of the mons pubis.

Labia majora

The labia majora form the lateral boundary of the vulva and extend from the mons pubis to

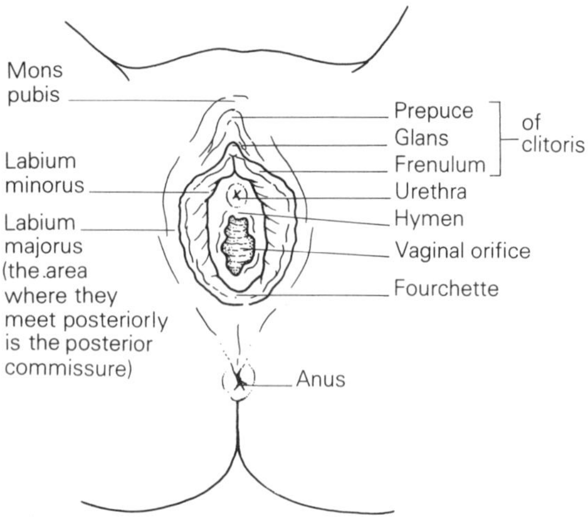

Fig. 2.2 *Anatomy of the vulva.*

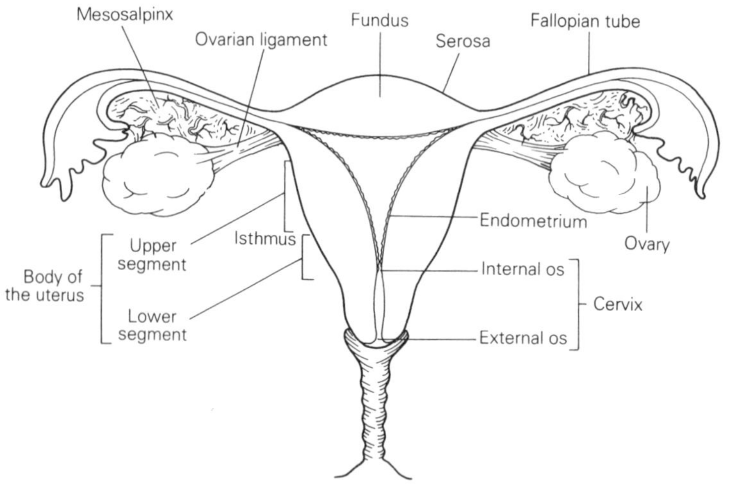

Fig. 2.1 *Anatomy of the uterus.*

the perineum. Their medial aspects consist of stratified squamous epithelium with hair follicles, a thin layer of smooth muscle (tunica dartos), a layer of fascia, adipose tissue and large numbers of sweat and sebaceous glands. They contain numerous nerve endings, some of which are free (pain sensitive), while others are in the form of corpuscles (e.g. Meissner). The nerve supply comes from the abdomen by the ilioinguinal and genitofemoral nerves; the buttocks by the posterior femoral cutaneous nerves; and the pelvis by the pudendal nerves. The arterial supply comes from the internal and external pudendal arteries which form a circular rete.

The venous drainage forms a plexus with extensive anastomoses to surrounding areas During pregnancy, these veins can become very distended, causing a vulval varicocoele. If damaged at delivery, severe haemorrhage will occur.

The lymphatic drainage is to the superficial subinguinal nodes, thence to the deep subinguinal nodes and the external iliac chain. The deeper tissues of the labia majora, together with the posterior third of the skin drain both anteriorly along the route described and posteriorly to the rectal lymphatic plexus and thence to the internal iliac chain.

The lymphatic drainage of squamous carcinoma of the vulva, and its spread to the inguinal glands should allow it to be readily detected. A radical vulvectomy for treatment of carcinoma of the vulva involves block dissection of the inguinal and occasionally the external iliac glands.

Labia minora

Labia minora are the folds of skin that overlap the vaginal vestibule. They split anteriorly to form two portions: one forming a hood or covering for the clitoris (prepuce) and the other passing ventrally to the clitoris as the frenulum. Posteriorly, the two labia minora meet at the fourchette. They consist of stratified squamous epithelium with hair follicles, sebaceous and sweat glands, and a thin layer of smooth muscle continuous with the tunica dartos. The epithelium is keratinised on the lateral surface, but changes to a mucous membrane on the medial side. The nerve endings are similar to but less abundant than those of the labia majora and the nerve supply similar to that described. The arterial supply again comes from the rete of the labia majora with an additional component from the dorsal artery of the clitoris. The venous drainage is again the same as that for the labia majora, with an additional superior connection to the vaginal plexus.

Clitoris

The clitoris consists of a small body of erectile tissue (the crura of the clitoris) covered by the prepuce. The nerve endings are similar to those of the labia, and the nerve supply arises from the terminal branch of the pudendal nerve. The arterial supply is the dorsal artery of the clitoris, which is a branch of the internal pudendal artery. Both labia minora and clitoris are highly sensitive with a rich vascular and nerve supply. They are, therefore, important erogenous areas for stimulation before and during intercourse. Ritual circumcision as practised still in some parts of Africa involves the removal of both labia and the clitoris during infancy.

Perineum

The perineum is bounded by the levatores ani muscles above, by the vulva and anus below and the pelvic outlet (subpubic arch, ischiopubic rami, ischial tuberosities and coccyx laterally. It is divided into a urogenital triangle anteriorly and an anal triangle posteriorly. There is a superficial fascia of fat, and a deep membranous fascia (Colles) which extends over the pubis and into the anterior abdominal wall as the fascia of Scarpa.

Urogenital triangle

The urogenital triangle contains the the vagina and urethra, the crura of the clitoris (erectile tissue) surrounded by the ischiocavernosus muscles, the bulb of the vestibule (erectile

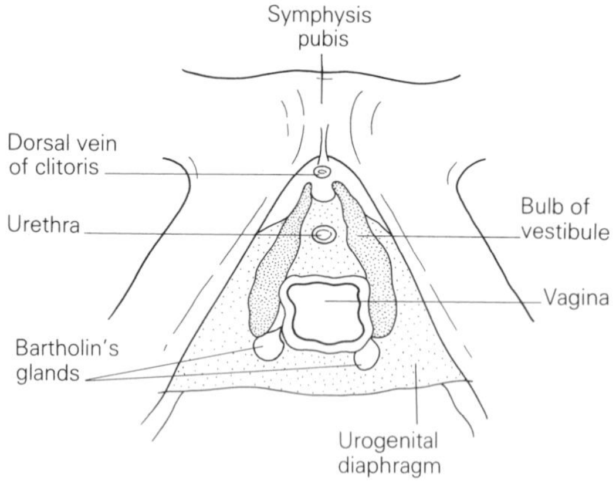

Fig. 2.3 *The urogenital diaphragm viewed from below. The urogenital diaphragm lies in the urogenital triangle which is the anterior portion of the perineum.*

tissue), surrounded by the bulbocavernosus muscles, Bartholin's glands, the urogenital diaphragm and the superficial and deep perineal pouches.

Urogenital diaphragm (triangular ligament). The urogenital diaphragm is a sheath of muscle enclosed between two triangular fascial membranes. The muscle is formed by the deep transverse perineal muscle and fibres from the sphincter urethrae. The superior fascial layer is the thin fascia bridging the gap between the anterior portions of the levatores ani. The inferior fascial layer is tough and fibrous. The urogenital diaphragm is penetrated by the urethra and vagina and the glands and bulb of the vestibule lie inferior (superficial) to it (Fig. 2.3).

The ability to contract this muscle is important in preventing stress incontinence of urine. Young women who develop mild stress incontinence after childbirth are often helped by pelvic floor exercises which strengthen all the muscles, but particularly the perineal muscles.

Muscles of the perineum

The ischiocavernosus muscle arises from the medial aspect of the inferior ischial ramus and ensheaths the crus clitoris. It compresses the crus and by blocking the venous outflow so promotes erection of the clitoris.

The bulbocavernosus muscle originates in the perineal body, where it interdigitates with the external anal shincter. It surrounds the bulb of the vestibule and is inserted into the body of the clitoris.

The superficial transverse perineal muscle radiates from the perineal body to the ischial ramus. The deep transverse perineal muscle has the same origin and insertion, but lies deep to the inferior fascia of the urogenital diaphragm.

Perineal body

This is a fibromuscular mass into which the bulbocavernosus, transverse perineal, external anal sphincter and levator ani muscles insert. The integrity of the perineum is important in maintaining the distance between vagina and anus, and in preventing prolapse of the posterior vaginal wall (rectocoele). It is damaged at childbirth by incision (episiotomy) or by tears. Failure to repair these adequately leads to an inadequate perineum, with consequent faecal soiling of the vagina and encouragement of rectocoele. The deep transverse perineal muscle has the same origin and insertion, but lies deep to the inferior fascia of the urogenital diaphragm.

Superficial perineal pouch

This is a potential space between the inferior fascia of the urogenital diaphragm and the fascia of Colles. It contains the Bartholin's glands and superficial transverse perineal muscles.

Deep perineal pouch

This is a potential space between the two fascial layers of the urogenital diaphragm and contains the membranous urethra surrounded by the external sphincter and deep transverse perineal muscles.

Damage to the urogenital diaphragm and deep perineal pouch can contribute to shortening of the urethra. Ascending urinary tract infection, particularly cystitis, can become common, especially after intercourse. A short urethra also contributes to stress incontinence of urine.

The blood supply of the perineum is largely from the internal pudendal artery and vein. Motor and sensory nerve supply is by the pudendal nerve, and anteriorly the genitofemoral nerve.

Vestibule, Bartholin's Glands and Vagina

Vestibule

The vestibule lies between the labia minora and the hymen. The hymen is a perforated membrane which after rupture consists of skin tags (carunculae hymenales). Anteriorly the vestibule includes the urethral orifice around which the periurethral glands of Skene open. The duct openings of the larger vestibular or Bartholin's glands are at 5 and 7 o'clock. The latter are arranged as lobules consisting of alveoli lined by a columnar epithelium. They produce a mucoid secretion in response to sexual stimulation. Blockage of the ducts following infection leads to mucoid retention cysts (Bartholin's cysts) or, if infected, an abscess which is very painful.

Deep to the vestibule on either side of the commencement of the vagina lies the bulb of the vestibule which is a flask-shaped mass of erectile tissue covered by the bulbocavernosus muscles.

The skin of the vestibule is stratified squamous epithelium without hair follicles. The nerve endings are mostly free and the blood supply is an anastomosisis between branches of the pudendal artery, the inferior haemorrhoidal artery and the azygous artery of the vagina.

Vagina

The vagina is 7–10 cm long; the posterior wall being 2 cm longer than the anterior. The anterior vaginal wall is in direct relation to the bladder and urethra throughout its length. Surgery of the anterior vaginal wall, therefore, always carries a risk of urethral and vesical damage. At the level of the junction between urethra and bladder are the pubocervical ligaments.

The upper quarter of the posterior vaginal wall is related to the intraperitoneal cavity or pouch of Douglas. The middle half of the posterior vaginal wall is related to the rectum, while the lower quarter is separated from the anal canal by the anal sphincters and perineal body. The lateral relations of the vagina are shown in Fig. 2.4.

The vagina has an extensive blood supply with contributions from the uterine artery, the

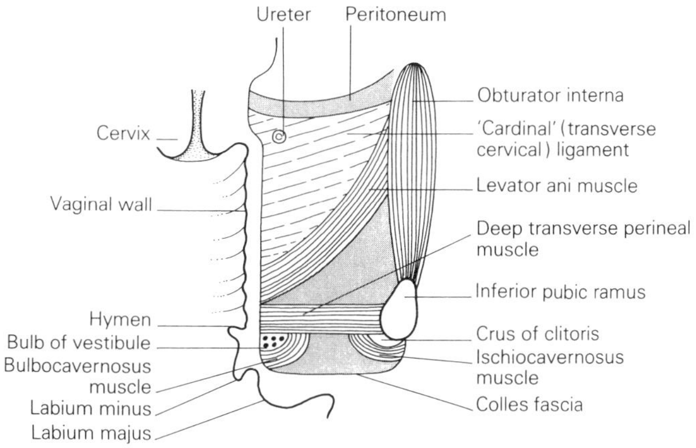

Fig. 2.4 *Lateral relations of the vagina. Superolaterally, the vagina is supported by transverse cervical ligaments. In its midposition it is surroounded by the medial fibres of the levator ani muscle. Inferiorly, it penetrates the urogenital diaphragm.*

inferior vesical arteries, the terminal branch of the internal iliac artery, the haemorrhoidal arteries and the dorsal artery of the clitoris. All of the above anastomose to form the anterior and posterior azygous arteries which pass down the midline of the vagina. The good blood supply helps to provide vaginal lubrication by means of exudate. The vagina is also a distensible structure allowing the passage of the fetal head without excessive trauma.

Lymphatic drainage of the vagina is as follows:

1. *Upper*: via the cervical channels to the external iliac nodes;
2. *Middle*: to the hypogastric nodes;
3. *Lower*: to the hypogastric nodes and via the vulva to the inguinal nodes. Those nodes are affected in the spread of carcinoma of the vagina or carcinoma of the cervix in volving the vagina.

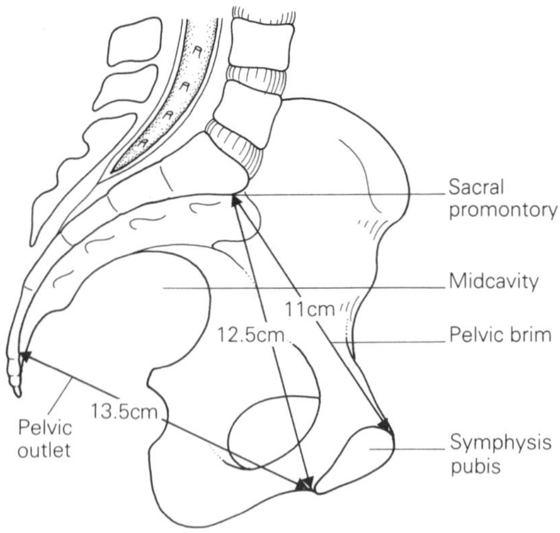

Fig. 2.5 *Saggital view of the bony pelvis. The true conjugate from the sacral promontory to the top of the symphysis pubis measures 11 cm. The diagonal conjugate (12.5cm) is measured to the bottom of the symphysis. The anteroposterior diameter of the outlet is shown.*

Bony Pelvis

The pelvis consists of a saucer-shaped false pelvis, which is situated above the pelvic cavity (true pelvis). The latter is of great significance and it is through here that the fetus passes during delivery. The true pelvis is a curved bony canal, the posterior wall (the sacrum) being considerably longer than the anterior wall (pubic symphysis) (Fig. 2.5).

The pelvic inlet is oval in shape with a shorter antero-posterior diameter between the sacral promontory and the back of the pubic symphysis (11 cm) and a longer transverse diameter (13.5 cm) (Fig. 2.6). The pelvic brim forms the inlet of the true pelvis and the fetal head passes through this when it engages in late pregnancy or early labour. Engagement of the fetal head is said to have occurred when the widest diameter of the fetal skull (biparietal) has passed through the pelvic brim. The transverse diameter (13.5 cm) is the maximum diameter of the pelvic brim and thus the largest diameter of the fetal head passes through this easily.

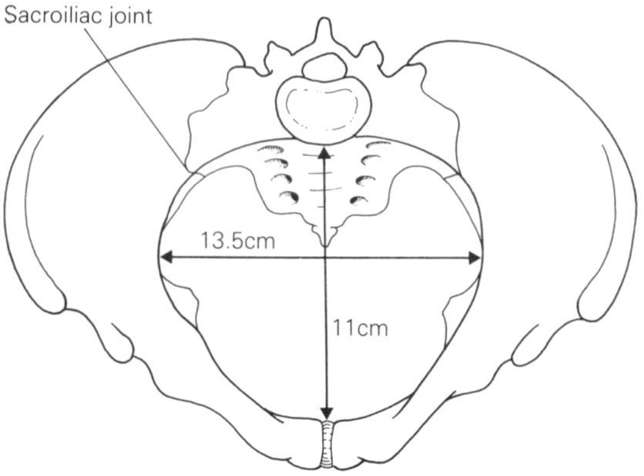

Fig. 2.6 *Mean diameters of the pelvic inlet.*

The curve of the sacrum allows the midcavity of the pelvis to be capacious and circular in outline with a diameter of 12 cm in all directions.

The pelvic outlet is diamond-shaped and is bound by the ischiopubic rami anteriorly and the sacrotuberous ligaments and sacral tuberosities posteriorly. The antero-posterior diameter of the outlet is taken from the lower border of the symphysis pubis to the bottom of the sacrum and the transverse diameter is between the ischial tuberosities (Fig. 2.7). Thus, the pelvis is wider from side to side at the brim

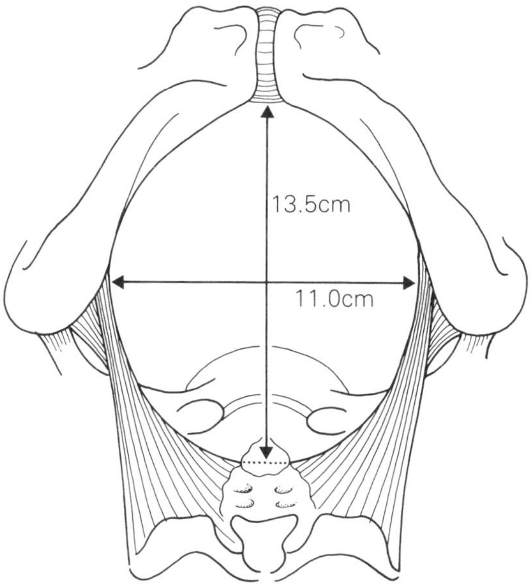

Fig. 2.7 *Dimensions of the diamond-shaped pelvic outlet. The anteroposterior diameter is measured from the bottom of the symphysis to the end of the sacrum and not to the end of the coccyx.*

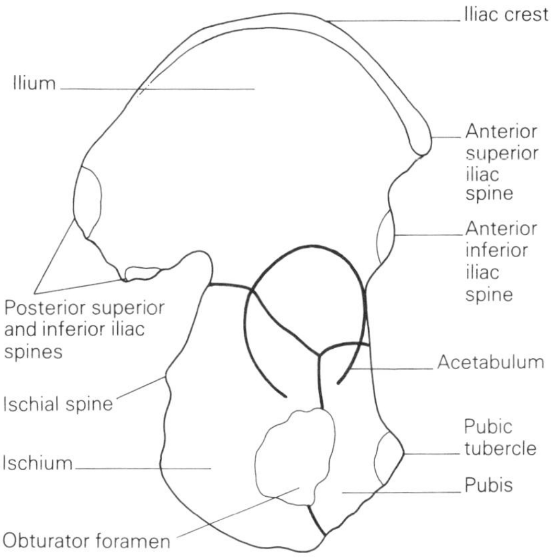

Fig. 2.8 *Lateral view of the innominte (hip bone).*

than from front to back at the outlet. The relationship of pelvic shape and size to the passage of the fetus during labour is described in Chapter 12.

The bony pelvis is made up of the hip bone and the sacrum. The hip bone itself consists of three separate bones: the ilium, the ischium and the pubis. These are joined by bone in the adult, but they are separated by cartilage in children. These three bones converge on the acetabulum (Fig. 2.8). It can be seen that the ilium forms the false pelvis and iliac crest and this bone articulates with the sacrum, forming the major non-mobile sacroiliac joint. The pubic bone consists of a body and two rami as does the ischium. The rami of these two bones fuse to form the obturator foramen. The sacrum consists of five vertebrae joined by bone in the adult and cartilage in children. There are four sacral foramina communicating with the sacral canal. The upper border of the pelvic surface is the sacral promontory. During pregnancy, the angle of the pelvis increases and there is a lordosis to compensate for the anterior shift of the woman's centre of gravity. Ligaments become looser, and so sacroiliac discomfort, and less commonly discomfort at the pubic symphysis, particularly on movement, can be troublesome. The laxity is designed to facilitate childbirth and is brought about by oestrogen and relaxin induced changes in collagen structure and density.

Uterus

The uterus is about 7.5 cm long and consists of a body, a constricted portion known as the isthmus (which includes the internal os) and a narrow terminal part called the cervix. The portion lying above the opening of the fallopian tubes is known as the fundus. The cervix penetrates the vaginal vault and is thereby divided into a supra- and infra-vaginal portion. The uterus lies between the bladder and the rectum in the peritoneal cavity. Removal of the uterus always involves dissection of the bladder from its lower part and cervix, so the operation carries risks of trauma to the bladder. It is separated from the rectum by the upper part of the pouch of Douglas.

The external cervical orifice (external os), circular in nulliparous women, becomes transverse and fissured as a result of childbirth. The axis of the cervical canal is directed obliquely, posteriorly and inferiorly, while the uterus is anteflexed and anteverted. Laterally the uterus is related to the broad ligaments and the uterine arteries.

The uterus has a remarkable capacity for enlargement during pregnancy. The isthmus elongates and its cavity becomes absorbed into the general uterine cavity to form the lower uterine segment. As further enlargement takes place, the upper part of the cervix is also incorporated into the thin lower segment. The uterus increases in weight only during the first half of pregnancy and its further enlargement in volume is achieved by thinning of the uterine walls.

The main blood supply to the uterus is from the uterine arteries which may arise directly from the internal iliac arteries, or in common with another of its branches, usually the superior vesical artery. The uterine artery crosses the transverse cervical ligament (see below) and thereafter passes anterior to and above the ureter at about 1.5 cm from the lateral vaginal fornix. Care must be taken when clamping the uterine artery during hysterectomy not to clamp or cut the ureter. The uterine artery then ascends in a tortuous course between the two layers of the broad ligament on the lateral border of the uterus, giving out branches to the myometrium and anastomosing at the superior angle of the vagina with the terminal portion of the ovarian artery. As mentioned above, the uterine artery also gives off a branch to the upper part of the vagina.

The main lymphatic drainage of the uterus is to the external and internal iliac group of lymph nodes, although some lymphatics in the upper part of the uterus pass directly to the lateral aortic nodes following the ovarian blood supply. A few small branches run with the round ligament to the superficial inguinal nodes.

Fallopian Tubes

The fallopian tubes lie in the upper margin of the broad ligament and are 10 cm long. The abdominal opening is at the base of a trumpet-shaped expansion with a fimbriated edge, the infundibulum; one of the fimbriae of the infundibulum may form a small vesicle or hydatid. From the infundibulum, the succeeding parts of the tube are the relatively wide tortuous ampulla, the cord-like isthmus and the uterine or intramural portion. The blood supply is from the uterine and ovarian arteries through the mesosalpinx. Sterilisation procedures and reversal of these are most effective if performed in the isthmic portions of the tubes. There is some form of physiological sphincter at the ampullary-isthmic junction which is thought to regulate the passage of the ovum through the tube. Tubal ectopic pregnancies frequently occur in the ampulla or ampullary-isthmic region of the tube. Rupture of the tube is less likely in the ampulla than if the pregnancy is in the narrow isthmus. Tubal occlusion for sterilisation purposes is best done at the isthmus.

Ovaries

The ovary is an almond-shaped organ attached to the posterior surface of the broad ligament by a fold of the ligament called the mesovarium and occupies the ovarian fossa on the wall of the pelvis. The fossa is bound anteriorly by the lateral umbilical ligament (obliterated umbilical artery) and posteriorly by the ureter and internal iliac vessels. In early fetal life, the ovaries lie in the lumbar region near the kidney.

The surface of the ovaries is covered with a layer of cuboidal cells, which is the germinal epithelium, and beneath this there is a thin layer of condensed connective tissue, the tunica albuginea. The cortex contains the primordial follicles, corpora lutea and corpora albicans.

The primordial follicles consist of a central oocyte surrounded by a single layer of flattened follicular cells. After puberty some follicles develop each month to form primary, secondary and tertiary follicles.

The blood supply is from the ovarian artery, which is a branch of the descending aorta reaching the ovary in the infundibulo-pelvic ligament. There is a venous pampiniform plexus at the hilum of the ovary draining to the ovarian vein and then to the inferior vena cava on the right and the renal vein on the left.

Female Urinary Tract

The female reproductive system cannot be fully understood without some mention of the urinary tract to which it is intimately connected.

Ureter

Each ureter is 30 cm in length and the abdominal part descends over the psoas muscle and is crossed by the ovarian vessels. It enters the pelvis in front of the external iliac vessels and the pelvic part follows the anterior border of the sacroiliac notch and runs above the levator ani muscle in the base of the broad ligament (parametrium) to the base of the bladder. In the parametrium, the ureter lies below the uterine artery and above the lateral fornix of the vagina. It passes 2 cm lateral to the cervix (a point of importance in radiotherapy), and then turns medially in front of the vagina to follow an oblique course through the bladder wall. The ureter is most liable to surgical trauma close to (1) the angle of the vagina, (2) the uterine artery in the base of the broad ligament and (3) the external iliac vessels at the postero-lateral margin of the broad ligament.

Bladder

The bladder is a three-layered hollow, muscular organ with a peritoneal covering on the superior surface. The three layers consist of serous, muscular and mucous coats and the smooth muscle itself has internal and external longitudinal layers and a larger middle circular layer. The mucosa is a transitional epithelium which is loosely attached to the muscle, except over the trigone (the triangular area bounded by the orifices of the ureters and the urethra) where it is firmly attached. The trigone lies against the anterior vaginal wall and the cervix, and, consequently, at hysterectomy and anterior colporrhaphy, the bladder must be carefully separated from the underlying structures.

Descent of the bladder through inadequate pubocervical fascia causes stretching of the anterior vaginal wall and the presence of a bulge or lump in the vagina (cystocoele).

Urethra

The female urethra is 4 cm long and is embedded in the anterior wall of the vagina running below and behind the pubic symphysis.

Its opening is between the labia minora and behind the clitoris. The muscle layer is continuous with that of the bladder and there is no anatomical internal sphincter at this junction. As it traverses the deep perineal pouch, it is surrounded by the voluntary external sphincter, which is supplied by the perineal branch of the pudendal nerve. Between the muscle and the mucosa is a thin layer of connective tissue, which may play a part in maintaining continence.

Peritoneum and Ligaments of the Pelvis

The peritoneum covers the uterus with the exception of the anterior part of the supravaginal cervix and the intra-vaginal cervix. From the anterior surface of the uterus, the peritoneum is reflected onto the superior surface of the bladder, forming the uterovesical pouch. From the posterior surface of the uterus, the peritoneum continues onto the upper-third of the vagina before it is reflected onto the anterior rectal surface, forming the recto-vaginal pouch (or pouch of Douglas). The lower extremity of this pouch is attached to the perineal body by connective tissue of the recto-vaginal septum (Fig. 2.9).

Broad ligament

From the lateral borders of the uterus, two layers of peritoneum on each side are reflected to the lateral pelvic walls forming the broad ligaments. These peritoneal folds include loose connective tissue referred to as parametrium which merge inferiorly with extraperitoneal

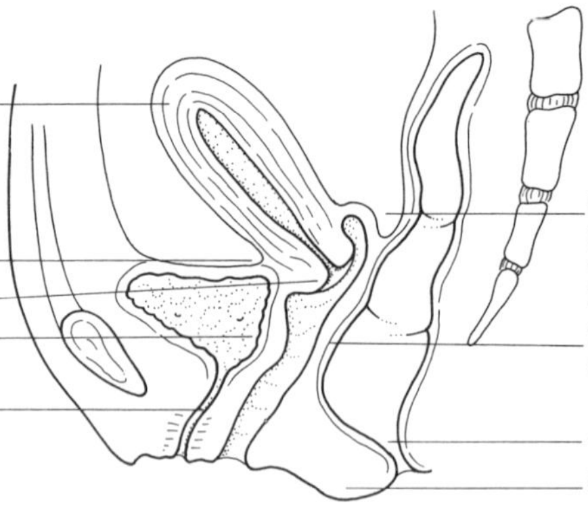

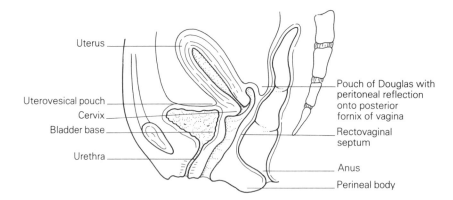

Fig. 2.9 *Saggital section of the pelvis to show the peritoneal reflections over the blader, uterus, posterior vaginal fornix and rectum.*

connective tissue. The upper lateral border of the broad ligament forms the infundibulo-pelvic fold and contains the ovarian vessels in their course from the side wall of the pelvis. The ovary is attached to the posterior layer of the broad ligament by a short double fold of the peritoneum — the mesovarium — and the portion of the broad ligament above this is the mesosalpinx. The top of the broad ligament envelops the fallopian tubes. Below and in front of the fallopian tube is the round ligament, and below and behind it is the ovarian ligament connecting the ovary to the uterine cornu, which are all enclosed within the broad ligament.

Vestigial remnants of the mesonephric bodies and ducts (wolffian ducts, duct of Gartner) are contained within the broad ligament. Remnants of the mesonephric body lie above and lateral to the ovary (epoophoron and hydatid of Morgagni) and between the ovary and uterus (paroophoron).

Round ligament

The round ligament attaches to the uterine body below and in front of the fallopian tube. It is 12 cm long and passes through the broad ligament to the lateral wall of the pelvis, where it crosses the psoas muscle and external iliac vessels. It hooks round the inferior epigastric artery to the deep inguinal ring, passes through the inguinal canal and fans out into the labium majora. It is composed mainly of fibrous tissue with some smooth muscle at the uterine end and some striated muscle at the labial end. It undergoes considerable hypertrophy during pregnancy, often causing mild pain on movement within the inguinal canal.

Ligaments formed from pelvic fascia

The connective tissue covering the levator ani is condensed into musculofibrous bands in three areas: (1) the transverse cervical ligament (cardinal ligament) arising from the arcuate line on the side wall of the pelvis; (2) the pubocervical ligaments arising from the fascia over the pubic bone and passing around the bladder neck; and (3) the uterosacral ligaments (posterior part of the cardinal ligaments) arising from the sacral promontory. All three ligaments insert into the upper vagina and supra-vaginal cervix and are important in supporting the pelvic viscera and the uterus. The cardinal ligaments are very important. Their apposition in front of the amputated cervix, to support and antevert the uterus, is the main part of the Manchester repair operation. Buttressing of the pubocervical fascia to raise and support the urethro-vesical angle, initially by sutures and subsequently by fibrous tissue, is the purpose of the anterior vaginal surgical approach to stress incontinence.

Blood, Lymphatic and Nerve Supply

Blood supply

The blood supply of the pelvis is shown in Fig. 2.10. The aorta divides at the level of the fourth lumbar vertebra, and the common iliac artery at the level of the lumbosacral inter-vertebral disc. Continuing vessels leave the pelvis through the obturator foramen (obturator artery); behind the inguinal ligament (femoral artery); and through the greater sciatic foramen (superior and inferior gluteal arteries — pudendal artery). The internal pudendal artery curves around the back of the ischial spine and enters the perineum through the lesser sciatic foramen and pudendal canal.

Lymphatic drainage

The lymphatic drainage of the pelvis begins as plexuses in the individual organs and generally follows the line of the blood vessels. Major and fairly constant groups of nodes include the common iliac, the external iliac, which drain the inguinal group; the internal iliac, the obturator, and the median and lateral sacral nodes.

Lymphatic drainage of the ovary is to the para-aortic nodes; of the body of the uterus to para-aortic iliac nodes and inguinal nodes; of the cervix to the iliac nodes and para-rectal nodes; and of the vagina to iliac and inguinal nodes.

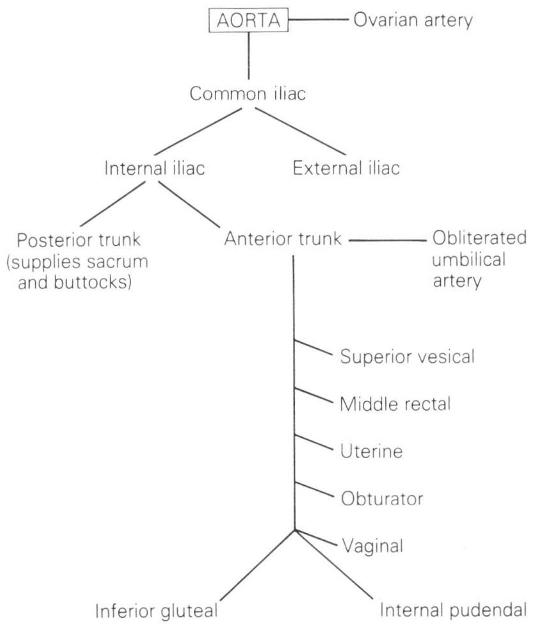

Fig. 2.10 *The arterial supply of the pelvis — diagrammatic.*

Nerve supply

The parasympathetic nerve supply to the pelvis emerges as myelinated, pre-ganglionic nerves with ventral rami of S 2 and 3 or S 3 and 4 to constitute the pelvic splanchnic nerves. The ganglia are situated in the walls of the organs supplied. Motor or inhibitory fibres supply the rectum, bladder and erectile tissue of the clitoris; vasodilator fibres supply the ovary and uterus.

The sympathetic nerve supply to the pelvis arises from the sympathetic nerve trunks, which have four ganglia in the lumbar region and a similar number anterior to the sacrum. The origin of the pelvic sympathetic fibres is from T 11 to L 2. From the ganglia, grey rami communicantes pass to the lumbar and sacral spinal nerves, while other fibres form the hypogastric plexus from which further plexuses radiate to the various pelvic organs. Stimulation of somatic afferent fibres from the external genitalia or adjacent skin causes vasodilatation through the parasympathetic fibres of the pelvic splanchnic nerves.

Muscles of the Pelvis

We have already dealt with the muscles of the perineum (p. 12). The remaining muscle mass — the levator ani — is extremely important in obstetrics and gynaecology, as this forms the pelvic floor or diaphragm. The levator ani muscles arise on each side of the pelvis from the line which passes backwards from the posterior surface to the superior ramus of the pubis. This line then passes over the internal surface of the obturator foramen (arcus tendineus) to the ischial spine, forming the origin of the levator muscle and from here the fibres sweep inferiorly and posteriorly to interdigitate with each other in the midline. As they sweep downwards and backwards, they surround the vagina and then insert into: (1) the pre-anal raphe where some fibres make a contribution to the perineal body; (2) the wall of the anal canal where fibres blend with the deep external sphincter muscle; (3) the post-anal or anococcygeal raphe, where again the muscle meets its fellow from the opposite side, and (4) the lower part of the coccyx (Fig. 2.11). The medial borders of each levator muscle have sphincteric action, and contraction partially occludes the vagina. The most medial portion of the levator ani is referred to as pubococcygeus muscle and it is this portion that is inserted in front of the rectum. The next portion is the puborectalis and this is inserted into the rectum and into the first part of the raphe behind the rectum. The most posterior portion is the iliococcy geus and this is inserted into the remainder of the posterior raphe and into the coccyx itself. Because the fibres of the levator ani run downwards as well as backwards, the pelvic diaphragm as a whole is funnel-shaped. Paradoxically, contraction of the abdominal wall with increased abdominal pressure, as in straining or coughing, relaxes the levator

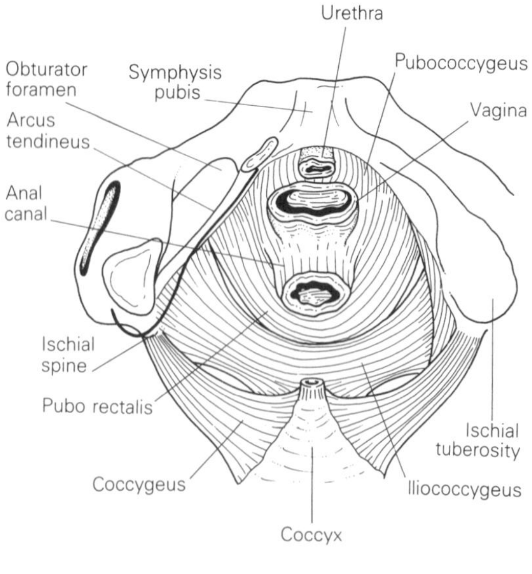

Fig. 2.11 *Inferior view of the levator ani muscles.*

muscles. Thus during straining, the puborectalis muscle is relaxed and the angle between the rectum and anus is diminished.

The nerve supply to the levator ani muscles is from the third and fourth sacral nerves.

MICROSTRUCTURE OF THE REPRODUCTIVE TRACT
(Excluding pregnancy)

Mucosa of the Fallopian Tube

The fallopian tubes are lined by a single layer of columnar epithelium with three types of cells — ciliated, secretory and resting (peg). The secretory cells are found throughout the tube, but they are most numerous at the isthmic end; they develop microvilli and become secretory at midcycle. Pelvic inflammatory disease leads to deciliation, particularly in the ampullary portion. This retards tubal transport of the fertilised oocyte and leads to an increased incidence of tubal ectopic pregnancy.

Fallopian tube secretions contain pyruvate, which is an important substrate for the embryo. They contain less glucose, protein and potassium than serum. Further understanding of the biochemistry of oviduct fluid is important in relationship to failure of implantation.

Endometrium

The endometrium is composed of a basal layer and a stroma covered by columnar epithelium. The latter forms uterine glands which extend through the stroma into the basal layer. The columnar epithelium includes ciliated cells, which are most numerous near the opening of the glands, and secretory cells with microvilli which are fully developed during the secretory phase. After menstruation, regeneration of the epithelium takes place from the base of the endometrial glands.

Following menstruation, the endometrium enters the proliferative phase. Under the influence of oestrogen, the epithelium proliferates and reaches a thickness of 5 mm. Towards midcycle the arterioles take on a spiral form and subnuclear aggregates of glycogen appear in the epithelium. During the luteal phase, there is slight further thickening of the endometrium due to vascular proliferation, oedema of the stroma and accumulation of secretion in uterine glands. The glands become tortuous and vacuoles of glycogen push the nuclei to the luminal surface. After about Day 20, these vacuoles move to the surface and are discharged. Pre-decidual changes occur in the stroma; the stellate cells become rounder and accumulate lysosomes.

In the final stage of the cycle, the coiled arterioles constrict and the superficial zone becomes avascular. There is a loss of interstitial fluid, leucocytic infltration of the stroma and extravasation of blood as the superficial layers become necrotic.

The blood enters the uterus, but does not clot. The underlying basal layer remains intact, as do the bases of the glands. Levels of PGF2α in the endometrium rise during the luteal phase and exceed levels of PGE2 by 25 : 1 at the time of menstruation. The former constricts spiral arterioles while the latter relaxes them. An altered ratio in favour of vasodilatory compounds such as PGE2 may be a factor in the aetiology of menorrhagia.

Cervix

The cervix is lined by secretory columnar epithelium arranged as branched glands. This epithelium undergoes only minor changes during the menstrual cycle. The cervical mucus becomes profuse and clear under the action of oestrogen before ovulation. It produces a ferning pattern on drying, exhibits "spinnbarkeit" (by Day 14 of the menstrual cycle a single thread may be drawn out to 8 cm) and has an alkaline pH. Towards midcycle the cervical fluid becomes more hydrated. The macromolecules of glycoprotein condense into "micelles" which form a network of channels through which sperm swim. Once progesterone secretion begins, the cervical mucus becomes thick, opaque, highly cellular and less abundant, as a result of increased binding between the glycoprotein filaments.

Vagina

The wall of the vagina consists of three layers: a mucous membrane, a muscular coat (circular and longitudinal) and a thin connective tissue covering. Striated fibres of the bulbocavernosus and levator ani muscles form sphincters. The stratified squamous epithelium has three layers: a basal layer of cuboidal cells, an intermediate layer, which is rich in glycogen, and a superficial zone of flat cornified cells (with small nuclei). The underlying lamina propria contains collagen and elastic fibres and a rich nerve and blood supply. The superficial zone is best developed at midcycle, as reflected by a high karyopyknotic index. This is much lower during the luteal phase when the vaginal smear contains many more leucocytes.

The pH is normally acid due to conversion of glycogen to lactic acid by Doderlein's lactobacillus. Increase in vaginal pH to 5 or more is often associated with pathogenic infection, presumably due to reduction in numbers of lactobacillus. Vaginal fluid has a higher potassium and lower sodium concentration than plasma.

FUNCTION

Sexual Intercourse

Vaginismus

This is a psychologically induced spasm of perineal muscles and vagina, making penetration difficult and painful or impossible. It may have had its origins in physical pain, such as an episiotomy scar, but often it is psychological, and sympathetic counselling may be of benefit.

Failure of orgasm

This has no effect on reproductive function. It is usually due to an unharmonious relationship, lack of adequate stimulation or general debility. In many women, vaginal intercourse without clitoral stimulation will not lead to orgasm. Manual stimulation of the clitoris by the partner or masturbation will lead to orgasm in most women. If it becomes a real problem, the couple should seek counselling.

Premature ejaculation

This is quite a common male problem, usually due to sexual inexperience, anxiety or, occasionally to some more deep-seated psychological problem.

Failure of ejaculation

This is usually psychological in origin. Both this and premature ejaculation are amenable to treatment using appropriate stimulating techniques.

Impotence

This can be primary due to a physical or congenital disorder, or secondarily due to physical or psychological stress. Identification of these causes can lead to cure. Occasionally, temporary inflatable splints can be used to allow intercourse to take place. Drug therapy to increase temporarily the arterial flow into the penis and reduce venous outflow is now available and is efficacious.

Sexual assault

Occasionally, doctors other than police surgeons are asked to see a woman who claims to have been sexually assaulted. Such women are usually deeply emotionally shocked and should be treated with great sympathy and gentleness, but also with frankness.

After a history has been taken, a thorough examination of all clothing and all parts of the body, in a good light, is essential. All parts of the body should be examined for signs of violence, with particular attention to the thighs, buttocks, introitus and vagina. Swabs and aspirates should be taken for the presence of seminal fluid and for infection. Finally a prescription of a postcoital contraceptive in the form of a double dose of a combined oral contraceptive on two consecutive days should be considered. Detailed notes must be taken of the entire examination, in case these are later legally required.

Micturition

This involves a complex interaction of bladder and pelvic muscles. As the bladder fills, it maintains a relatively constant tone in the muscle wall. Ultimately the increased intravesical pressure stimulates the sensory fibres in the pelvic splanchnic nerves. Through the efferent fibres of the same nerves, the bladder contracts while the urethra relaxes. Relaxation of the perineal muscles is caused by the pudendal nerve arising from the same segment of the spinal cord. Urine in the urethra stimulates sensory fibres in the pudendal nerve, which maintain the reflex until the bladder is empty. In addition to this basic spinal process, sensory impulses via the pelvic and hypogastric plexuses reach the thalamus and cerebral cortex. The higher centres exert inhibitory control of micturition.

Defecation

Defecation is similar in its control to micturition. Sensory fibres accompany the pelvic splanchnic nerves and carry afferent impulses from a distended rectum. This stimulates the parasympathetic fibres of the same nerves arising from S 2, 3 and 4, which causes a peristaltic wave to pass through the descending colon. Simultaneously, the anal sphincters relax unless there is cortical inhibition.

FURTHER READING

Philipp E., Barnes J., Newton M., eds. (1980). *Scientific Foundations of Obstetrics and Gynaecology*, 3rd edn. pp. 86–176. London: Heinemann Medical.

Smout C.F.V., Jacob E., Lillie E.W. (1969). *Gynaecological and Obstetrical Anatomy*, 4th edn. London: H. K. Lewis.

3

The Menstrual Cycle

The menstrual cycle is the term used to describe the monthly physiological events, which prepare the female for pregnancy and culminates in endometrial shedding and bleeding should this fail to occur. The average duration of the normal menstrual cycle is 28 days, but may range from 21–35 days.

Hormones from the hypothalamus, pituitary gland and ovaries mediate the regulation of the menstrual cycle. This is achieved by the production of trophic hormones at each level of the hypothalamic-pituitary-gonadal axis, which are in turn controlled by negative and positive feedback mechanisms. Feedback mechanisms are described as long, short or ultra-short depending on the site of production of the regulating hormone, i.e. whether from the ovary, pituitary or the hypothalamus. Negative feedback occurs when a rising level of induced hormone progressively inhibits further production of the stimulatory hormone, whereas positive feedback causes a further secretion.

The first part of this chapter will consider the hormonal control of menstruation, ovarian function, and the hormonal and histological changes in the female reproductive tract. The second part will describe the common disorders of the menstrual cycle, with the exception of abnormal uterine bleeding which is covered in Chapter 19.

THE HORMONES OF THE HYPOTHALAMIC-PITUITARY-OVARIAN AXIS (FIGS. 3.1–3.3)

The hypothalamus is the part of the brain that forms the floor and part of the lateral walls of the third ventricle. It secretes a decapeptide, gonadotrophin-releasing hormone (GnRH). This hormone has a half-life of only a few minutes and is secreted in pulses with a variable amplitude and frequency. During the normal menstrual cycle, the variable GnRH secretion causes luteinising hormone (LH) pulses every 90 minutes in the early follicular phase, increasing in frequency to 60-minute intervals at

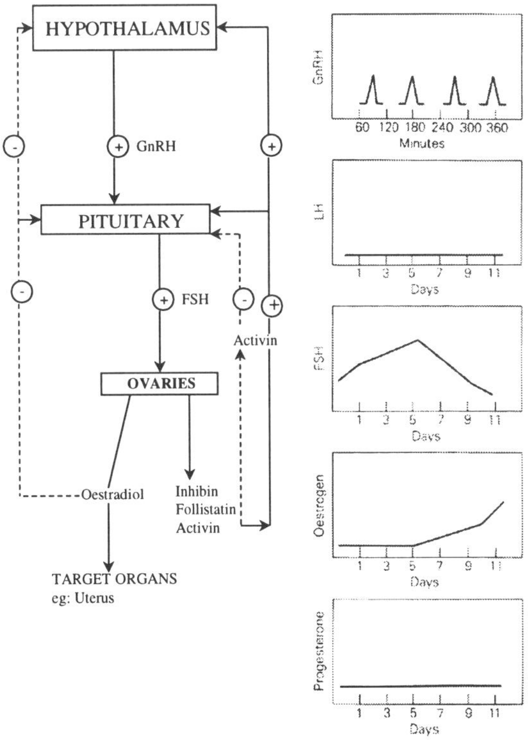

Fig. 3.1 ***The Hypothalamus-Pituitary-Ovarian Axis: Follicular Phase.***

Low oestrogens from the luteal-follicular menstrual interphase, and activin initially enhances GnRH and FSH secretion from days 1–5. The resulting oestradiol and inhibin rise from days 6–9 inhibit FSH in a negative feedback fashion.

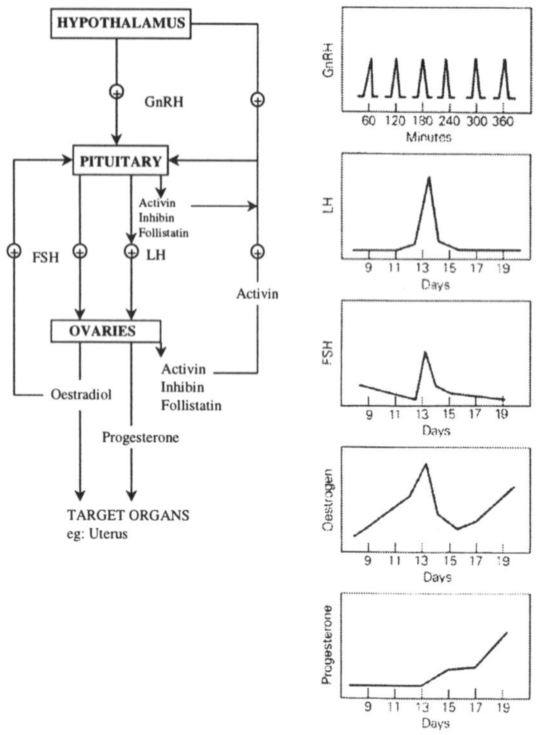

Fig. 3.2 ***The Hypothalamus-Pituitary-Ovarian Axis: Pre-Ovulatory Phase.***

Rising oestradiol and activin from day 10 exact a positive feedback on the pituitary gland. The LH surge is now thought to be due to the positive feedback exacted at the pituitary and not the hypothalamic level.

midcycle, and slowing to about 120 minutes in the luteal phase. GnRH secretion is under the influence of the catecholaminergic neurones, those with dopamine as the neurotransmitter are inhibitory, while those with noradrenaline are thought to be facilitatory. GnRH exerts its effect on the anterior pituitary, arriving by means of the hypophyseal-pituitary portal vasculature. It acts to increase synthesis, storage, activation and secretion of the gonadotrophins — LH and follicle stimulating hormone (FSH). GnRH activity is modulated at several levels, which include: (i) stimulating the formation of its own receptors, (ii) the ultra-short negative feedback loop within the hypothalamus, (iii) the short feedback loops from the pituitary, but (iv) largely by the ovarian steroids — oestrogen and progesterone, via the long feedback loops (see below).

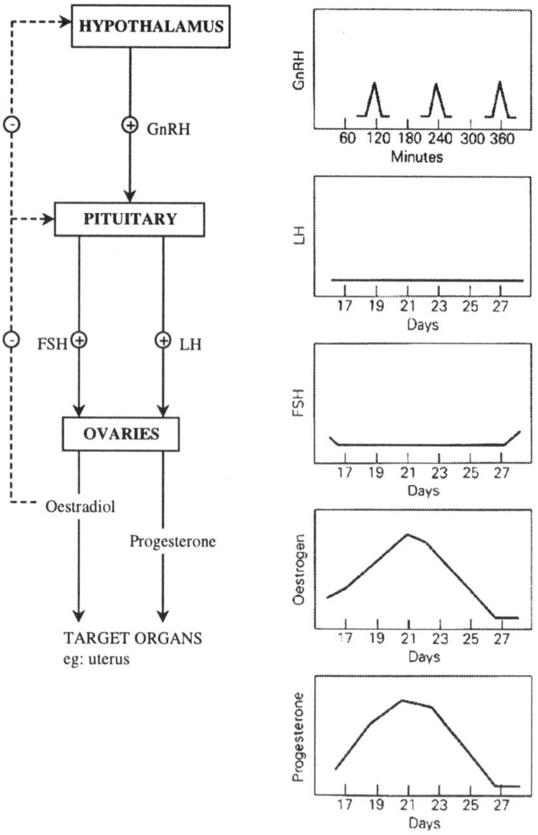

Fig. 3.3 ***The Hypothalamus-Pituitary-Ovarian Axis: Luteal Phase.***

Oestradiol and progesterone inhibit FSH and LH secretion. At the end of this phase, levels of oestradiol and progesterone have declined, allowing a rise in FSH, activin, inhibin and folistatin.

The anterior pituitary secretes LH and FSH from the gonadotrophic cells in a pulsatile fashion in response to GnRH. They act to stimulate ovarian activity directly. LH and FSH secretion are modulated by the pattern of GnRH secretion, by oestrogen and progesterone secreted by the ovary, and by activin, inhibin and follistatin produced by the pituitary and the ovary. Rising oestrogen secreted from the developing follicles acts on the hypothalamic-pituitary unit by inhibiting FSH secretion (negative feedback), while having little effect on LH secretion, in the first nine days (Fig. 3.2). In the pre-ovulatory period however, high levels of oestrogen acting on the *pituitary* by positive feedback effect, induce the

LH surge. Although the presence of GnRH is necessary for this surge, it is no longer believed that ovarian steroids mediate this positive feedback effect via an incremental production of GnRH. The pre-ovulatory rise in progesterone enhances the positive feedback of oestradiol, and may also be responsible for the FSH peak. In the luteal phase, high levels of progesterone act with oestrogen to inhibit gonadotrophin secretion (negative feedback) (Fig. 3.3).

Other hormones affect this axis, but mainly in pathological states. Prolactin has not been found to have any function in the normal menstrual cycle. It is under hypothalamic inhibitory control via dopamine, also called the prolactin inhibitory factor (PIF). Prolactin is responsible for its own regulation via positive feedback on the hypothalamus causing further dopamine release. It is subject to marked diurnal variation; highest concentrations are found during sleep and lowest levels during the late morning. Its secretion is also enhanced by stress. Thyrotrophin releasing factor also stimulates prolactin secretion. Although the physiological significance of this is unclear in *normal* menstrual cycle, it may explain why hypo- and hyperthyroidism are often implicated in the aetiology of menstrual disorders.

Cathecolamines and Endogenous Opioids

Dopamine, noradrenaline, serotonin and endogenous opioids are neurotransmitters also found from experiments, to have communication roles in the normal menstrual cycle.

1. *Noradrenaline* receptors in the anterior hypothalamus are stimulatory in action, and were thought to be involved in the mediation of the pre-ovulatory LH surge.
2. *Dopamine* (PIF) is the neurotransmitter delivered via the hypothalamic-hypophyseal portal system to inhibit pituitary prolactin secretion.
3. Endogenous opiate-like peptides or opioids include *endorphins*, *enkephalins* and *dynorphins*. They are believed to mediate inhibitory actions on gonadotrophin secretion by suppressing GnRH.

Paracrine and Autocrine Substances

Hormone-like peptides: activin, inhibin and follistatin

It is now known that ***hormone-like peptides*** act locally and at various levels of the hypothalamic-pituitary-ovarian axis (Figs. 3.1–3.2) where they function as endocrine, paracrine or autocrine substances. ***Paracrine*** peptides diffuse from cell to cell, across cellular membranes to mediate local tissue or organ functions. ***Autocrine*** substances on the other hand, act locally within a cell, to regulate intracellular functions. This knowledge is changing the way we have understood the control of normal menstruation for decades. Inhibin, activin and follistatin belong to the same family of peptides produced in tissues throughout the body where they serve as autocrine, paracrine and also endocrine regulators.

In the pituitary gland, GnRH is believed to induce the secretion of activin, inhibin and follistatin.

1. *Activin* in turn stimulates GnRH and enhances the gonadotrophin response to GnRH, whereas
2. *Inhibin* selectively inhibits FSH synthesis without affecting LH.
3. *Follistatin* is believed to suppress GnRH activity possibly by binding to activin.

In the ovary, the granulosa cells under the influence of FSH secrete the paracrine/autocrine peptides into the follicular fluid and the circulation.

1. *Activin* stimulates FSH secretion and also enhances its actions on the ovary in the follicular phase.
2. *Inhibin* is now believed to increase the activity of LH-mediated androgen production in the theca cells. The androgens, mainly in the forms of androstenedione and testosterone are then aromatised to oestrogens in the granulosa cells. Inhibin also suppresses FSH secretion from the pituitary gland in a negative feedback manner.

3. *Follistatin* is thought to suppress FSH activity by binding to activin, thereby inactivating it.
4. *Gonadotrophin surge attenuating factor* (GnSAF) is a new ovarian peptide, different from inhibin, produced under the stimulatory effect of FSH on a cohort of small super-ovulated follicles. It is believed to have an amino acid sequence as the C-terminal fragment of human serum albumin. Its function is to attenuate the pre-ovulatory LH surge in super-ovulated women.

Growth factors

Growth factors are polypeptides produced in many tissues where they mediate cell proliferation and differentiation. Whereas they cannot be regarded as typical hormones, they function similarly to autocrine and paracrine peptides. The follicular fluid is now known to contain an admixture of growth peptides. Only a few of them will be mentioned here:

1. *Insulin-like growth factors* (IGFs) are produced by granulosa, theca and luteinised granulosa cells. IGFs stimulate the proliferation of granulosa cells and enhance the LH-mediated production of androgens in theca cells. It is also believed to enhance progesterone synthesis. Insulin and IGFs are now implicated in the excessive androgen production associated with polycystic ovary disease (PCOD).
2. *Insulin-like growth factor binding proteins* (IGFBPs). These are peptides produced in the liver. Their function is to carry IGFs in the serum. By binding to IGFs, they prolong the half-life, thereby regulating their effects on tissues. Reduced hepatic production of IGFBPs and sex hormone binding globulins (SHBGs) are implicated in polycystic ovary disease (PCOD), causing increased serum levels of IGF which in turn contribute to excessive androgen production.
3. *Vascular endothelial growth factor* (VEGF) is an angiogenic factor produced into the follicular fluid in response to LH. It enhances vascularisation of the follicle and may increase vascular permeability. It is now believed to play an important role in the formation of the corpus luteum and is implicated in ovarian hyperstimulation syndrome (OHSS), a complication arising from ovarian stimulation (super-ovulation) during assisted conception. This endothelial mitogenic factor is also involved in endometrial repair during normal menstruation.
4. *Oocyte maturation inhibitor* (OMI) is a peptide produced by the granulosa cells of antral follicles. This peptide is believed to inhibit premature ovulation by preventing resumption of first meiosis until the LH surge.
5. *Endothelins* are also known as luteinisation inhibitors and may be involved in luteolysis, the process of corpus luteum degeneration. They are peptides produced by vascularised endothelial cells.
6. *Platelet-derived growth factor* (PDGF) is present in many tissues where it mediates local production of prostaglandins. It is involved in platelet plug formation and vasoconstriction during menstruation.

Cytokines

These are polypeptides that mediate inflammatory responses. They are produced by tissue macrophages.

1. *Tumour necrosis factor* (TNF-α) is a cytokine now thought to play a role in follicular atresia (apoptosis) and degeneration of the corpus luteum (luteolysis).

MECHANISM OF ACTION OF STEROID AND TROPHIC HORMONES

The mechanism of action of steroid hormones is similar irrespective of the target organ. The steroid crosses the cell membrane, binds to a cytoplasmic receptor protein to form a complex, which is then transferred across the nuclear membrane to the nucleus. The complex then binds to nuclear DNA, resulting in synthesis of specific messenger RNAs. These are then transported to the ribosomes where protein synthesis takes place. The major regulator of the process is the activity of intracellular receptors. The target cells of the ovarian steroids contain oestrogen receptors. Oestrogen stimulation causes the proliferation of further oestrogen receptors (*upregulation*) as well as the synthesis of progesterone and androgen receptors (*priming*). Progesterone and androgens cause a decrease in intracellular oestrogen receptors (*down-regulation*).

The trophic hormones, such as the gonadotrophins may act via the cyclic-adenyl monophosphate (c-AMP) pathway. This is a process whereby hormones bind with specific receptors in the cell membrane, thereby activating the enzyme adenyl cyclase, which increases conversion of adenyl triphosphate (ATP) to cyclic-AMP. The cyclic-AMP-gonadotrophin complex in turn activates a protein kinase, which in turn, catalyses the phosphorylation of several cellular enzymes. These cellular enzymes in turn, modulate the rate of catalytic activity. For example, phosphorylation of cholesterol esterase results in increased rates of release of cholesterol (the precursor of the steroid hormones) from cholesterol esters. Growth factors, paracrine and autocrine peptides also modulate the actions of gonadotrophins as described above.

OVARIAN CYCLE

The ovarian cycle usually culminates in the maturity of one egg, nurtured prior to ovulation within a follicle. Following ovulation, this same follicle becomes a different functional unit, the corpus luteum, which serves to maintain the hormonal environment necessary to allow implantation and very early development of the embryo. To understand the ovarian cycle, it would be divided into:

1. The phase of follicular development.
2. The ovulatory process.
3. The luteal phase.

Follicular Development

Most of what we knew about follicular development and the interactions of glycoprotein and steroid hormones that control it were derived from experiments in rodents. Experiments on monkeys and human ovarian tissues have now shown that paracrine and autocrine peptides inhibin, activin and follistatin play key roles in folliculogenesis. Although a continuous process, it can for the purposes of description be considered in three stages.

Very early follicular development (recruitment)

Primordial germ cells originating in the embryonic endoderm around the yolk sac, allantois and hindgut migrate to the germinal ridge and multiply rapidly by mitosis to form oogonia. Oogonia become primary oocytes after entry into the first meiotic division. By 20 weeks, there is a maximum of about 7 million primary oocytes in both ovaries. At birth only 2 million remain, reduced further to 400,000 at puberty. A primordial follicle, first recognisable in the fetal ovary at about the 25th week of gestation, is a primary oocyte arrested in the diplotene stage of the first meiotic prophase, surrounded by a single layer of granulosa cells.

The stimulus for the continuing development of a pool of primordial follicles is unknown, although it seems to be independent of pituitary control. It takes about 10 weeks for a primordial follicle to develop into an antral follicle. This is a follicle capable of undergoing

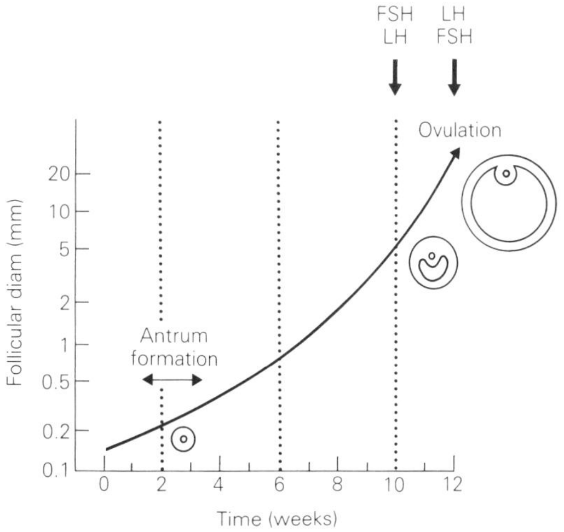

Fig. 3.4 *Development of a follicle destined to ovulated.*

complete maturation, provided it receives appropriate gonadotrophic stimulation (Fig. 3.4).

Each month, hundreds of primordial follicles will start to grow. Most will however undergo a process of programmed cell death called *apoptosis*, commonly referred to as atresia. It is now believed that the cytokine TNF-α plays a key role in follicular atresia. Only a few follicles will *escape* from apoptosis, and at the menstrual luteal-follicular interphase become *recruited* by rising basal FSH to progress to the next phase.

Early follicular development (selection)

By this stage, the follicles undergo several morphological changes. Fluid appears between the granulosa cells and coalesces to form a fluid-filled antrum. The oocytes enlarge and each separates itself from the granulosa cells by the zona pellucida, a porous non-cellular layer of glycoprotein. The granulosa cells proliferate; forming a dense layer called the cumulus oophorus, which surrounds each oocyte. The surrounding stroma, external to the basement membrane, differentiates into the theca interna, which is well vascularised and the theca externa that forms a fibrous layer.

The relatively avascular granulosa cells are the only unit to contain FSH receptors, and hence the only layer able to respond to this hormone. The theca interna contains LH receptors, and since it is well vascularised, responds to the relatively low, but ever present, circulating LH. Under LH stimulation, the theca is able to synthesise androgens, mainly androstenedione and testosterone from cholesterol. Continued follicular development is dependent upon basal FSH secretion, which acts via the c-AMP pathway. This is a process whereby hormones bind with specific receptors on the cell surface, thereby activating the enzyme adenyl cyclase, which increases conversion of ATP to cyclic-AMP. The cyclic-AMP-gonadotrophin complex in the granulosa cells in turn catalyses the aromatisation of androgens derived from theca cells to oestrogens (Fig. 3.5). These form the basis of the two-cell, two-gonadotrophin theory of steroid synthesis in developing ovarian follicles. The cyclic-AMP-gonadotrophin complex also amplifies both FSH and LH receptor contents.

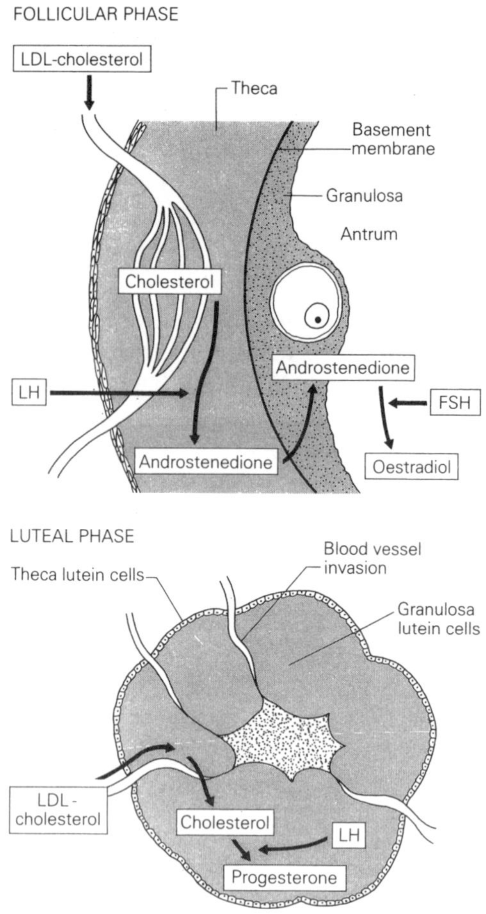

Fig. 3.5 *Ovarian steroidogenesis in the follicular and luteal phases. (Adapted from S.G. Hillier and E.J. Wickings, 1985. In The Luteal Phase. S.L. Jeffcoate, ed. Chichester, New York: Wiley.)*

Late follicular development

It has already been stated that there are a cohort of follicles developing of which only one is destined to be selected as the ovulatory follicle. Because of negative feedback on the hypothalamic-pituitary axis, FSH secretion rapidly diminishes. Only one dominant follicle is able to continue to respond to the decreasing FSH stimulation, because it has the largest number of granulosa cells, and hence the largest number of FSH receptors, increased intrafollicular oestrogen and paracrine/ autocrine peptides. The lead follicle also contains the largest number of the recently acquired LH receptors and so is able to respond to LH stimulation. Thecal vascularity is markedly increased, thereby allowing more gonadotrophins to permeate through and reach the receptors.

The dominant follicle is recognised as the largest follicle present in either ovary, measuring about 2 cm in diameter and containing about 6 ml of follicular fluid, just prior to ovulation. While the main function of the follicular phase is to allow these intraovarian events to take place, the secretion of oestrogen is the primary stimulus for a number of target organs, particularly the uterus.

The events of follicular development can be summarised as shown below:

1. FSH rise commencing at the menstrual luteal-follicular interphase stimulates follicular development and the formation of antra in the selected cohort of follicles.
2. The developing cohort of follicles secretes oestrogen, which exerts a negative feedback on follicular development and FSH secretion, causing a mild decline from day 6–9.
3. The dominant follicle is however not similarly affected because it protects itself by increased FSH receptors, a very high intrafollicular oestrogen concentration, or as shown by recent experiments in primates, the effects of paracrin and autocrine peptides.

Ovulation

Pre-ovulatory phase

LH is the chief hormone responsible for initiating the ovulatory process. The lead follicle has had prior priming with LH receptors in response to FSH stimulation.

The onset of the LH surge is the trigger that programmes the pre-ovulatory follicle into a timed and orderly sequence of events culminating in ovulation. Concomitant with the LH surge is a smaller FSH surge. After the gonadotrophin surge has been initiated, there is a dramatic and precipitate drop in serum oestradiol levels. This is probably due to down-regulation by LH of its own receptors in the theca cells, thus depriving the granulosa cells of the necessary androgen substrate. Progesterone also inhibits further granulosa cell proliferation.

The signal for the initiation of the midcycle gonadotrophin surge is unclear. It may be related to the pattern of oestradiol secretion, which under these circumstances assumes a form of positive feedback on LH secretion. Serum oestradiol rises steadily and reaches a peak. The LH surge is triggered as the oestradiol level approaches or attains its maximum (Fig. 3.2). It appears that LH production in order to reach a surge requires 2–3 days of sustained and incremental oestradiol priming at a critical level. Progesterone at low, but increasing, levels may act synergistically with oestrogen to enhance the surge. It seems likely that other factors are also involved.

As a result of the LH surge, specific cytoplasmic and nuclear events take place. Cytoplasmic changes include a marked increase in protein synthesis, particularly the proteolytic enzymes involved in lysis of the follicular wall. $PGF_{2\alpha}$ levels in follicular fluid also increase. Oestrogen levels decline and progesterone increases as the granulosa cells, under the influence of LH, switch to progesterone production. Nuclear maturation involves the progression of the chromosomes through the remainder of the first meiotic division, culminating in equal chromosomal, but unequal cytoplasmic division, with one cell (the secondary oocyte) taking nearly all the cytoplasm. The remaining chromosomes are discarded as the first polar body. The chromosomes are then arrested for a second time, this time in metaphase of the second meiotic division. Ovulation will occur with the oocyte in this state.

Premature oocyte maturation is prevented by local inhibitory factors in the follicular fluid, particularly the oocyte maturation inhibitor (OMI). The LH surge must overcome this local inhibitory factor for ovulation to take place.

Ovulation

Follicular rupture with escape of the oocyte depends upon degenerative changes in the expanding and thin follicular wall. There is enhancement of the activity of the proteolytic enzymes, such as collagenase. Plasminogen activators produced in granulosa and theca cells in response to the LH surge, and prostaglandins, particularly $PGF_{2\alpha}$, are believed to play significant roles in the activation of these enzymes. Prostaglandins also increase ovarian contractions that could increase the intra-follicular pressure. The site of follicular rupture is called the stigma. Tubal and ovarian motility ensure that the tubal fimbriae sweep over the ovarian surface to take in the freshly ovulated egg.

It is imperative that follicular maturation and the gonadotrophin surge coincide appropriately. The trigger for ovulation occurs as a result of hormonal feedback from the developing follicle. Only after the follicle has reached the appropriate stage of maturity will the positive oestrogenic feedback trigger the LH surge, thereby ensuring precise synchrony.

It is unclear how the LH surge is terminated. This may be as a result of one or a combination of factors including: depletion of pituitary LH, a negative feedback of LH on the hypothalamus, the loss of the positive feedback of oestradiol on the pituitary gland following its precipitate fall, or an increasing negative feedback of rising levels of progesterone.

Luteal Phase

Progesterone is the main hormone of the luteal phase. Normal luteal function is dependent upon optimal follicular development. The formation of sufficient numbers of LH receptors pre-determines the degree of luteinisation and hence its subsequent functional capacity. It is also dependent upon adequate vascularisation so that cholesterol substrate can be transported in order to synthesise progesterone.

Luteinisation of the developing follicle occurs before ovulation in response to the LH surge. This is reflected in a significant rise in serum progesterone prior to ovulation. Luteinisation may even occur in the absence of follicular rupture, with entrapment of the egg — the so-called luteinised unruptured follicle syndrome.

After ovulation, the follicle gives rise to a new anatomical structure, the corpus luteum. The granulosa cells become larger and stained with a yellow pigment (lutein) and are now known as the granulosa-lutein cells. The theca also differentiates to contribute to the corpus luteum, the theca-lutein cells. Proliferation of new capillaries into the granulosa layer is an essential feature of luteinisation. This is initiated by LH, enhanced by paracrine substances like the vascular endothelial growth factor (VEGF). Neovascularisation of the granulosa layer ultimately reaches the central cavity, now vacated by the follicular fluid after ovulation, often filling it with blood. Cholesterol, carried mainly within low-density lipoproteins (LDL), combines with specific receptors to be taken up by the granulosa-lutein cells. It is now available as substrate for progesterone synthesis (Fig. 3.5). This process along with the synthesis of both oestrogen and progesterone is dependent on continued gonadotrophic stimulation.

Oestrogen is synthesised in the corpus luteum in a manner comparable to the follicular phase, as FSH reaches the granulosa-lutein cells in significant quantities due to the increased vascularity. Corpus luteum function is twofold — it provides the hormonal stimulus for the target organs, specifically the uterus, and also regulates the ovarian cycle. Progesterone depletes local oestrogen receptors. It also acts synergistically with oestradiol to inhibit, by negative feedback, gonadotrophin secretion. As a result, FSH and oestradiol-dependent follicular growth is inhibited.

The corpus luteum reaches peak activity about 7 days post-ovulation. This is coincident with peak vascularisation, and is therefore reflected in peak serum progesterone and oestradiol levels in the luteal phase. The corpus luteum declines rapidly 9–11 days post-ovulation. Variability in cycle length is due mainly to differences in the length of the follicular phase.

Luteal regression or luteolysis involves ischaemia and cell death, resulting in a fall in progesterone secretion. The whitish scar tissue thus formed is called the corpus albicans. The main hormone responsible for luteolysis is probably oestrogen, but the mechanism is uncertain. Oxytocin, $PGF_{2\alpha}$, and endothelins can be detected in the late corpus luteum, and each may have a role. Luteolysis may involve inhibition of the conversion of cholesterol to pregnenolone, thus switching off progesterone production, and a reduction in the luteal blood flow, leading to ischaemia. However, the exact mechanism for initiation of luteolysis in the human is still poorly understood.

Regression of the corpus luteum is inevitable unless pregnancy supervenes. Should pregnancy occur however, rising beta-HCG levels are detectable around 12 days post-ovulation. HCG maintains the corpus luteum steroid output until about the 10th week of pregnancy after which the placenta takes over.

OVARIAN FUNCTION

Menarche

Follicles are first seen in the fetal ovary during the 25th week of gestation. From its inception, the follicles in the ovary are continuously undergoing development and atresia, though the steroid output of the ovary is minimal. Prior to puberty the ovary grows slowly in size. The menarche is defined as the age at which the first menstrual bleed takes place. It indicates that there is sufficient ovarian activity to have secreted some oestrogen to induce uterine development, and to have caused bleeding. It does not signify fertility, as during the first two years, the cycles are mainly anovulatory.

The menarche occurs fairly late in the pubertal process. Puberty starts initially with a growth spurt, followed by the development of the secondary sex characteristics, such as breast development, pubic hair and the development of external genitalia.

The onset of menarche requires the prior maturation of the hypothalamic-pituitary-ovarian axis. At birth, there are low plasma levels of gonadotrophins as a result of the high levels of circulating maternal steroids. This is followed by a rebound rise in the gonadotrophin levels, until about 2 years of age. FSH thereafter becomes very sensitive to the negative feedback effect of oestrogen. This coupled with an inherent repression of GnRH secretion leading to low levels of gonadotrophins until the age of 8 years.

The first changes in this pre-pubertal low endocrine balance occur between the ages of 8 and 11 years. This is a marked increase in magnitude and frequency of GnRH pulses at night, leading to similar pulses of the gonadotrophins. In late puberty, daytime pulses also become apparent, until gradually the adult pattern of GnRH pulsatility is reached. A maturation of the feedback mechanisms is also involved, as the negative feedback effect of oestrogen diminishes during puberty, allowing increased FSH and LH secretion for the same amount of oestrogen. The pituitary's sensitivity to GnRH also increases during puberty. This may be due in part to a self-priming effect, and in part to the rising oestrogen levels. The positive feedback effect of oestrogen and the ability to have a gonadotrophin surge is a relatively late process.

Over the past 150 years, the average age of the menarche has declined from 17 to 13 years, the normal range now being between 10–16 years. This decline can be attributed to improved healthcare and a rise in socio-economic standards, as the body weight at menarche has remained remarkably constant, 45–47 kg. It had been widely held that a critical body weight needed to be attained to allow activation of the hypothalamic-pituitary axis. This issue is now debatable. It appears that the proportion of body fat, rather than total body weight, or interplay of physical, social and genetic factors is responsible.

Menopause

The menopause is defined as the last menstrual period, a diagnosis usually made retrospectively after 12 months of secondary amenorrhoea, supported by very high serum FSH and low oestradiol levels. The average age at menopause is 51 years. When it occurs below the age of 40 years, this is termed premature menopause.

UTERINE CYCLE

The ovarian cycle determines the pattern of ovarian hormones measurable in the blood. The most important, but by no means the only target organ of these hormones, is the uterus.

Changes in the Uterine Body

Myometrium

Myometrial activity is inversely related to progesterone secretion. During menstruation, the uterus actively contracts with a greater frequency and strength than found in labour as a result of stimulation by locally released prostaglandins. After menstruation, there is a slow decline in activity during the follicular phase until there is almost no spontaneous activity at midcycle. This quiescence is maintained until the late luteal phase. If pregnancy supervenes, the myometrium remains inactive.

Uterine blood flow

Uterine blood flow correlates positively with the pattern of oestrogen secretion. Blood flow through the uterus is least during menstruation and the early follicular phase. There is then a marked increase with a peak just before ovulation, followed by a slight decrease and a secondary peak in the luteal phase. The flow then decreases prior to menstruation.

Endometrial changes (Figs. 3.6–3.10)

The proliferative phase. This is under oestrogenic control. Oestrogen stimulates the production of its own receptors, thus enhancing its own effect (upregulation). It also causes production of progesterone receptors, priming the endometrium, to enable it to respond to progesterone in the luteal phase. Without oestrogen priming, progesterone has no influence on the endometrium.

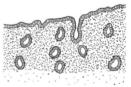

Within 48 hours of menstruation ceasing, the surface of the endometrium is covered by epithelial outgrowths from the remnants of glands in the basal part of the tissue. The rapid growth of the endometrium is seen mostly in the glands, which start as straight tubular structures (Fig. 3.6), but become increasingly long and convoluted. The gland cells are low columnar cells with centrally placed nuclei showing considerable mitotic activity (Fig. 3.7). The stromal cells similarly increase in number. These are small, spindle-shaped cells with very little cytoplasm. Except for a brief period of transient stromal oedema in the mid-follicular phase, the glandular epithelium thus extends onto the surface to link one segment with another, showing pseudostratification.

The blood supply to the endometrium is twofold: the basal layer is supplied by straight arteries; the glands are supplied by coiled spiral arteries, forming three capillary plexuses — one just below the surface epithelium, a second surrounding the glands and a third within the stroma. A network of veins drains into the venous sinuses.

During proliferation, the endometrium grows from approximately 0.5 mm to 5 mm in height — a tenfold increase. This is in

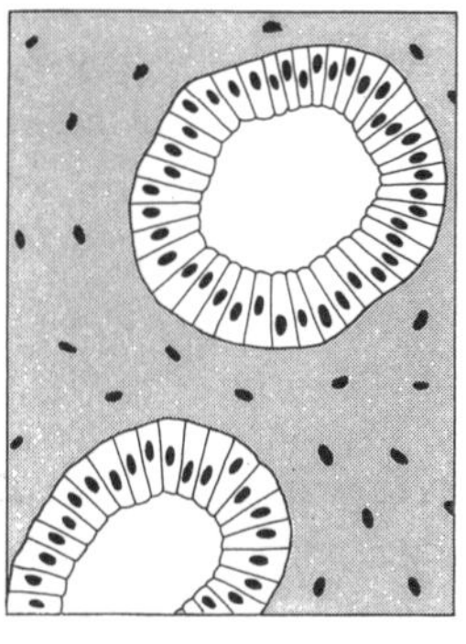

Fig. 3.6 *The endometrium in the early proliferative phase.*

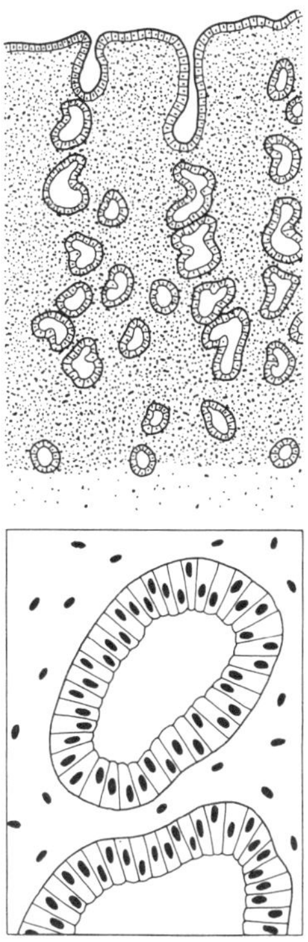

Fig. 3.7 *The endometrium in the late proliferative phase.*

part due to new tissue growth and in part to stromal expansion.

The secretory phase. Following ovulation, progesterone becomes the dominant hormone, although oestrogen is secreted in levels comparable to the follicular phase. Under the influence of progesterone, endometrial growth ceases, and the tissue now enters its functional stage as it prepares to accept the embryo.

The glands are convoluted and dilated with secretions. They commence secretory activity with subnuclear vacuoles appearing (Fig. 3.8). These gradually come to lie in the apical part of the gland before discharging their contents into the lumen of the gland. The secretions consist mainly of glycogen, sugars, amino acids, mucus and enzymes, such as alkaline phosphatase. By the end of the week following ovulation, the secretory process is finished and the glands appear exhausted (Fig. 3.9). Meanwhile, nuclear mitotic activity has declined considerably.

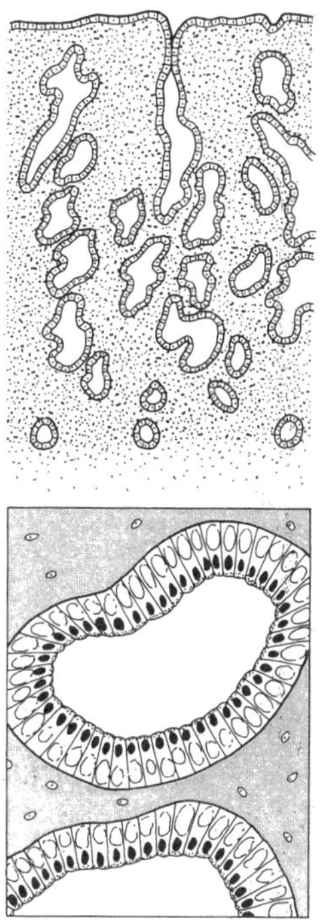

Cells have apical nuclei and basal vacuoles

Fig. 3.8 *The endometrium in the early secretory phase.*

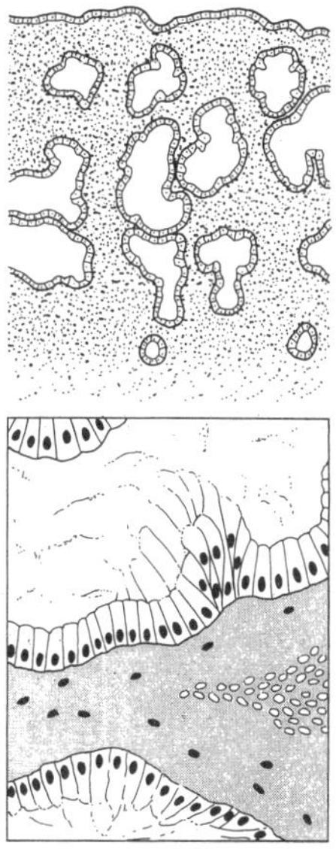

Marked decrease in tissue height. Glands exhausted of secretions
Cells show basal nuclei. Vacuoles have discharged their contents into the lumen. Breakdown of spiral arteries in the stroma

Fig. 3.9 *The endometrium in the late secretory phase.*

The spiral arteries are more prominent, becoming increasingly corkscrew in appearance. This is mainly due to their continuing growth, while the endometrial height has remained relatively static. The changes in the late secretory phase will depend on whether implantation has taken place.

Implantation. Glandular secretory activity is re-awakened, while the superficial stromal cells become large and polyhedral with cytoplasmic extensions, forming a strong compact layer, the stratum compactum. This overlies loose oedematous stroma, surrounding the tightly coiled spiral arteries, the stratum spongiosum. The basal layer remains unchanged with the spindle-shaped stromal cells surrounding the straight arteries, stratum basalis.

Non-implantation. A similar histological pattern is seen initially (pseudo-decidualisation). However, in the absence of implantation and continued gonadotrophic support to maintain the steroid output of the corpus luteum, there is first a modest, then a marked reduction in tissue height. This causes a tighter coiling of the spiral arteries, similar to a spring being compressed. This buckling causes stasis and ischaemia. The spiral arteries undergo rhythmic constriction and relaxation, each wave longer and more profound than the previous one, eventually leading to blanching of the endometrium. This activity is probably under local prostaglandin control. PGE_2 causes relaxation of vascular smooth muscle and $PGF_{2\alpha}$ causes vasoconstriction. Even more powerful are prostacyclin (PGI_2) as a vasodilator and inhibitor of platelet aggregation, and thromboxane A_2 as a vasoconstrictor. These substances are all synthesised in the endometrium and in the spiral arteries themselves. Their balance may be important in causing vasospasm.

In the 24 hours prior to menstruation, there is marked ischaemia and stasis. These stimuli further increase the local release of prostaglandins. White cells migrate into the stroma, red cells leak into the interstitial spaces, and thrombin-platelet plugs appear. Further thromboxane release occurs from the platelet plugs.

Menstruation. Interstitial haemorrhage occurs as a result of the breakdown of the superficial arterioles and capillaries. The generalised ischaemia weakens the structure of the superficial layers of the endometrium. The non-viable tissue formed as a result of cell and vascular necrosis is extruded into the endometrial cavity and contributes to the menstrual flow. This process continues until the basal layer is reached, where a natural cleavage plane is formed. Here the straight arteries maintain the blood supply and hence integrity of the basal layer, and in this way the layers superficial to the basal layer are shed (Fig. 3.10). Menstrual blood does not normally coagulate, and does not contain fibrin, probably as a result of proteolytic and fibrinolytic enzymes secreted by the damaged endometrial cells. Within 12 hours the endometrial height has shrunk from 4 mm to about 1 mm.

Menstrual flow is limited by *endometrial repair.* Resumption of oestrogen secretion by the developing follicle induces healing and new tissue growth, probably mediated by local epidermal and fibroblast growth factors, platelet-activated growth factor, vascular endothelial growth factor and endothelins. Menstruation eventually stops due to the formation of thrombin-platelet plugs, vascular stasis and prolonged vasoconstriction

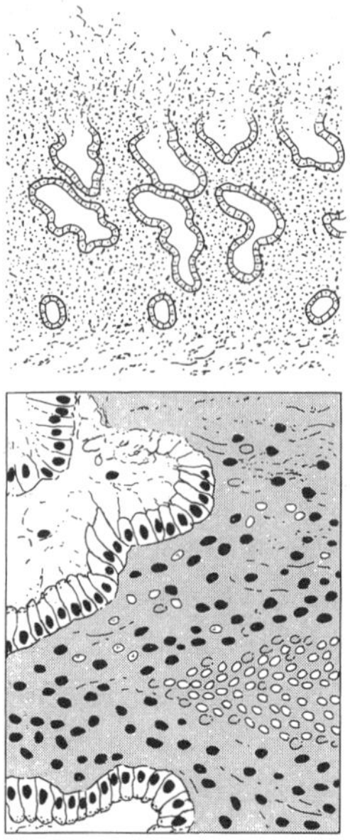

Fig. 3.10 *The endometrium during menstruation.*

of the spiral arteries — processes that involve local prostaglandins.

Changes in the Uterine Cervix

Oestrogen causes relaxation of the muscles of the cervix and increased stromal vascularity and oedema. Collagenase is activated and the tightly bound collagen bundles are largely dispersed into a loose matrix of collagen and stroma. It is softer to the touch, and eversion of the external os can be seen prior to ovulation. Under progesterone influence, the muscles retract and the stroma becomes more compact and the collagen matrix reforms. The cervix is therefore firmer and the external os becomes tighter.

Cervical epithelium

The endocervical canal is about 3 cm long and is lined with columnar epithelium. The epithelium is thrown into complex folds, with extensive gland formation, known as crypts. Groups of cells in each crypt secrete different types of mucus. The mucus produced in response to oestrogenic stimulation has a very high water content (98%), and a network of long polypeptide macromolecules, lying parallel to each other and linked by carbohydrate side chains. The channels thus formed are up to 5 microns in width and allow easy sperm migration. The type produced under progesterone influence consists of a meshwork of polypeptide strands with increased carbohydrate linkages, with much smaller spaces between the macromolecules, and with reduced water content.

Clinically, oestrogenised mucus is seen as a copious, clear watery secretion, which stretches easily for up to 8 cm between two glass surfaces (spinnbarkeit test). Under the microscope, the mucus is acellular, and on drying, the dehydration reveals strands of mucus forming a ferning pattern. Cervical mucus under progesterone effect is scanty, cloudy and tacky. Microscopy reveals the presence of cells and the absence of ferning. The function of the cervical mucus is to assist the passage of sperm deposited in the vagina at the appropriate time. It, along with the uterine isthmus, acts as a major reservoir for sperm. The mucus plug would also seem to serve to protect against the passage of infection.

Other Physiological Changes During the Menstrual Cycle

Fallopian tube

Oestrogen increases epithelial activity with increased ciliation and secretory activity. Progestogenic effects are the reverse of this. Progesterone also decreases muscle activity.

Vagina

Oestrogens increase mitotic activity in the surface columnar epithelium and cause keratinisation. These cells have a small pyknotic nucleus and abundant cytoplasm. Under progesterone influence, the nucleus becomes larger and vesicular. A vaginal smear shows cells clumped together and folded in on themselves, as opposed to the single flat cells seen during oestrogen stimulation.

Breast

Although oestrogenic and progestogenic changes have been shown, these are not marked until the premenstrual period. At this time, there is connective tissue oedema and hyperaemia. This is responsible for the increase in breast size and breast tenderness experienced during this period.

Skin

Changes are sometimes seen during the premenstruum. There is an increase in skin pigmentation, especially around the mouth, forehead, the nipple areolae and the linea nigra. Progesterone also causes constriction of the sebaceous gland ducts, thus exacerbating acne in sufferers.

Body temperature

Small rises in progesterone will cause a rise in basal body temperature. Progesterone or its metabolites act directly on the thermoregulatory centre in the hypothalamus to raise the temperature between 0.2°C and 0.6°C.

Thyroid function

The only change is the expected slight rise in the basal metabolic rate secondary to the rise in temperature in the luteal phase.

Adrenal function

Aldosterone is secreted in larger amounts during the luteal phase, probably in direct response to progesterone.

Symptomatic changes

During the premenstrual phase, from ovulation to the onset of menstruation, many women experience a feeling of bloatedness, breast tenderness, and a change of affect, particularly depression and irritability. It seems that up to 90% of women experience at least one of these symptoms to some degree.

DISORDERS OF THE MENSTRUAL CYCLE

Menstruation depends upon an intact hypothalamic-pituitary axis, normal ovarian function, a functionally responsive uterus and an intact outflow tract, i.e. cervix and vagina. A disturbance of any one of these components may result in disordered menstrual function.

The main symptom groups are:

1. Absent or scanty bleeding.
2. Heavy and/or frequent bleeding (discussed in Chapter 18).
3. Painful periods.
4. Premenstrual syndrome.

Symptoms related to the menstrual cycle often have considerable emotional and psychological overlay, which may be due to a central effect on the hypothalamus, altering its function, or to a colouring of the perception of the symptoms.

Primary Amenorrhoea

Primary amenorrhoea means that a woman has never had a period, while secondary amenorrhoea is defined as the absence of menstrual bleeding for 6 or more months in a woman who has had a normal period before. Oligomenorrhoea occurs in women with scanty, infrequent menstrual bleeding every 6 weeks or more, most having less than 6 periods in a year. If menstruation has not occurred by the age of 14 in the absence of growth and secondary sexual characteristics, particularly breast development, this is abnormal and should be investigated. If it has not occurred at the age of 16, irrespective of breast development or other signs of secondary sexual characteristics, the patient should also be investigated.

Amenorrhoea implies either a problem with the uterus and outflow tract, or profound depression of the ovarian steroids. The aetiology and diagnosis of primary amenorrhoea can seem complicated. The process of making a diagnosis can be simplified if, by a physical examination, patients can be divided into three categories. These are:

1. Primary amenorrhoea with *no* breast development, but *normal female genitalia.*
2. Primary amenorrhoea with *normal* breast development, but *absent uterus.*
3. Primary amenorrhoea with *normal* breast development, and an apparently *normal genital tract.*

The causes of the first two categories, together with the diagnostic steps needed to arrive at a conclusion are shown in Fig. 3.11.

Abnormal karyotypes

For women without, or with only streak ovaries due to an abnormal karyotype, hormone replacement therapy (HRT) from the age of 12–14 years is usually needed to start and maintain secondary sexual development and to protect the bones from osteoporotic thinning. If HRT is started too early however, it may lead to premature closure of the epiphyses, causing

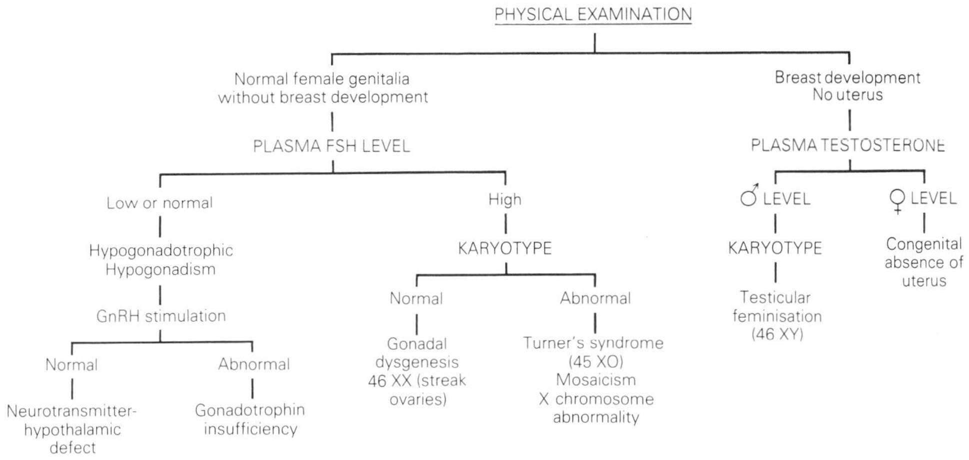

Fig. 3.11 *Scheme for establishing the cause of certain types of primary amenorrhoea. (By courtesy of D.R. Mishell, Jr. and V. Davajan, eds., 1979. Reproductive Endocrinology in Fertility and Contraception. Philadelphia: Davis.)*

short stature. Removal of intra-abdominal testes in complete androgen insensitivity should be undertaken at puberty. Immediate removal of streak ovaries in mixed gonadal dysgenesis is necessary, as soon as the presence of a Y chromosome is demonstrated on the karyotype because of the risk of early onset gonadal malignancy (gonadoblastoma or dysgerminoma). Patients with pure gonadal dysgenesis 46XX or Turner's syndrome, 45X however do not need to have gonadectomy.

Cryptomenorrhoea

Failure to expel menstrual blood occurs when there is an imperforate hymen or a transverse septum just above the hymen closing off the vagina completely. This is easily detected on physical examination or on ultrasound genital examination. The patient will be otherwise anatomically normal. Treatment is by surgical incision and drainage of the retained menstrual blood. Care must be taken to avoid introducing infection.

Congenital absence of the uterus

This may or may not be accompanied by other abnormalities of the genital tract, such as an absent vagina. Congenital uterine and vaginal abnormalities are associated with up to 40% incidence of minor urinary tract anomalies, and 10–15% of skeletal defects.

If the initial physical examination is unremarkable, then the cause of primary amenorrhoea can arise from the hypothalamus or pituitary.

Hypothalamic causes

Primary hypothalamic dysfunction prevents a normal interaction between GnRH and gonadotrophins, and there is usually evidence of other hormonal abnormalities. Hypothalamic dysfunction commonly arises from tumour-like craniopharyngiomas or gliomas. Craniopharyngiomas are cystic tumours with calcifications arising from the remnants of Rathke's pouch. They are the most common hypothalamic tumours causing primary amenorrhoea associated with delayed puberty, and *must* always be borne in mind. Craniopharyngiomas most commonly present before the age of 14 years, but may also cause secondary amenorrhoea in young women. Primary hypothalamic dysfunction can also occasionally follow trauma or infection such as encephalitis in childhood.

In many cases, FSH and oestradiol levels will be low, resulting in poor uterine development. In others, FSH assay may be normal. This is because such molecules are immunologically active, and therefore detectable normally by immunoassays, however they have increased sialic acids in the carbohydrate components which renders them biologically non-functional. Consequently, this later group will be hypoestrogenic and show no withdrawal uterine bleeding following 5 days of oral progestogen therapy, until the uterus is first primed with oestrogen. Diagnosing craniopharyngiomas requires a high index of suspicion, which can easily be confirmed by imaging (computerised tomography — CT scan, or magnetic resonance imaging — MRI) of the head. Patients with primary amenorrhoea due to hypothalamic causes will usually require prolonged GnRH administration.

Isolated GnRH deficiency may result from a malfunction of the rhinencephalon causing variable degrees of inability to smell (e.g. distinguish smell of coffee from tea) as well as primary amenorrhoea and infantile sexual development. It is known as Kallman's syndrome and responds to GnRH treatment. Colour blindness and mental retardation are sometimes associated.

Pituitary causes

Pituitary tumours are also easily diagnosed by imaging of the head. Sometimes there are altered visual fields due to pressure on the optic chiasma, therefore neurological and ophthalmic examinations are essential. Classically, a pituitary tumour is said to cause bitemporal hemianopia. Treatment of pituitary tumours is by surgical removal or ablation by radioactive implants. Small prolactinomas will usually respond to suppression by dopamine agonists like bromocriptine and cabergoline.

Patients with congenital hypopituitarism will present with other signs of pituitary dysfunction, such as failure to grow. The treatment of hypopituitarism is hormone replacement therapy.

Secondary Amenorrhoea

Secondary amenorrhoea is said to occur if menstruation ceases for 6 months or more, in a patient who had previously menstruated normally. This interval is usually necessary to distinguish it from oligomenorrhoea, which is defined as scanty, infrequent periods occurring not less than every 42 days. The most common causes of secondary amenorrhoea are physiological (pregnancy, breastfeeding and menopause), and these should always be considered first.

It is helpful to consider the possible causes of secondary amenorrhoea in two groups:

1. Acquired disorders of the uterus and lower genital tract.
2. Anovulation.

Acquired disorders of the uterus and lower genital tract

Asherman's syndrome is secondary amenorrhoea caused by uterine adhesions or synechiae following sharp curettage of the uterus for incomplete miscarriage or secondary postpartum haemorrhage. Cervical or vaginal stenosis caused by surgical, infective, neoplastic, or chemical injuries are very uncommon in developed countries. The diagnoses are usually obvious from the history and physical examination. The diagnosis of uterine adhesions or synechiae is confirmed by hysterosalpingography (HSG) or at hysteroscopy. Treatment by hysteroscopic division of uterine adhesions is performed if the patient wishes to conceive. Acquired cervical or vaginal stenosis have to be surgically corrected to relieve dammed-back menstruum (cryptomenorrhoea), alleviate cyclical abdominal pain or treat dyspareunia.

Anovulation

It follows that if the uterus and outflow tract are functionally intact, then the problem lies with the lack of appropriate sex steroid stimulation, as a result of anovulation. Failure to ovulate may be due to hypothalamic-pituitary-ovarian hypofunction or dysfunction.

Hypothalamic failure. Hypothalamic failure is diagnosed by finding low circulating gonadotrophin levels, although occasionally biologically inactive FSH may be detectable at normal levels by immunoassay. The causes of secondary hypothalamic failure include:

1. *Stress, severe weight loss* and *anorexia nervosa.* This group has disordered GnRH pulsatile secretion. Normal function is usually restored when the underlying cause is treated.
2. *Tumours* include hamartomas, gliomas or craniopharyngiomas.
3. *Miscellaneous causes* including tuberculosis and sarcoidosis. Irradiation may also cause hypothalamic failure.

Pituitary failure. Pituitary failure is characterised by low levels of pituitary hormones and lack of response to hypothalamic releasing factors. Low gonadotrophin levels will result in atrophy of the ovaries and uterus — hence the term 'hypogonadotrophic hypogonadism'. Hypopituitarism may involve only the gonadotrophin secreting cells, which are usually the first cells to be affected by the presence of a space-occupying lesion, except in children, when growth hormone is the first to suffer. When other aspects of pituitary function are involved, the condition is called 'panyhypopituitarism'. As for hypothalamic failure, FSH may be immunologically active but biologically inert.

Causes of secondary pituitary failure include:

1. *Pituitary tumours.* This is the most common cause of secondary hypopituitarism. The most common tumour is a chromophobe adenoma, although functional tumours also occur. Craniopharyngiomas may extend into, and present as a pituitary tumour.
2. *Empty sella syndrome.* This is a radiological finding. It is due to leakage of cerebrospinal fluid into the sella tursica, exerting pressure on the pituitary gland, thus flattening it against other structures, and also onto the sella itself, causing bony erosion. Endocrine problems are usually very mild, despite the fact that gonadotrophin secretion is usually very sensitive to outside influences.
3. *Sheehan's syndrome.* Pituitary failure developing, following obstetric shock. The pituitary is particularly vulnerable to circulatory collapse in pregnancy. This condition is rare as almost total destruction of the gland is needed before pituitary failure ensues.
4. *Miscellaneous causes,* including internal carotid artery aneurysm, tumours of the 3rd ventricle, radical ablative therapy following surgery or radiotherapy of a pituitary tumour, and infections such as meningitis or tuberculosis.

Ovarian failure. Physiological ovarian failure occurs at the menopause. If it occurs before the age of 40, it is known as 'premature ovarian failure'. The diagnosis is made on finding elevated gonadotrophin levels in the post-menopausal range, due to the lack of negative feedback by oestrogen. The cause is unknown, but there is a genetic pre-disposition. It may occur as an autoimmune phenomenon. Histological examination of ovarian tissue may reveal the presence or absence of primordial follicles. In the former case, the condition is known as the 'resistant ovary syndrome', presumably resistant to FSH. The rare occurrence of spontaneous resumption of ovulation has been recorded in this group. There is no cure for this distressing condition and treatment is aimed at relieving the 'menopausal symptoms', with cyclical hormone replacement therapy.

Hyperprolactinaemia, hyperadrenalism, hyperthyroidism and polycystic ovary disease (PCOD).

Hyperprolactinaemia inhibits both LH and FSH release, although LH to a much greater extent. It acts at the hypothalamic level, probably by disrupting the hypothalamic dopamine system. A raised prolactin will feedback to stimulate dopamine release (prolactin inhibitory factor). As a result, GnRH and gona-dotrophin pulsatility is lost. Clinically, there is probably a spectrum of effect, ranging from an inadequate LH and progesterone production to complete suppression of the gonadotrophin levels and resultant amenorrhoea.

Physiological causes of raised prolactin levels include:

1. Pregnancy.
2. Lactation.

3. Stress.
4. Marked diurnal variation (highest levels are seen during sleep).
5. Idiopathic.

Pathological causes of raised prolactin levels include:

1. *Prolactinomas.* These are prolactin secreting pituitary tumours. They may be either macro- or micro-adenomas depending on their size (< 10 mm in diameter is defined as a micro-adenoma). Like all pituitary tumours, they should be investigated as previously described. Treatment is either by ablative surgery, radiotherapy or with dopamine agonists. Bromocriptine is a lysergic acid derivative. It binds specifically to dopamine receptors, thereby mimicking the inhibitory dopamine effects. Cabergoline has similar actions and clinical indications as bromocriptine. It however has milder side-effects and because it is long-acting, weekly or twice weekly dosing is possible.
2. *Drugs.* The most common group of drugs that may cause hyperprolactinaemia are the phenothiazines. Others are methyldopa, reserpine, opiates and benzodiazepines. They act either to deplete dopamine levels or to block dopamine receptors. Treatment is either to stop the drug or to add bromocriptine or cabergoline.
3. *Hypothyroidism* causes raised prolactin levels indirectly. The subsequent raised hypothalamic thyroid-releasing hormone (TRH) acts as a prolactin releasing factor. Correcting the hypothyroid state promptly returns the prolactin to normal.
4. *Other causes* include tumours compressing the pituitary stalk, which may interfere with delivery of dopamine. The incidence of amenorrhoea is not increased after stopping combined oral contraceptive pills. There is also no association between pill use and raised prolactin level.

Hyperadrenalism may result in sufficiently high circulating androgen levels to inhibit menstruation, as a result of feedback at the hypothalamic-pituitary level, though the precise mechanism is unclear. Biochemical confirmation of hyperadrenalism is by finding a raised dehydroepiandrosterone sulphate (DHEA-S) level, as the ovary (the only other site of androgen secretion) does not have the necessary sulphatase enzyme to convert DHEA to DHEA-S.

There are two usual clinical presentations:

1. *Late onset congenital adrenal hyperplasia* most commonly due to 21-hydroxylase enzyme deficiency, thereby preventing the conversion of 19-hydroxyprogesterone to cortisol, causing it to be converted to androgens instead.
2. *Cushing's syndrome.* This arises from overactivity of the adrenal cortex, whether due to hyperactivity or tumour. The patient is obese and hirsute, with a plethoric complexion, in addition to the menstrual disturbance. She may complain of bruising and muscle weakness. The diagnosis is confirmed by detecting elevated urinary free cortisol, loss of diurnal rhythm of ACTH. There is an inability to suppress the morning peaks of ACTH and cortisol with a midnight dose of dexamethasone.

Hyperthyroidism may also cause amenorrhoea, although the mechanism is unclear. Treatment will cause resumption of normal menstruation in majority of cases.

Oligomenorrhoea and Polycystic Ovary Disease

Oligomenorrhoea is an anovulatory disorder; therefore it usually leads to prolonged, unopposed oestrogen stimulation of the endometrium. The resulting prolonged endometrial proliferation may result in hyperplasia. When breakthrough bleeding eventually occurs, it is patchy and incoordinate, resulting in a prolonged, variable volume of menstrual shedding. The most common cause of oligomenorrhoea is polycystic ovary disease (PCOD) originally known as the Stein-Leventhal syndrome. The earliest description of the syndrome included obesity, hirsutism, amenorrhoea and enlarged polycystic ovaries. Oligomenorrhoea, insulin resistance and hyper-insulinaemia are now well-recognised additional components of this disease. The pathophysiology of this condition is still not clearly understood. A familial tendency has been proposed to be present probably through autosomal dominant and sex-linked modes of inheritance.

Poor follicular development leads to decreased conversion of androgen substrate to oestradiol in the granulosa cells. This results in increased circulating androgens (testosterone, androstenedione and DHEA). It is now believed that in most women with PCOD, hyper-insulinaemia is the trigger for increased androgen levels, by inhibiting production of sex hormone binding globulin (SHBG) and IGF-binding proteins from the liver. There are many possible causes of hyperinsulinaemia and non-insulin dependent diabetes mellitus (NIDDM), including: obesity, insulin receptor defects, drugs, insulinomas and genetic pre-dispositions to hypersecretion of insulin.

The resulting circulating androgens are peripherally converted to oestrogens (mainly oestrone) in fat. The high levels of circulating oestrone and the increased free oestradiol resulting from the effects of suppressed SHBG act to increase GnRH pulsatile rhythm. This increased rhythm selectively raises LH levels without affecting FSH secretion. The increased pulsatile LH stimulates further ovarian androgen production, while aromatisation is depressed (Fig. 3.12).

The clinical picture will depend upon the severity and the duration of the dysfunction.

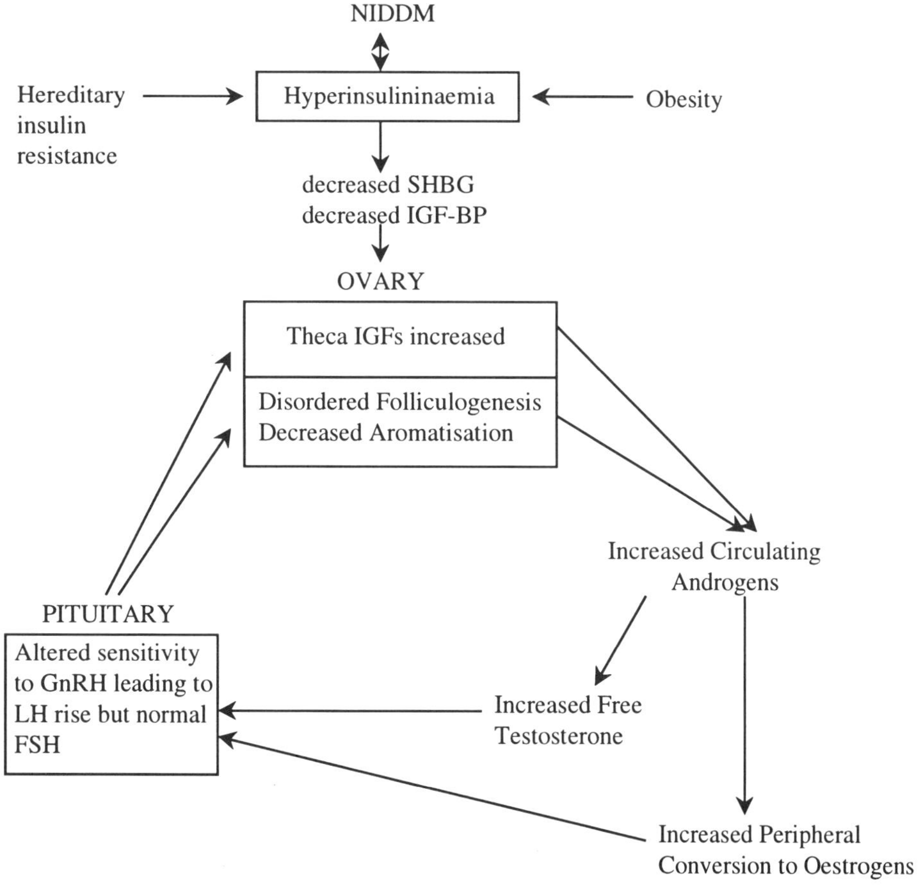

Fig. 3.12 ***Pathogenesis of Polycystic Ovary Disease.***
A vicious cycle of disordered hormone metabolism.

The patient may be hirsute because of the raised androgen levels. Anovulation results in the menstrual disturbance and infertility seen in the majority. The increased circulating oestrogen level causes the patient to be prone to endometrial cancer and cardiovascular disease. The cause/effect relationship between NIDDM and PCOD is not well understood (see below). If insulin resistance is present, the patient would be prone to diabetes mellitus. Endocrine investigations usually show raised LH, normal FSH and raised free testosterone levels. Transvaginal ultrasound scanning will usually show large ovaries with a hyper-echoic centre and multiple small peripheral cysts appearing like a necklace. Up to 25% of endocrinologically normal and ovulating women will have polycystic ovaries at ultrasound scanning.

Differential diagnoses of PCOD include late onset congenital adrenal hyperplasia, hyperprolactinaemia, Cushing's syndrome and androgen-producing tumours.

Treatment of PCOD depends on whether or not the patient wishes to conceive.

1. To treat anovulation, the principle is to raise FSH levels in order to stimulate follicular development. This is usually achieved with clomiphene citrate, an anti-oestrogen that prevents oestrogenic feedback on the hypothalamic-pituitary axis, or by giving exogenous FSH, usually in the pure form.
2. Diabetic drugs that improve insulin sensitivity have been found to be effective in treating overweight patients with PCOD. Metformin, a biguanide, reduces hyperinsulinaemia, LH and free testosterone levels. It has also been found to enhance the ovulation-inducing effect of clomiphene citrate when used concurrently. In normal doses, there is no risk of dangerous hypoglycaemia in non-diabetic PCOD patients.
3. Laparoscopic ovarian needle diathermy can also be used to treat PCOD effectively. It is thought to act by destroying part of the androgen producing ovarian stroma, thereby breaking the vicious cycle. Ovarian wedge resection is an old and effective treatment that has fallen out of favour, mainly because of the risk of adhesion formation.
4. If pregnancy is not desired, then cyclic progesterone therapy should be given to counteract the unopposed oestrogenic stimulation of the endometrium, which carries the theoretical risk of malignant change.
5. Hirsutism may be specifically treated with a choice of anti-androgens like cyproterone acetate, combined for example, with ethinyl oestradiol in the oral contraceptive pill called Dianette, or with glucocorticoids in the form of dexamethasone. Cosmetic treatment may be adequate for mild–moderate hirsutism.

Abnormal Uterine Bleeding

This will be dealt with in Chapter 18.

Dysmenorrhoea

Dysmenorrhoea means painful periods of which there are two main forms. This will be dealt with in Chapter 18.

Premenstrual Syndrome

The premenstrual syndrome (PMS) is a collection of a wide spectrum of symptoms and signs occurring after ovulation and relieved by menstruation. It is a psychological and somatic disorder defined as being *characterised by one or more of a very wide spectrum of symptoms occurring before menstruation, of sufficient severity to disrupt lifestyle or work, and followed by a period of relief after menstruation.* It is of unknown aetiology, and can be extremely debilitating and distressing, not only to the patient, but to live-in relatives, causing sufferers to believe that they possess a Jekyll and Hyde (oscillating good-evil) personality. PMS is very common, and most women at some time or other will have experienced one or more premenstrual symptoms. It is usually first reported by women in their mid-thirties.

The diagnosis is that of exclusion of other pathologies like anaemia, hypothyroidism, hyperthyroidism, causes of secondary dysmenorrhoea like endometriosis, the menopause and psychiatric disorders. Once these

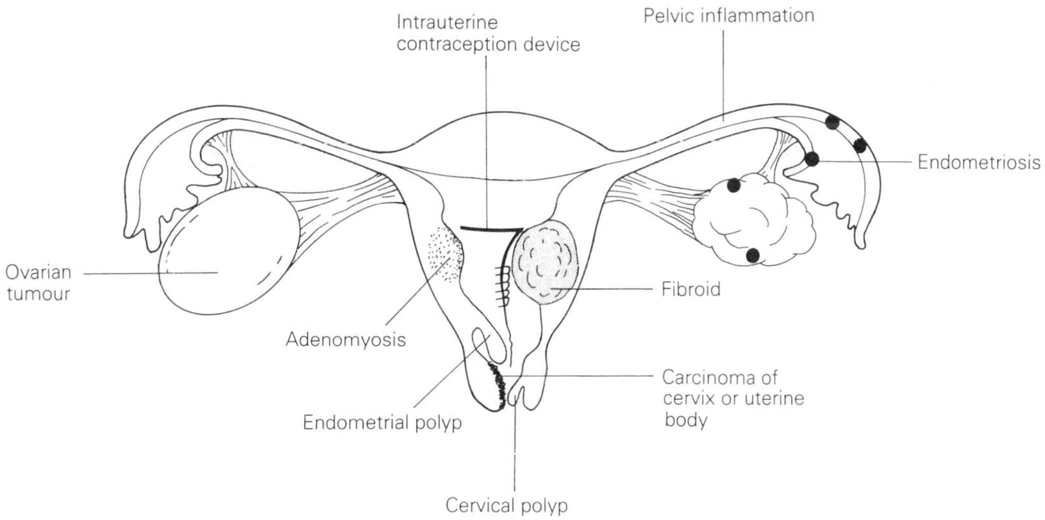

Fig. 3.13 *Causes of abnormal uterine bleeding.*

differential diagnoses have been excluded, definitive diagnosis is based mainly on an accurate prospective charting of symptoms over a period of at least three menstrual cycles (Fig. 3.13). The spectrum of symptoms include:

1. Wide swings in mood, e.g. tearfulness, sadness, anger, fluctuating with brief periods of happiness.
2. Depression, hopelessness and feelings of lack of control.
3. Fatigue and lack of interest in usual chores and activities.
4. Lack of concentration, forgetfulness, and being accident prone.
5. Anxiety and tension.
6. Suicidal and self-harm tendencies.
7. Loss of libido, increased libido.
8. Anti-social behaviours like shoplifting, aggression and assault.
9. Lack of sleep, or excessive somnolence.
10. Fluctuations in appetite.
11. Somatic symptoms, including bloatedness, weight gain, constipation or diarrhoea, flushes, breast swelling and tenderness, pelvic pain, or headache.

Aetiology

The aetiology of this multi-symptomatic condition is not understood. Although various theories have been put forward, none of these have been substantiated:

1. Oestrogen/progesterone imbalance: oestrogen lack, oestrogen excess and a relative progesterone deficiency have all been variously postulated.
2. Fluid retention due to raised aldosterone levels in the luteal phase.
3. Increased renin-angiotensin activity has also been incriminated.
4. Raised prolactin levels, particularly regarding breast symptoms.
5. Deficiencies of vitamin B6.
6. Prostaglandins, due to their ubiquitous nature, have also been implicated.
7. Changes in CNS cathecolamine activity.
8. Endogenous opioid levels decline in the premenstuum. One theory puts forward a withdrawal-like effect.
9. A neurotic personality.

Investigations

Where diagnostic doubts exist, particularly when bilateral oophorectomies are contemplated, a therapeutic trial of GnRH analogue for a period of 3 months (the Goserelin test) should confirm PMS, if symptoms are alleviated.

Treatments

This is largely empirical and is frequently no better than the placebo response, which occurs in an average of 40% of patients. It cannot be emphasised too strongly that there is a major need for psychological support, reassurance and explanation of the condition. Treatment can be considered under non-medication/supportive therapy, drug therapy and surgical treatment.

Non-medication/supportive treatments:

1. Support, explanation, education and counselling, preferably through self-help groups.
2. Exercising.
3. Dietary advice.
4. Psychotherapy.
5. Physiotherapy.
6. Alternative therapy, like acupuncture, hypnosis and yoga.

Drug therapy:

1. Placebo has been reported to be effective in up to 90% of cases by some researchers.
2. Pyridoxine (vitamin B6), a co-factor in neurotransmitter synthesis, is not significantly better than placebo.
3. Calcium supplementation has been found to be beneficial by some, although response rates are similar to that of placebo.
4. Diuretics like spironolactone may be helpful when there is objective fluid retention, and not just for subjective complaints of bloatedness.
5. Oil of evening primrose contains linolenic and gammalinolenic acids, which are precursors of prostaglandins.
6. Selective serotonin re-uptake inhibitors (SSRIs) like fluoxetine and paroxetine are antidepressant drugs shown also to be of benefit in many of the psychological symptoms of PMS.
7. The contraceptive pill has been prescribed to inhibit ovulation and relieve dysmenorrhoea. It is not as effective as was previously hoped and the symptoms may return during the pill-free week, although it can be given continuously.
8. Vaginal or rectal progesterone or oral synthetic progestogens such as dydrogesterone are frequently used. Treatment is usually started on day 12 of the cycle and continues for 2 weeks. In some cases therapy can be very effective.
9. Bromocriptine or cabergoline may be effective for breast symptoms.
10. Danazol may be beneficial for breast symptoms but does not improve other complaints. Patients should be warned of side-effects. Although it may cause amenorrhoea, contraception is not guaranteed, therefore barrier contraception should be advised.
11. GnRH agonists will reduce ovarian function and hence abolish PMS symptoms. It is used in some quarters over a few months as a diagnostic test. Sadly it does not render a permanent cure, as symptoms may recur with a rebound effect once the hormone is stopped. GnRH may however be given over a long period with an add-back therapy of oestrogen and progesterone replacement to prevent osteoporosis.
12. Oestrogen, testosterone implants and transdermal patches have been found to be beneficial for many of the symptoms of PMS, including loss of libido.

Surgical treatments:

1. Patients should not be subjected to hysterectomy and bilateral salpingo-oophorectomy unless diagnosis is certain, and there is objective proof that medical ovulation suppression can abolish the PMS symptoms. The Goserelin test should be used for this purpose.

ACKNOWLEDGEMENTS

We thank our colleagues, Spyros Papaioannou (MRCOG), Nahed Hammadieh (MRCOG) for proof reading this manuscript and their helpful criticisms, Julia Arnold [personal assistant to Masoud Afnan (FRCOG)] and Diane Blackmore (Medical Illustration Department, University of Birmingham, UK) for their valuable input in preparing Figs. 3.1–3.3 and 3.12.

FURTHER READING

Johnson M.H., Everitt B.J. (1996). Reproductive messengers. In *Essential Reproduction*, 4th edn. Johnson M.H., Everitt B.J. (eds). pp. 25–44. Blackwell Science Ltd.

Johnson M.H., Everitt B.J. (1996). Ovarian function. In *Essential Reproduction*, 4th edn. Johnson M.H., Everitt B.J. (eds). pp. 60–78. Blackwell Science Ltd.

Ojeda S.R. (1996). Female reproductive function. In *Textbook of Endocrine Physiology*, 3rd edn. Griffin J.E., Ojeda S.R. (eds). pp. 164–200. Oxford University Press.

Shaw R.W. (1997). Control of the hypothalamic-pituitary ovarian function. In *Gynaecology*. Shaw R.W., Soutter W.P., Stanton S.L. (eds). pp. 171–84. Churchill Livingstone.

Sharif K.., Afnan M. (1997). Ovarian function and ovulation induction. In *Gynaecology*, 2nd edn. Shaw R.W., Soutter W.P., Stanton S.L. (eds). pp. 223–36. Churchill Livingstone.

Speroff L., Glass R.H., Kase N.G. (1999). Regulation of the menstrual cycle. In *Clinical Gynecologic Endocrinology and Infertility*, 6th edn. Speroff L., Glass R.H., Kase N.G. (eds). pp. 201–46. Lippincott Williams and Wilkins.

4

Early Development

The development of the fetus begins with the process of fertilisation, a complex process involving the penetration of the oocyte by the spermatozoon.

FERTILISATION

Spermatozoa undergo a number of physiological changes during their course through the female genital tract before they are able to penetrate oocytes. The initial change is known as capacitation which involves changes in the plasma membrane induced by enzymes located in the acrosome region (Fig. 4.1).

This leads to the acrosome reaction, a process essential for fertilisation. The acrosome reaction involves structural changes, which start with swelling of the sperm head, followed by the fusion of the two outer membranes, releasing enzymes, which results in vesicle formation and loss of integrity of the acrosomal cap. As this degenerates, the acrosomal cap is lost, leaving the inner acrosomal membrane and nucleus exposed. The acrosome reaction usually occurs in the ampulla of the fallopian tube, where the oocyte is found soon after ovulation. There is an increase in motility of the sperm after the acrosome reaction has occurred.

The sperm (Fig. 4.2) now has to penetrate through several layers of the oocyte (Figs. 4.3 and 4.4). The outer layer of cumulus (corona radiata) is enzymatically penetrated by hyaluronidase and this exposes the zona pellucida to which the sperm loosely binds. The zona is also penetrated with the aid of an enzyme, a

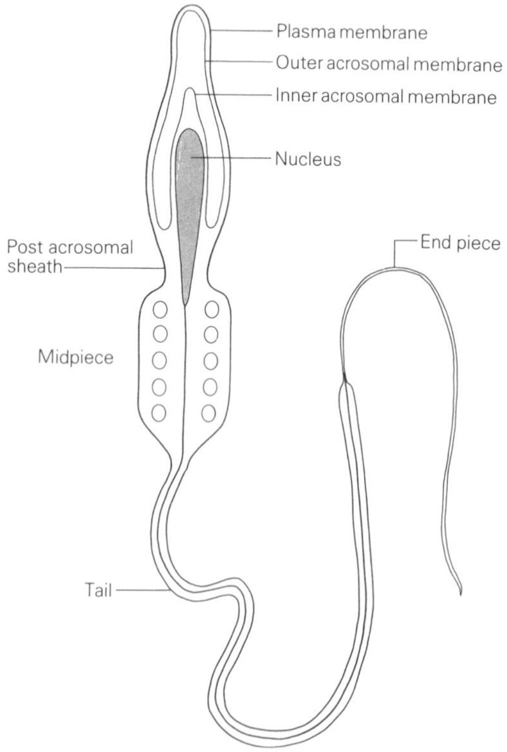

Fig. 4.1 *Diagram of human sperm.*

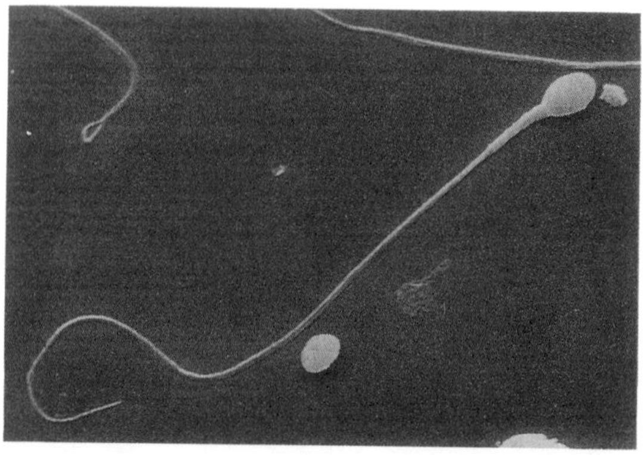

Fig. 4.2 *Scanning electron microscope of human sperm.*

protease known as acrosin, and the sperm enters the perivitelline space between the zona pellucida and the oocyte. More than one sperm may reach this space, but only one fuses with the nucleus, activating the oocyte, and thereafter the development of the block to polyspermia (Fig 4.5). The activated oocyte undergoes a meiotic division and discards 23 chromosome as the 2nd polar body (having lost nuclear material as 1st polar body in early ovum formation). These chromosomes form the pronucleus, which fuses with the pronucleus from the sperm and the cell is ready to divide, with 46 chromosomes.

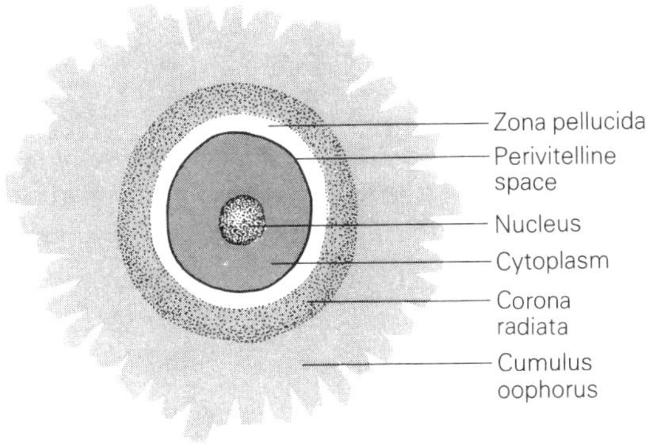

Fig. 4.3 *Oocyte and its surrounding layers.*

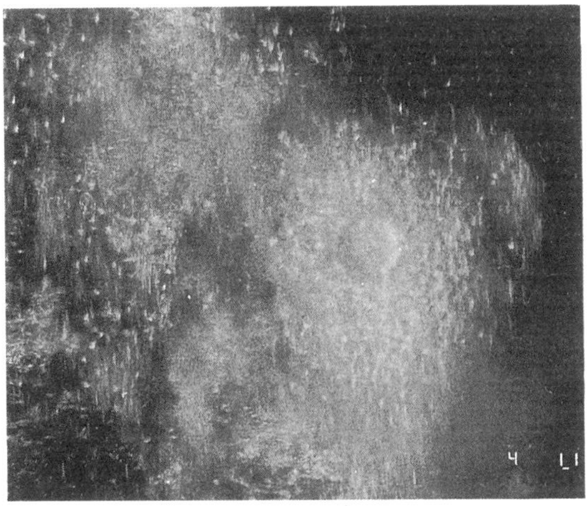

Fig. 4.4 *Human oocyte.*

CLEAVAGE

This first mitotic division of the embryo occurs about 36 h after fertilisation resulting in a 2-cell embryo. By 48 h, it has cleaved again to reach the 4-cell stage (Fig. 4.6) and by 72 h it is at the 16–32 cell stage.

During this time, the embryo is moving down the fallopian tube by a combination of tubal, ciliary and muscle action. The embryo is carried in tubal fluid which has a complex formulation of ions, proteins and steroid molecules, all of which are necessary to promote the ideal environment for embryo growth. Any damage to the fallopian tube, e.g. salpingitis, will interfere with tubal transport, as cilia will be destroyed, and the tubal environment may no longer be ideal. So, infertility can result from altered tubal physiology without tubal blockage.

The human embryo enters the uterus about 3–4 days after ovulation, at about the 16–32 cell stage.

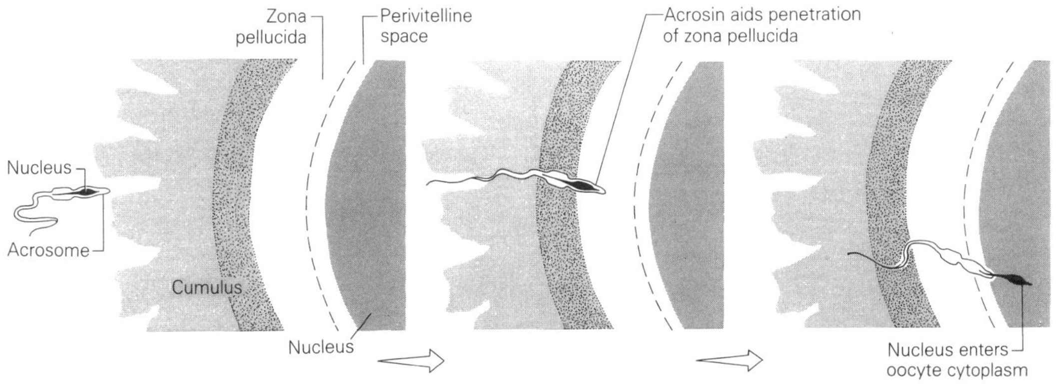

Fig. 4.5 *Fertilisation.*

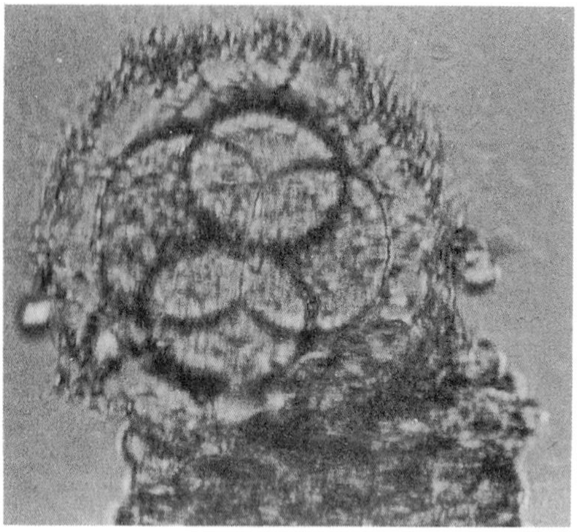

Fig. 4.6 *Four-cell human embryo.*

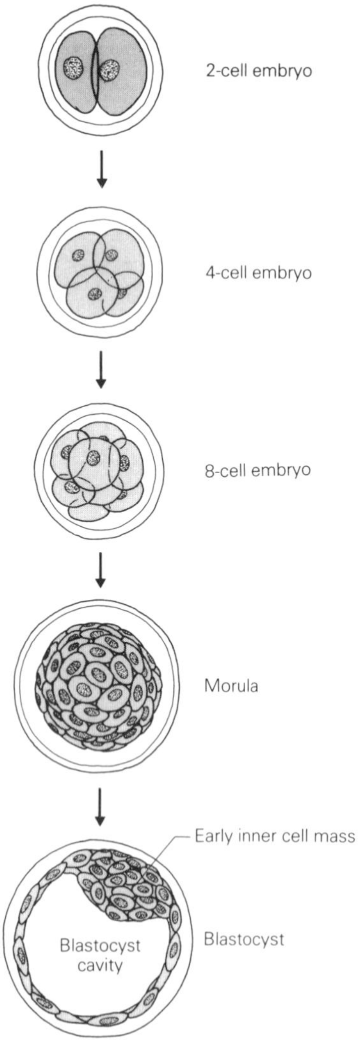

Fig. 4.7 *Embryonic cell division leading to blastocyst formation.*

The Morula and Blastocyst

Cell division continues in the uterus until the 32-cell (morula) to 64-cell (blastocyst) stage. Cleavage is synchronous in the early stages, but by the morula stage, the division is much more haphazard. Eventually, individual blastomeres become indistinct, a process called compaction. This results in the formation of an outer layer of cells (the future trophectoderm) and the inner cells which are destined to become the inner cell mass. This then leads to blastocyst formation with secretion of fluid into the morula and the inner cell mass becomes eccentrically placed (Fig. 4.7).

The zona pellucida persists until this stage and now the zona opens (hatching) and the blastocyst is expelled.

IMPLANTATION

The uterus is primed by steroid hormone changes during the follicular and early luteal phase of the cycle and the blastocyst is now lying free in the uterine cavity in close approximation to the endometrium.

The endometrium has undergone several biochemical and physiological changes, resulting in changes in the secretions of the uterine glands. There is an increase in the cellular content of the stroma, an increased uterine blood flow and endometrial oedema. These changes are brought about by the influence of progesterone and a receptive phase is created.

The embryo also plays an active role in implantation (Fig. 4.8) and there are changes in the membranes which result in receptor formation, enabling the blastocyst to respond to external stimuli. The time when an embryo can implant is probably restricted to 1 or 2 days, and the rise in oestrogen and progesterone in the luteal phase is critical. The endometrial receptor for these steroids must be primed in order to facilitate implantation, and the proteins produced in response to this (chemokines) probably stimulate the embryo directly.

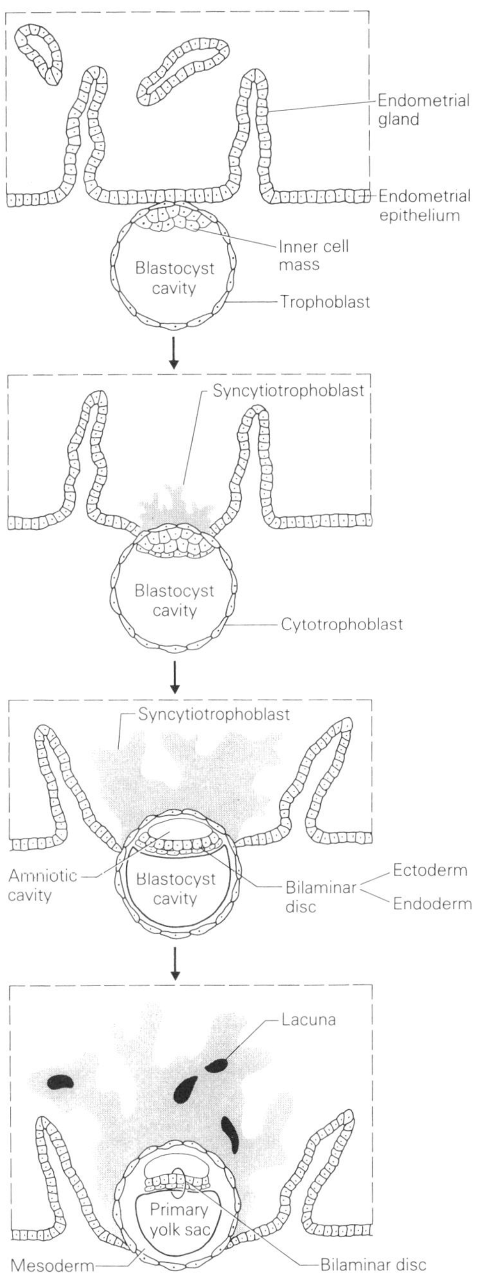

Fig. 4.8 *Implantation.*

The human embryo implants by a process called interstitial implantation, becoming apposed to and then invading the endometrium. At the site of implantation, there is a change in capillary permeability which occurs about 24 h before attachment occurs. These changes may be due to adhesion molecules, which change the endometrial cell's apoptosis pattern.

There are three steps in implantation:

Apposition
Adhesion
Penetration

During apposition, the blastocyst becomes closely orientated to the endometrium, facilitated by microvilli on both the trophoblast and the endometrium. The process of adhesion involves interdigitation of the endometrial and trophoblastic microvilli and adhesion is further enhanced by the secretion of glycoproteins which have a 'sticky' nature. The final process of penetration involves the trophoblast, now firmly attached, growing between the endometrial cells and invading the endometrium. The erosion of the surface of the endometrium means that 2 days after apposition, the blastocyst is completely implanted. From the time of entering the uterus, the embryo has been secreting proteins, especially human chorionic gonadotrophin (HCG) which is released into the maternal circulation to maintain the corpus luteum.

As invasion proceeds, the trophoblast cells enter the local capillaries and spaces (lacunae) appear, filled with blood, which are the primitive intervillous spaces. The development of the trophoblast is not uniform, being most marked toward the decidual base of the blastocyst, which will become the placenta.

DEVELOPMENT OF THE EMBRYO

There are changes within the blastocyst during implantation. By Day 7 after ovulation, the cells of the outer layer of the inner cell mass become ectodermal cells and the inner layer, endodermal cells. One day later, the ectodermal layer becomes split and the space becomes enlarged to form an amniotic cavity. So by Day 10 postovulation, there is a two-layered inner cell mass, and two cavities, the amniotic cavity and the primary yolk sac.

By Day 11, there is active proliferation of cells from the inner surface of the trophoblast, which leads to separation of the ectoderm and the endoderm and the formation of an intermediate, mesodermal layer.

The surrounding tissue is called the mesoblast; vacuolation occurs and two layers form, one lining the trophoblast and the other lining the embryo and yolk sac. The cavity is called the extra embryonic disc from the trophoblast except for the body stalk. The embryonic disc, by Day 16, is trilaminar (Fig. 4.9). The amniotic cavity continues to expand and by Day 50 completely surrounds the embryo and fuses with the chorion.

From this point, there are two separate entities to consider, the placenta and the fetus. The former will be described in Chapter 7.

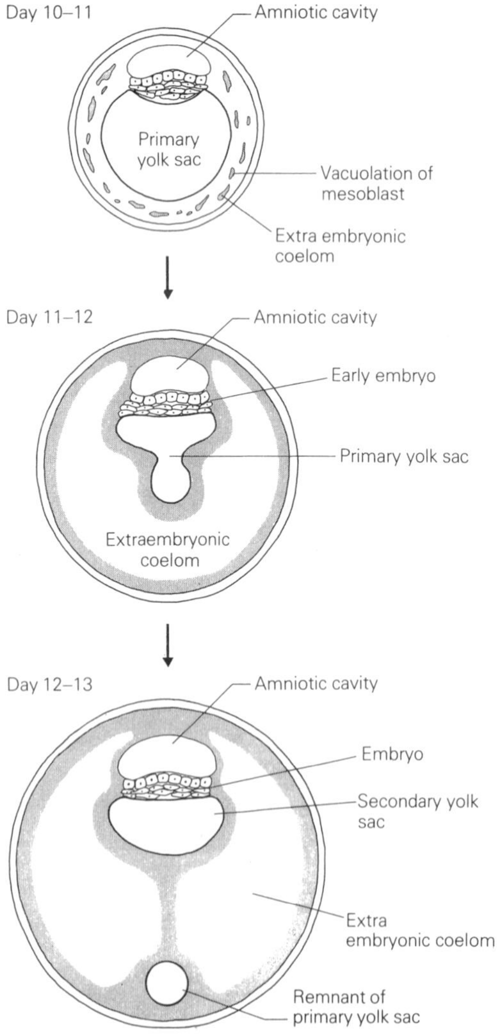

Fig. 4.9 *Early embryonic development.*

LATER DEVELOPMENT OF THE EMBRYO

By Day 21, the embryo is ready to enter the somite stage of development which lasts 10 days. At this point, it is a trilaminar disc consisting of layers of ectoderm, mesoderm and endoderm. The endoderm and mesoderm only remain in contact at two areas, the oral and cloacal membranes. During the invasion by mesoderm, an area of intense mitotic activity, called Henson's node, arises in the endoderm and ectoderm to form the notochord. The ectoderm spreads laterally on both sides and moves anteriorly to fuse in the midline, taking the mesoderm with it. The ectodermal tube forms the basis of the nervous system and the endoderm forms somites which become the vertebral column. There are usually a total of 25.

By the 7 somite stage, closure of the neural plate and cephalic enlargement have begun, and by the 10 somite stage, three ventricles can be discerned. From this point onwards, differentiation and growth are rapid and embryogenesis occurs in a very fixed time scale.

The somite stage closes with the fusion of the distal ends of the neuropores and the formation of a well-defined umbilical cord and tail. The embryo is comma shaped at this stage.

The external changes from now on are much less rapid. During weeks 6–8, there is the development of forelimb buds and the arms, hindlimb buds and the legs, expansion of the brain, modifications to the tail, development of the face and eyes, so that by 8 weeks, the embryo has a human form and is now called a fetus.

CONGENITAL MALFORMATIONS

The fetus may be born with an anatomical abnormality, which may be microscopic or macroscopic, as a result of either primary maldevelopment or disordered normal development due to interference from an external influence. It is estimated that 10% of human developmental abnormalities result from drugs, viruses and other environmental factors, and 20% of deaths in the perinatal period are attributed to congenital malformations.

Causes of congenital abnormalities are divided into genetic and environmental factors, although some abnormalities may occur as a result of genetic and environmental factors occurring together. This is called multifactorial inheritance.

Genetic Disorders

These are the largest group of anomalies and are present in 1: 200 newborn infants in some form or other. The chromosomes can be subjected to two kinds of change, numerical and structural. Either of these two types of alteration in chromosomes will initiate developmental changes which result in a characteristic phenotype, such as Down's syndrome.

Numerical disorders usually arise as a result of non-disjunction. Chromosomes normally exist in pairs and, if at the time of cell division the paired chromosomes fail to separate (or disjoin), then there is depletion of the total number of chromosomes. Normally, females have 22 autosomes (non-sex chromosomes) plus two X chromosomes, and males have 22 autosomes plus one one X and one Y chromosome. Any deviation from the normal 46 chromosomes is called aneuploidy and the most common problem is non-disjunction, such as Turner's Syndrome where the chromosome complement is 45 with one X chromosome missing. If a chromosome is missing, then the condition is called monosomy; for instance Turner's syndrome is called Monosomy X. If an autosome is missing, the embryo almost always dies.

If three chromosomes are present instead of two, the condition is called trisomy and again the cause is usually non-disjunction, resulting in a germ cell with 24 instead of 23 chromosomes. The most common condition is trisomy 21 or Down's syndrome, in which three chromosome 21s are present. Other chromosomes are susceptible to trisomy; for instance, 18, 13 and 22, but they are less common. Trisomy may occur in the sex chromosomes and this is much more common. The incidence of these disorders, e.g. 47,XXX, 47,XXY (Klinefelter's syndrome) or 47,XYY is about 1:1000. Usually the greater the number of X chromosomes present, the greater the mental retardation; there is no effect of extra sex chromosomes on male or female characteristics.

It is possible for an individual to have a combination of cell lines and this is known as mosaicism. The malformations are usually less severe than the monosomy or trisomy forms, for example Turner Mosaic 45,X0/46,XX.

If a complete extra set of chromosomes is incorporated into the embryo, then it is known as triploidy and these embryos all spontaneously abort.

Structural abnormalities, on the other hand, are the result of chromosome breaks which may be induced by environmental factors, such as drugs, viruses, radiation, etc. The type of abnormality depends on what happens to the broken pieces.

Translocation is the transfer of a piece of one chromosome to a different chromosome. It does not necessarily result in abnormal development; for example translocation between chromosome 21 and 14 (Robertsonian translocation) is phenotypically normal. Persons who have a normal phenotype, but have a translocation anomaly are called translocation carriers.

If a chromosome breaks and the piece is lost, this is known as deletion, e.g. deletion of the short arm of chromosome 5 results in cri-du-chat syndrome.

Malformations can be caused by mutant genes, such as achondroplasia, polydactyly, or they may occur *only* if these abnormal genes are present on both of the paired chromosomes, known as an autosomal recessive disorder, for example congenital adrenal hyperplasia. As these disorders are only manifest when two sets of chromosomes with a mutant gene unite, many carriers remain undetected.

Environmental Causes

Certain agents, called teratogens, may be responsible for inducing congenital malformations when the tissues and organs are growing, and they are most sensitive during the time of rapid differentiation. The critical period of human development depends on the tissue or organ concerned, e.g. the brain grows rapidly from the start of its development and for the first two years of life, but other organs are only rapidly developing from Days 15 to 60, and during this time teratogens may be lethal. Each organ has a critical time during which its development may be altered, and a teratogen may affect different developing systems at the same time (Fig. 4.10).

Drugs and chemicals as teratogens

Drugs vary greatly in their teratogenicity from severe, for example thalidomide, to mild, smoking. While few drugs have been positively implicated in congenital abnormalities, the use of all drugs in pregnancy should be avoided if possible. Some examples of teratogens are shown in Table 4.1.

Infectious agents

Three viruses are known to be teratogenic in man (Table 4.2).

Table 4.1

Teratogen	Congenital malformation
Alcohol	Growth retardation Mental retardation Microcephaly
Androgens	Masculinisation of female fetus
Busulfan	Stunted growth, cleft palate, skeletal abnormalities
Lithium carbonate	Cardiovascular abnormalities
Methotrexate and other cytotoxic drugs	Multiple congenital abnormalities
Phenytoin Tetracyclines Warfarin	Mental retardation, growth retardation, bone and teeth abnormalities, cartilagenous abnormalities

Table 4.2

Virus	Onset	Condition
Rubella virus	Early	Cataract Cardiac anomalies Deafness
Cytomegalovirus	Early Late	Most pregnancies abort Growth retardation Mental retardation Deafness Cerebral calcification
Herpes simplex virus	Late	Microcephaly Mental retardation

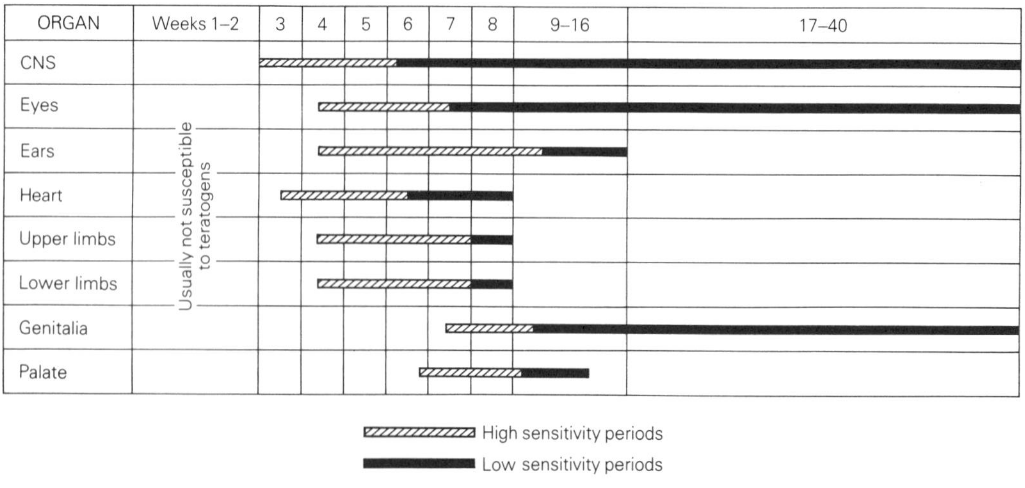

Fig. 4.10 *Critical periods of teratogenicity.*

Table 4.3

Micro-organism	Condition
Toxoplasma gondii	Microcephaly Microphthalmia Hydrocephaly
Treponema pallidum (syphilis)	Deafness Hydrocephalus Mental retardation

Two other micro-organisms are known to be teratogens (Table 4.3).

Radiation

Large amounts of ionising radiation can produce congenital malformations and if the exposure during early pregnancy is over 0.25 Gy, over a short space of time, it is recommended that the pregnancy be terminated. There is no evidence that human congenital malformations have resulted from exposure to diagnostic levels of radiation. However, it is prudent to minimise X-ray examination of the pelvic region in pregnant women.

Multifactorial Inheritance

Most common congenital malformations are the result of a subject who is susceptible to a disorder being exposed to some co-factor which predisposes to the condition. These traits tend to run in families, such as cleft lip, neural tube defects, congenital dislocation of the hip. What the co-factors are in these cases remains unclear, but one theory is exemplified by the use of folic acid to prevent neural tube defects recurring, the co-factor thought to be the lack of folic acid during development in susceptible subjects.

FURTHER READING

Edwards R.G., Fischel S. (1986). Ovulation, fertilitsation, embryo damage and early development. In *Scientific Foundations of Obstetrics and Gynaecology*, 3rd edn. Philipp E., Barnes J., Newton M. (eds). pp. 212–23. London: Heinemann Medical.

Jones O.W. (1984). Reproductive genetics. In *Maternal Fetal Medicine*. Creasy R.K., Resnik R. (eds). pp. 3–92. Philadelphia: W.B. Saunders.

5

Abortion: Spontaneous and Therapeutic

ABORTION

The *Concise Oxford Dictionary* defines abortion as the 'act of giving untimely birth to offspring, premature delivery, miscarriage; the procuring of premature delivery so as to destroy offspring' (L. *abortus* — an untimely birth). The World Health Organisation defined abortion as 'the loss of a fetus or embryo weighing 500 g or less which corresponds to a gestational age of 20–22 weeks, the irreducible age for fetal well being'. Since October 1992, spontaneous abortion is defined in the UK as 'a pregnancy loss occurring before 24 completed weeks of gestation'.

To the physician, the terms 'abortion' and 'miscarriage' are synonymous, but to the patient the terms have different implications: abortion is an operation deliberately to end a pregnancy (termination to the physician), miscarriage is an accidental, unwanted event in a woman's reproductive life (abortion to the physician).

Both abortion (miscarriage) and termination are hugely traumatic and emotional events for any woman and can have long term emotional sequelae. Physicians should take great care and compassion to manage these women with understanding and sympathy, and use appropriate terminology.

SPONTANEOUS ABORTION

Spontaneous abortion is the loss of a pregnancy prior to 24 weeks gestation, without prior intervention which aims to end that pregnancy. It can occur in the first trimester (up to 12 weeks amenorrhoea) or in the second trimester (12–24 weeks gestation). However, now that neonatal intensive care units are increasingly skilled at resuscitating and managing extremely premature infants, consideration should be given to administering antenatal steroids to a mother threatening to miscarry in the 23rd week of gestation and a paediatric team should be present at the delivery of these late abortions in case the infant shows signs of life and resuscitation is appropriate.

Incidence

The true incidence of spontaneous abortion is unknown, but up to 25% of women will bleed in early pregnancy and the loss rate among clinically recognised pregnancies is accepted as 15%. To assess the incidence of pregnancy loss prior to 6 weeks gestation, levels of serum human chorionic gonadotrophin (HCG) have been monitored and suggest very early miscarriage rates of 22–45%. Of course this method will not detect losses of pre-embryos or blastocysts which have failed to implant (Table 5.1)

Table 5.1
Predicted Future of an Individual Ovum

16% of ova do not divide.
15% of ova are lost during various preimplantation stages in the first postovulatory week.
27% of ova abort during implantation in the second postovulatory week.
10.5% of ova surviving the first missed menstrual period, subsequently abort spontanteously.

(After Opitz *et al.*, 1979. Postgraduate Medicine; **65**, 247.)

Table 5.2
Aetiology of Spontaneous Abortion

Feto-placental cause	Maternal cause
Chromosomal abnormality	Infection
Morphological abnormality	Uterine abnormality — congenital or acquired
Placental abnormalities	Endocrine or auto-immune problems Drug ingestion

Note: 25% of spontaneous abortions are of unknown cause.

It is estimated that up to 12% of miscarriages occur in the second trimester.

Aetiology of Spontaneous Abortion

This is summarised in Table 5.2.

Chromosomal and morphological abnormality

Fifty percent of first trimester losses are chromosomally abnormal — 30% of abortuses have an extra chromosome (trisomy) which is usually an autosome.

Structural defects have also been discovered in increased numbers in abortuses and although many of these are related to chromosomal defects, major structural abnormalities are more frequent in abortuses than in ongoing pregnancies.

Placental abnormality

The role of the placenta in maintaining a pregnancy is paramount, and although poorly understood, the process of abnormal placentation may be of great importance in the aetiology of spontaneous abortion. With normal placental development, the blastocyst with syncytiotrophoblast at the embryonic pole, erodes the secretory endometrium to form an implantation cavity in the decidua. Cytotrophoblast and mesoderm containing fetal blood vessels grow into the syncytiotrophoblast, in which the lacunae containing maternal blood have formed. The lacunae become the intervillous spaces, and the

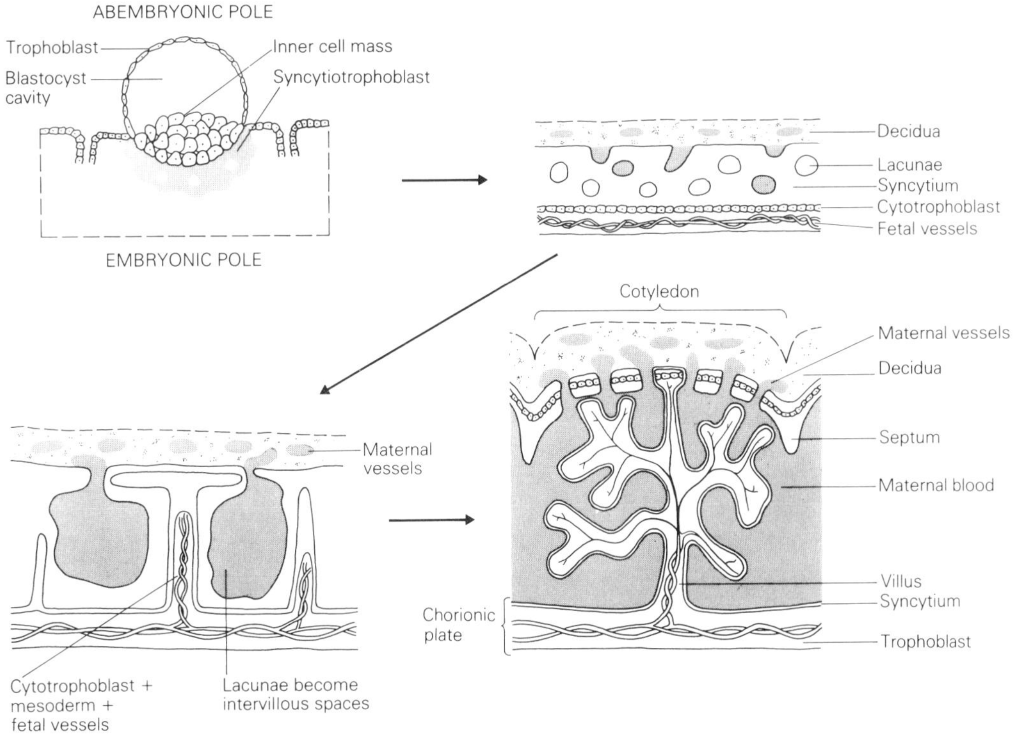

Fig. 5.1 *The development of the placenta.*

in-growths containing the fetal blood vessels become the villi (see Fig. 5.1).

Haemorrhage during miscarriage is due to separation of the syncytiotrophoblast, and later the placenta from the uterine wall. Abnormalities such as retro-placental haemorrhage, uteroplacental ischaemia and choriomanionitis are the most common histological placental findings in spontaneous abortion.

Infection

Infections, especially those which cause a high temperature (malaria), can cause spontaneous abortion. Bacterial and viral infections can also cause abortion by killing or severely damaging the developing embryo/fetus. Syphylis, cytomegalovirus (CMV), rubella, toxoplasmosis and listeriosis are all known to cause sporadic abortion.

Unknown aetiology

About 25% of spontaneous abortions are of undetermined aetiology, though this could be because the majority of sporadic miscarriages are not investigated. Women who experience three or more spontaneous abortions are regarded to be a recurrent aborters and warrant further investigation as outlined in Chapter 6.

Management of Spontaneous Miscarriage

Management of any clinical problem involves making a correct diagnosis and treating the patient. To make a diagnosis the patient needs to have a history taken, be examined and investigated appropriately.

History

Vaginal bleeding in pregnancy is a common presenting complaint. It can be light (often associated with a threatened or missed abortion) or much heavier (often indicative of an inevitable abortion). The bleeding is frequently associated with pain. Pain associated with miscarriage tends to be located centrally, suprapubically, or in the low back. Uterine pain is referred to areas of skin supplied by branches of the first lumbar nerve. It can be a mild ache (minimal pain is associated with a threatened abortion) or much more severe and crampy (likened to severe period or even labour pains, more common with an inevitable abortion). *It is important to always suspect the possibility of ectopic pregnancy in any woman in early pregnancy with pain and bleeding.*

As well as taking a full history of the presenting complaint, the duration, amount and colour of the bleeding and the severity, duration and location of the pain, it is also important to ask:

- Date of 1st day of last menstrual period.
- Regularity of cycle prior to conception.
- Use of contraception.
- Presence or disappearance of signs or symp toms of pregnancy (women with a missed abortion often report they no longer feel nauseous or have breast tenderness).
- Previous pregnancies, miscarriages or terminations.
- Past medical history.
- Drug history and any known allergies.
- Social history including whether this was a planned or wanted pregnancy.

It is imperative to remember to adopt a sympathetic manner while taking the history. Although bleeding in pregnancy is common, for each individual woman the process is the cause of great anxiety and distress. Women often fear the worse and it is the responsibility of the clinician to offer an understanding, efficient and realistic approach to the management of these women.

Examination

Pulse rate, blood pressure and temperature should always be checked in any woman bleeding in pregnancy. Abdominal palpation will reveal the area of tenderness or pain. This is important to help exclude the possibility of an ectopic pregnancy.

Although some women show considerable anxiety at the thought of being examined vaginally there is no evidence that vaginal examination will precipitate miscarriage. This must be fully but sympathetically explained to the woman and if she still declines this must be respected. Cuscoe speculum examination will demonstrate the extent of vaginal bleeding, allow visualisation of the cervix to confirm its gross normality and any products within the os can be seen. Any products in the os should be removed with sponge holding forceps and sent to histopathology. This ensures clear documentation of the presence of products of conception and excludes trophoblastic disease. Digital vaginal examination demonstrates uterine size, tenderness, the presence of cervical excitation and whether the cervical os is open or closed.

IMPORTANT CLINICAL POINT

It is essential that any woman who is shocked or compromised by heavy vaginal bleeding be appropriately resuscitated:

— achieve IV access.
— send blood for haemoglobin concentration estimation and group and save or cross-matching as deemed clinically necessary.
— an intravenous infusion of crystalloid or colloid should be administered.
— ergometrine 500 mg can be administered to help stop the bleeding as can 20–40 iu of syntocinon.
— products of conception distending the cervical os can cause cervical shock — the treatment for this is immediate removal of products from the cervix with sponge-holding forceps.

Investigation

The use of ultrasound scanning (USS) has revolutionised the management of women with bleeding in early pregnancy. It is now the primary investigation for any woman suspected of suffering a threatened abortion, and the Royal College of Radiologists (RCR) and Royal College of Obstetricians and Gynaecologists (RCOG) have provided guidance on the use of USS in early pregnancy to avoid erroneous diagnosis of fetal death. Most units now use a written policy of procedure when early intrauterine death is suspected, to minimise the chances of evacuating the uterus in error. If there is any doubt about pregnancy viability, evacuation of the uterus must be delayed until non-viability is certain.

Ultrasound investigation allows all of the following to be clearly recorded:

- The number of gestational sacs.
- The mean gestational sac diameter — the mean of three perpendicular measurements within the sac.
- The regularity of the sac outline.
- The presence of a yolk sac.
- The presence of a fetal pole.
- The crown rump length measurement of the fetal pole.
- The presence or absence of fetal heart movements.
- Evidence of cause of bleed e.g. failure of one pregnancy in a twin gestation.

If any of the information is difficult to obtain clearly from an abdominal USS examination, a transvaginal scan should be performed, again reassuring the anxious woman of the safety of this procedure. This information should be clearly documented on a standard USS report.

The findings at USS in combination with the clinical picture will determine the management of the patient.

USS Findings and Subsequent Management

Viable fetus

If the USS demonstrates a fetal pole with cardiac activity, viability is confirmed and there is a 90–95% chance that the pregnancy will progress satisfactorily. Bed rest is of no therapeutic value but strenuous exercise and sexual intercourse should be avoided. Treatment with progestogens or HCG cannot be justified. This opportunity should be taken to counsel women to take 400 μg of folic acid for the first trimester, to stop smoking and to book with her general practitioner (GP) for antenatal care. Patients should always be advised of a 24-hour telephone advice line which they should contact if vaginal bleeding becomes heavy or if pain worsens.

Empty intrauterine gestational sac

If a gestational sac is demonstrated within the uterus without any evidence of a yolk sac or fetal pole, it is important to estimate the mean sac diameter (MSD), which is the mean of three perpendicular measurements within the sac.

If the MSD is greater than 20 mm, it is highly suggestive of a blighted ovum and these findings should be sympathetically conveyed to the patient. A blighted ovum can be managed by surgical evacuation of the uterus (see ERPC), by medical evacuation of the uterus, or by expectant management. Medical evacuation involves the administration of mifepristone 600 mg orally followed 36–48 h later by the administration of vaginal gemprost 1 mg or misoprostol 800 μg. The patient should then rest in a designated, appropriately staffed ward until she miscarries. If a woman is managed expectantly, she should be advised that she will eventually start to bleed and miscarry spontaneously, though this may be complicated by infection or incomplete miscarriage.

Embryo within gestational sac, but no fetal heart

If there is a fetal pole within the gestational sac, and it has a crown rump length of >6 mm, but there is no evidence of fetal heart pulsations, this is highly suggestive of a missed abortion and management can be as for a blighted ovum.

Inconclusive findings

If there is evidence of a gestational sac with the presence of a yolk sac within the uterus, but there is no significant fetal pole or a small pole without an FH, this is consistent with a pregnancy of about 5 weeks, and even when this does not correspond accurately with menstrual dates, a re-scan in 7–10 days is essential to confirm or negate viability.

Likewise, if the gestational sac is < 20 mm (MSD) or the fetal pole <6 mm without evidence of a fetal heart beating, a repeat USS in 7–10 days to assess growth and development of the pregnancy is essential.

Empty uterus

Any woman with a positive pregnancy test and an empty uterus on trans-vaginal (TV) USS must be considered to have an ectopic pregnancy until this is excluded. Other possible diagnoses include a complete miscarriage, and early intrauterine pregnancy, which may be viable or non-viable. It is essential to take a detailed history and examination from these women and management is very dependent on clinical signs and symptoms. Serum BHCG assessment serially (48 h apart) can also be helpful to make an accurate diagnosis. A serum BHCG concentration of 1000iu/l or greater indicates that an intrauterine pregnancy should be visible on TV USS. A serum BHCG concentration which falls over 48 h usually represents a failing pregnancy either intrauterine or ectopic, but a static or suboptimally rising BHCG (less than doubling in 48 h) may indicate an ectopic pregnancy.

Presence of retained products of conception (RPOC)

USS diagnosis of RPOC is by identifying mixed echogenic products within the uterus. It is no longer standard practice to offer all women with any RPOC an ERPC.

If RPOC are <15 mm on USS, i.e. minimal and the woman is clinically stable, conservative/expectant management is treatment of choice. Eighty percent of women with an inevitable abortion will have no USS evidence of RPOC within 3 days of onset of signs and symptoms. If RPOC are between 15 and 50 mm on USS women can be offered expectant management or surgical management (see ERPC). When RPOC are significant i.e. >50 mm on USS surgical evacuation or medical management (see ERPC and above) are appropriate.

Any woman managed conservatively should be fully counselled about the possibility of persistent bleeding, persistent RPOC, infection and eventual need for ERPC should clinical symptoms not settle. These women should be provided with an information leaflet and a 24-hour contact telephone number. Women with more than minimal RPOC on USS who are managed conservatively should also be offered a follow-up appointment in 7 days to assess symptoms and perform a repeat USS if clinically appropriate.

IMPORTANT CLINICAL POINT

Early intrauterine death should be regarded as of equal significance to fetal death occurring at a later stage of pregnancy and those performing early pregnancy USS must be sensitive to the emotional aspects of early pregnancy loss. It is important to deal with the situation in a supportive and sympathetic way and to recognise when more detailed counselling is appropriate.

Evacuation of Retained Products of Conception (ERPC)

Evacuation of retained products of conception is appropriate management for women with:

- a missed abortion.
- an anembryonic pregnancy.
- RPOC after an incomplete abortion.
- a septic abortion.
- persistent bleeding after expectant management of an incomplete abortion.

All women undergoing an ERPC should be fully counselled about the procedure (see below) and informed of the potential risks:

- risks associated with anaesthesia.
- risks of the procedure e.g. bleeding, uterine perforation, retained products of conception after the procedure, infection — which can be endometrial or pelvic.

They should also have their haemoglobin concentration, blood group and rhesus status checked.

In the case of a missed abortion or an anembryonic pregnancy, the use of misoprostol 400 mg vaginally or gemeprost 1 mg vaginally 1–2 h prior to ERPC causes softening of the cervix making dilatation of the cervix easier during the procedure. This avoids forcible dilatation of the cervix, which may have long-term consequences such as cervical incompetence.

In the main ERPC is performed under general anaesthetic (though it can be performed with regional anaesthesia such as a spinal anaesthetic or even local anaesthetic such as a paracervical block). The patient should be examined under sterile conditions when asleep to determine:

— if the uterus is anteverted or retroverted,
— if there are any adnexal masses,
— if the cervical os is open — likely in an incomplete abortion.

If the cervix is closed, cervical dilatation with a Hegar dilator will be necessary. Systematic suction curettage with a Berkley or Karman currette is then performed to remove retained products of conception. Products can also be removed using sponge-holding forceps. In each case, care is always taken to avoid perforation of the uterus. During evacuation, 10 u syntocinon given IV will decrease uterine bleeding and make the uterine muscle firm with a sustained contraction, reducing the risk of perforation. The uterine cavity can then be gently checked to be empty with a blunt curette, ensuring no vigorous evacuation is performed, as this can cause endometrial scarring, intrauterine adhesions and result in Aschermann's syndrome. It is sensible to use prophylactic antibiotics post-operatively. Metronidazole 1 g can be given rectally while the patient is still asleep and a 7-day course of doxycycline 100 mg twice daily should be prescribed to prevent post-op sepsis which can lead to salpingitis.

All women undergoing ERPC irrespective of gestational age who are non-sensitised RhD negative should be given anti-D IgG.

Although ERPC is one of the most common gynaecological procedures, it is essential to always remember that this is an enormously emotional time for any woman and sensitive, understanding, efficient management and counselling must be employed.

SEPTIC ABORTION

Septic abortion is a serious complication of spontaneous or induced abortion. It may also complicate procedures such as amniocentisis, cervical cerclage and ERPC. Necrotic products of conception provide good culture medium for organisms, the most commonly found being *Escherichia coli*, aerobic haemolytic and non-haemolytic plus anaerobic streptococci, *Staphylococcus aureus*, and the anaerobes bacteroides, *Clostridium welchii* and rarely now *Clostridium tetanii*. The infection is usually confined to the products and the uterine cavity and is manifested by an offensive purulent or pinkish discharge from the cervix and vagina, pelvic and abdominal pain, pelvic and supra-pubic tenderness, cervical excitation, signs of peritonitis and pyrexia which if severe is accompanied by rigors. Severe infections may be complicated by Gram-negative endotoxic shock secondary to the vasodilatation produced by the endotoxin. Severe endotoxic shock may be complicated by disseminated intravascular coagulation (DIC).

The priorities in the management of septic abortion are:

1. ressuscitate.
2. treat the infection.
3. empty the uterus.

Detailed description of treatment of endotoxic shock is beyond the remit of this Chapter. In the absence of septicaemia, i.v. cefuroxime and metronidazole are antibiotics which will provide adequate therapy until the bacterial sensitivities are available. Antibiotic therapy can be completed orally when the patient improves. A full blood count, blood cultures and swabs from the discharge should be sent for culture. Close monitoring of patient temperature and pulse are important.

Great care should be taken during evacuation of the septic uterus as the risks of perforation are greater as the septic uterus may be softer.

Anti-D Immunoglobulin for Rh Prophylaxis Following Abortion

Anti-D Ig should be given to all non-sensitised RhD negative women who have a spontaneous threatened, complete or incomplete abortion after 12 weeks gestation. Anti-D Ig should be given to all women who have had instrumentation to evacuate the uterus irrelevant of gestation, whereas the risk of immunisation by spontaneous miscarriage before 12 weeks gestation is negligible when there has been no uterine instrumentation and therefore anti-D Ig is not required in these circumstances. The dose of anti-D Ig prior to 20 weeks gestation is 250 iu. It is important that all women requiring anti-D Ig fully understand about Rh prophylaxis and that they also understand that anti-D Ig is a blood product.

Importance and Development of Early Pregnancy Assessment Units (EPAU)

The management of early pregnancy complications can be optimised by running a clinic dedicated to accurately diagnosing, treating and supporting women suffering from such problems. Outlined below are practical reasons why early pregnancy assessment clinics have transformed the management of women with problems in early pregnancy.

Most women with bleeding in early pregnancy contact their GP with symptoms. It is the role of the primary care doctor to decide if the woman needs to be seen immediately (if there is heavy bleeding, sepsis or suspicion of an ectopic pregnancy) or if the woman can be assessed the next day in the EPAU. If so, the GP can phone for a specific appointment time for the woman to be seen the next morning. This avoids the waiting times patients have to endure when being seen as an emergency in casualty or gynaecology emergency rooms.

EPAU is staffed by a trained gynaecologist, skilled in trans-abdominal and trans-vaginal USS. Each patient attending clinic has a history taken, often onto a pre-formatted history sheet and is examined. As a designated clinic, this reduces the number of invasive examinations the patient has to undergo (avoiding the casualty officer and gynaecology SHO examinations).

After examination, USS can be performed immediately. This further reduces the patient waiting time, thereby reducing patient anxiety and stress levels. USS findings should be clearly documented according to joint RCR RCOG guidelines and with all the information obtained, a management plan should be formulated for each individual patient.

The benefits of a daily, easily accessible, well run, well staffed and structured EPAC to GPs, patients and hospital staff are numerous:

1. The GP is provided with an easy referral system to offer patients prompt scanning in early pregnancy.
2. Patient waiting times are significantly reduced.
3. The workload on casualty and gynaecology emergency services is reduced.
4. The patient can be treated in a more sensitive and sympathetic way.
5. The patient avoids numerous vaginal examinations.
6. The patient is dealt with by a more experienced gynaecologist with skill in TV USS and counselling rather than 3–4 medical professionals along the way.
7. The counselling and psychological support essential to these women can be efficiently offered.
8. Blood tests and follow-up arrangements can be easily arranged.
9. If a patient needs an ERPC, this can be organised for the same day during working hours which is beneficially reducing hospital bed occupancy and overnight stays.
10. Anti-D prophylaxis can be organised as necessary.

THERAPEUTIC ABORTION

Induced abortion or termination is one of the most commonly performed gynaecological procedures in England and Wales (180,000 per year). In fact, greater than one-third of British women have had a termination by the age of 45 and 'threat to maternal mental or physical health' is the reason documented for termination in 98% cases. This is dubbed as the 'social' clause for termination. Recently, an RCOG guideline has been published on 'The care of women requesting induced abortion' and the recommendations of this will be considered below.

Ideally any woman requesting termination of pregnancy (TOP) should have prompt access to a service that provides information, medical assessment and counselling within 5 days of request for TOP or at most 2 weeks. It is the aim to undergo TOP within 7 days of the decision to proceed. This aimed to reduce the gestation at which TOPs are performed as complications are less the lower the gestation. Although most women can undergo a TOP as a day case procedure, 10% will require inpatient admission.

All women requesting TOP should be clinically assessed. Menstrual history is essential to estimate gestational age. Clinical examination should confirm dates, and if there is any discrepancy a USS may be necessary for accurate dating. The USS should be performed in a sensitive manner by shielding the screen from women and ensuring it is not performed in an antenatal clinic setting where there are many women with wanted pregnancies. The woman should have a check haemoglobin concentration, assessment of her ABO Rh status and sickle cell status if necessary. Depending on her gestation, the mode of termination should then be fully explained to the woman. Counselling any woman for TOP should include discussion and planning of contraceptive use.

Although sterilisation can safely be performed at the time of surgical TOP, it is associated with higher failure rates and higher levels of regret on the part of the woman and it is not recommended.

The time around TOP is difficult emotionally for women, and support in decision making, additional counselling or even social service input should always be made available. A sensitive, supportive attitude from hospital staff looking after these women is essential. Accurate verbal advice must be provided for all women requesting TOP, and this should be reinforced with impartial printed information which can be taken away for reading. These leaflets should be clear and be modified for non-English speakers or women with learning difficulties.

Complications of TOP

Haemorrhage — <1% risk and risk reduced further for TOPs <13/40 gestation.

Uterine perforation — <1% risk.

Cervical trauma — risk is no greater than 1%.

Failed abortion — risk for surgical procedureg 2.5/1000.
— risk for medical procedure: 6/1000.

Infection — can lead to endometritis in about 10% which can spread to pelvic inflammatory disease. This can be reduced which the use of prophylactic antibiotics.

Future reproductive outcome — there is no association between TOP and future infertility and pre-term labour.

Maternal death — there was only one maternal death reported after legal termination between 1994–1996.

There is of course a risk of psychological distress post procedure and the need for any extra counselling should be identified and offered. It is however rare for there to be long term psychological sequelae.

Suction Termination of Pregnancy (STOP)

This is an appropriate method of termination for women 7–14 weeks gestation, though in practice many practitioners prefer medical termination for those above 12 weeks gestation. STOP should be avoided when the gestation is less than 7 weeks. Cervical priming with 400 μg of misoprostol or 1 mg gemprost 2–3 h prior to STOP may be beneficial to assist cervical dilatation during the procedure, especially in women <18 years of age or > 10 weeks pregnant. Although most surgical terminations are performed under general anaesthetic, the use of local anaesthesia should be considered as it may be a safer option.

If greater than 14 weeks gestation, a dilatation and evacuation (D&E) is safe if preceded by adequate cervical priming and if performed by a medical practitioner who has a caseload large enough to maintain their skills. It is safe practice to perform a D&E with direct USS guidance in theatre.

During a STOP or D&E the use of oxytocin may decrease blood loss, and if a perforation is suspected, laparoscopy is necessary. Metronidazole 1 g PR and doxycycline 100 mg twice daily for 7 days should be prescribed to reduce the incidence of infection.

Medical Termination of Pregnancy

This form of termination is appropriate and recommended for TOP less than 7 weeks gestation and is a safe form of TOP up to 9 weeks gestation. The procedure involves the administration of 600 mg mifepristone orally followed by gemprost 1 mg vaginally 36–48 h later (other options include mifepristone 200 mg orally) followed 36–48 h later by misoprostol 800 μg vaginally or mifepristone 200 mg orally followed 36 h later by gemprost 0.5 mg vaginally (these regimens are unlicensed as described).

Medical TOP is also safe and effective for women greater than 12 weeks gestation. When at greater than 15 weeks gestation, cervical priming with gemprost or misoprostol is repeated 3-hourly until abortion occurs. Surgical evacuation is not routinely required after mid-trimester termination unless there is evidence that the abortion is incomplete.

Women undergoing medical TOP should ideally be cared for separately from other gynaecology patients and looked after by experienced nurses.

Post-TOP

After a termination, women should be provided with a written account of symptoms they may experience, and a 24-hour help line telephone number to use if they are concerned with any bleeding, pain or are feeling unwell.

Referral for further counselling should be available for women suspected of suffering from post-abortion distress and the GP should be communicated with regarding the procedure performed.

Anti-D IgG should be given to all non-sensitised RhD negative women following TOP regardless of gestation and regardless of mode of TOP.

FURTHER READING

The Royal College of Radiologists, The Royal College of Obstetricians and Gynaecologists (1995). *Guidance on Ultrasound Procedures in Early Pregnancy.*

The Royal College of Obstetricians and Gynaecologists (2000). *The Care of Women Requesting Induced Abortion.* Guideline No. 7.

Fox R., Richardson J., Sharma A. (2000). Early pregnancy assessment. *The Obstetrician and Gynaecologist,* **2:** 7–13.

The Royal College of Obstetricians and Gynaecologists (1999). *Use of Anti-D Immunoglobulin Prophylaxis.* Green Top Clinical Guidelines No. 22.

6

Recurrent Miscarriage

DEFINITIONS AND PREVALENCE

A pregnancy may be lost at any stage of development but the term miscarriage is used for all losses occurring up to 24 weeks gestation. The majority of sporadic (or one-off) miscarriages occur in the first trimester and are termed early pregnancy losses. Recurrent miscarriage is defined as the loss of three or more consecutive pregnancies irrespective of gestation and is a heterogeneous condition.

Sporadic miscarriage is the most common complication of pregnancy, affecting a quarter of all women during the course of their

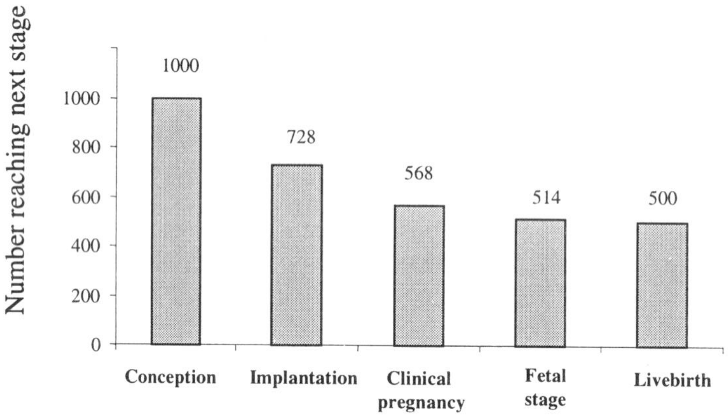

Fig. 6.1 *The fate of 1000 fertilised ova (after Kline et al., 1989).*

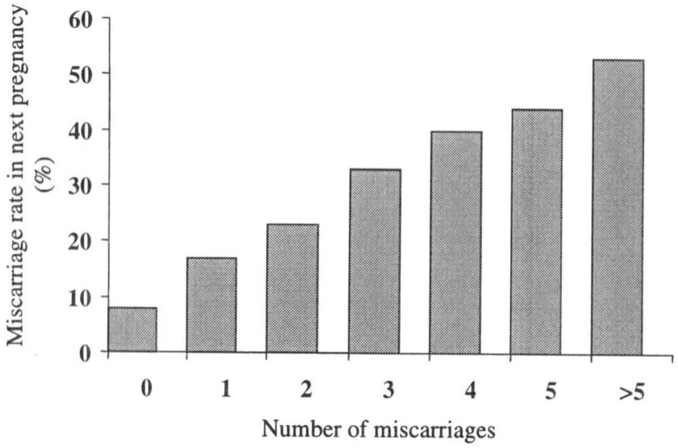

Fig. 6.2 *Likelihood of a miscarriage after successive pregnancy losses (derived from pooled data).*

reproductive lives. It is consistently reported that 12–15% of all clinically recognised pregnancies fail spontaneously, although the rate of subclinical loss, before the woman realises she is pregnant, is much higher than this figure. It has been estimated that for every 1000 conceptions, only 500 livebirths result (Fig. 6.1). Assuming that 15% of pregnancies fail, the likelihood of three consecutive losses would be expected to be 0.3% from chance alone. The observed rate of recurrent miscarriage of approximately 1% is higher than this calculation, and together with the finding that the risk of miscarriage increases with each successive loss (Fig. 6.2), it appears that a systematic abnormality underlies many cases of recurrent miscarriage.

AETIOLOGY OF RECURRENT MISCARRIAGE

Genetic Factors

Fetal chromosomal abnormalities are the most common cause of sporadic miscarriage, accounting for over 60% of losses. Although women with recurrent miscarriage can still experience sporadic-type losses, the majority of losses have a normal chromosome complement. However, in approximately 3–5% of couples with recurrent miscarriage one or other partner carries a chromosome anomaly and so are at risk of repeated miscarriages with the loss of pregnancies with an abnormal karyotype. The most common type of parental chromosome rearrangement is a balanced translocation. This is usually either a balanced reciprocal translocation, where the overall number of chromosomes is unchanged, or a Robertsonian translocation where there are only 45 chromosomes but the genetic information is intact. The conceptuses of such parents carry a high risk of an unbalanced translocation where the genetic information is altered and these pregnancies are usually lost in the first trimester. Although the prevalence of parental chromosome abnormalities is low, parental karyotyping is an important test when investigating recurrent miscarriage due to the profound effect of an abnormal parental karyotype on future pregnancy outcome. Affected couples should receive genetic counselling and in ongoing pregnancies, pre-natal diagnosis should be offered to detect the occasional ongoing pregnancy with an abnormal karyotype.

Structural Abnormalities of the Uterus

Mullerian duct defects

Congenital Mullerian duct anomalies have long been quoted as a cause of recurrent miscarriage, both in early pregnancy and in the mid-trimester. These arise from the abnormal development or incomplete fusion of the Mullerian (paramesonephric) ducts. The range of abnormalities include the normal differentiation of only one Mullerian duct (unicornuate uterus), the complete failure of midline fusion of the ducts resulting in a double system (uterus didelphys), and partial fusion of the ducts resulting in a bicornuate uterus or a subseptate uterus. The prevalence of structural abnormalities in women with normal reproductive histories identified at the time of laparoscopic sterilisation is approximately 4%, whereas the prevalence in recurrent miscarriers is in the region of 15%. Uterine abnormalities can be detected by hysterosalpingography, hysteroscopy and ultrasound (most recently 3D ultrasound), although the best method is not clear. It is important to understand that many women with congenital abnormalities of the uterus have normal pregnancies without treatment and there is no good evidence that surgical correction of the anomaly improves pregnancy outcome, as the livebirth rate without treatment is around 60–65%.

Cervical incompetence

Cervical incompetence is a condition in which painless dilatation of the cervix leads to miscarriage or premature delivery in the absence of uterine contractions or haemorrhage. Cervical incompetence is not a cause of recurrent early pregnancy loss and the role played by cervical incompetence in the aetiology of second trimester loss remains contentious. Traditionally, cervical cerclage has been considered on the basis of a past history of mid-trimester, painless cervical dilatation or rupture of the membranes, as diagnosis in the non-pregnant state is unreliable. Cervical cerclage involves insertion of a suture, usually of mersilene tape or nylon, around the top of the cervix (MacDonald suture). Higher placement of the suture can be obtained when the bladder is reflected upwards off the cervix (Shirodkar suture). The suture is usually inserted at about 14 weeks of pregnancy (after a viable pregnancy has been confirmed on ultrasound) and removed at 37 weeks. In the MRC/RCOG randomised controlled trial of cervical cerclage, 1 in 25 cases benefited from a cervical suture in terms of a reduction in premature deliveries, although a beneficial effect on miscarriage and perinatal mortality rates was not seen. The use of transvaginal ultrasound in pregnancy to look for progressive shortening of the cervix and funnelling of the upper cervix prior to overt cervical dilatation may improve the diagnostic accuracy and allow more selective use of cerclage. Transabdominal cervical cerclage, with the objective of closing the internal os at the junction with the isthmus of the uterus, has been advocated as a treatment for recurrent mid-trimester loss although as yet there is no good evidence of improved efficacy.

Genital Tract Infection

Many infections of the genital tract have been reported to cause sporadic miscarriage. However, the role played by infective organisms in the aetiology of recurrent miscarriage is unclear. The majority of organisms implicated do not persist for sufficient periods of time to produce repeated miscarriages or are found in high prevalence in the normal population. Bacterial vaginosis (BV), a polymicrobial anaerobic infection associated with a loss of the normal vaginal lactobacilli, has been implicated in the aetiology of pre-term labour and late miscarriage. To date, antibiotic treatment appears to benefit only those women with BV and a previous history of pre-term loss.

Social and Environmental Factors

Although some chemical and toxic agents have been associated with miscarriage, a history of exposure to such agents is rarely encountered in a clinical setting. Heavy alcohol consumption and smoking have both been associated with an increased risk of miscarriage in some studies. However the contribution that these habits make to the overall problem of recurrent miscarriage is small.

Autoimmune Causes

It is now well established that circulating antiphospholipid antibodies (aPL), the most important of which are the lupus anticoagulant (LA) and anticardiolipin antibodies (ACA), are associated with recurrent pregnancy failure at all stages of pregnancy. Although the adverse effects of aPL on the outcome of pregnancy were first noted in women with systemic lupus erythematosus, the primary antiphospholipid syndrome (PAPS) is now well documented as an important cause of recurrent miscarriage. The features of the syndrome are raised circulating aPL, in association with recurrent fetal loss, arterial or venous thrombosis or thrombocytopaenia. There may be other clinical features of the syndrome as detailed in Table 6.1. Fetal loss can occur at all stages of the pregnancy and there is an association with pre-eclampsia, intra-uterine growth restriction (IUGR) and placental abruption. The most common type of pregnancy loss is the loss of a fetus in the first trimester after the establishment of fetal heart activity.

The pathophysiology of aPL is uncertain. The adverse effects of aPL may be mediated via thrombosis and fibrin deposition in many vessels including the uteroplacental circulation, which may show signs of infarction. This may be due to inhibition of endothelial prostacyclin production, enhanced thromboxane release

Table 6.1
Clinical Features of the Primary Antiphospholipid Antibody Syndrome (PAPS)

Obstetrics and Gynaecology

Recurrent miscarriage
Infertility
Pre-eclampsia
Placental abruption
Intra-uterine growth restriction

Vascular

Venous thrombosis
Arterial thrombosis
Mitral valve disease
Thrombotic endocarditis

Neurological

Transient ischaemic attacks
Cerebrovascular disease
Migraine
Epilepsy
Multiple sclerosis

from platelets, reduced antithrombin III production or decreasing the activation of protein C.

The prevalence of aPL in women with recurrent miscarriage is 15%, compared to 2% in women with normal obstetric histories. The livebirth rate in women with recurrent miscarriage and aPL is only 10% without treatment. The mainstay of treatment for pregnant women with aPL is low-dose aspirin in combination with sub-cutaneous heparin, commenced at the beginning of pregnancy. It has been established that the livebirth rate amongst women with PAPS is improved to 40% when they are treated with low-dose aspirin alone, but that this is further and significantly increased to over 70% when treated with aspirin in combination with heparin (Fig. 6.3).

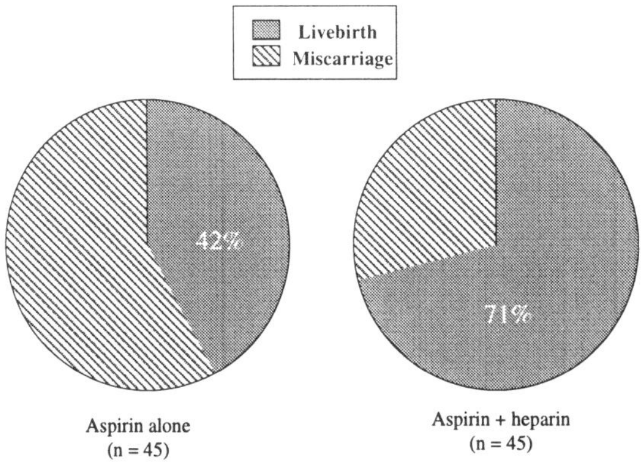

Fig. 6.3 *Outcome of pregnancy in women with recurrent miscarriage and anti-phospholipid antibodies treated with aspirin or aspirin + heparin (after Rai et al., 1997).*

Inherited Thrombophilia

Thrombophilic defects have recently been identified as potential causes of both early and late miscarriage and adverse pregnancy outcome. Many thrombophilias have recently been associated with recurrent pregnancy loss including activated protein C resistance (APCR), which is the most common inherited thrombophilia with a prevalence in the general population of 3–5%. In up to 90% of cases, it is due to a single point mutation in the factor V gene resulting in a mutated factor V, known as Factor V Leiden. Factor V Leiden is resistant to inactivation by activated protein C, a natural inhibitor of coagulation, and therefore a state of increased thrombin generation occurs. It remains to be established whether women with thrombophilias have a poor pregnancy outcome when studied prospectively, as direct evidence that they are causally related to pregnancy loss is still lacking. One of the possibilities is that it is only in the presence of more than one thrombophilic defect that pregnancy outcome is significantly influenced.

Endocrine Dysfunction

Generalised endocrine disease

Historically diabetes mellitus has been considered to be an important cause of recurrent miscarriage. Whilst poorly controlled diabetics do have an increased rate of early miscarriage, there is good evidence that well controlled diabetes is not associated with an increased risk of pregnancy loss.

Thyroid dysfunction has previously been cited as a cause of recurrent miscarriage but direct evidence is lacking and thyroid function tests are rarely abnormal in these women. There does appear to be an association between anti-thyroid antibodies and recurrent pregnancy loss although this may well reflect a generalised autoimmune abnormality rather than a specific endocrine dysfunction.

Hypersecretion of luteinising hormone

In the mid-1980s, studies suggested that hypersecretion of luteinising hormone (LH) had an adverse effect on fertility and pregnancy outcome. Women with recurrent miscarriage and infertility have a prevalence of ultrasound diagnosed polycystic ovaries (PCO) of about 50% compared to a background rate of PCO of 23% in a "normal" population of women of reproductive age. It appeared to be the presence of LH hypersecretion that was responsible for the poor reproductive outcome in these women rather than a polycystic ovarian morphology *per se.* Women with high LH levels have been reported to have reduced rates of fertilisation, lower conception rates and higher miscarriage rates when undergoing IVF or ovulation induction and, more importantly, the adverse effect of LH hypersecretion has also been documented in spontaneous, unstimulated cycles. An adverse effect on the oocyte and/or the endometrium has been suggested.

Following the hypothesis that high LH levels are detrimental to the establishment of early pregnancy, many workers have examined the reproductive outcome after suppression of elevated LH concentrations with analogues to LH releasing hormone. Several studies of women undergoing assisted conception have documented improved pregnancy and livebirth rates after LH suppression. However, this appears not to be the case for fertile women with recurrent miscarriage who hypersecrete LH. There is now good evidence that there is no benefit from LH suppression in these women and, importantly, the livebirth rate with supportive care alone is in the region of 76%. It is possible that factors other than LH (such as abnormal androgen or insulin secretion) influence the pregnancy outcome in women with PCO.

Unexplained Recurrent Miscarriage

In most series, the number of women with recurrent miscarriage who have no identifiable cause after thorough investigation is 50%. In the next pregnancy several factors appear to influence the pregnancy outcome. After unexplained recurrent miscarriage the number of previous losses has been shown to affect outcome. There is a steady increase in the risk of subsequent miscarriage for each previous loss — the risk of miscarriage rising from 30% after 3 losses to over 50% after 6 or more losses. Maternal age also influences the prognosis for the future. A pronounced effect is seen after the mid-thirties with more than 50% of women over 40 years losing the next pregnancy irrespective of the number of previous losses. Most studies report that a previous successful pregnancy in the past history does not appear to influence outcome, with a similar prognosis whether or not the woman has had a previous successful pregnancy.

The most striking observation is that early pregnancy clinics offering supportive therapy (or "tender loving care") confer a highly significant beneficial effect on pregnancy outcome in women with unexplained recurrent miscarriage. Women who receive supportive therapy in the first trimester have a 75% chance of a successful pregnancy without any pharmacological treatment, although the mechanism of action is not clear.

MANAGEMENT OF RECURRENT MISCARRIAGE

Women with recurrent miscarriage should ideally be seen in a specialist miscarriage clinic where there are established protocols for investigation and management. At the first appointment, the couple should be seen together and sufficient time should be allowed for a detailed discussion. Current

Table 6.2
Recurrent Miscarriage — Recommended Investigations

Evidence-based Investigations	Research-based Investigations
Karyotype both partners	Thrombophilia screen
Karyotype products of conception after a pregnancy loss	Assess ovarian morphology Mid follicular LH
Establish uterine morphology (ultrasound/hysteroscopy)	Screen for bacterial vaginosis
Antiphospholipid antibodies (lupus anticoagulant and anticardiolipin antibodies)	

evidence-based investigations for recurrent miscarriage are shown in Table 6.2.

In future pregnancies, direct access to a dedicated early pregnancy clinic is invaluable. If the next pregnancy fails, obtaining fetal tissue for karyotypic analysis is important. Not only is there an explanation for the miscarriage if the karyotype is abnormal, but the results are also important for guidance for future pregnancies.

CONCLUSION

Sporadic miscarriage is the most common complication of pregnancy and is associated with a good prognosis for future pregnancies. Recurrent miscarriage is less frequently encountered and is best managed in a specialist clinic. Such clinics have the opportunity to develop protocols for the investigation and management of the condition, audit the outcome of subsequent pregnancies, provide a comprehensive multi-disciplinary approach to the management of recurrent miscarriage and conduct research investigations into potential new treatments. Recent studies have identified that antiphospholipid antibodies and possibly thrombophilic defects are important causes of repeated pregnancy failure.

After thorough investigation, approximately 50% of women with a history of recurrent miscarriage will have no identifiable cause for their losses. The future pregnancy outcome for these women is good and supportive therapy alone is the treatment of choice in the next pregnancy. To avoid the pitfalls of the past, empirical treatment of women with recurrent miscarriage should be avoided and new therapies should only ever be tested in the setting of a randomised trial.

7

Anatomy and Physiology of Normal Pregnancy

The anatomical and physiological adjustments that occur in pregnancy are specifically designed to promote an environment that supports good fetal growth without jeopardising maternal well-being. The dependence of the fetus upon the mother means that there needs to be maternal changes to ensure the fetus receives adequate sustenance and also an ability to remove waste products of metabolic processes, including heat. Thus the main physiological systems which are affected are those of circulation, respiration and renal function. As a result of this haematological, biochemical and physiological indices alter during pregnancy and new normal ranges and values must be applied.

CARDIOVASCULAR SYSTEM (TABLE 7.1)

Blood Volume

The total blood volume increases by about 40% above non-pregnant levels, reaching a maximum at around 32 weeks of pregnancy. The retention of sodium and water during pregnancy accounts for a total body water increase of 6–8 litres and two-thirds of this is retained within the extra-vascular space. Plasma volume begins to rise around 6 weeks gestation and in singleton pregnancies the increase averages 50%, rising to 70% with twin gestations. Red cell mass begins to rise around the start of the second trimester and by term it is between 20–35% above non-pregnant levels. The disproportionate increase in plasma volume relative to that of red cell mass means there is a relative haemodilution known as physiological anaemia of pregnancy. Haemoglobin concentration will fall, only minimally in women with adequate iron stores, but in those with inadequate reserves there will be a considerable drop (2–3 g/l).

Cardiac Output

Cardiac output is one of the first changes in the cardiovascular system to occur in pregnancy and it rises to 4–5 l/min in response to the increase in blood volume. These changes begin early in the first trimester and by mid-pregnancy have increased by 40% above non-pregnant levels. The early increases in cardiac output are mainly brought about by an increase in stroke volume, but this falls in the latter half of pregnancy and so cardiac output

Table 7.1
Cardiovascular Changes in Pregnancy

Blood pressure		
Systolic	↓ 5 mm Hg	at mid-gestation returning
Diastolic	↓ 8–15 mm Hg	to pre-pregnancy levels at term
Heart rate	↑ 12–15 beats/min	
Stroke volume	↑ 25%	
Cardiac output	↑ 40%	

is maintained by an increase in heart rate. In twin and higher order pregnancies, cardiac output changes are greater than those seen in singleton pregnancies. Cardiac output is increased during the first trimester, continues to increase during the second and then remains relatively static thereafter. Cardiovascular response to exercise is altered during pregnancy and oxygen consumption is higher during exercise in the pregnant than in the non-pregnant woman. Cardiac output is also raised in comparison to the non-pregnant woman and maximum cardiac output is reached at lower levels of activity.

Blood Pressure

Paradoxically, despite the increase in both plasma volume and cardiac output, blood pressure does not rise during pregnancy, but in fact, diastolic blood pressure shows a fall. This fall in diastolic blood pressure is greatest during the second trimester, after which it rises progressively to reach non-pregnant values in the third trimester. This fall in diastolic blood pressure seems to be due to a decrease in peripheral vascular resistance, which may be due to local production of vasodilatory prostaglandins within the placental circulation. However, diastolic blood pressure has also been found to correlate with maternal plasma angiotensin II levels during pregnancy, indicating that the renin-angiotensin system may be very important in the regulation of blood pressure during pregnancy. The increase in cardiac output is distributed between the kidneys, skin, breasts, uterus, and to a lesser extent, other organs. The increase in blood flow to the kidneys is brought about in order to cope with the increased metabolic waste that occurs during pregnancy and the increased flow to the skin to dissipate increased heat loss. These two maternal adaptations require increased plasma volume rather than whole blood, thus explaining the increase in plasma volume over red blood cells in the haematological changes described above. Renal blood flow is increased by approximately 30% and skin blood flow accounts for approximately 12% of cardiac output.

Anatomical Changes

These physiological changes that occur lead to an increase in the size of the heart, which is a combination of hypertrophy and increased diastolic filling. The heart also changes position during pregnancy, being pushed upwards by the elevation of the diaphragm and rotated forwards. These changes lead to changes in the electrocardiograph with a shift of the electrical axis of the heart of approximately 15 degrees to the left.

Changes in peripheral blood flow may be brought about by mechanical displacement due to the enlarging uterus and this may have marked effects on blood flow through the iliac veins and the inferior vena cava. Pregnant women in the third trimester adopting a supine position may cause venous compression leading to a fall in venous return and hence decreased cardiac output. This occurs in approximately 10% of women and causes nausea, dizziness and feeling faint. This is known as supine hypotension and is relieved by a change of posture.

Venous compression by the uterus on veins which normally drain the legs and other pelvic organs leads to increased pressure, which in turn may lead to varicose veins in the legs and vulva and haemorrhoids. The rise in venous pressure is the major cause of peripheral oedema, which is so commonly characteristic of pregnant women. It must also be remembered that this reduced venous blood flow increases the risk of deep and superficial venous thrombosis.

Haemostasis

Bleeding time and prothrombin time are shortened during pregnancy and this is accompanied by an increase in fibrinogen, as well as factors VII, VIII and X with smaller increases in factors IX and XII and prothrombin. At the same time, there are decreases in fibrinolytic

Table 7.2
Changes in Respiratory Function in Pregnancy

	Before Pregnancy	Late Pregnancy
Ventilation rate (l/min)	8	10
Tidal volume (ml)	500	600
Respiratory rate (/min)	16	16
Vital capacity (l)	3200	3200
Residual volume (ml)	1000	800

substances. Platelet numbers and function are thought to be unchanged by pregnancy. These quantitative increases in factors do not imply a hypercoagulable state, although the coagulation system is activated more swiftly during pregnancy and this probably contributes to the shorter bleeding time.

RESPIRATORY SYSTEM (TABLE 7.2)

There is an increase in ventilation rate in pregnancy, which is principally due to an increase in tidal volume with little change in respiratory frequency. The increase in tidal volume may be caused by the central action of progesterone on central and/or peripheral chemoreceptors. In the latter half of pregnancy, there is a decrease in the expiratory reserve volume, residual volume and thus functional residual capacity of approximately 20%. As a consequence of this, mixing and distribution of gas in the lungs is more efficient during pregnancy leading to increased efficiency in gaseous exchange. Various other tests of pulmonary function, such as maximum breathing capacity, timed vital capacity and pulmonary diffusing capacity are unchanged by pregnancy.

If the changes in respiration are indeed attributable to the actions of progesterones, they would be expected to start from the point of the first missed period, and women in early pregnancy often comment on changes in respiratory pattern. The growth of the fetus and placenta account for almost half of the increased demand for oxygen in the latter stages of pregnancy. The rest of the increased oxygen consumption is due to an increase in cardiac and respiratory work and an increase in uterine muscle and breast tissue.

Due to hyperventilation, arterial and alveolar PCO_2 falls to a level of 28–32 mmHg compared with the non-pregnant mean of 37–39 mmHg. Plasma pH is maintained by a fall in the levels of plasma bicarbonate.

Anatomical Changes

There is an increase in chest size during pregnancy, which most pregnant women notice as a flaring of their lower ribs. The sub-costal angle increases during pregnancy from a value of approximately 68° in early pregnancy to 103° in late pregnancy. The diaphragm is elevated by about 4 cm and this is accompanied by breathing becoming more diaphragmatic than costal as pregnancy progresses.

RENAL SYSTEM

Anatomical Changes

The major anatomical change in the urinary tract during pregnancy is dilatation of the ureters, which can occur as early as the tenth week. The right side becomes more affected and the dilatation may extend to the renal pelvices. The dilatation is most likely due to mechanical compression of the ureters by the dilated ovarian vein plexus, the iliac artery and the increasing size of the uterus. This is more likely than the previously held belief that it was due to smooth muscle relaxing effect of progesterone. Vesicoureteric reflux is more common during pregnancy and this increases the risk of pyelonephritis.

Renal Function

Effective renal plasma flow, blood flow and glomerular filtration rate are all increased from early in pregnancy to a value approximately 40–50% greater than the non-pregnant values and this change is achieved by mid-gestation. In response to water load or deprivation, pregnant women are able to produce dilute or concentrated urine to the same extent as the non-pregnant woman, but plasma osmolality is maintained at approximately 9 mosmol/kg lower than in the non-pregnant woman.

Pregnant women excrete greater quantities of amino acids and sugars (glucose, lactose, fructose, ribose and xylose) than non-pregnant women and the incidence of pregnant women displaying glycosuria increases during gestation. The glycosuria is caused by increased amounts of glucose entering the kidney tubules due to increased glomerular filtration rate and also to the decreased ability of the tubules to reabsorb glucose.

THE RENIN-ANGIOTENSIN SYSTEM

The renin-angiotensin system is markedly altered in pregnancy with concentrations of renin, renin substrate and angiotensin I and II being elevated. Renin levels remain elevated throughout pregnancy, although the exact role played by renin during pregnancy remains unclear.

ALIMENTARY SYSTEM

A change in appetite is one of the most common symptoms a woman will notice on becoming pregnant. Increase in appetite is more marked in the earlier stages of pregnancy and declines towards the end. The changes in appetite and food consumption may be under the same regulatory processes as those of thirst, although this remains still a little unclear. The threshold of taste in pregnancy has been found to be elevated when compared to non-pregnant women, although changes in dietary desires (pica) would seem to be an effect of HCG on the appetite centre in the hypothalamus.

There is a reduction in gastric secretion during pregnancy and gastric tone and motility are reduced, and consequently passage of food through the stomach is delayed. This process may contribute towards some of the nausea and vomiting in later pregnancy, although early nausea and vomiting, which is frequently encountered and may lead to the condition of hyperemesis gravidarum, would seem to be related to HCG production and again an abnormal response within the hypothalamus and the vomit centre. Hyperemesis gravidarum is characterised by dehydration, electrolyte imbalance and ketosis, due to excessive vomiting and decreased intake and may lead to serious metabolic disturbances.

There is also evidence to show that the ileum and colon have reduced motility during pregnancy and gut transit times are reduced. Absorption is not thought to be affected by pregnancy, except that greater quantities of iron are absorbed from the small intestine and greater quantities of water and sodium are absorbed in the colon. These latter changes are the pre-requisites to the increased problem of constipation in pregnancy.

ENDOCRINE SYSTEM

Pregnancy leads to an increased secretion in a number of pituitary hormones. TSH levels are raised, which in turn causes an increase in thyroxine secretion and the thyroid gland normally shows moderate enlargement during pregnancy. As a result of this, a pregnant woman's basal metabolic rate is increased by around 25%.

Adrenocorticotrophic hormone (ACTH) is also increased, and although this leads to an increased secretion of cortisol, most of this is bound in the circulation to corticosteroid binding globulin or transcortin, although some elevated free cortisol is detectable. Whether this change in cortisol level leads to changes such as striae gravidarum and impaired glucose tolerance in pregnancy remains unclear.

Increases in melanin stimulating hormone cause the increased skin pigmentation, which is characteristic of pregnancy. Prolactin, important in lactation, is produced in greater amounts, as is oxytocin, which rises significantly during the second half of pregnancy. Oestrogens and progesterone are produced in large quantities by the placenta, the predominant oestrogen being oestriol. These are the main stimuli for uterine growth and development and progesterone produced by the cytotrophoblast, is known to have an inhibitory action on the myometrium. Human placental lactogen is also produced by the placenta in the latter half of pregnancy and this alters glucose and insulin metabolism and may well be involved in the initiation of lactation. Chorionic gonadotrophins prolong corpus luteum function early in pregnancy and may be involved with progesterone metabolism in later pregnancy.

Table 7.3

Weight Gain at Term

Component	Weight (kg)
Fetus	3.3
Placenta	0.65
Amniotic fluid	0.8
Sub-total	4.75
Uterus	0.97
Breasts	0.4
Blood	1.2
Interstitial fluid	1.67
Fat	4.0
Sub-total	8.27
Total Wt Gain	13.02

WEIGHT GAIN IN PREGNANCY

The average weight gain in pregnancy is between 12 and 14 kg and this is made up of a number of components (see Table 7.3). As can be noted, the fetus and components of conception account for around 40% of the total maternal weight gain.

POSTURE AND PELVIC CHANGES

The changing centre of gravity of the pregnant woman leads to increasing lordosis. The effect of raised levels of oestrogen, progesterone, and possibly the effect of relaxin causes laxity of ligaments throughout the body. Slight movement in otherwise very firm joints, such as the sacroiliac joints and the pubic symphysis can cause discomfort on movement which in extreme cases can be severe. Laxity of the pelvic ligaments allows for maximum pelvic capacity during labour and delivery.

DIAGNOSIS OF PREGNANCY

There are many changes which occur during early pregnancy which enable the diagnosis of pregnancy to be made. These can be divided into clinical, biochemical and biophysical in nature.

Clinical

The symptoms of pregnancy begin with a missed menstrual period. The woman who becomes pregnant fails to menstruate at the expected time in the majority of cases, but some bleeding may occur (called an implantation bleed) and this may confuse the issue for both patient and doctor. The failure to menstruate is, of course, due to maintenance of the corpus luteum which continues to produce progesterone, thereby maintaining the endometrium. After pregnancy is established, the secretory endometrium undergoes changes and is known as decidua.

The mother may well complain of nausea, supposedly due to HCG production which affects the vomit centre in the hypothalamus. Her breasts become enlarged and tender due to the influence of progesterone. The rising progesterone levels will also increase the glomerular filtration rate, possibly causing the symptom of urinary frequency.

The signs of pregnancy begin with pigmentation due to increased production of melanin stimulating hormone (MSH) from the anterior pituitary. The pigmentation occurs in a number of areas, i.e. facial, in a butterfly distribution over the malar region, known as cloasma; the nipples with associated protruberance of Montgomery's tubercles; the mid-abdominal line, usually below the umbilicus, known as the linea nigra (black line). The vulva becomes engorged, and because of this, the labia majora may have a bluish appearance, as do the vagina and cervix. The uterus becomes enlarged (the size being appropriate to the gestation) and soft, and the body of the uterus and the cervix can almost be felt separately. The blood supply to the uterus is much increased, and on bimanual examination, the uterine arteries may be felt pulsating. The examination of the ovaries may reveal one or both to be enlarged by the corpus luteum, which by 6 weeks' gestation is often cystic, perhaps 3–5 cm in diameter.

Biochemical

A number of steroid and protein hormones are produced in pregnancy and the presence of these may be indicative of pregnancy. The most widely used diagnostically is HCG, which is produced from the time of implantation onwards throughout pregnancy. There is an increasing rate of production until about 10–12 weeks gestation, when it reaches its maximum and then declines by 14–18 weeks to reach a maintenance level for the rest of pregnancy. Detection of the presence of HCG in blood or urine of the woman confirms the presence of a pregnancy. HCG may be detected within two days of a missed period with modern enzyme colorimetric techniques, which have been added to the antigen/antibody concept in the detection of HCG.

Ultrasound

A gestation sac may be seen in the uterus from 5½ to 6 weeks' gestation with modern ultrasound equipment. The fetal parts may be identified at 7 weeks and the movement of the fetal heart seen using real time ultrasound. Crown-rump length can be measured very accurately from 7 weeks onwards and this gives an accurate estimate of gestation.

ANATOMICAL CHANGES IN THE UTERUS AND ANATOMY OF THE PLACENTA

The uterine vasculature undergoes quite remarkable and unique changes in the first half of pregnancy, specifically to accommodate increasing flows of blood to the placental intervillous space under conditions of low pressure. Maternal blood supply to the placenta is by way of up to 9–14 branches of the uterine artery on both sides of the uterus. These branches give rise to the arcuate arteries, which encircle the uterus in the basal third of the myometrium to form the stratum vasculare. The radial arteries, which come off the arcuate arteries, pass through the remainder of the myometrium and eventually lead to the spiral arteries with their branches, the basal arteries, supplying the superficial myometrium.

The changes in the spiral arteries during pregnancy are brought about by and are an extension of placental growth. The trophoblast of the placenta invades the uterine wall, migrating through the decidua of the placental bed and also within the lumen of the spiral arteries, where they can be seen on histological section to form cytotrophoblastic plugs. The trophoblast cells begin to invade the walls of the spiral arteries, which are gradually replaced by a mixture of trophoblast in a ground substance of fibrinoid. The spiral arteries become inert and widely expanded down to the level of the myometrial-decidual junction. A second migration of trophoblast early in the second trimester extends this 'physiological change' of the spiral arteries deep into the myometrium. Failure of this process is thought to play some part in the pathogenesis of pregnancy induced hypertension and fetal growth retardation.

Placentation

The placenta begins to form as soon as implantation takes place. The outer layer of the blastocyst (trophoblast) invades the endometrium and loses its form to become the syncytiotrophoblast. The outermost layer of this, called the chorion, forms projections or villi, some attached to the endometrium, but mainly lying free in the lacunae, filled with blood.

The maternal blood supply becomes concentrated on the deep surface of the embryo. The trophoblast grows most profusely here, forming the chorion laeve, which, in turn, forms a villous system called the chorion frondosum. The other areas of trophoblast tend to become less active. The chorion frondosum becomes the placenta proper and its formaton is completed by Day 70.

There are about 200 projections of trophoblastic cells which branch indefinitely, but there are about 10 main branches called cotyledons and many other smaller cotyledons of less significance.

By about Day 20, fetal blood vessels invade the villous trunks and by Day 23 there is a primitive circulation as these vessels join with the blood vessels in the inner cell mass which becomes the heart.

The intervillous spaces are formed by septae from the maternal surface and these are filled with arterial blood from the uterine arteries, and drained by the uterine veins, bathing the fetal surface in maternal blood. The maternal blood flow through the placenta is estimated to reach 600 ml/min at term, over a surface area of villi of about 11 m^2.

Blood supply

Two umbilical arteries supply one half of the placenta each, although this functional arrangement is not entirely discrete due to an anastomosis of the arteries (Hyrtle's anastomosis) prior to the point of insertion into the placenta. The umbilical arteries divide at the point of insertion to give rise to first order chorionic vessels, which travel along the surface of the placenta, branching up to three more times to give chorionic vessels of the 2nd, 3rd and 4th order. The chorionic veins (1st, 2nd, 3rd and 4th order) sometimes travel in conjunction with the arteries in an inferior position, but can also be seen to meet the artery only at the point at which they descend into the placenta. First order villous vessels (2–3) branch off from chorionic arteries of the 2nd, 3rd and 4th order and descend into villous stems. First order villous arteries subsequently divide to give 4–8 vessels of the 2nd order, which run parallel to the fetal surface of the placenta. The 2nd order vessels then curve in the direction of the basal plate, at which point they are termed villous vessels of the 3rd order. Third order villous vessels pierce the basal plate to return in a retrograde course to the chorionic plate (fetal surface of the placenta).

The capillary network of the placental villi arises from branches of 3rd order villous vessels. The capillaries of a single villous anastomose by way of short connecting parts and quite often show wide, sinusoidal dilatations, the syncytiotrophoblastic covering of the villous thins and appears almost to fuse with the endothelial lining of the capillary to form the vasculosyncytial membranes.

A placental cotyledon is defined as the villous 'tree', which is supplied by a single villous artery of the 1st order. The intervillous space is loosely divided into 10–38 lobules by foldings of the basal plate (placental septa). Each lobule may contain 1–3 cotyledons, individually supplied by one, or less often two, spiral arteries which are thought to open into the centre of the cotyledons. Drainage of the intervillous space is by way of a complex of venous sinusoids, which may have their openings located around the periphery of each cotyledon. A cotyledon may thus be viewed as a functional unit of the placenta, comprising a fetal part, which is the villous tree, and a maternal part, which is the immediate surrounding portion of the intervillous space and the vessels which supply it. Loss of one of these units due to blockage of a spiral artery, therefore, does not compromise the overall function of the placenta as an organ of exchange.

The widening of the spiral arteries leads to large amounts of blood entering the intervillous space at low pressure which is less than 20 mmHg in the primate placenta and low velocities (0.1–10 mm/s in the primate placenta). The direction of flow is probably from the centre of the cotyledon outwards and by way of thin capillary-like spaces formed by the high density of the branching villi. The low velocites of flow safeguard this loose arrangement of the placental villi and reduces transit time through the placenta, allowing longer times for exchange. Exchange is further facilitated by a gradual reduction in the diameters of the villi and, as a consequence, the closer apposition of the fetal villous capillaries with the syncytiotrophoblastic layer. This development is epitomised by the formation of the vasculosyncytial membranes which decreases the diffusional barrier of the villi (Fig. 7.1).

Clinical Aspects

The shape of the placenta is determined at the time of implantation and there are considerable variations, none of which are of any functional significance.

Generally, the cord enters at the midpoint, but it may enter at the placental edge (marginal) or the vessels may divide some distance from the placenta and traverse its surface (velamentous insertion).

As regards implantation, the decidual plate and the chorionic plate are of similar sizes, but if the chorionic plate is reduced, the lateral invasion is reduced and thus is poorly supplied with blood and so villi die. The resulting outer

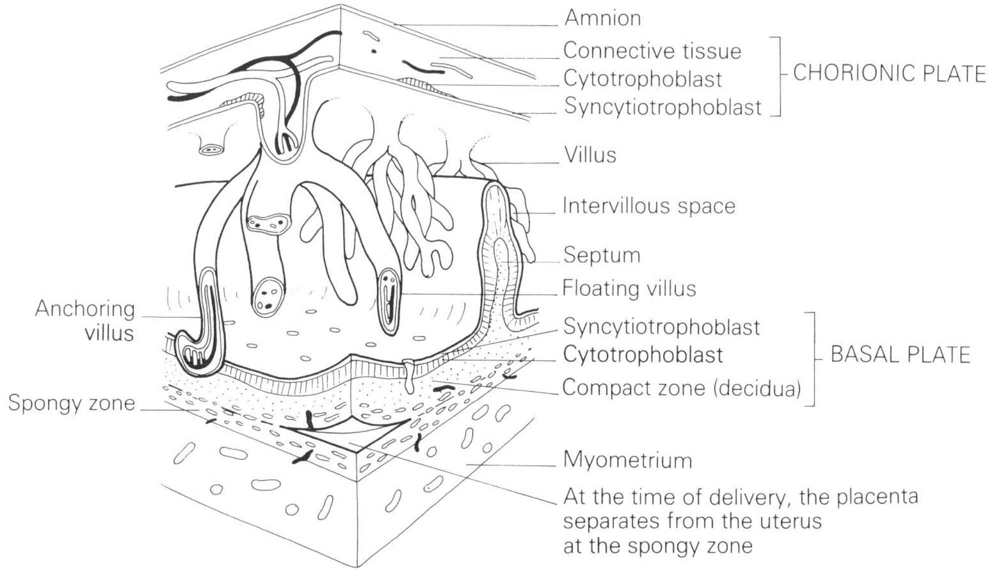

Fig. 7.1 *Structure of the placenta. Villous tissue consists of an outer continuous layer of multinucleate syncytiotrophoblast with an inner layer of mononucleate germinative cytotrophoblast cells. The cytotrophoblast cells are less prevalent in the later stages of pregnancy, but will reform syncytiotrophoblast damaged by hypoxia. (Adapted from H. Tuchmann-Duplessis, G. David and P. Haegel, 1972. Illustrated Human Embryology, Vol. 1 Embryogenesis. Paris: Masson et Cie Editeurs.)*

ring of the placenta tends to have its membranes unfolded (circumvalate placenta).

Occasionally, a lobe of placental tissue develops separately from the main placenta (succentruriate lobe) and remains within the uterus after delivery.

In rare instances, invasion of the uterus is so deep that there is a morbid attachment of the placenta (accreta) onto the myometrium, into the myometrial cells (increta) or through the serosal surface (percreta). This condition may well necessitate hysterectomy.

THE BREASTS

The breast is made up of numerous lobules, which are collections of hollow spheres called alveoli that are the secretory units of mammary gland. Each alveolus consists of secretory cells surrounded by contractile myopithelial cells. Small ducts connect the alveoli to a lactiferous sinus from which 10–15 ducts extend to the openings in the surface of the nipple.

During early pregnancy, the breasts receive an increased blood flow and hypertrophy. The increase in size, under the regulation of steroid hormones and human placental lactogen, is due to the full development of lobules with the alveoli and ducts becoming dilated. The cells of the alveoli differentiate, so that by the fourth month of pregnancy they are capable of producing milk. Colostrum, a concentrated yellow fatty substance, is usually secreted in small quantities during the last few weeks of pregnancy.

Further information on lactation can be found in Chapter 15.

FURTHER READING

Chard T., Lilford R., eds. (1986). *Basic Sciences for Obstetrics and Gynaecology*, 2nd edn. London: Springer-Verlag.

Hytten F.E., Chamberlain G.V.P. (1980). *Clinical Physiology in Obstetrics.* Oxford: Blackwell Scientific Publications.

Panigel M. (1986). Anatomy and morphology of human placenta. In *Clinics in Obstetrics and Gynaecology*, 2nd edn. Chard T. (ed.) London: Saunders.

8

Antenatal Care

Antenatal care is a form of preventive medicine by which risk factors are recognised and specific intervention instituted when necessary. Structured access to medical attention is provided for this purpose. This also allows common symptoms of pregnancy to be dealt with promptly and provides an ideal opportunity for population screening measures, such as cervical cytology, and testing for rubella immunity. Above all, perhaps, antenatal care fulfils a psychological role in which the woman prepares for childbirth and motherhood. This chapter is mainly concerned with the most ostensible aim: recognition of factors which may harm the mother or her baby. A detailed knowledge of the conditions involved encompasses most of obstetrics and forms the subject matter of much of this book. Here, we are concerned with the methods by which antenatal care is implemented, rather than the conditions themselves.

THE BOOKING VISIT

This is important as at this time the medical risk factors are ascertained (Table 8.1). It consists of three components: the history, examination and special investigations.

Timing of the Booking Visit

Traditionally, women have been asked to book by 16–18 weeks of gestation. This is the ideal

Table 8.1

Some Medical Disorders that Constitute Risk Factors

	Risk Factor	Action
1.	Oral anticoagulants for deep vein thrombosis or prosthetic heart valve	Consider changing to heparin in first and third trimesters
2.	TB contact	Chest X-ray
3.	Recurrent cystitis	Serial midstream urine examination
4.	Idiopathic thrombocytopenic purpura	Observe baby for coagulation disorder
5.	Endocrine disorder	Check fetus and baby for neonatal thyrotoxicosis
6.	Myasthenia gravis	Observe newborn for myasthenia (transient)
7.	Steroid therapy within 6 months	Cover labour with steroids
8.	Poliomyelities with persistent deformity or congenital defect of spine or pelvis	Pelvimetry in third trimester
9.	Allergies	Avoid allergenic drugs
10.	Hyperprolactinaemia	Serial visual fields; Repeat X-ray after delivery
11.	Hyperprolactinaemia with adenoma	The above, plus bromocryptine after delivery
12.	Epilepsy	Monitor dose of anticonvulsant required Special instructions for breast feeding

time for maternal alpha fetoprotein screening, assessment of gestational age by ultrasound and amniocentesis if required.

Early booking has always been desirable, but more so now as some obstetric interventions are required at an earlier gestational age (chorion villus biopsy at 8–12 weeks, nuchal translucency scanning at 10–12 weeks, cervical encerclage at 12–14 weeks). There is also a move towards preconception counselling. In this way, rubella immunity can be confirmed and patients on some potentially teratogenic drugs, such as coumarin, may be changed to alternative treatment such as heparin. It has been shown that among juvenile diabetics, optimal control reduces the incidence of congenital abnormality, and it is suggested that periconceptual vitamins, especially folate, 400 μg, may reduce the risk of neural tube defects. Preconceptual counselling also enables couples to be screened for carrier status to certain diseases such as Tay-Sachs and to discuss issues that may be worrying for them.

Booking History

The booking history may be divided into identification factors, the psycho-social history, the menstrual/contraceptive history, past obstetric history, maternal conditions, factors suggesting an increased risk of congenital abnormalities and miscellaneous.

Identification details

Some of the information recorded under this section, which includes the patient's name and date of birth, patient's address, and that of her general practitioner and next of kin, is also of medical importance. Thus a history that the patient is unmarried or that she and her husband/partner are unemployed is associated with a higher perinatal mortality and calls for more rigorous assessment of fetal well-being in later pregnancy.

Social history

A general assessment of the patient's social circumstances is appropriate. This should include details of whether she is married or single, supported or unsupported, and what is her attitude and that of her partner's to the pregnancy. Details of her occupation and housing should be recorded as this may influence the antenatal period. Her partner's occupation is also noted. Where relevant, advice about availability and eligibility for the various social services and benefits is of value. Consumption of alcohol should be stopped or restricted to 1 or 2 units per day, while cigarette smoking should also be stopped or restricted to less than 5 per day. Any current drug medication should be recorded in detail.

Menstrual and contraceptive history

One of the most difficult, but nevertheless important, items to acquire accurately at the booking clinic is an estimate of the patient's gestational age. This calculation requires the following data:

1. The date of the last menstrual period.
2. The degree of certainty of the above.
3. The regularity of the menstrual cycle.
4. The average length of the menstrual cycle.
5. Whether the last menstrual period was abnormal.
6. If it was abnormal, date of previous menstrual period.
7. Whether this menstrual period was normal.
8. Presence of bleeding in the first 3 months after the apparent last menstrual period.
9. Date of ovulation induction, if applicable
10. Date of stopping an ovulation inhibitor.
11. Whether a withdrawal bleed followed the stopping of an ovulation inhibitor.

In some cases, no relevant menstrual history can be obtained. These include pregnancy after a previous confinement with no intervening menstruation, pregnancy after a long period of secondary amenorrhoea and even pregnancy before the first period.

It is important to ascertain, while obtaining the contraceptive history, whether an intrauterine device was in use at the time of conception. Such a device should be removed if possible and, if the patient is less than 10 weeks pregnant, an ectopic gestation should be excluded.

Obstetric history

This is the most important source of risk factors for the current pregnancy. A history of a previous unexplained stillbirth or severe growth retardation is an indication for more careful monitoring of fetal well-being in the third trimester. A history of recurrent mid-trimester miscarriage in the absence of fetal growth retardation or infection may call for cervical encerclage. This is described in Chapter 6. A history of previous caesarean section should lead to further questions about the type of caesarean section and the indication, as it is on these factors that a decision to perform elective surgery or encourage a trial of labour will depend. If necessary, this information must be obtained by writing to the hospital where the previous confinement took place. A history of postpartum haemorrhage, retained placenta or third degree tear should be sought, as this is an indication for the obstetrician to attend the subsequent delivery. A history of a baby weighing over 4.0 kg suggests gestational diabetes and is an indication for a glucose tolerance test in centres where this is not routine.

Medical history

Most patients volunteer any history of previous illnesses, but this is one area where direct questioning is of value to achieve completeness and save time. Current medication should be clearly recorded and specific medical conditions enquired about, e.g. diabetes mellitus, epilepsy, anaemia, chest disease, tuberculosis, hypertension, rheumatic fever, cardiac disease — congenital or acquired — renal disease, venereal disease, rubella and previous blood transfusion. Conditions such as heart disease and diabetes mellitus have extremely wide implications for subsequent management of the pregnancy and a history of these should be sought by specific questions. A history of chronic hypertension or renal disease increases the chance of subsequent pre-eclampsia and calls for more frequent assessment in the second half of pregnancy. Other maternal conditions with specific obstetric implications are listed in Table 8.1. Previous surgical procedures may be relevant to the current pregnancy, especially gynaecological operations such as dilatation and curettage, cervical cone biopsy and pelvic-floor repair. Any previous psychiatric disorder should be recorded. Allergies, especially to previous drug treatment, require clear annotation.

Additional gynaecological history

The following features in the gynaecological history may prove relevant to the present pregnancy in greater or lesser degree:

Postcoital bleeding.

Intermenstrual bleeding.

Vaginal discharge; colour, consistency, odour, blood-stained, irritative.

Previous or current contraception; pregnancy occurring with an intrauterine contraceptive device *in situ*; continued use of an oral contraceptive in the early weeks of any unrecognised pregnancy.

Primary or secondary infertility and the details of any treatment.

Previous abortions, spontaneous and therapeutic, including the period of gestation attained and any subsequent complications, such as vaginal bleeding and pelvic infection.

Date and result of last cervical smear.

Other questions

The patient should be asked about her present complaints. Some of these, such as backache, are indications for general advice, i.e. the use of a firm mattress, while others, such as heartburn, require specific medication. Heartburn in pregnancy is due to oesophagitis resulting from regurgitation of stomach contents due to a relatively incompetent cardiac sphincter and increased pressure on the stomach from the gravid uterus. These contents are usually acid and respond to alkalis and often elevation of the head of the bed to reduce reflux. Occasionally, there is incompetence of the pyloric sphincter resulting in biliary reflux causing gastritis and sometimes oesophagitis. These rare cases respond to ingestion of dilute hydrochloric acid.

A history of insulin-dependent diabetes in the patient's parents should be sought, as a glucose tolerance test is then indicated if this is not the routine policy of the clinic. Some questionnaires include a family history of twins, but as this does not significantly increase the chance of multiple pregnancy, a possibility which should always be considered, this question is unnecessary. Similarly, a history of consanguinity should not be sought, as nothing can be done to pre-empt the increased risk of an autosomal recessive disease.

Factors pertaining to genetic risk

Risk of chromosomal trisomy rises with maternal age and is an indication to offer amniocentesis or chorion biopsy if the patient is aged 37 or more. Ultrasound assessment of nuchal translucency at 10–12 weeks gestation has become a very important and useful screening method for the assessment of the risk of trisomy 21 (Down's syndrome). In addition, serum screening at about 15–16 weeks using measurements of alpha-feto protein, HCG and oestriol is widely used to identify those at high risk of Down's syndrome (< 1 in 250). Certain racial groups are at increased risk of specific diseases; for example, Negroes of West African stock should be screened for sickle trait, Ashkenazy Jews for Tay-Sachs disease and people of Mediterranean and Eastern origin for haemoglobinopathies. In all these cases, prenatal diagnosis is available if both parents are found to be carriers.

A history of recent rubella contact, especially in an unimmunised person, is an indication for several specific IgM estimations. Patients with previous 'multifactorial' conditions, such as neural tube defects, congenital heart disease and cleft lip/palate, have a higher incidence of recurrence which calls for specific diagnostic methods. In addition, couples should be asked about any known inherited diseases, such as haemophilia or muscular dystrophy, in their family.

Examination of the Obstetric Patient

The patient is weighed and her height and development recorded, including any abnormal gait or deformity. The heart and lungs are examined and blood pressure is recorded. The breasts are examined for any discreet mass or inverted nipples. Historically, a pelvic examination was performed at the booking visit to assess uterine size in order to confirm gestational age and to perform a cervical smear. However, the advent of early ultrasound scanning provides a much more accurate and reliable assessment of gestational age. Pelvic examination is therefore now rarely performed at the booking visit and usually when pelvic pathology is suspected and requires assessment, e.g. fibroids, ovarian cyst and cervical pathology.

During the second trimester, the uterus becomes palpable on abdominal examination. The position of the uterine fundus within the abdominal cavity is used to estimate the duration of pregnancy, but is misleading in the

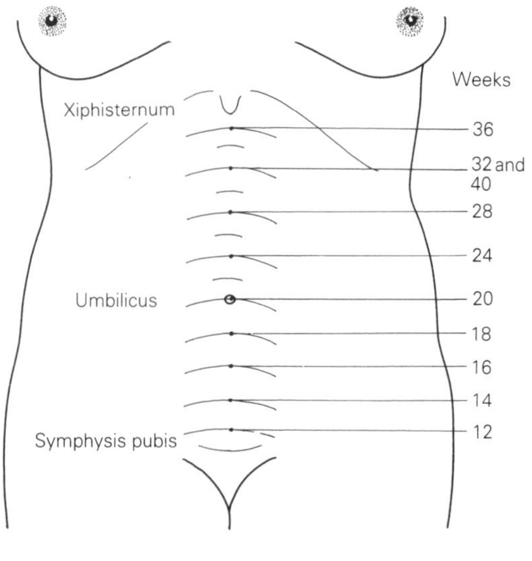

Fig. 8.1 *Fundal position and gestation.*

presence of fibroids, hydramnios or multiple pregnancy. Traditionally, the umbilicus is taken as a reference point (Fig. 8.1), but its position varies from one patient to another and it is not always midway between the xiphisternum and symphysis pubis. However, such an estimate does reflect the progression of pregnancy and its accuracy and reproducibility is enhanced by measuring fundal height from the symphysis pubis in centimetres.

Palpation

Abdominal palpation. The woman lies supine, arms by her side, with her head and shoulders slightly raised. The examiner stands on the right side and gently palpates the abdomen in a routine sequence.

Fundal palpation. (Fig. 8.2) The uterine fundus may be located by applying light pressure either with the ulnar border of the left hand or by the parted fingers of the left hand placed flat in the region of the uterine fundus. The height of the fundus above the symphysis pubis can thus be determined. Both hands are then applied to each side of the fundus and the polarity of the fetus (breech or head) ascertained.

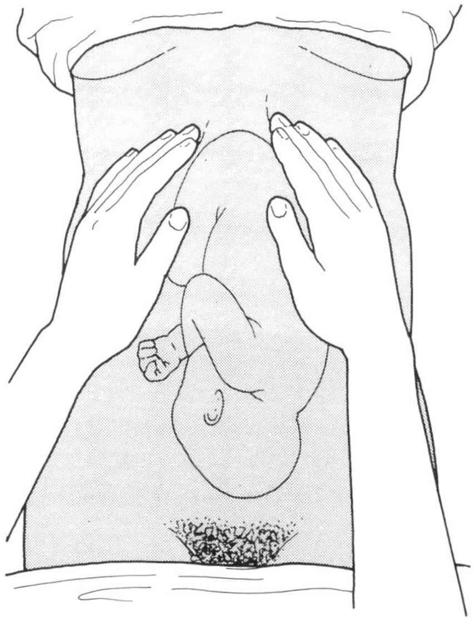

Fig. 8.2 *Abdominal palpation. Step 1 — fundal palpation.*

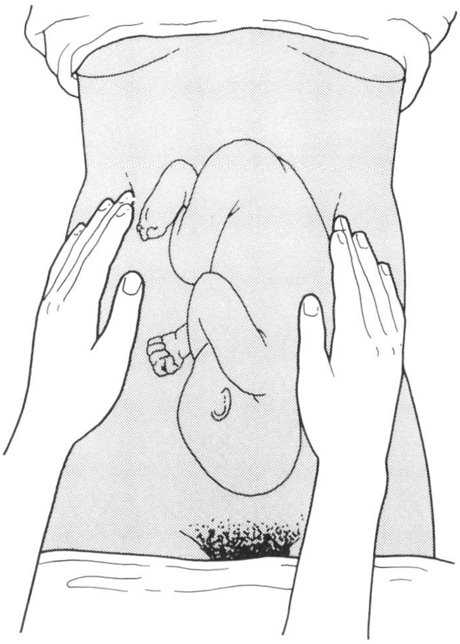

Fig. 8.3 *Abdominal palpation. Step 2 — lateral palpation.*

Lateral palpation. (Fig. 8.3). The hands are then gently moved along the contour of the uterus. The lie of the fetus is thus determined. When the presentation is cephalic and in the usual lateral or anterolateral position, the fetal spine is identified as a continuous firmness on one side, and the limbs as irregular shapes on the other side, giving a softer impression to the examining hand. Fetal movements are often felt at this stage. When the fetus has adopted a posterior position, the findings are slightly different. The fetal spine lies over the maternal spine giving a characteristic flattening below the mother's umbilicus and, if not obviously visible, may be realised by placing the hand flat across the abdomen below the umbilicus. Fetal limbs are usually palpable on both sides of the midline.

Pelvic palpation. The examiner now faces the patient's feet, placing his/her hands on either side of the lower portion of the uterus (Fig. 8.4). Gentle pressure is applied with the distal phalanges of the fingers and the presenting part identified. The presenting part is usually the fetal head and is identifiable by its hard, rounded character. If unengaged, it

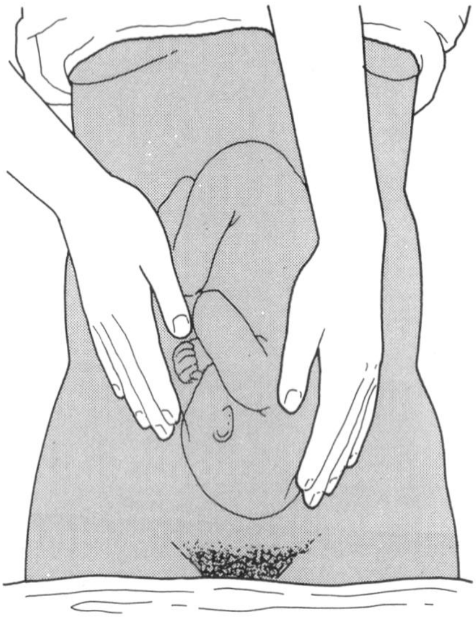

Fig. 8.4 *Abdominal palpation. Step 3 — pelvic palpation.*

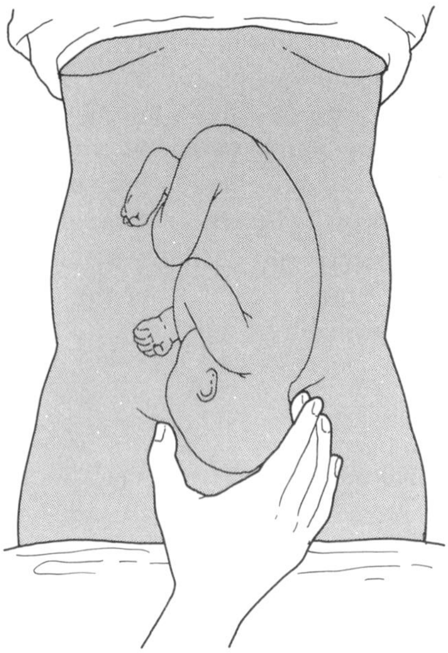

Fig. 8.5 *The Pawlik manoeuvre.*

will be easily ballotable. Engagement has occurred when the widest diameter of the presenting part has passed through the pelvic brim. As the fingers of each hand are moved towards the pelvis, the impression will be of the head becoming wider until the pubic rami are touched. However, when the head is unengaged, the impression will be of the head becoming wider and then narrower again as the fingers are advanced towards the pelvic brim. If the head is deeply engaged, it may be completely impalpable. Vaginal examination will confirm a cephalic presentation.

The Pawlik grip. This stage of the palpation is not always required, but should be left to last as it is the most uncomfortable part (Fig. 8.5). The examiner faces the woman and, spreading the fingers and thumb of the right hand, places them suprapubically. With gentle fundal pressure from above, the fingers and thumb are approximated across the presenting part and its mobility either above or within the pelvic brim is assessed.

To complete the examination of the fetus, the fetal heart is auscultated with a Pinard fetal heart stethoscope or battery operated sonicaid. Its presence, rate and rhythm are noted.

At this stage, the examiner should have a clear impression of: (1) the height of the fundus (interpreted as gestational age equivalent); (2) the lie of the fetus; (3) the position of the fetus; (4) the presentation; (5) whether the presenting part is engaged or unengaged; and (6) the rate and character of the fetal heart.

Special Investigations

The blood group is determined and an antibody screen carried out. The latter is performed irrespective of the patient's Rhesus group, in case antibodies against other red blood cell antigens are present. A base line haemoglobin estimation is performed and Negro patients and those of Mediterranean origin are screened for haemoglobinopathies by electrophoresis. The serological tests for syphilis are carried out and rubella titre investigated so that vaccination can be offered in the puerperium if the patient is not immune. In many clinics, the serum is examined for alpha-fetoprotein as a screening test for neural tube defects and this is most reliable between the 16th and 18th week. Some clinics screen all patients for the hepatitis β surface antigen. If this is present and the patient has the e antigen (or lacks anti-e antibodies), she may infect staff. Precautions are needed at delivery or when taking blood samples. Such patients are also likely to transmit the virus to the fetus at birth, and some authorities recommend immediate vaccination of the newborn to prevent a chronic infection and later hepatoma. Many clinics routinely offer a modified glucose tolerance test in which only fasting and 1 hour glucose estimations are measured. In recent years, HIV status has become increasingly important. With the advent of effective drug treatment for the baby born of a HIV positive mother offers of testing mothers antenatally are now routine. Careful, sensitive counselling is required.

Routine ultrasound scans are now performed in early pregnancy. A first trimester ultrasound between 10–12 weeks is very useful and accurate in estimating gestational age and confirming the number of fetuses. Measurement of the thickness of the pad of fat at the base of the cervical spine allows a reasonably accurate assessment of the risk of Down's syndrome (trisomy 21). This is known as the Nuchal Translucency Measurement. A second ultrasound scan is carried out at 20 weeks gestation and is particularly useful in assessing fetal anatomy, e.g. spinal, cardiac, renal and gastrointestinal anomalies. Some patients may decline this investigation on the basis of unconfirmed reports of harmful effects. Animal and human studies on the effects of *diagnostic* sonar have been reassuring, and doses a hundred times greater than those in current use are required to produce any biological effect. Most patients, therefore, consider the following concrete advantages to outweigh any hypothetical disadvantage:

1. It forms an accurate assessment of gestational age. Thirty per cent of patients have menstrual ambiguities. Even among those patients who are sure of their last menstrual period, ultrasound has been shown in some series to provide a more reliable indication of the due birthdate. Furthermore, randomised trials have shown that the induction rate for presumed post-maturity may be reduced by means of early ultrasound dating.
2. The maternal alpha-fetoprotein estimation is a more specific index of spina bifida when the gestational age is calculated on the basis of the biparietal diameter.
3. It provides a firm and objective baseline against which further growth assessment may be judged. (This is a by-product of the first advantage.)
4. Twins, one-sixth of whom would otherwise remain undiagnosed by the start of labour, will be detected (Fig. 8.6).

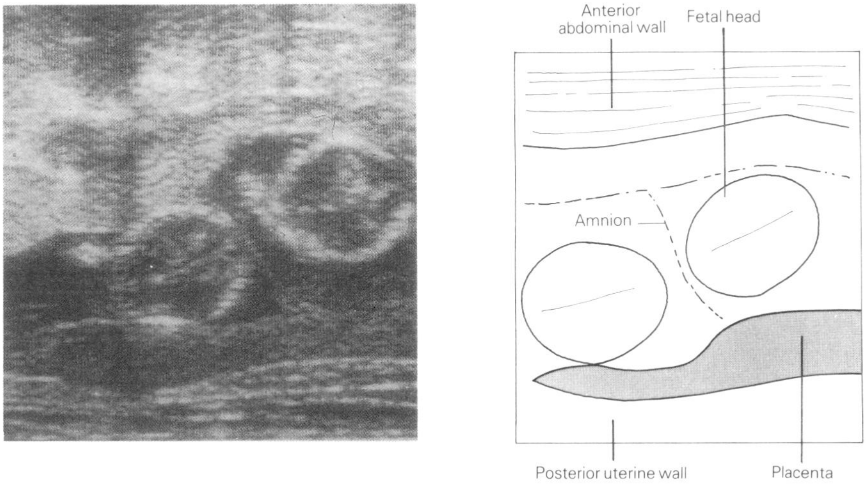

Fig. 8.6 *Detection of twin fetal heads by ultrasound.*

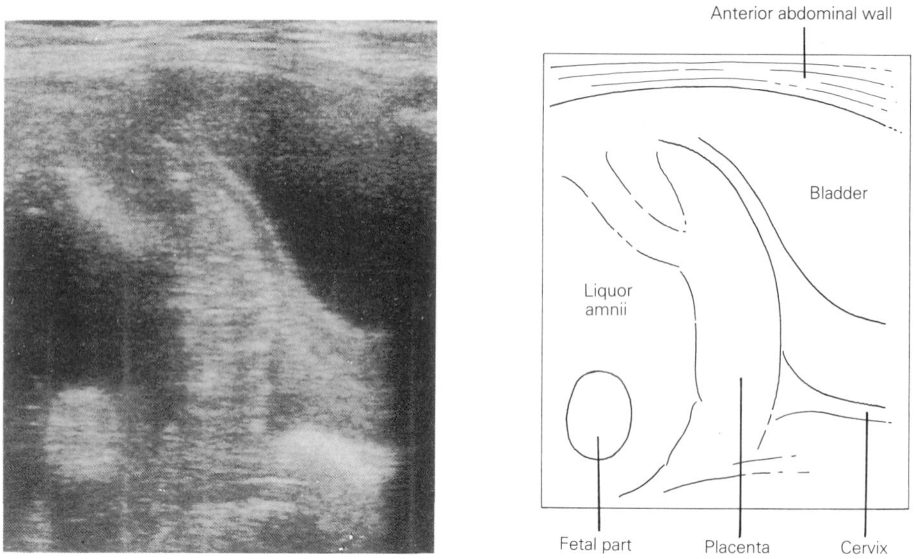

Fig. 8.7 *Recognition of low placenta by ultrasound.*

5. A large number of congenital abnormalities, the proportion of which will be determined by the expertise of the individual ultrasonographer, may be observed.
6. Recognition of the low placenta (Fig. 8.7); 5–10% of the scans at 20 weeks will demonstrate a low-lying placenta and, in 5% of these, placenta praevia can be confirmed by a subsequent scan in the third trimester. This information may warrant hospital admission in order to pre-empt a severe haemorrhage in the case of a major degree of placenta praevia. In addition, subsequent management of antepartum haemorrhage is easier if a low placenta has been diagnosed or excluded by an early scan.
7. A psychological benefit has been claimed, and there is no doubt that most mothers and fathers enjoy the experience of seeing their unborn child on the ultrasound screen.

It is only fair to point out that this technology also has some disadvantages (apart from the hypothetical dangers of high frequency sound waves), in that the discovery of self-correcting conditions, such as minor dilatation of the renal tract and small cysts of the choroid plexus, will engender unnecessary anxiety.

SUBSEQUENT ANTENATAL VISITS

At every subsequent visit, the mother's weight and blood pressure are measured, and the urine checked for protein and glucose. Weight gain should average about 10 kg during pregnancy. Blood pressure should be considered abnormal if, in a previously normotensive patient, it reaches 140/90 mmHg or if there is a rise in systolic and diastolic pressure of 20 mmHg or more between visits.

Proteinuria in an ordinary specimen of urine usually represents contamination of the urine by vaginal discharge. If present in an MSU, it is either due to infection, chronic renal disease or, occasionally, orthostasis. In the presence of hypertension occurring during pregnancy, it indicates renal and placental pathology which warrant urgent admission.

Glycosuria can indicate gestational diabetes, or merely the lowered renal threshold for tubular reabsorption of glucose, the latter being more common. An oral glucose tolerance test should be carried out to make the diagnosis.

On each visit, the fetal size is assessed and the distance from the symphysis pubis to the uterine fundus may be recorded. From the 32nd week onwards, the presentation of the fetus is also recorded. After the 36th week, it is customary to determine whether the fetal head is engaged or will engage in the pelvis.

The amount of liquor should also be determined from the 32nd week onwards and a general impression obtained of fetal size, so that any suspicion of inadequate fetal growth can be confirmed by ultrasonic measurements. From 24 weeks onwards, the mother should be asked about fetal movements as any sudden diminution warrants further investigation.

The haemoglobin concentration is re-estimated at 30 and 36 weeks, and antibody titres are obtained at this time from Rhesus negative mothers and those with other pre-existing antibodies. It is becoming increasingly common to offer Rhesus negative mothers an anti-D γ-globulin injection at 28 and 34 weeks. This reduces the chance of sensitisation prior to delivery which otherwise occurs in 1% of mothers.

The number of times that such antenatal examinations should be carried out varies according to the patient's history. Where there are no specific risk factors, the patient should be seen every 4 weeks until 28 weeks, fortnightly until the 36th week, and thereafter every week until the onset of labour. Many patients and general practitioners prefer a policy of shared care, and this is usually carried out on an agreed basis between the hospital and referring general practitioners. A 'shared care' card facilitates information exchange in such circumstances, and in many obstetric units, the mothers carry their own notes which comprise the entire medical record of this pregnancy.

Engagement of the Fetal Head

In primigravida, the head may be engaged by 38 complete weeks. Some of the causes of non-engagement are shown in Table 8.2 but cephalopelvic disproportion must be actively excluded. In multi-gravida, the head may not become engaged until the onset of labour, but cephalopelvic disproportion should, nevertheless, be excluded even though the pelvis has already been tested by a previous delivery.

Table 8.2

Causes of Non-Engagement of the Presenting Part

1.	Full bladder or rectum
2.	Mistaken dates
3.	Occipitoposterior position
4.	Cephalopelvic disproportion
5.	Hydramnios
6.	Multiple pregnancy
7.	Placenta praevia
8.	Pelvic tumours
9.	Fetal malpresentation, e.g. brow, face
10.	Short umbilical cord
11.	Fetal abnormality, e.g. hydrocephalus
12.	High assimilation pelvis

Three clinical methods of assessing the capacity of the pelvis to allow the presenting part to engage will be considered. If there is any doubt, X-ray lateral pelvimetry should be carried out.

Abdominal palpation

The mother is placed supine and gentle pressure is applied to the fundus with the left hand to push the fetal head towards the pelvis. The right hand is placed flat across the suprapubic region with the ring finger overlying the symphysis pubis. The fetal head is gently pressed backwards and will normally enter the pelvis easily. Should there be doubt, the assessment may be aided by asking the mother to sit up partially by supporting herself on the elbows and placing the forearms by the side of her chest. By raising the upper portion of her body in this manner, the rise in intra-abdominal pressure assists descent of the head.

Combined abdomino-vaginal palpation

This is the Munro-Kerr method and is depicted in Fig. 8.8. The left hand, placed suprapubically, pushes the head downwards and backwards into the pelvis to meet the fingers in the vagina at the level of the ischial spines. The thumb of the right hand may be used to assess the degree of any overlap. This

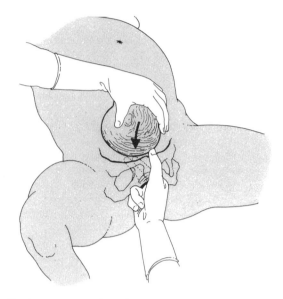

Fig. 8.8 *Estimating the relative size of the fetal head and the maternal pelvis by the Munro-Kerr 'head fitting' test.*

method also allows an assessment of the bony pelvis and will detect any soft tissue pelvic tumour. Placenta praevia as a reason for non-engagement of the presenting part must be excluded before this manoeuvre is performed.

Vaginal examination

Pelvic assessment by vaginal examination is employed to predict the possibility of cephalopelvic disproportion. The sacrum is gently palpated and its anterior surface should be concave with the coccyx following the line of the curve. The fingers are then moved to the lateral borders of the sacrum, in turn, and placed on the sacrospinous ligament allowing assessment of the greater sciatic notch, which should accept two fingers' breadth with ease. The sacrospinous ligaments are attached anteriorly to the ischial spines which should lack prominence and, therefore, not encroach into the pelvic cavity. The pelvic outlet is now assessed. The subpubic angle should easily accept two fingers' breadths, but must be assessed gently. The transverse diameter of the outlet is reflected by the distance between the ischial tuberosities and normally four knuckles of the hand will fit between them. Such manocuvrcs providc an impression of pelvic capacity which can prove useful. The student is well advised to practise the examination on a pelvic model, when the technique of the assessment will be better appreciated.

GENERAL ADVICE TO THE PATIENT IN PREGNANCY

Counselling is an essential part of the antenatal care, and helps the mother to prepare for childbirth and cope with some of the common symptoms of pregnancy. It is axiomatic, therefore, that a relaxed atmosphere should be created, although this ideal is sometimes compromised by the tempo of busy antenatal clinics. It is important that each patient should be given a booklet in which the policies of the hospital and general practice are laid out, and explanations of the events of pregnancy and labour can be found. This booklet should also explain the purpose and possible hazards of various investigations which the woman may be offered. Specific issues which may be discussed include the following.

Diet

The pregnant woman requires extra energy to supply the needs of the growing fetus and to keep pace with her own increased metabolic rate and weight gain (Fig. 8.9). The average person requires 2500 calories a day and this is not greatly increased from her daily non-pregnancy food consumption. The total increased calorie requirement of pregnancy is relatively small and a balanced diet should be able to supply all the extra protein and fat required, together with most of the minerals such as zinc, a deficiency of which may be associated with congenital abnormalities, and calcium. The question of iron supplements is more controversial and, again, may be unnecessary provided the mother is not vegetarian. If the mother is not given iron, her iron stores will inevitably decline during pregnancy. This is not a cause for concern provided she was not anaemic to start with and did not become

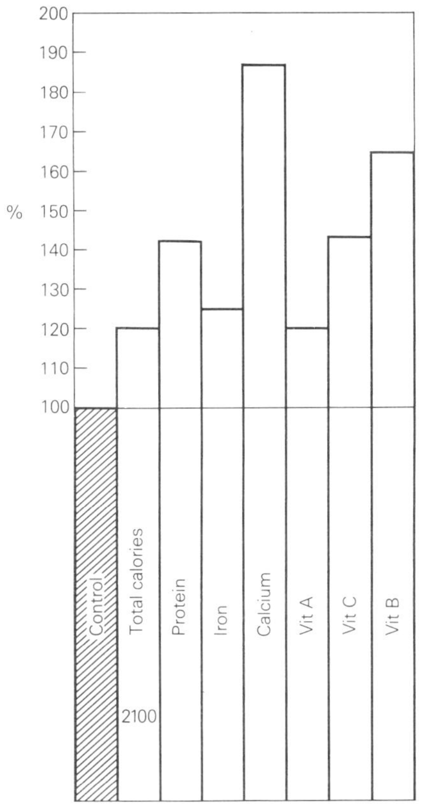

Fig. 8.9 *Approximate increases in daily requirements of important dietary constituents during pregnancy expressed as a percentage above non-pregnant needs.*

pregnant with already depleted iron stores. Iron supplements combined with folic acid should be given in the case of multiple pregnancy. Folic acid without iron should be the treatment for otherwise uncomplicated haemogloginopathies. Doses of iron and folic acid vary considerably from one preparation to another. The average requirements for prophylaxis are 50–100 mg elemental iron and 350–500 mg folic acid per day. Intolerance to iron is very variable, usually causing diarrhoea or constipation.

Rest and Exercise

It has been shown by Doppler studies that violent exercise causes increased femoral artery flow at the expense of the uterine supply and competitive running is, therefore, inadvisable. Furthermore, body temperature rises during strenuous exercise, especially in fit people and, as the fetus is unable to control its own heat loss, any extreme form of physical exertion is contraindicated during pregnancy. It is, nevertheless, important for a sense of well-being and in preparation for labour that gentle exercise is taken. Swimming, cycling and walking are all beneficial during pregnancy.

Sexual Activity

The bulk of evidence seems to indicate that coitus is not harmful during pregnancy. Nevertheless, most obstetricians would counsel patients with repeated miscarriages against having sexual intercourse during the critical period of up to 14 weeks.

Preparation for Lactation

No single measure would cut down on mortality throughout the world as much as the widespread resumption of breast feeding. The best preparation for this is to ensure that the mother is aware of the normal course of events following delivery and is mentally prepared for breast feeding. Inverted nipples usually correct themselves spontaneously during pregnancy and can be made to protrude by means of gentle manipulation, or occasionally by the use of a nipple shield.

General Education and Instruction

This varies from specific instruction on items such as the preparation of the baby's clothes and the advantages of breast feeding to a discussion of what to expect during labour and the provision of breathing exercises during labour to help cope with pain. Analgesia should be discussed in order to give the mother a deeper appreciation of the options open to her. These discussions should include the husband, who should be encouraged to be present during the labour which is, after all, a family event. It is also important that the patient should have a tour of the labour ward, so that this is not a frightening or strange place when the big day arrives. A number of patients will have specific requests about issues such as birth position which will be discussed later in this book.

THE ISSUE OF HOME BIRTH

Many women will wish to discuss this possibility with their doctors and it is, therefore, important to have an appreciation of this issue. Arguments for and against home births often evolve around overall perinatal mortality associated with hospital and domiciliary confinement. This is inappropriate; the overall perinatal mortality of home births is slightly higher than that of the country as a whole, but it is quite fairly pointed out by proponents of this method that these figures include many premature and precipitate labours and a number of unbooked deliveries among high risk patients. The perinatal mortality which is defined as stillbirths and neonatal deaths occurring during the first 7 days of life among low risk patients especially selected for home birth is 4 per 1000 births. This, however, cannot be compared with the perinatal death rate in hospital, as many patients booked for home births will be transferred to a hospital as an emergency, and fetal deaths among these patients will appear in hospital statistics which, of course, also include all other high risk patients. The 0.4% perinatal mortality quoted above, therefore, constitutes the intrapartum and early neonatal death rate. The proportion of this accounted for by intrapartum asphyxia is not known, but is unlikely to compare favourably with intrapartum death rates quoted by hospitals of 0.1–0.2%. It seems reasonable to conclude, therefore that women electing to have a home birth, because of the emotional warmth and comfort of their own surroundings, do so at the cost of a small increase in the risk of fetal death. Perhaps of greater importance, however, is the observation that such losses represent only the tip of the iceberg and permanent damage is a more likely and, in a sense, more serious sequel of unrecognised intrapartum hypoxia. A compromise for women wishing to be at home during childbirth is to conduct the early labour at home, transferring to hospital for the delivery of the baby and transferring back home, if all is well, within 2–6 hours after delivery of the baby.

9

Ultrasound in Obstetrics and Gynaecology and Prenatal Diagnosis

BASIC PRINCIPLES

Ultrasound scanning permits real time imaging, by utilising high frequency sound waves which travel through most human tissues with a degree of reflection of these sound waves at tissue interfaces. Sound waves are transmitted from a transducer which also receives the reflected waves or echoes. These echoes are then converted into a grey scale image which is displayed on a screen. The higher the frequency of the sound waves, the greater the resolution although the depth of penetration is less. Thus, to scan an organ which is near the transducer, a high frequency can be used whereas if the target organ is deep, a lower frequency will be required. For example, when scanning a non-pregnant uterus or ovaries by transvaginal sonography, a high frequency (7.5 MHz) transducer is used. When scanning the fetus in the third trimester, lower frequencies will be required (3.5 MHz).

Sound waves are a form of energy. Although there has never been any harm to the fetus demonstrated by the use of ultrasound, it is prudent to minimise exposure and use the lowest amount of energy that is reasonable (the so-called ALARA principle — as low as reasonably achievable). Thus, scans should only be performed when clinically indicated.

In order for the ultrasound waves to be transmitted from the transducer to the body, there needs to be an interface of water or gel, as sound waves do not travel well through air. For this reason, gel is applied to the skin before an ultrasound examination is performed.

In addition to B-mode scanning (real time), a different type of ultrasound, Doppler ultrasound, can be used to examine blood flow. This relies on the Doppler effect (*the frequency of oscillation an observer measures is affected by relative movement between the observer and the source of oscillation*). The best known example of the Doppler effect (or shift) is the change of pitch of the sound of a train as it approaches then passes a stationary observer. Thus, as ultrasound waves hit a red blood cell moving in a stream of blood, the frequency of the reflected waveform when received by the transducer will be different from the original frequency. This change in frequency can be displayed on a screen to give a spectral image of flow, from which calculations regarding blood flow rates etc. can be made. Further developments have lead to the introduction of colour and power Doppler. These permit identification and examination of flow direction (colour — used extensively in echocardiography) and perfusion at low flow rates (power).

The introduction of ultrasound has revolutionised many aspects of both obstetric and gynaecological practice. However, it must be appreciated that all imaging techniques have limitations. Even with the most sophisticated machines, scanning women who are very fat, or who have extensive scarring of their abdominal walls, provides a challenge for the sonographer. In skilled hands, ultrasound can provide impressive structural detail but limited information regarding function. Whenever a scan is requested, the person requesting it must know what information they hope to glean, and what clinical value there is to the scan. Ultrasound is an adjunct to the basic tenets of clinical practice: history taking and clinical examination. It must never be seen as an alternative to these.

APPLICATIONS IN GYNAECOLOGY

Imaging Pelvic Organs

Imaging of the pelvis has been enhanced by the introduction of transvaginal transducers. Previously, the pelvis could only be examined by transabdominal scanning with a full bladder permitting a window through which the ultrasound waves could pass, and also lifting the uterus up out of the pelvis. By scanning much closer to the target organs, transvaginal sonography permits the use of higher frequencies and thus enhanced resolution.

The uterus and cervix can be easily visualised and measured. Figure 9.1 demonstrates a longitudinal section through a normal uterus with the endometrial cavity clearly defined. Ultrasound permits investigation of the size, shape and consistency of the pelvic organs, with pathology such as ovarian cysts and fibroids being clearly defined. The presence of free fluid in the pelvis, usually seen in the Pouch of Douglas, is easily detected.

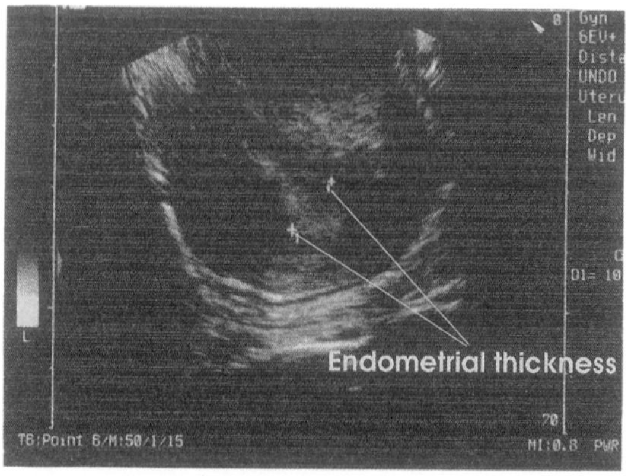

Fig. 9.1 *Longitudinal section of normal uterus.*

Abnormalities which may be detected using ultrasound include ovarian cysts, tubal abscesses, etc. The addition of Doppler to examine blood flow, in particular perfusion of the ovaries, may be of help in the diagnosis and management of malignant disease.

The function of the ovaries can be examined using ultrasound, with the follicular development being easily monitored. This is of particular value in assisted reproductive techniques involving ovulation induction.

APPLICATIONS IN OBSTETRICS

Introduction

The pregnant uterus is an organ particularly well suited to ultrasound examination as the fetus is surrounded by amniotic fluid which acts as a window through which ultrasound waves can freely pass. As the fetus moves independently within the uterus, real time imaging is essential. Ultrasound permits detailed examination of fetal structure, assessment of fetal growth by serial measurements, investigation of fetal well-being and guidance for invasive procedures used in diagnosis and treatment of congenital abnormalities and diseases. The information which can be obtained from an ultrasound scan depends on the gestation at which it is performed.

First Trimester

Most women booking for antenatal care are offered what is referred to as a booking scan. This will usually be performed between 10 and 14 weeks gestation, and its purpose is to confirm that the pregnancy is in the uterine cavity, that the fetus is alive, to count how many fetuses there are and to measure the fetus to confirm the gestational age.

From 5 weeks of pregnancy (taken from the first day of the last menstrual period or LMP), the gestation sac can be identified within the uterine cavity. From 6 weeks, it is possible to identify the fetal pole and the fetal heart beating. It is also possible to count the number of fetuses and gestation sacs. Measurement of the gestation sac diameters gives an estimation of gestational age which is accurate to within a week. From 7 to 11 weeks, it is possible to accurately measure the crown rump length of the fetus which again is accurate to within a week. By eleven weeks, it is possible to examine certain details of fetal anatomy.

First trimester complications

Complications of early pregnancy include sspontaneous abortions, or miscarriages, and ectopic pregnancies. Ultrasound examination is of value in confirming the diagnosis in such cases. If a woman presents with abdominal pain, bleeding and a history of amenorrhoea or a positive pregnancy test, it is necessary to confirm whether or not the pregnancy is in the uterine cavity and whether or not the fetus is alive. The uterus is clearly delineated using ultrasound, thus permitting confirmation of the location of a pregnancy within the cavity. If the scan fails to demonstrate an intrauterine gestation sac or if there is free fluid in the pouch of Douglas or a "pseudogestation" sac present, a laparoscopy should be performed to exclude an ectopic. If there is bleeding and the cervix is closed, confirmation of the presence of fetal heart activity will make the diagnosis of a threatened miscarriage. If there is no fetal heart activity, then the diagnosis of a missed abortion is made, and uterine evacuation is performed.

Sometimes, the size of the gestation sac is less than expected, and no fetal pole is seen. This may be because the dates are not correct or that the pregnancy is anembryonic, a so-called blighted ovum. In such cases, repeating the scan in a week will confirm the diagnosis.

Multiple pregnancy

Early diagnosis of multiple pregnancies is important, not only to allow the parents to come to terms with the situation, but also in permitting accurate identification of the

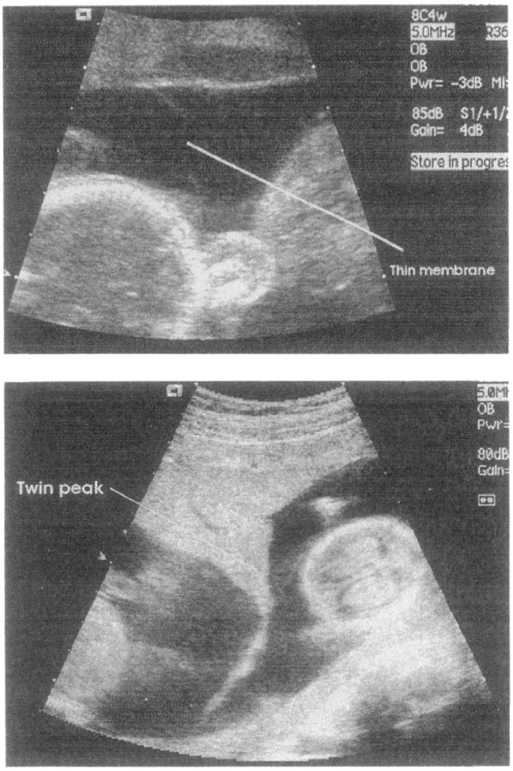

Fig. 9.2 *Top: Monochorionic diamniotic twins with thin membrane; Bottom: Dichorionic twins with twin peak sign.*

chorionicity. If twins share a placenta, i.e. monochorionic, the pregnancy is at risk of twin to twin transfusion syndrome which carries a significant risk of fetal loss. Similarly, higher order multiples carry increased risks of loss. It is easier to identify chorionicity during the first trimester than later. If there are two placentas, there is a so-called "twin peak" sign where the membranes meet the placenta. If there is only one placenta, the single inter-amniotic membrane meets the placenta effectively at right angles (Fig. 9.2).

Dating

Traditionally, pregnancy is dated from the first day of the last period. This assumes a regular 28-day cycle, with ovulation occurring 14 days after the commencement of the last period. In many cases, women cannot remember the LMP and in others, irregular cycles mean that the dates are not reliable. It is essential to know the exact gestation of a pregnancy in order that screening tests for Down syndrome may be interpreted accurately. If a woman goes into premature labour, it is very important for the paediatricians to have an accurate assessment of gestation in order to give an accurate prognosis. Similarly, if the pregnancy is prolonged (i.e. more than 42 weeks) induction of labour may be considered. If the dates are wrong, such intervention can lead to the delivery of a premature baby. The majority of women undergo at least one scan during pregnancy which permits measurement of the fetus to assess the gestation. Crown rump length measurement between 7 and 11 weeks is accurate to within 7 days. Until 24 weeks, measurement of the biparietal diameter, head circumference, abdominal circumference and femur length will provide an estimation of gestational age which is accurate to within 10 days. However, after 24 weeks, ultrasound dating is only accurate to within 2 weeks.

Nuchal translucency

A recent development in screening for Down syndrome (or trisomy 21) is nuchal translucency measurement. As any woman's risk of having a baby with a chromosome problem such as trisomy 21 increases with her age, diagnostic tests such as amniocentesis were previously only offered to women over the age of 35–38 years. In the 1980s, the relationship between maternal serum alpha-fetoprotein and human chorionic gonadotrophin levels was defined and maternal serum screening became the standard screening procedure, invasive testing being offered to women with a high risk (i.e. greater than 1:250) result. However, because serum screening was only performed in the mid-trimester (between 14 and 20 weeks gestation), attempts to find an earlier screening test were pursued. Between 11 and 14 weeks, there is a transient small collection of fluid behind the fetal neck which can be detected on ultrasound (Fig. 9.3). The greater the thickness of this fluid, the greater the risk of aneuploidy. The measurement of the nuchal translucency, crown rump length, maternal age and any history of aneuploidy contribute to the calculation of risk for the index pregnancy, with women with risk in excess of 1:300 being judged high risk and offered invasive testing. An increased nuchal translucency with a normal karyotype is a marker for other fetal abnormalities such as congenital heart disease.

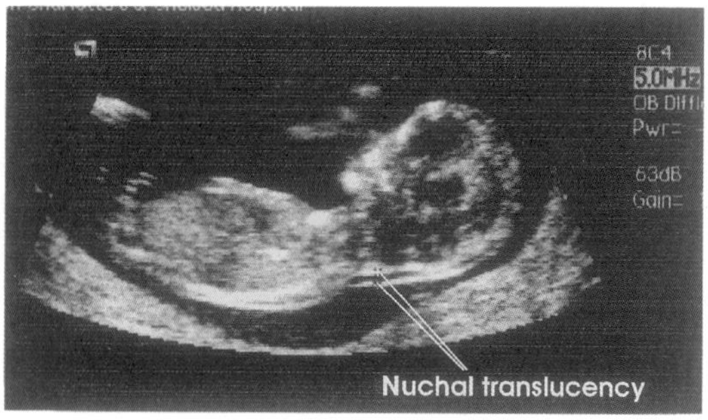

Fig. 9.3 *Nuchal translucency measurement.*

Structural abnormalities

First trimester scanning for the detection of structural abnormalities is not widely practised but it is possible, with high resolution equipment, to detect a number of major abnormalities such as anencephaly, holoprosencephaly, exomphalos and some skeletal dysplasias before 14 weeks gestation. The approach used may be either transabdominal or transvaginal, depending on the quality of image obtained.

Second Trimester

The RCOG recommends that all pregnant women be offered an ultrasound scan at around 20 weeks gestation, the routine anomaly or level 2 scan. At this time, fetal biometry is measured to confirm dates, and most structural abnormalities can be detected. If resources are such that only one scan can be offered during the pregnancy, this presents the best opportunity to maximise the information obtained. The timing permits detection of major anomalies with time available for further investigation such as karyotyping to permit termination of pregnancy under the Abortion Act 1967 (amended 1991) if appropriate.

Dating

At around 20 weeks, accurate dating is possible by measurement of various anatomical parameters. The standard measurements made are the biparietal diameter (BPD), head circumference (HC), abdominal circumference (AC) and femur length (FL). If there is a discrepancy of more than 10 days between the ultrasound assessment of gestation and that from the menstrual dates, then the ultrasound dates are adopted. If the fetus is much smaller than expected, a further scan should be performed after 2 to 4 weeks to confirm that the growth rate is normal.

Anomalies

By 20 weeks gestation, it is possible to obtain clear anatomical information of all major organ systems. The list of abnormalities which can be detected by ultrasound is very long. Table 9.1 shows the details which are examined in a standard 20 weeks anomaly scan.

Prenatal detection of structural abnormalities permits further investigations such as karyotyping, if appropriate, and also allows the parents to be counselled about the probable outcome. For example, when a gastroschisis is diagnosed, the parents can be informed of the need for, and outcome of, postnatal surgery.

Some abnormalities have a significant association with aneuploidy (e.g. atrioventricular septal defect (AVSD) and trisomy 21) whereas others are virtually never found in association with an abnormal karyotype (e.g. gastroschisis). Other abnormalities have a loose association with aneuploidy, and are often described as markers for aneuploidy. Examples include hydronephrosis, choroid plexus cysts and talipes. The risk of any fetus being aneuploid will increase with maternal age, high risk on screening test and with increasing number of markers present. Following the diagnosis of a structural abnormality, the parents will be counselled about the risk of aneuploidy and offered fetal karyotyping when appropriate.

Table 9.1

Examples of Fetal Anomalies Which can be Detected by Ultrasound

Organ system	Structures examined	Examples of abnormalities detectable
Central nervous	Cranium	Anencephaly
	Brain	Hydrocephaly
	Spine	Holoprosencephaly
		Spina bifida
Cardiovascular	Heart and great vessels	Tetralogy of Fallot
		AVSD, VSD
		Aortic and pulmonary stenosis/atresia
		Hypoplastic left heart
Gastrointestinal	Stomach	Duodenal atresia
	Bowel	Bowel atresia
	Diaphragm	Diaphragmatic hernia
Urogenital	Kidneys	Bladder outflow obstruction
	Bladder	Renal agenesis
		Hydronephrosis
		Cystic dysplasia
Face	Orbits	Cleft lip
	Lips	
Skeletal	Long bones	Dwarfism
	Extremities	Talipes
Abdominal wall	Integrity	Gastroschisis
		Exomphalos

Fetal growth

There are many reasons why fetal growth may be abnormal. Intrauterine growth restriction (IUGR) is best defined as a failure to fulfill growth potential, and is diagnosed by serial ultrasound scans. It is unusual for fetal growth to be abnormal in the first half of pregnancy, and if the early growth velocity is markedly reduced, there is a high risk of aneuploidy (e.g. triploidy), fetal infection or abnormality.

The most common reason for reduced fetal growth is uteroplacental insufficiency. This usually presents in the late second or third trimester. In women with risk factors for IUGR (previous history, maternal disease e.g. hypertension, etc.) serial scans for growth are recommended from 24 weeks. The frequency of such scans should be no more than fortnightly. The standard fetal biometry is performed and plotted on charts demonstrating the 50th, 90th and 10th (or 50th, 95th and 5th) centiles. The most important measurement for assessment of fetal growth is the abdominal circumference which effectively measures the fetal liver, the site of fetal energy stores. In addition, the amniotic fluid volume and placenta are assessed, with Doppler evaluation of the fetal and uteroplacental circulation as necessary. If an abnormal growth velocity is detected, increased fetal surveillance is instigated, by Doppler examination of the fetal blood flows, cardiotocographs and biophysical profile. This is aimed at detecting fetal compromise. If this occurs, then delivery is usually effected, depending on the gestation.

Whilst the exact mechanisms involved in IUGR remain unclear, reduced placental blood flow and transfer certainly contribute. Trophoblast invasion of the myometrium occurs in two waves, the second occurring between 20 and 24 weeks gestation. During this process, the muscular walls of the spiral arteries within the myometrium are invaded by the trophoblast leading to a low resistance, high flow circulation through the placental bed. If this process is incomplete, the resistance within the uterine blood vessels remains high, with a resultant increase in the resistance to the blood flow on the fetal side of the placental circulation.

Maternal blood flow is commonly assessed by Doppler interrogation of the uterine arteries. In a normal pregnancy, the blood flow demonstrates a large volume flow, with a smooth systolic peak and constant plentiful flow during the whole of diastole. However, if the trophoblast invasion is inadequate, there is a high resistance to flow with a marked systolic peak followed by an early diastolic reduction (or notch) followed by increased but low constant forward flow during diastole. The presence of notches in the uterine arteries after 24 weeks increases the risks of a pregnancy being complicated by IUGR and pre-eclampsia.

When the maternal resistance is increased, there is a corresponding increase in the resistance in the umbilical arteries. In a normal pregnancy, there is constant forward flow during the whole of the cardiac cycle, with a smooth increase in systole. With an increased placental resistance, there may be absent flow during the end of diastole, and in severe cases, the end-diastolic flow may be reversed. Abnormalities of flow in the umbilical arteries indicate a fetus that is either at risk of compromise or is already compromised. If umbilical blood flow is normal, there is a low risk of fetal hypoxia. If end-diastolic flow is absent, the fetus is at risk of hypoxia whereas if the flow is reduced, there is a very high risk of hypoxia (Fig. 9.4).

When a fetus becomes compromised *in utero*, with a reduction in oxygen supply, it preferentially supplies oxygenated blood to its brain, myocardium and adrenals — so-called central redistribution. This can be detected using Doppler, by examining the blood flow in the middle cerebral artery. Whilst redistribution is indicative of fetal compromise, it does not equate with hypoxia.

The fetal heart rate will show a reduction in short-term variability as a fetus becomes compromised, with the onset of decelerations as the situation worsens.

Growth restricted fetuses tend to demonstrate a reduction in amniotic fluid volume.

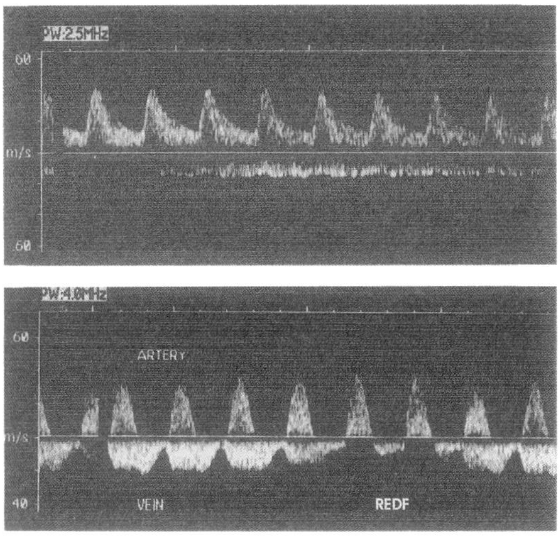

Fig. 9.4 *Top: Normal umbilical artery; Bottom: Reversed end diastolic flow (REDF)*

This is likely to be partly due to a reduction in water transfer across the placenta and membranes but primarily due to a reduction in renal blood flow secondary to redistribution. The amniotic fluid volume is assessed on ultrasound by measuring the amniotic fluid index (AFI). This involves measuring the deepest vertical pool in each of the quadrants of the uterus. When the liquor is markedly reduced, there may be only one measurable pool. It is essential to ensure, using colour Doppler, that the pools of liquor do not contain loops of umbilical cord.

If the uterine artery Dopplers are abnormal, it is very likely that the umbilical artery Dopplers will show evidence of increased resistance. Umbilical artery Dopplers are of proven value in the management of fetuses at risk of hypoxia, but there is no place for routine Doppler assessment of umbilical artery blood flow in an uncomplicated pregnancy either at, or post, term.

Biophysical assessment

The biophysical profile is an ultrasound-based method of assessing fetal well-being. The components are:

- Fetal biometry
- Amniotic fluid index
- Fetal movements
- Fetal tone
- Cardiotocogram.

Many units do not offer formal biophysical profiles because they are time-consuming, and expensive in terms of ultrasound time. However, most sonographers assess all aspects of the profile, with the exception of the CTG, each time they perform a scan. Of all the components, the most reliable is assessing the risk of fetal distress is the amniotic fluid volume, whether assessed by the AFI or deepest pool.

Scanning in the Third Trimester

The main indications for scanning late in pregnancy are:

- Fetal growth
- Amniotic fluid volume
- Presentation
- Placental localisation.

Fetal growth scans should be performed in any woman in whom there is a clinical suspicion of IUGR based on measurement of the symphysis fundal height or palpation. In addition, women with known risk factors and multiple pregnancies should be offered regular growth scans. In the presence of normal growth, the scans should be repeated every 4 weeks, i.e. 24, 28, 32 and 36 weeks. If there is concern about the growth rate, then fortnightly scans are indicated.

Although abdominal palpation, in experienced hands, is reliable for determining the presentation of a fetus, there are times when it may be very difficult to confirm the presentation, e.g. in cases of polyhydramnios, multiple pregnancy, excessive adiposity, etc. In such circumstances, it is reasonable and sensible to use ultrasound to confirm whether it is the head or breech presenting. With a breech presentation either at term, or if preterm delivery is contemplated, an estimated fetal weight will assist in management decision-making.

One cause for abnormal presentations is an abnormally sited placenta. If the placenta lies wholly or partially within the lower segment of the uterus, it may obstruct descent of the presenting part into the pelvis. A low-lying placenta may also present with bleeding. The definition of placenta praevia is reserved for cases where the placenta lies within the lower segment when it has formed, i.e. towards the end of the third trimester. Thus, if a placenta is seen to be low within the uterus earlier in pregnancy, it is correctly described as low lying rather than praevia. Placenta praevia is described as major or minor. A minor degree of placenta praevia is defined as the placenta lying within the lower segment, but the leading edge not encroaching on the internal cervical os. If the placenta encroaches on or covers the os, it is a major degree. When a low-lying placenta is discovered at routine 20-week scan, it is recommended that a scan be performed between 32 and 36 weeks to confirm the placental site. Transvaginal sonography is perfectly safe in cases of placenta praevia, and may be preferable to transabdominal scanning particularly when the placenta is posterior. In minor degrees of placenta praevia, it is possible to measure the distance between the leading edge and the internal os, and to define whether or not the presenting part lies below the leading edge. This is important in clinical decision-making in terms of mode of delivery.

PRENATAL DIAGNOSIS

The detection and prevention of congenital disorders is the most rapidly expanding area in obstetric practice. The relative importance of this topic has become greater as perinatal mortality due to all causes has diminished to around 10/1000 births. Single gene defects alone occur this frequently (Table 9.2). Structural congenital abnormalities are now 3 or 4 times as common as perinatal loss from other causes. With a birth prevalence of 2/1000, serious chromosomal abnormalities are as common as intrapartum death and have more serious long-term consequences. In developed countries, 30% of stillbirths, 20% of neonatal deaths and 30% of all paediatric admissions are the result of congenital disorders. The genetics of single gene defects and structural abnormalities are, summarised in Table 9.3.

The fetus is not amenable to traditional methods of physical examination, and prenatal diagnosis, therefore, involves the use of specific technology. Detection of abnormalities is dependent on 1 of 3 basic methods:

1. **Imaging techniques.** In practice, ultrasound is much the most important, although conventional radiology still has a place, and

Table 9.2

Contribution of Different Categories of Congenital Abnormality to Overall Incidence

Category of defect	Incidence per thousand	
	Detectable abnormality	Serious' abnormality i.e. with permanent life-threatening implications
Chromosomal	5 (includes balanced translocations and sex chromosome abnormalities)	2
Single gene defects	10	10
Structural abnormalities*	30–40 (includes talipes and congenital dislocation of hip)	10–20 (includes congenital heart disease)
Congenital infection	4–8	1–2

*A small proportion of structural abnormalities are the result of chromosomal, single gene or infective causes. Thus, duodenal atresia is sometimes caused by Down's syndrome; many forms of dwarfism have autosomal inheritance; and microcephaly may have an autosomal recessive or infective basis. Most structural abnormalities, however, are caused by a combination of many genes and environmental agents. We call these conditions multifactional or polygenetic and they include the majority of organ defects such as congenital heart disease, neural tube defects, cleft-lip and palate and gastrointestinal and renal anomalies.

Table 9.3
Mechanisms of Genetic Inheritance

Type of inheritance	Recurrence risk	Other features	Examples
Autosomal dominant	1:2 if present in a parent	May be new mutation (with very low recurrence risk) if no family history. The more lethal the condition, the more frequently it is caused by a new mutation. Penetrance also varies for some conditions.	Achondroplasia Huntington's chorea Tuberose sclerosis Neurofibromatosis Von Willebrand's disease Congenital spherocytosis Multiple endocrine adenomatosis
Autosomal recessive	1:4	Includes most inborn errors of metabolism. Prenatal diagnosis frequently available.	Cystic fibrosis Thalassaemia Tay Sach's disease Phenylketonuria
Sex-linked recessive	1:2 males affected 1:2 female carriers (the female is an obligatory carrier if she is the daughter of an affected man)	The probability that a female is a carrier can often be increased or decreased by specific testing, e.g. creatinine phosphokinase for Duchenne dystrophy and factor VIII for Haemophilia.	Haemophilia Christmas disease Duchenne and Becker dystrophies Lesch-Nyhan syndrome Ornithine carbamyl transferase deficiency
'Polygenetic' (multifactorial)	1:20 where the condition is common to 1:100 where it is rare	A number of genes and environmental agents (usually unidentified combine to produce the abnormality. Concurrence rate in identical twins is 50%.	This group includes most of the major structural abnormalities such as congenital heart disease, intestinal atresia, cleft lip and palate, Sometimes, however, these are caused by single gene defects, e.g. the Meckel syndrome (*see text*) or as part of a chromosomal abnormality, or as a result of infection or drugs.

nuclear magnetic resonance may be useful in the future.

2. **Measurement of fetal products in maternal blood.** In practice, this involves measurement of the fetal protein, alpha-fetoprotein, but techniques to harvest minute numbers of fetal cells from the maternal circulation have exciting implications for the future.
3. **Analysis of fetal tissue or fluids.** Prenatal diagnosis has great potential in reducing the total of suffering and the economic consequences of congenital disease. The incidence of the world's most common and one of the most serious autosomal recessive disorders, beta-thalassaemia, has been reduced by 70% in Sardinia by means of fetal tissue sampling and gene probe diagnosis. Similarly, the incidence of Tay Sachs disease has been reduced by an even greater amount in the state of New York, where a specific enzyme assay is carried out on pregnancies at risk.

Congenital Malformations

The majority of structural malformations occur in individuals without any known risk factors. Some are associated with pregnancy complications e.g. duodenal atresia with polyhydramnios, whereas many others would remain undetected without routine sonography.

When a structural malformation is detected, the parents need to be counselled regarding the nature of the defect, any associated problems such as aneuploidy, the prognosis for normal development and the need for postnatal treatment. A multidisciplinary approach is essential, including obstetricians, neonatologists, geneticists and paediatric surgeons. In some malformations, it is necessary to consider the best place for delivery, e.g. babies with congenital diaphragmatic hernia should be delivered in a unit with neonatal intensive care facilities, ideally with paediatric surgery on site. In the presence of a cleft lip, which although amenable to postnatal repair with excellent cosmetic results can be devastating at the time of birth, parents will require counselling to enable them to accept the very obvious facial features evident immediately on delivery. Other disorders, including hydrocephalus and other intracranial abnormalities, are associated with a risk of abnormal neurodevelopment and handicap, and termination of pregnancy may be considered by the parents. There is also a group of lethal abnormalities, which include bilateral renal agenesis and anencephaly. In some cases, parents will seek termination of pregnancy whereas others will be content to allow nature to take its course. Religious and cultural factors will be very important in such decision-making.

If an abnormality is suspected on routine scan, most women are referred to a fetal medicine unit for confirmation, counselling and further tests as appropriate.

Chromosome Anomalies

Down syndrome (trisomy 21) is the most common chromosome disorder seen, and is a significant cause of handicap. However, many other chromosome anomalies occur, in particular the other autosomal trisomies (trisomy 13 or Patau's syndrome and trisomy 18 or Edward's syndrome) and sex chromosome anomalies. Patau's and Edward's syndromes are described as lethal with the majority dying before birth and if born alive, very few surviving more than a few hours. Other trisomies are usually lethal *in utero* and account for many spontaneous abortions.

In order to diagnose a chromosome anomaly, a sample of fetal cells must be obtained. This requires an invasive procedure, although research into the identification of fetal cells in the maternal circulation is very active. There are three possible tests for obtaining a fetal karyotype:

- Chorion villus sampling
- Amniocentesis
- Fetal blood sampling.

All these tests are carried out under continuous ultrasound guidance.

Chorion villus sampling

This involves taking a small piece of placenta, and may be performed from 11 weeks gestation. Although it is possible to perform a CVS at any stage until term, this test is usually performed in the first trimester. CVS may be performed by the transabdominal or transcervical route, and involves inserting a needle or biopsy forceps into the placenta under continuous ultrasound visualisation. The sample is then either aspirated or grasped within the forceps.

Villi have many rapidly dividing cells, and it is possible to obtain a chromosome count within 48 hours using short-term culture techniques. Full culture is also performed to obtain a full karyotype, which involves banding of the chromosomes and examination of each one. A placental biopsy is also an excellent source of fetal DNA which is required for testing for many genetic syndromes such as sickle cell disease and cystic fibrosis. Once the sample reaches the laboratory, it is examined under a microscope to permit dissection of any decidual tissue which may be attached to the villi. Obviously, decidua is maternal tissue, and must be removed before any further testing to avoid the risk of an ambiguous result.

The risk of miscarriage after CVS is between 1–2%. The mechanism for pregnancy loss relates primarily to the risk of infection following the procedure. It is possible for the placenta to have a different chromosome count from the fetus, so-called confined placental mosaicism. This occurs in approximately 1% of CVS tests. A further test may be necessary to confirm the accurate fetal karyotype.

Amniocentesis

This is the traditional and most commonly performed test for determining the fetal karyotype. It involves passing a fine needle into the amniotic cavity under continuous ultrasound guidance and aspirating a small volume of liquor. Amniocentesis can be performed at any gestation from 14 weeks onwards. The liquor obtained (usually 1 ml per week gestation) is less than 10% of the total volume and is rapidly replaced. Once in the laboratory, the amniotic fluid is centrifuged to obtain a pellet of cells which are mainly fibroblasts from the fetal skin. These cells are then grown by cell culture techniques, and eventually arrested in metaphase so that the chromosomes can be examined. This process takes between 12 and 14 days in most modern laboratories.

Newer laboratory techniques are being developed to achieve a more rapid result. Fluorescent *in situ* hybridisation (*FISH*) stains a locus on a specific chromosome, and the cell is examined to count the number of fluorescent signals obtained. Probes exist for many chromosomes, and the technique is mainly used for the common trisomies. Advantages of the technique include a rapid result (within 24 hours) with no need for cell culture. Polymerase chain reaction (PCR) has also been developed, when the DNA on particular chromosomes is multiplied and quantified, enabling detection of the trisomies. This technique also obviates the need for cell culture, and provides a result within 24–48 hours. However, both of these techniques provide limited information, only pertaining to the specific chromosomes examined. Thus, the rarer aneuploidies would not be detectable, unless full culture and cytogenetic techniques were applied.

Amniocentesis carries a risk of miscarriage of approximately 1%, although this is less in later gestations. The disadvantages of this test are the late gestation at which results become available. If the test is performed at 16 weeks, the result is not available until 18 weeks, which is quite late if termination of pregnancy is to be considered.

The same procedure is used in other clinical situations, e.g. monitoring of bilirubin levels in the amniotic fluid in pregnancies affected by Rhesus isoimmunisation.

Fetal blood sampling

Using an adaptation of the above ultrasound guided techniques, it is possible to aspirate fetal blood from the umbilical vein either in the cord or from its intrahepatic portion. This technique is rarely applied before 20 weeks gestation, as the vessels are too small. However, by culture of fetal lymphocytes, it is possible to obtain a full karyotype within 48 hours. In addition, any tests which can be performed on postnatal blood samples may be performed on fetal blood, although the volume available will be very limited.

Fetal blood sampling is particularly valuable in providing a rapid karyotype in cases of fetal abnormality detected at the 20-week scan. It is also essential in investigating some forms of abnormality such as hydrops (or intrauterine cardiac failure) where fetal anaemia (which is treatable by transfusion) may be a cause. The risk of miscarriage is approximately 1%, although it is higher if the fetus demonstrates signs of compromise such as abnormal Dopplers or hydrops. Fetal blood sampling may be employed in the investigation of some cases of severe IUGR, when blood gas analysis may provide valuable extra information to assist in the management of the case.

LABORATORY PROCEDURES

These are carried out on fetal tissue obtained from one of the above methods and consist of:

1. Chromosomal analysis.
2. Enzyme analysis.
3. Haematological tests.
4. Recombinant DNA technology.

Chromosomal analysis detects a large number of anomalies but the most important of these are the aneuploidies (abnormalities in chromosome number). About 97% of cases of Down's syndrome and the other trisomies arise from non-dysjunction during the meiotic division of the oocyte. A small number arise from a balanced translocation in a parent. Abnormalities of the sex chromosomes are also important. These include: Turner's syndrome (XO) with phenotypic abnormalities but no mental abnormalities, Triple X syndrome with the opposite, and Fragile X syndrome which leads to mental abnormalities in males.

Enzyme defects can be diagnosed by incubating fetal tissue with a specific substrate. In addition, a small number of conditions may be diagnosed by the measurement of an accumulating metabolite in amniotic fluid supernate. This type of diagnosis is applicable when parents have already had an affected child or are known carriers.

Haematological tests on fetal blood will detect deficiencies of factor VIII and IX, and beta-thalassaemia may be diagnosed by specific assay for the beta-globin chains.

Recombinant DNA technology is providing a valuable and more accurate tool to detect defects at a molecular level in genes. Genes are expressed in fetal fibroblasts obtained from skin biopsy. Provided there is a specific gene probe which has been identified, then the presence or absence of that gene can be detected. Gene probes are available for the haemoglobinopathies, Duchene muscular dystrophy, Haemophilia A, Christmas disease (factor IX deficiency), Huntington's chorea, and an increasing number of others. Diagnosis is easier when there is a whole gene deleted, but in many cases, more detailed family studies are needed. Linkage analysis of the presence or absence of various endonuclease cutting sites (restriction fragment length polymorphisms) in the DNA between genes are required.

Therapeutic Procedures

There are a number of fetal conditions which are amenable to prenatal therapy. This may involve maternal administration of drugs (e.g. spiramycin in toxoplasmosis infection), direct fetal administration of drugs (e.g. digoxin in fetal supraventricular tachycardia), blood transfusion and other procedures such as insertion of vesico-amniotic shunts in bladder outflow obstruction. The majority of therapeutic procedures are rarely required, and should be performed in a tertiary referral unit. The majority involve ultrasound-guided insertion of a needle or trochar into the relevant organ. Some endoscopic procedures are being developed including laser ablation of placental anastamoses in twin-twin transfusion syndrome, a complication of monochorionic diamniotic twins.

In America, open fetal surgery has been performed for repair of congenital diaphragmatic hernias. This involves maternal general anaesthesia and hysterotomy, with a high risk of preterm labour and rather disappointing overall results.

There are few situations in which fetal therapy is indicated and in many where it has been attempted, the value of such intervention in improving the outcome is unclear. However, the oldest therapeutic intervention, intrauterine transfusion in the management of Rhesus affected pregnancies, has dramatically improved the outcome.

What Happens When an Abnormality is Found?

If an abnormality is suspected on the grounds of screening, known risk factors or previous ultrasound examination, the parents must be informed and referred as appropriate for confirmation of the diagnosis and other tests as indicated. Although informing parents of a fetal abnormality is devastating for them, it is essential to be honest, however distressing. Such news may be greeted by anger and resentment at the person who made the diagnosis, but the couple must be given time to assimilate the information, ask any questions and come to terms with the situation.

When an abnormality is confirmed, some people will make an immediate request for termination of pregnancy. Whilst this may be an appropriate option, it is essential that the couple are given time to make sure that this is the right decision for them. Obviously, although the later a termination is performed the more stressful it is, there is no need for unseemly hurry.

Termination of pregnancy after 14 or 16 weeks will usually involve induction of labour, with the woman delivering the fetus vaginally. If over 22 weeks, it is recommended that feticide is performed before labour is induced, to ensure that the baby is not born alive. This is usually achieved by intracardiac injection of potassium chloride, which needs to be done in a fetal medicine unit.

It is very important that the maximum amount of information is obtained concerning the diagnosis and any other anomalies, so that the parents can be accurately counselled regarding reasons why the problem arose and the risks of it happening again. This usually necessitates post-mortem examination of the fetus, which should be performed by a perinatal pathologist. Limited post-mortem examination, using photographs, X-rays and MRI scans may be valuable when parents decline full post-mortem and should be encouraged.

Some parents will decide to continue with a pregnancy, whatever the diagnosis and prognosis. Such decisions must be respected and supported, even if they seem illogical to the doctors and other carers involved. The aim of prenatal diagnosis is to provide information to enable the parents to make informed decisions regarding the management of their pregnancy.

Support after termination or other fetal or neonatal loss is essential, and the majority of units have a dedicated midwife who is trained in such bereavement counselling.

FURTHER READING

Romero R., Pilu G., Jeanty P., Ghidini A., Hobbins J.C., eds. (1988). *Prenatal Diagnosis of Congenital Anomalies.* Appleton & Lang.

Nicolaides K.H., Sebire N.J., Snijders R.J.M. (1999). *The 11–14 Week Scan.* Parthenon Publishing.

Chudleigh P., Pearce J.M. (1992). *Obstetric Ultrasound: How, Why and When,* 2nd edn. 1992.

10

Medical Disorders and Pregnancy

The principle of management of pregnant women with medical disorders is to achieve the most effective control of the medical disorder, and then to deal with subsequent problems along standard obstetric lines. The principle is best applied if the patient is seen before she conceives. This enables review of the medical disorder, adjustment of treatment, appraisal of risks, and achievement of the understanding and co-operation of the patient. She can then start her pregnancy with the best chance of success. In order that preconception review can become routine in patients with medical disorders, it is still necessary to convince physicians that almost any woman between 12 and 50 years of age may become pregnant, regardless of her apparent circumstances.

HYPERTENSION IN PREGNANCY

Arterial blood pressure is a continuously distributed variable in the general population. The difference between normal blood pressure and hypertension is an arbitrary level. It is generally accepted that a blood pressure of 140/90 mmHg or above is abnormal in women of reproductive age.

Measurement of blood pressure

When taking blood pressure in a pregnant woman, the patient's position should be consistent. Semi-prone with lateral tilt is best, but the sitting position is convenient. The first phase of the Korotkoff sounds defines the systolic pressure. In pregnancy, the diastolic pressure is best recorded when the Korotkoff sound becomes muffled (fourth phase), and errors then tend to cause an overestimation. Obese women should have their blood pressure taken with a large cuff.

Hypertension Occurring Before Pregnancy

Hypertension can be classified into primary or essential hypertension where there is no apparent precipitating factor, and secondary hypertension, which is much less common, and where there is some identifiable cause. Malignant hypertension occurs in a minority of patients with essential hypertension and is characterised by the rapid development of severe hypertension and the presence of papilloedema.

Essential hypertension tends to occur in older parous and obese women, often with a family history of hypertension. The blood pressure is usually raised in the first half of pregnancy, but may be masked by the physiological decline in blood pressure during the middle trimester. Patients with intermittent hypertension in early pregnancy have an approximately five-fold increased risk of developing significant hypertension in the third trimester.

Causes of secondary hypertension are:

1. Renal disorders, whether ischaemic, infective, congenital or an infiltration such as amyloid.

2. Endocrine disorders such as thyrotoxicosis, Cushing's syndrome, Conn's syndrome or phaeochromocytoma.
3. Congenital heart disease such as coarctation of the aorta or aortic regurgitation.
4. Collagen disorders such as systemic lupus erythematosus.

The approach to secondary hypertension is to obtain the best therapeutic control of the underlying condition, and then to treat any residual hypertension.

Diagnosis of hypertension antedating pregnancy

If the blood pressure is 140/90 mmHg or higher in the first 24 weeks of pregnancy, chronic hypertension can be inferred, and this is most likely to be due to essential hypertension, although the possibility of secondary hypertension must be borne in mind. In the latter half of pregnancy, diagnosis can be a problem because pre-eclamptic symptoms may superimpose on pre-existing hypertension.

Physical signs. Displacement of the apex beat to the left and its prominence may indicate left ventricular hypertrophy, suggesting long-standing hypertension. Renal enlargement such as occurs in polycystic disease, or a renal systolic bruit, as in renal artery stenosis, suggests hypertension secondary to renal causes. Examination of the optic fundi may show arteriolar tortuosity, silver wiring and arteriovenous nipping in long-standing hypertension. In most women who develop pre-eclampsia, there is no abnormality in the optic fundi. Asymmetrical blood pressure in the arms or diminished or absent femoral pulses may reveal coarctation of the aorta.

Investigations. In pregnancy, levels of plasma urea above 5 mmol/l and plasma creatinine above 100 μmol/l suggest an underlying renal problem.

Measurement of creatinine clearance will establish any degree of renal failure.

Platelet counts tend to fall to 100×10^9/l or less with severe hypertension associated with placental insufficiency and intra-uterine growth restriction. Occasionally, severe exacerbations are associated with coagulopathy and should be investigated appropriately.

In essential hypertension, plasma uric acid is usually below 0.35 mmol/l. It rises in pre-eclampsia. In the absence of urinary tract infection (bacterial count of $<10^5/\text{mm}^3$), proteinuria of 0.5 g/l or more in a 24-hour urine collection is significant. Progressive rise of proteinuria to more than 4–5 g/day suggests severe pre-eclampsia and may indicate serious renal impairment.

Urinary vanillyl-mandelic acid is raised in phaeochromocytoma. This condition is rare, but can have fatal consequences to mother and baby. It should be remembered that in pregnancy, phaeochromocytoma presents more commonly with sustained than with unstable hypertension, and the most common misdiagnoses are diabetes mellitus and Cushing's syndrome.

Management of chronic hypertension

Patients who are having antihypertensive treatment should be advised to seek advice before becoming pregnant. Revision of the drug regimen may be appropriate. Elimination of cigarette smoking and of obesity before becoming pregnant is helpful. The patient should be advised that rest, and perhaps hospital rest, may be necessary during pregnancy, and that controlled weight gain is desirable. Low dose aspirin, 75 mg/day should be considered for patients with a history of intra-uterine growth restriction, and planned to start at 10–12 weeks.

Methyldopa is well established as a safe basic drug for treatment of hypertension in pregnancy, and transfer to this agent should be considered, particularly in women who have had a perinatal loss on other drugs. Side effects of postural hypertension or depression are uncommon in pregnancy. A combination of a β-blocking drug and a diuretic is not ideal for pregnancy, as both components may impair utero-placental blood flow. β-blockers including atenolol, propanolol and labetalol, and also nifedipine, are associated with fetal intra-uterine growth restriction, and should be avoided for management throughout pregnancy. If they are used, fetal growth should be monitored with serial ultrasound scans. Long-term use of hydralazine alone should be avoided, as increased doses may be needed and the maternal side effects include a lupus erythematosus-like syndrome. Angiotensin converting enzyme (ACE) inhibitors such as captopril or enalapril should be stopped as soon as pregnancy is diagnosed and should not be used during pregnancy — they are known to have caused cases of defective fetal skull bone formation, fetal oliguria and consequent oligohydramnios, and impaired newborn renal function.

Close control of hypertension is best instituted with divided doses of methyldopa. Should it not be possible to achieve daytime and overnight control with this drug alone, doses of nifedipine or atenolol may have to be added.

Patients who present during the first 20 weeks of pregnancy with a blood pressure of more than 150/90 mmHg need admission for observation and investigation. If the blood pressure settles to completely normal, management without antihypertensive drugs is reasonable until such time as the blood pressure rises again. Some obstetricians feel that these patients should be treated from the start, even though doses required in the middle trimester may be small, to protect the placental bed circulation from irreversible structural damage. Other obstetricians prefer to wait until the need for treatment becomes obvious.

The object of treatment is to control hypertension, thereby protecting the mother against cerebral haemorrhage, kidney damage, eclampsia and placental abruption as well as maintaining uteroplacental circulation and preventing placental infarction. In general, achievement of a maternal blood pressure consistently at or below 140/90 mmHg is good.

Control to levels below 120/80 may impair uteroplacental perfusion.

Oral antihypertensive agents

Methyldopa. The metabolite α-methylnoradrenaline acts by decreasing sympathetic outflow from the central nervous system, with a reduction in arteriolar resistance, but with little or no effect on heart rate or cardiac output. Initially, an oral dose of 250 mg twice or three times daily is given and adjusted at intervals of not less than two days. If 2 g/day proves inadequate to control hypertension, the addition of small doses of nifedipine, a β-blocker or oral hydralazine should be considered.

β-Adrenergic blocking agents. Propranolol was the first of these to be used in pregnancy and was thought to be responsible for cases of fetal bradycardia, neonatal hypoglycaemia and perinatal loss. Modest doses are actually reasonably safe, and in severe hypertension, the fetus is at risk anyway. The risks are increased by attempts to secure rapid control of acute situations with propranolol. In general, β-blockers take two or more days of consistent administration before their effects are stabilised.

Both atenolol (50–75 mg at night) and oxprenolol (40–120 mg twice daily) have been used in pregnancy, either alone or in combination with methyldopa.

Labetalol (100–400 mg twice daily) is said to act by peripheral vasodilatation without change in cardiac output or uteroplacental blood flow. It has been used without harm in cases of mild hypertension in pregnancy. When it is used intravenously in acute situations to control severe hypertension, some patients do not respond to the first dose, and some not to a subsequent administration.

Nifedipine is a calcium-channel blocker which reduces blood pressure by peripheral vasodilatation. It causes coronary artery vasodilatation and a reflex tachycardia but has no direct action on the heart. For controlling chronic hypertension, either alone or in conjunction with methyldopa, it is used as a long-acting preparation, 10–40 mg once or twice daily. The short acting preparation, 5–10 mg, the capsule crushed in the mouth and swallowed, may cause abrupt hypotension, flushing and dizziness and is only used in the initial management of a severe episode of hypertension.

Hydralazine is a vasodilator and reduces blood pressure by decreasing peripheral resistance. It tends to improve renal, uteroplacental and cerebral blood flow. Oral hydralazine combined with another antihypertensive drug can be useful in controlling blood pressure. The dose is 25–50 mg by mouth every 6 hours. It is safe in pregnancy, although prolonged use may cause skin rashes and headaches. The parenteral dose is considerably lower (10–15 mg i.m.).

Adrenergic neurone blockers. Bethanidine, guanethidine and debrisoquine are not commonly used, as their effects in pregnancy are not well understood. They convey a risk of impairing autonomic responses which may be needed in emergency obstetric situations.

Diuretics are not recommended as components of antihypertensive regimens in pregnancy except in emergency situations, such as heart failure.

HEART DISEASE IN PREGNANCY

Pregnancy imposes an extra haemodynamic burden on the cardiovascular system. Although the incidence of organic heart disease in pregnancy is less than 1%, symptoms of breathlessness and haemodynamic murmurs may occur in a majority of women with normal hearts.

Preconception counselling is of importance. Cardiac status can be fully assessed, risks discussed with the patient and future co-operation secured. Anaemia can be corrected and drug treatment modified. Cardiac surgery can make the difference between a risk to the mother's life and an uncomplicated pregnancy. With severe aortic valve lesions, operation may permit a successful pregnancy.

Physiological changes in pregnancy

These are described in Chapter 7.

With the onset of labour, cardiac output, already increased by 40%, increases further by 10–20%, especially in the lateral position, and reaches a peak immediately after delivery with values as high as 80% greater than before labour began. This peak increase in reduced by caudal and spinal anaesthesia, and to a greater extent by epidural anaesthesia.

Incidence of heart disease in pregnancy

There has been a steady decline in the incidence of rheumatic disease and an apparent increase in the incidence of congenital heart disease in pregnancy. The most important rheumatic lesion is mitral stenosis, accounting for 90% of cases. Mitral regurgitation, aortic regurgitation and aortic stenosis account for most of the rest. The more common forms of congenital heart disease are atrial septal defect, patent ductus arteriosus, ventricular septal defect, pulmonary stenosis, aortic stenosis, Fallot's tetralogy, and coarctation of the aorta.

Maternal mortality is low in rheumatic heart disease and highest in conditions where there is pulmonary hypertension, such as Eisenmenger's syndrome. Perinatal mortality in patients with rheumatic heart disease in pregnancy is comparable to that in normal patients, although babies tend to be lighter. With cyanotic congenital heart disease, babies are usually growth restricted, and perinatal mortality may be as high as 40–50%.

Diagnosis during pregnancy

Some cases of heart disease are not diagnosed until the patient has become pregnant. Some symptoms and signs of normal pregnancy may mimic heart disease. Complaints of breathlessness, palpitations, syncope and ankle swelling are all consistent with a normal heart in pregnancy; chest pain and haemoptysis suggest heart disease. Again, increased pulse volume, forceful apex beat, ectopic beats, a systolic ejection murmur, an internal mammary murmur at the second left intercostal space and peripheral oedema may be simple consequences of pregnancy. An apex beat more than 2 cm lateral to the midclavicular line, a raised jugular venous pressure, a diastolic, pansystolic or late systolic murmur, ejection clicks, and signs such as cyanosis, finger clubbing or splinter haemorrhages, all suggest heart disease.

Investigations

Chest X-ray. Significant cardiac enlargement may be detected, although this investigation is unhelpful in the diagnosis of minor degrees of heart disease.

Electrocardiography is more helpful in diagnosis of arrhythmias than in demonstration of an anatomical abnormality.

Echocardiography. The majority of structural cardiac abnormalities may be demonstrated and this is the investigation of choice.

Antenatal Care

At each visit, pregnant cardiac patients should be seen if possible by both an obstetrician and a cardiologist so that the nature and severity of their heart disease can be assessed. Assessments include a decision as to whether the pregnancy should continue and if there is a need for cardiac surgery.

Congenital mitral valve prolapse is now recognised as benign in pregnancy. There are no haemodynamic problems and outcome is good. At the other extreme, primary pulmonary hypertension and Eisenmenger's syndrome are definite indications for legal abortion as there is a maternal mortality rate of about 30%; the abortion itself conveys some risk to life. The indication for closed mitral valve surgery in pregnancy is usually deteriorating pulmonary oedema not responding to medical treatment. These patients do well during pregnancy. If a life-threatening situation arises, for example with an aortic valve defect, it is difficult to establish and maintain a bypass circulation during surgery adequate to sustain the fetus, which usually succumbs unless caesarean section precedes the heart surgery.

The aim of antenatal care with cardiac patients is to reduce the risk of heart failure.

1. Obesity and excessive weight gain during pregnancy should be avoided.
2. Dental treatment with antibiotic cover should be advised early in pregnancy to prevent any dental sepsis and reduce the risk of subacute bacterial endocarditis.
3. Anaemia should be prevented with iron and folic acid supplements.
4. Upper respiratory tract infections may be an indication for hospital admission. At each visit, the patients should be examined to detect arrhythmias and raised jugular venous pressure and for evidence of pulmonary oedema at the lung bases.
5. Over-exertion and stress should be avoided.

Hospital admission for bed rest

Between 28 and 32 weeks of pregnancy, the load on the heart has usually reached its height, and any patient with deterioration will benefit from hospital rest for the remainder of the pregnancy. It is a mistake to consider that the strain on the heart diminishes after 32 weeks; the risk of failure remains or increases throughout the third trimester. The development of pre-eclampsia indicates urgent hospital admission and control of hypertension, not only because of the increased burden on the heart, but also because of fluid retention.

All patients with signs of heart failure must be treated in hospital.

Treatment of Heart Failure in Pregnancy

The principles of management are similar to those of heart failure developing at any other time.

Increase the oxygen supply. Supplemental oxygen may be given by face mask or nasal cannula. Anaemia may be corrected by iron supplements. If the haemocrit is less than 30%, transfusion of packed red blood cells may be given after initiating a diuresis with a modest dose of frusemide.

Decrease peripheral circulatory demand. Bed rest is important, especially after meals. Any infection must be treated and fever must be suppressed as pyrexia increases cardiac workload. Drugs and food additives which increase cardiac output, such as sympathomimetics like ritodrine, terbutaline, salbutamol, and theophylline compounds and caffeine should be avoided as should psychological stress and anxiety.

Augmentation of myocardial contractility. Digoxin is used to control the heart rate in atrial fibrillation and to increase the force of myocardial contraction. Digoxin crosses the placenta, but there is no associated fetal toxicity or reported teratogenicity. Myocardial depressants such as alcohol, or large doses of β-sympatholytics should be avoided.

Reduction of intravascular volume. Treatment with diuretics such as oral thiazides or frusemide may be necessary. Hypokalaemia should be avoided. Excess salt intake should be restricted and intravenous overload avoided.

Decrease in left ventricular afterload is achieved by controlling hypertension. Methyldopa is the best drug available, but moderate doses of β-blockers can be used.

Anticoagulation

Treatment with anticoagulants is necessary in patients with atrial fibrillation or pulmonary hypertension from congenital heart disease. In an acute situation, intravenous heparin may be necessary but, subsequently, subcutaneous low molecular weight heparin is adequate. There is a small risk of alopecia and of demineralisation of bone with prolonged heparin treatment and X-ray bone density in a hand, and serum calcium and phosphate, should be checked each month or two after 3 months.

Patients with artificial plastic heart valves must be fully anticoagulated. There are small risks of abortion with heparin in the first trimester, of warfarin embryopathy at 6–9 weeks after conception, and of warfarin fetal central nervous system damage in the second and third trimesters. Heparin may be used during the first trimester to avoid possible teratogenicity. The best regimen for anticoagulation is then an oral anticoagulant throughout most of pregnancy, with a change to heparin for the last 2–3 weeks. Oral anticoagulants cross the placenta and so there are risks of fetal haemorrhage during labour. Heparin is safe for the fetus as the large molecule does not cross the placenta, but overdose can result in placental damage.

Management in Labour

The patient who has no obstetric complication is best allowed to go into spontaneous labour. Nevertheless, induction should not be withheld if there is an obstetric indication.

During labour, a sitting or semi-reclining position is most comfortable. Aorto-caval compression should be avoided. Respiratory support, frusemide, digoxin and aminophylline should be readily available.

Dyspnoea may be avoided by administration of oxygen and, if analgesia is required in the second stage, nitrous oxide and oxygen can be used. Breathlessness may be due to anxiety and the discomfort of labour, so effective analgesia must be provided, either with narcotic analgesics, or with epidural anaesthesia, provided hypotension is avoided and there is neither a cardiac outflow obstructive lesion nor anticoagulation. Strict fluid balance is very important, as patients with heart disease cannot cope with an increase in intravascular volume and easily develop pulmonary oedema.

It is wise to keep the second stage of labour short to reduce maternal effort. If the patient is likely to deliver herself, an episiotomy may reduce the effort at delivery. If forceps are to be applied, it is better to wait for the fetal head to descend to the pelvic floor provided that the patient is not seriously distressed.

There has been debate as the use of oxytocic drugs in cardiac patients in the third stage of labour, but a postpartum haemorrhage is a disaster. Oxytocin is generally safer than ergometrine and is the drug of choice. In patients with heart failure, an oxytocin infusion may be given with intravenous frusemide.

There should be no reluctance to deliver cardiac patients by caesarean section for the usual obstetric indications.

Antibiotic prophylaxis

The basis of antibiotic cover in labour is to prevent the development of subacute bacterial endocarditis. Women with valvular disease, particularly those with septal defects, should be given antibiotic prophylaxis. Amoxicillin 500 mg and gentamicin 80 mg i.m., 8-hourly, is a suitable regimen.

Management of the puerperium

The first 12 hours after delivery are the most critical, as venous return is increased. Signs of pulmonary congestion and oedema must be carefully sought. If oral anticoagulants have been used antenatally, these should be recommenced. Warfarin is not contraindicated with breast feeding, but phenindione does pass into breast milk. If there are no signs of heart failure, the patient is not restricted to bed and graduated activity is allowed before she returns home. Domestic assistance may be required when the patient is at home.

Specific Heart Conditions in Pregnancy

Mitral stenosis

Pregnant women with mitral stenosis are particularly prone to develop pulmonary oedema but, with good conservative management, mitral valvotomy is only rarely needed in pregnancy. Patients considered for closed valvotomy should have no significant mitral regurgitation in conjunction with mitral stenosis. The mitral valve should not be calcified and there should be no other significant valve involvement. Echocardiography is valuable to discover the severity of the lesion and assess the state of the valve cusps.

Artificial heart valves

Patients who have had a successful isolated mitral or aortic valve replacement do not usually have haemodynamic problems in pregnancy. Patients with biological heart valves usually do not require anticoagulation.

Cyanotic heart disease

The incidence of premature delivery and intra-uterine death is increased because of the development of severe placental insufficiency. When ultrasound measurements show that the fetus has failed to grow, there should be no hesitation about delivering the baby, if necessary by caesarean section, especially after 34 weeks.

Eisenmenger's syndrome is a severe form of cyanotic heart disease. It consists of pulmonary hypertension with a raised pulmonary vascular resistance together with a congenital cardiovascular lesion that allows shunting from the right to the left side of the heart. Pregnancy should be avoided in this condition and early surgical abortion is recommended if it does occur. The risk to the mother is high in those with pre-eclampsia and in the puerperium. Fetal loss has been quoted as between 30% and 80%.

Arrhythmias

Most of the agents used to prevent or treat cardiac arrhythmias during pregnancy appear to be harmless to the fetus. In particular, modest doses of β-blockers, digoxin, quinidine, adenosine, lignocaine and verapamil appear to be harmless, though the last drug may inhibit uterine contractions. Amiodarone should not be used in pregnancy as it can cause fetal hypothyroidism and goitre. Cardioversion has been successfully accomplished in pregnancy many times, without harm to the fetus, but anticoagulation is required to prevent embolism.

VENOUS THROMBOEMBOLISM AND PREGNANCY

Deep vein thrombosis is more common in pregnancy and the puerperium. It is important because it predisposes to pulmonary embolism, which is an important cause of maternal mortality. Pregnancy increases the risk of thromboembolism by five to six times compared to non-pregnant women who are not on oral contraceptives. The incidence of deep vein thrombosis is about 0.2% and that of pulmonary embolism about 0.03% of all pregnancies.

Aetiology

Clotting factors. In pregnancy there are increases in clotting factors VII, VIII and X, together with an increased fibrinogen level and decreased fibrinolytic activity. This contributes to haemostatic efficiency when placental separation occurs. There is thus an increased tendency to thrombosis.

Venous stasis. The pregnant uterus compresses the inferior vena cava and reduces venous return from the legs. There is also reduced venous tone. Restriction of activity and prolonged bed rest promote venous stasis, and all pregnant patients confined to bed should wear support stockings.

Operative procedures. The incidence of fatal pulmonary embolism is about ten times greater after caesarean section than after vaginal delivery. Difficult forceps deliveries and prolonged labour also increase the risk of thromboembolism. Surgical procedures during pregnancy and tubal ligation in the puerperium convey an increased risk of thromboembolism. Patients with risk factors should have prophylaxis with subcutaneous heparin for caesarean section, started either before or shortly after the operation.

Age and parity. The risk of fatal pulmonary embolism is greater with a fourth or subsequent pregnancy and in women over 30 years of age.

Obesity. Excessively obese women are especially at risk.

Other factors. There was an association with the use of oestrogen to suppress lactation and thromboembolism. Women with blood group O are less likely to develop thromboembolic disease in pregnancy; women with sickle cell anaemia are at risk of developing pulmonary embolism. Women who are severely anaemic in the puerperium are thought to be at increased risk of thrombosis.

Prophylaxis of Venous Thromboembolism

When a woman has had thromboembolism in the previous pregnancy, she will be at increased risk during the present pregnancy and in the puerperium, though the risk of recurrence is now recognised as small. Prophylactic measures are:

1. Elastic stockings worn regularly.
2. Calf muscle exercises.
3. Anticoagulants — heparin subcutaneously.

Prophylaxis with warfarin may be given for 6 weeks after delivery.

Diagnosis of Deep Vein Thrombosis

Symptoms and signs are calf pain and tenderness, with a positive Homan's sign; unilateral oedema, a difference of 2 cm or more in circumference between identical sites on the legs being significant; and increase in warmth of the leg.

Many patients who have an acutely tender swollen calf do not necessarily have deep vein thrombosis. Thus an objective technique should be used whenever diagnosis is in doubt.

Objective tests

Tests that are safe in pregnancy and reasonably effective are:

1. *Doppler ultrasound* examination of flow in the femoral vein. The sound of blood flow may be absent if the vein is completely

obstructed, or altered compared with the opposite side if there is a partial obstruction.

2. *Isotope venography*. Albumin macroaggregates labelled with technetium ($^{99}Tc^{m}$) concentrate around the thrombus to form a 'hot spot'. An accuracy of 85–98% may be obtained.
3. *Limb impedance plethysmography* is accurate in only about 50% of cases.

Treatment

This is with heparin initially, usually followed by warfarin (see pp. 109 and 113). The patient may be mobilised after 24 hours of heparin anticoagulation.

Thrombectomy may be indicated in major iliofemoral deep vein thrombosis.

Diagnosis of Pulmonary Embolism

In the first place, the diagnosis of pulmonary embolism is clinical. A major embolism presents with a sudden onset of chest pain, usually pleural in character, dyspnoea, cough, hypotension, cyanosis and collapse. There may be haemoptysis, a parasternal heave, a raised jugular venous pressure and a third heart sound. Blood P_{O_2} is usually reduced and P_{CO_2} is sometimes low. In many cases, pain may be absent or minimal and the main symptom is dyspnoea. Pulmonary embolism should be considered in all cases of such unexplained dyspnoea in pregnancy. The most important differential diagnoses are myocardial infarction, pulmonary atelectasis, aspiration, or viral or bacterial pneumonia. To this extent, an electrocardiogram and a chest X-ray may be of some value. Definitive diagnosis of pulmonary embolism is made by prompt echocardiography and a perfusion lung scan. In late pregnancy or in relation to a confinement, the additional important differential diagnosis is amniotic fluid infusion, which is nearly always related to a clinical event such as rupture of the membranes, placental abruption, violent uterine contractions, rupture of the uterus, or delivery, the most prominent clinical sign being dyspnoea. The other important early diagnostic features of a major amniotic fluid embolism are a normal chest X-ray soon after the initial episode, diffuse floccular shadows all over the lung fields 2 to 4 hours later and a prompt response to intravenous heparin (given in the absence of acute bleeding). Subsequently, the consequences of a consumption coagulopathy will make the diagnosis clear.

Treatment of Pulmonary Embolism

Management of massive pulmonary embolism includes elevation of the legs to increase venous return; oxygen inhalation; if the patient is unconscious, external cardiac massage to help break up the clot; if respiration has ceased, full cardio-pulmonary resuscitation; intravenous fluid; heparin 10,000 units intravenously; and alteplase or streptokinase as an adjunct to assist clot dispersion, though they may cause bleeding from the placental site. Pulmonary embolectomy may be indicated if severe hypotension persists and pulmonary peripheral perfusion is reduced by 75%, but mechanical clot dispersion with a cardiac catheter is preferable.

Early phase of management

Heparin is effective in arresting active thrombosis and does not cross the placenta. It is best given as a continuous infusion of 25,000–40,000 units of heparin in saline per day, adjusted to an activated partial thomboplastin time increase of about 2-fold. Intravenous heparin should be given initially for 48 hours, but may be continued for 7 days in severe cases. Bleeding is the most important complication, and stopping a heparin infusion for 2 to 3 hours will usually allow haemostasis to recover. In urgent situations, protamine sulphate will rapidly reverse the action of heparin.

Later management

Coumarin derivatives such as warfarin are the most commonly used oral anticoagulants in pregnancy. They act by depressing the hepatic vitamin K-dependent synthesis of coagulation factors. Warfarin is best for chronic treatment in the non-pregnant patient but, as it crosses the placenta, it can cause fetal abnormalities if given between 6 and 11 weeks of pregnancy and, occasionally, central nervous system abnormalities in the fetus if given in the second or third trimester. The main fetal abnormalities that can arise from first trimester use are saddle nose, nasal hypoplasia, frontal bossing and short stature with stippled epiphyses. Late in pregnancy or in labour intracerebral bleeding can occasionally occur in the fetus, especially if premature, and may cause mental retardation and blindness. For these reasons, it has been recommended that, if there is a real need to continue full anticoagulation after the initial treatment with heparin, although there is some risk of abortion, this drug should be continued for the first trimester and, if necessary, followed by warfarin between 13 and 36 weeks of pregnancy, reverting to heparin in the last few weeks of pregnancy.

Long-term treatment with subcutaneous, self-administered heparin is the method of choice in pregnancy. Between 5000 and 10,000 units of heparin 12-hourly given in 0.2–0.4 ml into the lateral aspect of the subcutaneous abdominal wall fat is usually adequate. Ideally, heparin levels should be checked frequently; peak levels should not exceed 0.2 iu/ml. Use of single daily subcutaneous doses of low molecular weight heparins is being studied. After delivery, treatment with subcutaneous heparin or warfarin should be continued for 5 to 6 weeks. Demineralisation of bone or alopecia may result from long-term heparin treatment.

If thromboembolism occurs in the puerperium, anticoagulant treatment should be continued for a total of 6 weeks.

Superficial Vein Thrombosis, Thrombophlebitis

A superficial vein cannulated for transfusion or varicose veins in the leg are usually affected. There is pain and swelling along an inflamed and tender superficial vein. In such cases, the thrombus is firmly attached to the vein wall, so there is little risk of pulmonary embolism. In the calves, there is often an undetected deep extension of the thrombosis and a period of anticoagulation is wise.

Pelvic thrombophlebitis may occur following caesarean section, and treatment involves antibiotics and a course of heparin.

HAEMATOLOGICAL DISORDERS

Physiological Changes in Pregnancy

The increases in plasma volume and red cell mass are described in Chapter 7.

As the expansion of plasma volume is greater than that of red cell mass, red cell count, haematocrit and haemoglobin concentrations tend to fall during pregnancy. Nevertheless, total circulating haemoglobin is higher than before pregnancy.

Iron Deficiency Anaemia

In pregnancy, nutritional iron deficiency anaemia is the most common haematological problem. It is found in between 20% and 30% of pregnancies, being more common with lower social grade, multiparity, a previous history of menorrhagia and in women whose nutrition is poor. Chronic infection, particularly urinary tract infection, is an important cause. The World Health Organization has suggested that, in pregnancy, the minimum acceptable haemoglobin concentration is 11.0 g/dl.

Iron metabolism

Iron is required mainly for the expanding red cell mass and for the fetus and placenta. The requirement for pregnancy is about 4 mg of iron per day. A normal daily diet contains 10–20 mg, but of this only 1–2 mg may be absorbed. Approximately 120 mg of iron is conserved by amenorrhoea, so an extra 800–1300 mg of iron are required during pregnancy.

Table 10.1
Diagnosis for Iron Deficient Anaemia in Pregnancy

Red cell indices			**Normal range**	**Iron deficiency**
Mean Corpuscular Volume (MCV)	=	Packed Cell Volume (PVC) / Red Cell Count (RBC)	75–99 fl	Decreased
Mean Corpuscular Haemoglobin (MCH)	=	Haemoglobin concentration (Hb) / Red Cell Count (RBC)	27–31 pg	Decreased
Mean Corpuscular Haemoglobin Concentration (MCMH)	=	Haemoglobin concentration (Hb) / Packed Cell Volume (PVC)	32–36 g/dl	Decreased
Biochemistry				
Serum iron			13–27 μmol/l	<9 μmol/l
Total iron binding capacity			45–72 μmol/l	>98.5 μmol/l
Ferritin			10–150 μg/l	<10 μg/l

Diagnosis

Iron deficiency is most often diagnosed from the results of a peripheral blood count. When iron stores are depleted, there is a reduction in serum iron; this is followed by a reduction in haemoglobin concentration (Table 10.1).

Marrow biopsy. Marrow aspiration is rarely indicated in pregnancy. If required, a sample obtained from the iliac crest or the sternum is reliable in assessing iron stores.

Prophylaxis and treatment

The World Health Organization recommends that supplements of 30 to 60 mg of elemental iron per day be given to pregnant women with normal iron stores, and 120 to 240 mg to women with low stores. Supplementation with a daily dose of iron from about 16 weeks of pregnancy until delivery will maintain the stores and prevent iron deficiency anaemia. Side-effects of oral administration of iron, such as nausea, epigastric pain, diarrhoea and constipation occur in about 20% of women. Most preparations used commonly in pregnancy now contain small amounts of folic acid.

There is a risk that folate deficiency will occur in the anaemic patient who is responding to iron treatment, and in patients who have an antepartum haemorrhage.

Megaloblastic Anaemia

Megaloblastic anaemia should be suspected when the expected response to adequate iron treatment is not achieved. Sometimes, after an initial haemopoietic response to iron, no further increase in haemoglobin occurs until folic acid supplements are given.

Diagnosis

In megaloblastic anaemia, haemoglobin concentration is usually below 10.0 g/dl and films of the buffy coat layer show hypersegmented neutrophils, Howell-Jolly nuclear inclusion bodies, nucleated red cells, orthochromatic macrocytes and giant polymorphs. Serum and red cell folate are decreased. It is important to exclude vitamin B_{12} deficiency in patients from the Indian subcontinent and in vegetarians.

In the puerperium, folate levels are often low, sometimes being depleted by the haemopoietic response to blood loss at delivery. Lactation increases the demand on folate, while on the other hand, the diminished folic acid absorption of pregnancy and the requirements of the fetus have been relieved. If megaloblastic anaemia has been undiagnosed and untreated in late pregnancy, it may persist and need management in the puerperium. Megaloblastic anaemia arising *de novo* in the puerperium is rare, and the response of puerperal anaemia to iron treatment alone is usually as good as if folic acid supplements were given as well.

Prophylaxis and treatment

For prophylaxis in pregnancy, folic acid 300 to 500 μg is given daily, usually in the form of iron and folic acid preparations. Prophylaxis is particularly important in the grand multipara, in multiple pregnancy, in patients with a malabsorption syndrome, in those taking anticonvulsants or sulfasalazine, during treatment with co-trimoxazole or antimalarial drugs, and in patients with haemolytic anaemia (who do not need iron). In all these groups, folic acid, 5 mg daily is an appropriate dose.

For the treatment of proven folic acid deficiency, 5 mg orally, three times daily, should be prescribed. Reticulocytosis usually occurs about 5 days after initiation of treatment.

In malabsorption states, i.m. injections of folic acid, 3 mg each week, may be needed and, by implication, should be accompanied with mixed parenteral B vitamins.

Vitamin B_{12} deficiency

Megaloblastic anaemia of pregnancy from B_{12} deficiency is rare in the United Kingdom and is due to inadequate diet, malabsorption syndrome and, rarely, true pernicious anaemia.

When macrocytic anaemia and low serum vitamin B_{12} levels are found, hydroxycobalamin should be given i.m., 1 mg every 2 months.

Haemolytic Anaemias

Red cell survival span is shortened either by an intrinsic red cell abnormality or by an extrinsic factor. Reticulocyte counts are usually increased. Iron treatment is only indicated if serum iron levels are low, and then it should be oral, as otherwise there is a risk of iron overload.

Intrinsic red cell defects

Hereditary spherocytosis and elliptocytosis. This condition is diagnosed by appearances of a blood film. Inheritance is dominant, hence the baby should be investigated when parents are affected. Treatment is usually with folic acid and, if necessary, by blood transfusion.

Haemoglobinopathies. These are inherited defects in haemoglobin resulting from impaired globin synthesis.

β-chain haemoglobin variants such as HbS and HbC are common in black Africans and white Mediterranean women. Clinical manifestations occur mainly in the homozygous patient. If the sickle cell test is positive, electrophoresis is performed. In homozygous sickle cell disease, the patients are particularly prone to infection; thrombotic episodes or bone crises which may be precipitated by infection and dehydration. Fetal loss is increased in pregnant women with sickle cell disease, but not in the heterozygous form. Many cases do not need treatment other than folic acid and, if a patient has already had a successful pregnancy without haemolytic crises, it is a mistake to submit her to intensive treatment. In patients who do need treatment, repeated blood transfusions may be required to maintain HbA levels at 60–70%.

During labour, hypoxia, acidosis and hypotension must be avoided and prophylactic antibiotics should be given. It may be considered that the best way of achieving this is caesarean section, but this is unreasonable in a woman who has previously had a normal confinement without complications.

Thalassaemia. Homozygous α-thalassaemia is incompatible with life and the fetus becomes hydropic *in utero* or shortly after birth. Patients with homozygous β-thalassaemia (Cooley's anaemia) often die in childhood. If they do survive and conceive, pregnancy does not seem to affect the disease process adversely.

Heterozygous thalassaemia patients are usually healthy apart from mild anaemia, and normal pregnancy is possible.

Antenatal diagnosis of the status of the fetus is important if both parents carry the trait. Fetal blood sampling can be performed by cordocentesis and legal abortion may be requested. Methods of DNA analysis on chorion biopsies convey less risk.

In maternal thalassaemia in pregnancy, the red cells have a reduced haemoglobin content, and anaemia may be severe. There is a large decrease in MCV and MCH values, but the MCHC is within the normal range. In pregnancy, the haemoglobin concentration should be maintained above 8 g/dl, and routine treatment is with folic acid, 5 mg orally, three times a day. Blood transfusion may be necessary. Iron supplementation is contraindicated unless there is iron deficiency.

Glucose-6-phosphate dehydrogenase deficiency has a sex-linked inheritance. Oxidation of haemoglobin leads to formation of methaemoglobin, and drugs like sulphonamides, salicylates, nitrofurantoin, nalidixic acid, antimalarials and vitamin K may precipitate a haemolytic crisis. If these drugs are being given to the mother in late pregnancy, transplacental passage may lead to haemolytic problems in the newborn.

Extrinsic haemolytic anaemias

Auto-immune haemolytic disease can be divided into warm antibody and cold antibody types. About 50% of patients with warm antibody haemolytic anaemia have demonstrable underlying disorders, such as systemic lupus erythematosus or lymphoma. The blood shows polychromasia with spherocytes and a reticulocytosis and Coombs' test is positive. Treatment is with corticosteroids. The cold antibody type is associated with infections, particularly with *Mycoplasma pneumoniae.* Red cells undergo autoagglutination at 4°C, which is dispersed at 37°C. The direct Coombs' test is positive. Treatment is not usually required. Many drugs can, rarely, cause haemolysis.

Coagulation Disorders

Immune thrombocytopenic purpura

This auto-immune disorder tends to occur in women during the childbearing years. With careful management, prognosis for mother and baby is fairly good.

When patients are in remission at the onset of pregnancy, two-thirds of them will have uneventful pregnancies. A short course of steroids (prednisolone 10 mg/day) started a day or two before labour is anticipated and continued with parenteral hydrocortisone during the confinement may prevent neonatal thrombocytopenia. The latter condition is usually self-limiting over the first few weeks of life, if it does occur. Patients not in remission at the start of pregnancy, those having recurrences during pregnancy, and those where the disease develops during pregnancy need full doses of steroids (prednisolone 20–40 mg/day, increased to 60–100 mg/day before a planned delivery). Intravenous normal immunoglobulin may also be needed.

The objective should be a planned vaginal delivery, avoiding episiotomy, with good control of the third stage, including i.v. ergometrine, controlled cord traction, and immediate manual removal of the placenta if the cord breaks. Platelet transfusions may be needed before caesarean section or if haemorrhage occurs.

Von Willebrand's disease

This is the most common clinically significant abnormality of blood coagulation in women. It is characterised by a prolonged bleeding time, decreased levels of factor VIII and defective platelet function.

In general, factor VIII levels of more than 30% do not require treatment in pregnancy. Levels of 60% or more are associated with safe vaginal delivery, 100% levels are recommended for caesarean section. One transfusion of fresh frozen plasma daily will maintain levels of factor VIII, three units of fresh frozen plasma or six units of cryoprecipitate produce a maximal level.

Disseminated intravascular coagulation

This term is used to indicate a range of consumption coagulopathies associated with prolonged retention of a dead fetus, severe pre-eclampsia, placental abruption, amniotic fluid infusion, Gram-negative sepsis and prolonged shock of any aetiology. The features of the full syndrome are a coagulopathy, a low platelet count and the presence of fragmented red cells in the peripheral blood. Fibrin degradation products in the plasma are elevated, but the use of this as a diagnostic feature is limited, as all the associated conditions can also have this effect. With abruptio placentae, the predominant characteristic is hypofibrinogenaemia. Sometimes, there is considerable activation of fibrinolytic enzymes.

In the serious acute situation with bleeding, management is with fresh blood, fresh frozen plasma and cryoprecipitate with central venous pressure monitoring; and sometimes platelet infusions. The definitive manoeuvre is to deliver the baby, when improvement will ensue. Even if there is evidence of fibrinolysis, antifibrinolytic agents are best avoided, as renal infarction and other ischaemic organ damage can occur. Sepsis must be treated vigorously with broad spectrum antibiotics and the patient managed by maintenance of cardiovascular, respiratory and renal systems in an intensive care situation.

In less acute situations where there is no active bleeding, heparin infusions are of value and may protect the kidney from deposition of fibrin and red cell fragments in the glomeruli. Response is monitored by platelet counts and fibrin degradation product levels. Dipyridamole infusions, low dose oral aspirin and prostacyclin infusions have also been used.

DISEASES OF THE RESPIRATORY SYSTEM

The respiratory system adapts to the physiological stress of pregnancy more easily than does the cardiovascular system. Nevertheless, as many as 70% of previously normal women experience dyspnoea at some time during pregnancy, this being most common at term.

Physiological Changes in Pregnancy

Oxygen consumption rises by an average of 18% from 250 ml/min to about 300 ml/min. About one-third of the increased oxygen consumption is required by the fetus and placenta, the remainder is for maternal metabolism.

Pulmonary function testing in the normal pregnant patient shows an increased minute ventilation due to an increased tidal volume, with no change in respiratory rate. Tidal volume increases by about 40% from 500 to 700 ml. In the second half of pregnancy, functional residual capacity and total lung capacity are reduced, but vital capacity is unchanged.

Ventilation increases twice as much as oxygen consumption and so arterial P_{CO_2} falls, with an equivalent fall in plasma bicarbonate, while arterial P_{O_2} remains fairly constant. The increased progesterone influence in pregnancy affects the respiratory centre, and there is also an increased sensitivity to carbon dioxidc, resulting in the increase in ventilation.

Bronchial Asthma

About 1% of pregnancies are complicated by acute asthma, but the risk to the fetus is very small. Asthma is not generally affected by pregnancy, though a few patients deteriorate symptomatically in every pregnancy. If one parent has asthma, the risk of the child having asthma is doubled compared to the general population.

Classically, asthmatics have been divided into two clinical groups, extrinsic and intrinsic.

Extrinsic

Affected individuals are usually younger and have had their disease since childhood. Their attacks are often seasonal, precipitated by allergens and accompanied by a history of hay fever or atopic dermatitis.

Intrinsic

Intrinsic asthma is an adult onset illness without an atopic history and requires long-term treatment. Associated bronchitis is common.

Treatment

The presence of green or yellow purulent sputum is evidence of chest infection, and an appropriate broad spectrum antibiotic should be prescribed. Tetracycline should not be used after 16 weeks, because it colours fetal teeth brown.

A rational principle is to use as little as possible of the safest drug required to keep the patient free from symptoms. For occasional attacks, selective β_2-sympathomimetic bronchodilators, salbutamol or terbutaline inhalers are used. It should be noted that ritodrine is devoid of bronchodilator activity. When there are more frequent attacks, prophylactic treatment is with sodium cromoglicate inhaled 6 to 8 times a day, reducing to 4 times a day to maintain control. If cromoglicate fails, steroid aerosols like beclometasone dipropionate or fluticasone dipropionate may be used. Theophylline or aminophylline may be added to the regimen. If there is no improvement in the patient's condition, corticosteroids in a titrated dose are used to control asthma, beginning for example, with a high dose of 20–30 mg prednisolone for 2–3 days and reducing progressively until symptoms begin to recur. Once steroid treatment is initiated in pregnancy, it is better to continue a maintenance dose until the pregnancy is over.

Objective measurement of airway obstruction using a peak flowmeter or a spirometer is important in the management of asthma. This is useful to establish the severity and to confirm objectively that treatment is effective.

When the asthmatic goes into labour, treatment with inhaled β-sympathomimetic agents should be used first. The corticosteroid-dependent asthmatic should be given hydrocortisone 100 mg i.m., every 8 hours to cover the course of labour. Epidural analgesia is preferable to narcotic analgesics but when general anaesthesia is required, it is not contraindicated.

Respiratory Infections

Influenza

In relation to pregnancy, influenza is associated with a higher fatality rate than in non-pregnant women. In general, the condition is self-limiting and the patient improves with symptomatic treatment, such as bed rest, antipyretics, and increase in fluid intake. The influenza virus can cross the placenta. No definite congenital defects have been attributed to it, but there is some evidence of a slightly increased rate of childhood leukaemia in the offspring (4/1000). Effective vaccination is with a live attenuated virus, and is best delayed until the second trimester, but it is desirable when an epidemic is anticipated.

Bacterial pneumonia

Bacterial pneumonias are commonly due to *Streptococcus pneumoniae, Haemophilus influenzae, Mycoplasma* and the haemolytic streptococcus. Pneumococcal pneumonia classically begins with a shaking chill, pleuritic chest pain, fever, cough and dyspnoea. Chest X-ray evidence of lobar consolidation may help to distinguish it from pulmonary embolism and infarction. A sample of sputum should be sent for culture and antibiotics such as amoxicillin, erythromycin or a cephalosporin prescribed. As premature labour is a definite risk associated with pyrexia, antipyretic measures, such as tepid sponging and paracetamol, should be used in addition to aggressive antibiotic treatment.

Bronchitis and bronchiectasis

Management is as with non-pregnant patients, except that the use of iodine containing expectorants and tetracyclines is contraindicated.

Pulmonary tuberculosis

Pulmonary tuberculosis in pregnancy is becoming less common. Chest radiography in pregnancy should be performed in those populations at significant risk and in those in contact with the disease.

In general, with treatment, pregnancy has no unfavourable effect upon the course of the disease. There is no good evidence that the outcome of pregnancy is adversely affected by tuberculosis, although transplacental passage of the tubercle bacilli to the fetus has been reported.

Cough, purulent sputum, fever, weight loss and chest pain occur in pulmonary tuberculosis. Diagnosis is usually made from chest X-ray findings and the presence of acid-fast bacilli on examination and culture of the sputum. The Mantoux test becomes positive 1 to 3 months after a primary infecton. Treatment of the mother should in general be as if she were not pregnant. There are still lingering doubts about the safety of rifampicin for the developing fetus and treatment with this drug is sometimes postponed until after the first trimester. Actual hearing loss in the infant due to streptomycin given to the mother is uncommon. Ethionamide may be teratogenic and is not used in pregnancy.

There is a risk of the neonate being infected by the mother with sputum positive active disease, although the risk is minimal a few days after chemotherapy has been initiated. Exposed babies may be protected with isoniazid and tuberculin tested after 3 to 6 months. There is no need to separate the baby from the mother.

Cystic Fibrosis

This is an inherited disease with between 1 in 20 and 1 in 50 carrying the gene. Heterozygous people are asymptomatic, but homozygous people are affected, the incidence being 1 in 2300 births. Fertility is markedly impaired, particularly in males. In pregnancy, maternal mortality is the same as the general rate for women with the disease. Pulmonary hypertension and pancreatic insufficiency are adverse prognostic factors. Perinatal mortality is increased, and related to degree of dyspnoea and cyanosis before pregnancy. Maternal weight gain in pregnancy is poor, but the fetus grows normally.

Management in pregnancy includes monitoring of pulmonary function and continued physiotherapy. Any suggestion of infection is treated promptly with hospital admission and antibiotics. Vaginal delivery is preferred; epidural analgesia is useful and general anaesthesia is avoided if possible. The risk of occurrence of pneumothorax in the second stage of labour may be reduced by elective forceps delivery.

GASTROINTESTINAL DISORDERS

Vomiting and Heartburn

The vomiting centre in the reticular formation of the medulla controls vomiting. Irritation of the mucosa of the upper gastrointestinal tract generates impulses which are relayed by the sympathetic nerves and the vagi to the vomiting centre. Emotionally charged stimuli causing emesis are also conducted to the vomiting centre from the diencephalon and limbic system. Circulating chemical agents may stimulate the chemoreceptor trigger zone in the medulla which can initiate vomiting.

Morning sickness

The term 'morning sickness' is used to describe mild symptoms of nausea and vomiting, often occurring at other times in the day, between 6 and 14 weeks of pregnancy. The incidence is between 50% and 80%. Usually there is some disturbance of appetite, but in general there are no signs of disturbed nutrition. The aetiology of morning sickness is uncertain, but oestrogen has been suggested to be a cause, as has excess human chorionic gonadotrophin. Cultural attitudes and social disturbance during pregnancy may also be associated.

It is important to exclude medical and surgical causes before attributing vomiting to pregnancy alone. Following explanation of the possible aetiology, all that may then be required is to stop any oral iron treatment and to give simple advice on taking small frequent meals containing a lot of carbohydrate. When an antiemetic is indicated, an antihistamine with or without pyridoxine should be selected initially. Promethazine has been widely used for many years.

Hyperemesis gravidarum

Hyperemesis gravidarum is a term applied when the patient develops intractable vomiting with ketosis, acetonuria, alteration of electrolyte imbalance and weight loss of 5% or more. If untreated, renal and liver damage and neurological disturbances may occur. This condition may be associated with hydatidiform mole, multiple pregnancy and hydramnios.

The immediate management of hyperemesis involves correction of fluid and electrolyte balance, parenteral vitamins, bed rest and sometimes sedation. Phenothiazines and related drugs have antiemetic and sedative properties and are suitable for use parenterally for 1 to 3 days at a time. Promethazine, 25 mg, promazine, 50 mg or chlorpromazine 25 to 50 mg, may be given i.m. three times a day, or prochlorperazine, 5 or 25 mg rectally, 8-hourly for up to 24 hours. Metoclopramide, 5–10 mg i.m., may also be useful. Steroids are occasionally useful in controlling recurrence. In certain cases, subsequent care may include psychiatric consultation.

Vomiting in late pregnancy

Vomiting sometimes recurs in the last few weeks of pregnancy in women who have had troublesome vomiting in the early months. Nevertheless, full investigations should be undertaken as it may be due to a serious condition. The vomiting often appears to be due to mechanical factors, such as gastro-oesophageal reflux, but the possibility of other conditions, such as urinary tract infections, pre-eclampsia, acute hydramnios, gastroenteritis and appendicitis, cholecystitis, pancreatitis or intestinal obstruction must also be considered.

Heartburn and hiatus hernia

Heartburn often accompanies nausea and vomiting and is especially common in late pregnancy. It is due to regurgitation of gastric contents into the oesophagus. The reflux of bile is even more irritant than reflux of gastric acid. The reduced tone in the muscle of the lower oesophagus is probably responsible for regurgitation. Other factors such as increased intragastric pressure, pyloric sphincter incompetence and hormone influences may be related.

In the first trimester, it is best to confine treatment to simple dietary measures, avoidance of lying flat and simple antacids. Magnesium trisilicate mixture or an antacid mixture with alginate are adequate for most purposes. Magnesium hydroxide mixture may be used in patients who have a tendency to constipation.

In late pregnancy, a gastric motility stimulant such as metoclopramine, preparations containing local anaesthetics such as oxetacaine, gastric antispasmodics such as belladonna alkaloids and their synthetic analogues, may all be given to alleviate symptoms.

Hiatus hernia is a well recognised cause of heartburn in pregnancy. It appears to be more common in women with advancing age and multiparity. Ten to twenty per cent of women in late pregnancy have been shown to have some degree of hiatus hernia. Severe heartburn with pain radiating to the neck is made worse by lying down, stooping or straining. An antacid at night and several pillows will help. Rarely, haematemesis may occur.

Ptyalism

Ptyalism, which is excessive salivation and compulsive expectoration is a rare complication of early pregnancy of neuropsychiatric origin. It sometimes results in mild hypokalaemia, but without systemic effects. The condition is self-limiting and no specific treatment is required.

Peptic Ulceration

The incidence of peptic ulceration during pregnancy is low. In nearly 23,000 deliveries, only 12 patients were admitted for ulcer-like symptoms and of these only 6 were thought to be active. Most women with a history of peptic ulceration seem to improve during pregnancy, probably due to reduction in gastric secretion of acid. Perforation is very rare in pregnancy. In the third trimester, acidity in the stomach may be increased with delayed gastric motility. This may explain the occasional complication of peptic ulceration occurring in pregnancy. Quiescent ulcers may suddenly become active in the puerperium, presenting with haemorrhage.

Management in pregnancy follows general principles in peptic ulcer treatment. Mucosal barrier strengtheners, such as carbenoxolone, have side-effects of salt and water retention, hypokalaemia and occasionally, raised blood pressure. Their use in pregnancy has been limited. Histamine H_2 receptor antagonists, cimetidine and ranitidine, may be used in late pregnancy for the treatment of peptic ulceration. Radical antibiotic treatment for *Heliobacter pylori* is best postponed until after pregnancy.

As a general rule, the pregnant woman with severe gastric haemorrhage or perforation should be treated as if the patient is not pregnant. Hesitation to operate on a pregnant patient with a perforated ulcer and peritonitis yields a high mortality.

Acute Appendicitis

Acute appendicitis is seen with equal frequency in the first two trimesters of pregnancy and only slightly less often in the third trimester.

Pregnancy confuses the clinical picture of acute appendicitis. The base of the appendix is pushed upwards and outwards by the enlarging uterus, causing the appendiceal inflammatory reaction to occur progressively higher and more laterally in the abdomen. The diagnosis becomes more difficult and peritoneal involvement occurs more readily in late pregnancy.

The normal leucocytosis of pregnancy (up to $15 \times 10^9/l$) makes this guide unreliable. Urinary tract symptoms and abnormalities of urine analysis are common during pregnancy and make the differentiation between appendicitis and urinary tract infection difficult. Other causes like cholecystitis, renal colic, or torsion of an ovarian cyst should be considered.

The mortality of appendicitis in pregnancy is the result of delay. Where real doubt exists, it is far better to perform a laparotomy. Appendicectomy performed during pregnancy for an appendix that is found to be normal carries only minimal risk for mother and fetus. Antibiotics should be used in all cases to reduce the chance of infection.

Intestinal Obstruction

The most common cause is strangulation by bands of adhesions from previous operations, which become stretched by the enlarging uterus. Vomiting secondary to bowel obstruction occurring in early pregnancy may be mistaken for morning sickness and the pain of obstruction late in pregnancy may be similar to that of labour pains. The presence of surgical abdominal scars, localised tenderness, a peristaltic rush and air-fluid levels in an upright X-ray film may help to diagnose intestinal obstruction. Volvulus may occur.

Adequate replacement of fluid and electrolytes should be achieved before surgery. The obstruction must be identified and relieved; necrotic bowel requires resection; obstruction of the colon requires colostomy. If the pregnancy is close to term, a caesarean section may be necessary to give access to the intestinal obstruction.

Non-Specific Inflammatory Intestinal Disorders

This group of intestinal disorders include ulcerative colitis, Crohn's disease and non-specific colitis. They occur almost equally between females and males and usually manifest before the age of 30 years. The incidence in developed countries is between 40 and 100 per 100,000 population and is probably lower in developing countries. Ulcerative colitis is more common than Crohn's disease, but this difference is becoming less marked.

Well-managed inflammatory bowel disease has a good fetal outcome in 70–90% of cases where the disease presents before pregnancy, even if a relapse occurs in pregnancy. There appears to be no overall increase in the incidence of congenital defects.

Between 40% and 50% of affected women have a clinical relapse during pregnancy. Relapse may occur at any time during pregnancy, but is more likely during the first trimester and early in the puerperium.

Management. Patients should be encouraged to embark on a pregnancy when their disease is clinically quiescent, and when taking a minimum number of drugs. When they are seen before conception, any anaemia should be treated and folic acid and B vitamin supplements should be prescribed to continue in pregnancy. Management during pregnancy should involve monthly monitoring with blood counts and estimations of serum iron, folic acid, calcium, phosphate and, in severe cases, magnesium. Hospital rest is a primary measure in treatment of exacerbations.

Ulcerative colitis

Medical treatment suppresses disease activity, but never cures. Mild attacks can be treated with sulfasalazine and topical steroids.

Sulfasalazine is considered safe for use throughout pregnancy and also in breast feeding mothers. It impairs absorption of folic acid and supplements of 5–10 mg/day will be required in pregnancy. There is a small risk of neonatal jaundice.

Local applications of corticosteroids in the form of prednisolone enemas are preferable in mild cases when the disease is confined to the lower bowel. Patients with severe bowel symptoms, and those who fail to respond to topical steroids, need bed rest, an adequate diet, correction of fluid and electrolyte deficits, especially potassium, the correction of anaemia and treatment with systemic steroids.

Oral broad-spectrum antibiotics aggravate ulcerative colitis and should be avoided. The value of intravenous antibiotics in severe attacks is not well established.

Crohn's disease

Simple measures should be tried before any treatment. Fluid stools can often be controlled by codeine phosphate and bulk-forming agents are helpful in colonic disease. Patients should be allowed a full diet with adequate protein. Diarrhoea may respond to eliminating milk from the diet. Supplementation with folic acid is advisable and vitamin B_{12} is essential in patients with ileal disease or after ileal resection.

Sulfasalazine may improve symptoms in patients with modestly active disease. Broad-spectrum antibiotics are indicated in patients with intra-abdominal or perianal sepsis. Corticosteroids are indicated in acutely ill patients or for persistent disabling disease which has failed to respond to simpler measures. Azathioprine may be used to maintain a steroid-induced remission. The clinical response often requires a latent period of several weeks.

Indications for surgery in ulcerative colitis and Crohn's disease during pregnancy are usually perforation, toxic megacolon and, rarely, intestinal obstruction.

Patients who have been on corticosteroids should have hydrocortisone 100 mg i.m. every 8 hours to cover general anaesthesia, a surgical procedure or labour.

Constipation

There is a tendency to constipation during pregnancy. This may be due to increased sodium and water absorption in the colon and general hypotonia of the intestine, caused by increased progesterone activity on smooth muscle, and constipation is sometimes aggravated by iron supplements given in pregnancy. Simple measures include advice on a diet containing a high fibre content, bran and adequate fluids. Cellulose-containing foodstuffs and hydrophilic stool bulking agents should be the initial treatment. If these fail, magnesium hydroxide mixture, senna, or bisacodyl may be used. Purgatives such as liquid paraffin should be avoided for they impair absorption of fat-soluble vitamins A, D and K.

Diseases of the Liver

Liver diseases can be caused by conditions which are associated with and peculiar to pregnancy or conditions which are unrelated to pregnancy.

Conditions peculiar to pregnancy

Hyperemesis gravidarum. In severe cases of hyperemesis gravidarum, jaundice may occur. If so, then the odds are strong that the diagnosis of viral or toxic hepatitis or, rarely, fatty degeneration, has been missed.

Pre-eclampsia and eclampsia. Liver dysfunction has been detected in about 18% of pre-eclamptic and eclamptic patients and is due to ischaemia. The right upper quadrant pain sometimes present in severe pre-eclampsia is traditionally due to hepatic oedema and haemorrhage, with distension of Glisson's capsule. Subcapsular haemorrhage is now uncommon and if haemorrhage into the liver occurs, it is usually parenchymal. Pruritus does not usually occur. The level of serum transaminase, usually slightly raised in pregnancy (50–300 iu/l), is a sensitive guide to hepatocellular involvement. Bilirubin elevations are usually mild and reflect both hepatic dysfunction and intravascular haemolysis.

Acute fatty liver. This is a rare, but serious, complication of unknown aetiology, characterised by the accumulation of microvesicular fat in the hepatic parenchyma. Patients present in the third trimester of pregnancy or in the puerperium with abdominal pain, nausea, vomiting and varying degrees of jaundice. Pruritus is unusual. The course of acute fatty liver of pregnancy is characterised by the rapid progression to acute hepatic failure, with coagulation disturbances and encephalopathy. In contrast to hepatitis, the disease has a short prodromal period, abdominal pain is a predominant feature, and serum transaminase and alkaline phosphatase levels are only moderately elevated. Complications include hypoglycaemia, gastrointestinal bleeding, renal failure and metabolic acidosis. Remission of the disease is frequently observed after the pregnancy; vaginal delivery is preferred.

Intrahepatic cholestasis of pregnancy. This condition, which is related to excess oestrogen influence, is due to an exaggeration of the difficulty in transport of bilirubin into the biliary canaliculi in pregnancy. The predominant symptom is pruritus due to accumulation of bile acids in the skin and jaundice is usually mild. Right upper quadrant abdominal pain is rarely present and the general health of the patient is usually unaffected. Liver enzymes, and particularly alkaline phosphatase, are elevated. Extrahepatic causes of cholestasis and drug toxicity must be excluded.

Antipruritic drugs, such as antihistamines, are only partly effective; potentially hepatotoxic agents must be avoided. Cholestyramine has been used to alleviate pruritus, but it is not very effective. Adiometionine, 800 mg twice daily, has produced symptomatic relief. Regular vitamin K injections should be given to the mother for 2 weeks before labour is anticipated to prevent fetal haemorrhage. Fetal outcome is generally good.

Patients with a history of intrahepatic cholestasis of pregnancy should avoid the oral contraceptive pill thereafter.

Conditions incidental to pregnancy

Acute viral hepatitis. This may be due to hepatitis A (infective hepatitis) or to hepatitis B (serum hepatitis).

In hepatitis A, the infective agent is found only in faeces and transmission is by the oral-faecal route. The onset is usually abrupt with gastrointestinal symptoms, low-grade fever and general influenza-like manifestations. Recent infection is confirmed by a rising titre of anti-HA IgM. Hepatitis A usually resolves within 2 to 3 weeks and chronic hepatitis is not observed.

In hepatitis B, the infective agent can be detected in the blood. Transmission is parenteral with a high incidence in drug addicts. Maternal-fetal transmission also occurs. The disease has a long incubation period with a prodrome of arthralgia and urticaria. In the acute period, hepatitis B antigen (Hb_sAg) is present in the serum. This may be followed by Hb_eAg in serum. When the 'e' or core antigen is present, there is a high incidence of neonatal hepatitis B infection.

Hepatitis B Carriage. The incidence of symptomless carriers of hepatitis B surface antigen among antenatal patients varies greatly from country to country. It is highest in Africa and South-East Asia. The incidence in Europe is about 0.5%, with most of the carriers coming from the higher incidence areas. Carriers of the 'e' antigen (mainly patients of Far East extraction) are by far the most infectious and are likely to transmit the infection to their babies. Hepatitis B antibody positive patients are usually immune and not infectious. The disease is blood-borne, and so it is desirable that medical and nursing staff should be immunised, but precautions should also be taken to prevent cross-infection. The babies of 'e' antigen positive mothers should be immunised with anti-hepatitis B immunoglobulin and a vaccine genetically engineered from yeast. The vaccine should also be given to staff when there is a possibility of infection.

Hepatitis C appears to infect as many as 0.6% of the pregnant population. Vertical transmission to the baby occurs in 7–8%. Breast feeding is contraindicated.

Acute pancreatitis. Although rare, acute pancreatitis in pregnancy has a maternal mortality of 20%. Biliary tract disease is a prominent cause. In pregnancy, it has been suggested that the actions of progesterone may promote bile reflux into the pancreatic duct, and that hyperlipidaemia, which occurs normally in pregnancy, may cause pancreatitis. About half the cases of pancreatitis in pregnancy occur during the third trimester.

NERVOUS SYSTEM DISORDERS

Epilepsy

The prevalence rates for epilepsy vary from about 5% of the population who will suffer a non-febrile epileptic seizure during their lifetime, to about 0.5% with chronic epilepsy. The risk of an epileptic adult having a child with epilepsy is small, about 1 in 30; but still 5 times that for the general population. The risk is greatest among those with an electroencephalographic pattern showing symmetrical three cycles per second spikes and slow wave discharges.

In pregnancy, it has been estimated that one-third of epileptics will suffer an increase in seizures, one-third a decrease and in one-third there will be no significant change. Factors responsible for the increased frequency of seizures may be a fall in the plasma concentrations of the anticonvulsant drugs. This can be due to decreased drug absorption, increased hepatic metabolism and impaired patient compliance.

Some patients develop seizures for the first time during pregnancy or the puerperium. Care should be taken to distinguish petit mal in particular from syncope in early pregnancy. A small number of patients suffer seizures only during pregnancy or the puerperium. It should be remembered that some cerebral tumours increase in size during pregnancy, and the development of seizures may be the first sign of this condition.

Clinical differentiation between epilepsy and eclampsia may be difficult. In eclampsia, there is usually a history of signs and symptoms of pre-eclampsia such as hypertension and proteinuria, and there may have been severe headache, visual disturbances, epigastric pain and vomiting.

In epilepsy, blood pressure is unchanged, and proteinuria and oliguria are not features.

Management

This should begin in a preconception clinic. The decision whether to treat in pregnancy is generally made on the same grounds as for non-pregnant patients. The risks of uncontrolled seizures to the fetus are greater than the risks of exposure to anticonvulsant drugs. If a woman having treatment for epilepsy is planning a pregnancy, it is best if she can be controlled on a single drug with monitoring of free plasma or salivary levels. Nevertheless, if a patient is on combination therapy to control seizures and is found to be pregnant, it can sometimes be best to continue on the same drug regimen. Sudden withdrawal or change of drug therapy may lead to status epilepticus.

In general, the choice of drugs in pregnancy should be governed by the same considerations as in the non-pregnant patient. Phenobarbitone may be best if epileptics can be managed on a barbiturate alone. If anticonvulsants are to be used in pregnancy, folic acid supplements (5 mg/day) should be started well before conception, as there is evidence that the teratogenicity of anticonvulsants is related to effects on folate absorption and metabolism. Rarely, the frequency of fits increases with folic acid, so there should be ample time to adjust anticonvulsant dose. Folic acid supplements also prevent development of megaloblastic anaemia. Prophylactic vitamin K tablets should be started 2 weeks before delivery is anticipated; 5 mg of phytomenadione i.m. should be given to the mother at the onset of labour and 0.5–1 mg i.m. to the newborn to reduce the risk of neonatal haemorrhage when phenytoin or barbiturates have been used at the end of pregnancy.

There is a two- to three-fold increase in the incidence of congenital malformations in the offspring of epileptic mothers treated with anticonvulsants, but not given preconception folic acid. It must be made clear to the potential mother that there is a 95% chance that she will have a normal baby.

Breast feeding is not in general contraindicated when mothers are on anticonvulsant drugs, though occasionally a "sleepy baby" may result.

Cerebrovascular Disease

Arterial occlusive disease

Ischaemic stroke presents with the sudden onset of deficits in the central nervous system function such as hemiplegia, hemianopia, aphasia and apraxia. The incidence of an arterial occlusion in pregnancy and the puerperium has been assessed at 1 per 20,000 live births, with a mortality rate about three times that in non-pregnant women. Middle cerebral artery occlusion is the most common finding in pregnancy and internal carotid artery occlusion in the puerperium. The differential diagnosis in late pregnancy is cerebral vascular spasm.

Cerebral phlebothrombosis

Aseptic cerebral venous thrombosis usually presents in the second or third week after delivery. It presents with severe headaches, usually culminating in generalised and focal seizures, which are followed by weakness, aphasia and other deficits in cerebral cortical function. If the patient survives the initial episode, long-term prognosis is good, but a progression of symptoms is a poor prognostic sign.

Subarachnoid haemorrhage

In normal pregnancy, the incidence of spontaneous subarachnoid haemorrhage is not increased. A majority of cases are due to ruptured berry aneurysms on the circle of Willis and less frequently to arteriovenous malformations, which have a tendency to rupture during labour. Patients may have hypertension, and may complain of a sudden onset of severe headach, neck stiffness and nausea. The finding of heavily and uniformly blood-stained cerebrospinal fluid at lumbar puncture confirms the diagnosis.

About a third of the patients die within 24 hours. In those who survive, initial treatment is sedation and bed rest. Delivery is by caesarean section or, in selected cases, vaginal delivery with full epidural anaesthesia to prevent bearing down. Diagnosis of cerebral vascular lesions involves cerebral angiography and computerised axial tomography (CAT) or nuclear magnetic resonance (NMR) scans.

Chorea Gravidarum

Jerky purposeless movements associated with limb hypotonia acquired during pregnancy usually begin after the first trimester and cease within 2 or 3 months after childbirth. There is a strong link with a history of rheumatic fever. These movements are absent during sleep. Severe chorea can lead to rhabdomyolysis, myoglobinuria and hyperthermia. Treatment is with chlorpromazine or haloperidol.

Brain Tumours

Brain tumours sometimes increase in size during the second half of pregnancy and temporarily remit after childbirth. Their neurosurgical treatment is frequently postponed until several weeks postpartum, when the tumour is less vascular. Exceptions include pituitary tumours, acoustic neuromas, metastatic chorioncarcinoma, and tumours such as supratentorial malignant gliomas and posterior fossa tumours which require prompt surgical intervention.

Prolactinoma

Hyperprolactinaemia may be due to prolactin-secreting pituitary adenomas. These may be macroadenomas (greater than 10 mm in diameter). Most women with hyperprolactinaemia are infertile until treated with bromocriptine to induce ovulation.

During pregnancy, the growth of pituitary adenomas is accelerated by the influence of oestrogen and may impair vision by pressure on the optic chiasma. It is not possible to predict which tumours will enlarge to cause symptoms. Nevertheless, women known to have macroadenomas who wish to become pregnant should have their tumours treated before starting a pregnancy. This can be with bromocriptine, radiation (yttrium implants) or neurosurgery. During pregnancy, visual fields and acuity should be determined monthly, and more frequently if any visual failure is observed. If there is deterioration, treatment with bromocriptine may be re-instituted and is safe for use in pregnancy. Progressive visual field defects at 38 weeks of pregnancy may be an indication for early delivery as visual defects improve afterwards.

Retinal Detachment

There is a case for delivering patients with a history of retinal detachment by caesarean section; alternatively, epidural anaesthesia and complete avoidance of bearing down in the second stage by means of a forceps delivery can be used.

Otosclerosis

A condition which is often progressive in women of reproductive age. Terminating a pregnancy will not affect its course.

Multiple Sclerosis

This is a condition susceptible to remission and exacerbation. Sometimes these changes occur in relation to a pregnancy. There is no medical case for legal abortion in a woman with multiple sclerosis who wants a baby.

Neuropathies

Bell's palsy

Bell's palsy is said to be associated with pregnancy. Usually, there is an isolated paralysis of the seventh cranial nerve, without apparent inciting cause. The palsy commonly occurs in the third trimester. Generally, the condition improves during the puerperium. Steroids (prednisolone, 40–60 mg daily) have been used for treatment starting within one week of the onset of symptoms. Electrodiagnostic techniques are valuable in assessment. Patients with conduction block have a good prognosis.

Carpal tunnel syndrome

This is one of the most common neurological causes of pain in the hand. It is thought to be due to compression of the median nerve in the carpal tunnel by oedema of its wall during pregnancy. The pain and tingling tend to occur at night and to wake the patient. The hand feels numb and swollen as well as painful. These symptoms usually disappear when the patient starts to move the hand and fingers. In the fully developed case, there is atrophy of the median-supplied thenar muscles and sensory loss of appropriate distribution. The condition usually responds well to elevation of the arm, splinting of the wrists and treatment with oral diuretics, but occasionally surgical relief of the compression may be indicated.

Meralgia paraesthetica

In this condition, there is entrapment of the lateral cutaneous nerve of the thigh under and sometimes through the lateral end of the inguinal ligament. This causes numbness and tingling on the anterolateral surface of the thigh. This condition appears to be more common in pregnancy due to lumbar lordosis. Pain may be precipitated by standing and relieved by recumbency. Weight gain should be restricted by dietary control. Treatment is with analgesics and sometimes infiltration of the nerve with local anaesthetic may be necessary. Surgical decompression is rarely required.

Foot drop

Paralysis of a lower limb of the mother after labour, or maternal obstetric palsy, has been considered to result from injury to the lumbosacral plexus by the fetal head or obstetric forceps. The most common form is unilateral foot drop. Generally, there is improvement within a few weeks. When paralysis is noted, lumbar disc protrusion must be considered. The presence of pain is associated with disc protrusion; pain with plexus injury rarely persists. Peroneal palsy, due to compression of the nerve around the neck of the fibula when the patient is placed in the lithotomy position, may also cause foot drop.

RENAL AND URINARY TRACT DISORDERS

Urinary Tract Infection

In pregnancy, the combined effects of increased progesterone secretion and pressure from the gravid uterus on the urinary tract cause a tendency to urinary stasis and ureteric dilatation and reflux. The result is an increased incidence of urinary tract infection. This can present as asymptomatic bacteriuria or as an overt infection.

Asymptomatic bacteriuria (>100, 000 bacteria/ml)

This occurs in 4–7% of pregnant women and a proportion of these patients may develop acute pyelonephritis later in pregnancy. *E. coli* is the organism responsible in most cases, but streptococci and proteus are not uncommon. By treating bacteriuria, the incidence of acute infection may be reduced to one-tenth, but the associated incidence of prematurity, pre-eclampsia and anaemia is unchanged.

With bacteriuria, blood urea or creatinine should be estimated to check renal function.

The aim of treatment is to maintain a sterile urine in pregnancy with a short course of appropriate antibiotics. Usually a 5-day course of amoxicillin or co-trimoxazole is the appropriate primary treatment. Sulphonamides are best avoided during the last 2 to 3 weeks of pregnancy because of the chance of neonatal jaundice if the patient goes into labour. If co-trimoxazole is used, then folic acid supplements, 5 mg daily, should be given by mouth. Alternative drugs useful with resistant infections include cephalosporins, nitrofurantoin and metronidazole. Tetracyclines are contraindicated after 16 weeks of pregnancy.

Where bacteriuria has recurred following initial treatment, a full urological assessment should be carried out 3 months after delivery to exclude any renal tract abnormality.

Acute urinary tract infection

Acute pyelonephritis is not confined to the woman with pre-existing bacteriuria; the incidence is about 2%. It is more common for the right kidney to be most affected, perhaps due to the dextro-rotation of the uterus in pregnancy. *E. coli* is the most common infective organism, but *Streptococcus faecalis,* staphylococci, proteus, klebsiella, pseudomonas and other Gram-negative bacteria can also be responsible.

In pregnancy, it is relatively uncommon to find a patient with the full clinical features of pyelonephritis, marked pyrexia, loin pain, severe renal angle tenderness, rigors and severe dysuria. More frequently, she has a slightly elevated temperature with vague symptoms of increased frequency, dysuria, backache, malaise and vomiting. There may be minimal loin tenderness and the diagnosis is made only from examination of the urine. Acute pyelonephritis must be distinguished with care from acute appendicitis.

Hospital admission is indicated in the severe case. Immediate antibiotic therapy, rehydration with intravenous fluids, analgesia to relieve pain, and tepid sponging to reduce pyrexia should be prescribed. The risks to the fetus from severe pyrexia are premature labour or intra-uterine death. Antibiotic treatment should be continued for 10 to 14 days, when a further specimen of urine should be examined.

It is desirable to perform midstream urine cultures at subsequent antenatal visits. After a recurrence, prophylactic treatment with amoxicillin or a cephalosporin for the remainder of the pregnancy should be considered. Renal tuberculosis is now rare, but should not be forgotten when there is a sterile pyuria.

Haematuria in Pregnancy

Haematuria in pregnancy is usually related to a contaminated specimen of urine, urinary tract infection or calculus. Nephrolithiasis causes diagnostic problems, because of the difficulty of distinguishing ureteric colic from obstetric causes of abdominal pain. There may be a predisposition to haematuria by the engorgement of veins in the renal pyramids. Haematuria may also be present after a difficult vaginal delivery, especially if the bladder is catheterised. Rupture of a caesarean section scar involving the bladder may be considered in the differential diagnosis.

Other causes of haematuria include renal tuberculosis, renal neoplasm, polycystic kidneys, hydronephrosis, bladder papilloma, viral urinary infection and acute and chronic nephritis.

Acute Renal Failure

Prerenal causes of reduced renal function include renal hypoperfusion due to hypotension associated with acute haemorrhage, including placental abruption, or due to reduced plasma volume, as in the severest forms of hyperemesis, pre-eclampsia or septic shock.

Intrinsic renal causes of renal failure include acute tubular necrosis and cortical necrosis. The distinction is not absolute — a proportion of glomeruli are often damaged in association with tubular necrosis. Complete cortical necrosis is now rare in obstetrics. These conditions may be due to prolonged renal hypoperfusion, disseminated intravascular coagulation, particularly associated with pre-eclampsia, amniotic fluid embolism or sepsis.

Postrenal causes of renal failure include ureteric or bladder outlet obstruction due to calculi, tumours or surgical trauma.

Diagnosis

The cause for the sudden decline in renal function should be sought, as early diagnosis is important. Acute onset of oliguria after haemorrhage, septicaemia or a hypotensive episode during operation suggests acute

Table 10.2
Differences Between Prerenal and Intrinsic Renal Failure

	Prerenal	Intrinsic
Urine osmolatity (m osm/kg)	>500	<400
Urine/plasma osmolal ratio	>1.5	<1.1
Urine sodium (mmol/l)	>20	<40
Urine/plasma urea ratio	>10	<10
Urine/plasma creatinine ratio	>10	<10

tubular nephropathy. When the cause is not obvious, obstruction of the urinary tract should be considered. Catheterisation will exclude bladder outlet obstruction. Ultrasound scanning of kidneys and ureters is particularly helpful. Plain abdominal films may reveal radio-opaque calculi. Differentiation of prerenal from intrinsic acute renal failure may be a problem. Comparison of electrolyte, urea and creatinine concentrations in the urine and plasma may be useful, but are not always accurate due to effects of therapeutic manoeuvres such as salt and fluid repletion and administration of diuretics. Response to plasma volume expansion or frusemide are more helpful in assessing intrinsic renal damage.

Differences between prerenal and intrinsic renal failure are shown in Table 10.2.

Management

The management of acute renal failure in association with obstetrical and gynaecological problems is the same as for any other precipitating factor.

Pregnancy and Chronic Renal Disease

Fertility and the ability to maintain a pregnancy depend on adequate renal function. Estimation of creatinine clearance gives a good guide to renal function. Adverse prognosis for mother and fetus is directly related to whether there is proteinuria alone, when the outlook is good; or in addition hypertension or nitrogen retention.

The incidence of intra-uterine growth restriction, prematurity and perinatal mortality is increased in mothers with chronic renal disease.

Some thousands of patients with renal transplants have now had successful pregnancies, taking steroids and azathioprine or cyclosporin. The prognosis is best if the transplant has been working well for 2 years, there is no hypertension, there have been no episodes of rejection and graft function is adequate and stable. The transplant seldom interferes with vaginal delivery, and if caesarean section is conducted, it is usually on obstetric grounds.

Few pregnancies occur in women on chronic renal dialysis. Abortion is common, but there have been some successful pregnancies.

DIABETES MELLITUS

Since the recognition of the importance of good diabetic control during pregnancy, there has been a dramatic improvement in maternal and fetal mortality and morbidity in these patients. The decline in perinatal mortality correlates with lower mean maternal blood glucose levels, and maternal and fetal mortality rates approaching those in non-diabetic pregnancies have been reported in recent studies. Fetal malformation now accounts for at least 50% of deaths among babies of diabetic mothers. It must be recognised that these defects have their own origin in the first trimester, and that they are related to lack of scrupulous control in the earliest weeks of pregnancy. It is, therefore, vital that diabetic patients be seen before they conceive and that optimal control, assessed by blood sugar and glycosylated haemoglobin measurements, be obtained before they embark on a pregnancy.

The incidence of diabetes is between 1% and 3% of the obstetric population, but much effort is involved in achieving success in this group of pregnant mothers. It is important for the patient to understand the need for the strict control of her diabetes, to comply with frequent hospital visits and to accept admission readily.

Terminology

Clinical diabetes. The glucose tolerance test is abnormal and the patient presents with symptoms or complications of diabetes.

Gestational diabetes. Glucose tolerance is abnormal in pregnancy and reverts to normal after delivery.

Potential diabetes. Certain features (Table 10.3) increase the likelihood of abnormal glucose tolerance in pregnancy.

Latent, chemical, borderline and asymptomatic diabetes are terms often used synonymously and with confusion. They are generally applied to asymptomatic individuals with an impaired glucose tolerance.

Diagnostic criteria

Random or fasting blood sugars are of little value for screening for diabetes in pregnancy.

The pregnant woman given a 50 g oral glucose tolerance test who has a 1 hour glucose level of greater than 7.8 mmol/l needs a full glucose tolerance test. When she is given a 100 g oral glucose test, she has gestational diabetes if two or more of the following values are exceeded:

Fasting	5.8 mmol/l
1 hour	10.6 mmol/l
2 hours	9.2 mmol/l
3 hours	8.1 mmol/l

Table 10.3
Risk Factors Indicating Potential Diabetics

Family history of diabetes in first degree relatives
Patient's own birth weight >4.5 kg
Obstetric history of recurrent miscarriages, unexplained perinatal deaths, fetal malformations, large babies (>4.0 kg), or hydramnios
Maternal obesity (body mass index >25), age >30, or parity >5

Table 10.4
White's Classification

A	Chemical diabetes or impaired glucose tolerance only
B	Maturity onset diabetes (age over 20 years at onset), duration less than 10 years
C1	Onset at age 10–19 years
C2	Duration 10–19 years
D1	Onset under 10 years of age
D2	Over 20 years of age
D3	Benign retinopathy
D4	Calcified leg vessels
D5	Hypertension
E	Calcification of pelvic arteries
F	Nephropathy
G	Recurrent fetal loss
H	Cardiomyopathy
R	Proliferative retinopathy
T	Renal transplant

Classification

The White classification of diabetes in pregnancy (Table 10.4) is of prognostic value as fetal mortality increases with duration of diabetes and presence of diabetic complications.

Effect of Pregnancy on Diabetes

There is no deterioration of glucose tolerance in pregnancy in normal women. The increased demand for insulin during pregnancy is probably related to increased metabolic rate, but the precise mechanism is far from clear. The hormone changes of pregnancy may be an important factor. The placental hormones, in particular oestrogen, progesterone, human chorionic gonadotrophin and placental lactogen, play an important role. Increased destruction of maternal insulin by placental insulinase has also been suggested as a causative factor.

The *instability* of diabetes in pregnancy is probably related to dietary changes, erratic absorption, a lowered vomiting threshold and infections.

Effect of Diabetes on Pregnancy

Fertility

When diabetes is well controlled and uncomplicated, there is no significant effect on fertility. Diabetics with severe nephropathy tend to be infertile.

Fetal development

There is an increased incidence (4 to 12%) of congenital, often multiple, malformations among the babies of diabetic mothers. There is an increase in major congenital abnormalities in the offspring of diabetic mothers with elevated glycosylated haemoglobin (HbA_1) in early pregnancy, indicating less than adequate control of the diabetes.

There is no evidence that there is an increased incidence of fetal malformations in women with potential or gestational diabetes or if the father is diabetic. There seems to be no increase in dysmorphic fetal abnormalities in women normally taking oral hypoglycaemic drugs.

Although fetal hyperinsulinism is unlikely to be a major contributory factor in malformation, it may cause 'unexplained' deaths in the later stages of pregnancy and perinatal complications from a macrosomic fetus. Inadequate production of surfactant, resulting in respiratory distress syndrome, used to be a more common complication of diabetic pregnancy than it seems to be now.

Infection

Common conditions such as vaginal thrush and urinary tract infections are more frequent among diabetics and require prompt treatment.

Pre-eclampsia

This occurs two to ten times more commonly in diabetic than in non-diabetic pregnancies. It is particularly associated with diabetic nephropathy and the presence of hydramnios.

Hydramnios

Excessive accumulation of amniotic fluid occurs in up to 1% of normal pregnancies, but in poorly controlled diabetic pregnancies the incidence may be as high as 30%. It is associated with fetal macrosomia. Hydramnios can provoke premature labour and pre-eclampsia, thus adding risks for the fetus. In well controlled diabetics, the presence of hydramnios may suggest gastrointestinal or neuroskeletal defects in the fetus.

Management

Before conception

Abnormal metabolic conditions for the fetus during organogenesis are a major cause of fetal malformation. One of the main aims of preconception management is to achieve normal diurnal blood glucose levels.

Ideally, the patient should be instructed in self-monitoring of her blood glucose levels, using a finger prick sample applied to a glucose oxidase impregnated strip, and read off by a portable reflectance meter. During pregnancy, urine glucose testing is generally unsuitable for monitoring diabetic control.

Estimations of glycosylated haemoglobin are good indicators of the quality of diabetic control over the preceding 4 to 6 weeks. The normal (non-diabetic) range of HbA_1 is between 4 and 7% of the total haemoglobin. HbA_1 contains three subfractions, HbA_{1a}, HbA_{1b} and HbA_{1c}. The level of the last is closely related to that of the total HbA_1. Serial estimations are useful for month to month monitoring of diabetic control before conception and during pregnancy.

Diabetics on oral hypoglycaemic drugs are best changed over to twice the daily doses of combined short and intermediate acting insulin.

Antenatal

The preprandial blood glucose levels should be maintained between 4 and 7 mmol/l and postprandial levels at 8 mmol/l without hypoglycaemic episodes. HbA_1 should be maintained within the normal range.

Gestational diabetics. In most instances, gestational diabetes will respond to a diet regimen alone. In the obese woman, calorie restriction to 1000–1200 kcal is advised. Failure to achieve optimal diabetic control is an indication for insulin.

Insulin dependent diabetics. In pregnancy, if insulin is required to control blood glucose, this often involves three pre-prandial injections of a short acting insulin and a bed-time injection of an intermediate or long-acting insulin. Human insulins are preferred.

Poorly controlled diabetics, with either frequent hyperglycaemia or severe hypoglycaemia, unresponsive to outpatient treatment, should be admitted to hospital. The problem may be poor motivation from, or lack of understanding by, the patient. If control remains poor, continuous insulin infusions may be considered. An assessment of fetal status can be made during the admission.

Diabetics do not frequently go into preterm labour; if they do, the best course may well be to allow them to deliver. If β-sympathomimetics or steroids are used, close monitoring of blood glucose is desirable.

Ultrasound monitoring of fetal biparietal diameters and abdominal girths is desirable not only to detect possible fetal growth restriction, but also macrosomia. The latter may indicate early delivery or caesarean section to avoid the risk of shoulder dystocia during vaginal delivery.

Admission and delivery

The optimal time for delivery in a diabetic pregnancy remains a dilemma. The fear of sudden intra-uterine death originally led to a policy of preterm delivery by elective caesarean section at 36 weeks of pregnancy in diabetic mothers. This resulted in some neonatal morbidity and mortality from respiratory distress syndrome. It is now clear that well controlled diabetics with normal fetal growth can be allowed to proceed to term and deliver vaginally without added risk to the fetus.

A bad obstetric history, pre-eclampsia, nephropathy, hydramnios, and fetal dysmaturity or macrosomia are indications for admission and early delivery. Delivery of the baby is indicated if hypertension becomes severe or the fetus is compromised by severe growth restriction or intra-uterine hypoxia. If delivery is planned before 38 weeks, it is important to assess fetal lung maturity by amniocentesis and estimation of both the amniotic fluid lecithin : sphingomyelin ratio and the phosphatidyl-glycerol content. Dexamethasone or betamethasone may be used to accelerate fetal lung maturity.

Planned vaginal delivery at 39 weeks is preferred, but management of patients who begin labour spontaneously is similar. Elective caesarean section is indicated between 38 and 39 weeks if there are predictable risks to the mother or the fetus, such as suspected disproportion, malpresentation or previous caesarean section.

During labour, it is essential to maintain normoglycaemia, 4–7 mmol/l. Maternal hyperglycaemia causes fetal hyperinsulinism, which can result in hypoglycaemia in the newborn.

The diabetic controlled by diet alone requires no special management during labour except monitoring of blood sugar. Insulin-dependent diabetics require control using intravenous dextrose and insulin only.

Postpartum

The gestational diabetic controlled on insulin during pregnancy should have her insulin stopped in the puerperium. Preprandial blood glucose estimations should continue into the puerperium. After 6 weeks, a 75 g oral glucose tolerance test is performed. If the result is impaired, she is referred to a physician for follow-up.

In the insulin-dependent diabetic, the maternal insulin requirements fall within hours of delivery and the patient is then at risk from hypoglycaemia. Frequent blood sugar estimations and close observation are necessary.

Perinatal complications

Fetal endogenous hyperinsulinism causes hypoglycaemia and may compromise the newborn, especially if macrosomia is present. The baby may have fits, apnoea, hypotonia, hypothermia, hypomagnesaemia, hypocalcaemia and hyperbilirubinaemia. For these reasons, the baby should be delivered and cared for in a unit with neonatal special care facilities.

THYROID DISORDERS

Thyrotoxicosis or hypothyroidism complicating pregnancy are relatively uncommon. In thyrotoxicosis of moderate severity, partial thyroidectomy can be considered before pregnancy, minimising the need for drugs. Goitres of significant size can be removed before they enlarge dangerously in pregnancy.

Physiological Changes in Pregnancy

The increased vascularity of the thyroid gland, increased renal excretion of iodide, increase in thyroxine binding globulin concentration and the production of placental thyroid stimulators contribute to enlargement of the thyroid gland in pregnancy. Despite this and the increase in basal metabolic rate, the normal pregnant woman is euthyroid.

Thyroxine is the main hormone detectable in the fetus. By term, the concentration of thyroxine is just less than the maternal level.

Thyroxine (T_4) and tri-iodothyronine (T_3) undergo metabolic change in the placenta and only small amounts cross to the fetus. Iodine and antithyroid drugs such as propylthiouracil and the imidazole derivatives cross the placenta readily.

Hyperthyroidism

The incidence of thyrotoxicosis complicating pregnancy is 0.5 to 1.0%. It is uncommon for untreated severe thyrotoxic patients to become pregnant, as they tend to have anovulatory cycles. In untreated cases of lesser severity, there is an increased incidence of spontaneous abortion and perinatal mortality. Premature delivery is also increased. With treatment, the perinatal outcome improves dramatically. In the majority of patients, the disease has been diagnosed before pregnancy and they are under treatment.

The normal pregnant woman exhibits many signs and symptoms of hyperthyroidism, but the presence of goitre with bruit, exopthalmos, myopathy, sleeping pulse greater than 90/min, as well as specific signs such as brisk deep tendon reflexes and pretibial myxoedema all suggest Graves' disease. Due to changes in protein binding, the most important diagnostic and monitoring test in pregnancy is the free thyroxine level (1st and 2nd trimesters 10–20, 3rd trimester 7–15 pmol/l).

Medical treatment in pregnancy is usually with propylthiouracil or carbimazole or its active metabolite, methimazole. Both iodine and radioactive iodine (^{131}I) are contraindicated, as they can cause fetal goitre. Propanolol is particularly associated with fetal growth retardation and should be avoided except parenterally for control of the acute situation of a thyroid crisis. Excellent results have been obtained in America with partial thyroidectomy in the second trimester.

Intra-uterine growth restriction is a fairly common complication. Management is along the usual obstetric lines.

In labour, problems specifically related to thyrotoxicosis are unusual if the patient has complied with treatment. Should a thyroid crisis occur, treatment is with intravenous propanolol.

The presence of thyroid-stimulating immunoglobulins in the mother seems to be associated with neonatal thyrotoxicosis. About 1 in 20 babies born to mothers treated with antithyroid drugs are affected by neonatal hypothyroidism or thyrotoxicosis, and investigation of the neonate is essential, for treatment is important, but not usually prolonged. About 1 in 20 babies have a goitre.

Treatment of the mother can be discontinued after delivery. She should then be monitored to see if further antithyroid drugs are necessary.

All antithyroid drugs pass into breast milk in significant quantities, although there is some evidence that this is less of a problem with propylthiouracil. If further treatment is indicated, it should be with propylthiouracil and the breast-fed baby should be monitored for any effects on its thyroid function.

Hypothyroidism

Hypothyroidism is often associated with infertility and a high fetal wastage. Symptoms of cold intolerance, excessive weight gain and skin changes together with a slow pulse rate and delayed tendon jerks should make one suspicious of a positive diagnosis. In most instances, thyroid hormone replacement will have been commenced before pregnancy and should be continued.

Serum-free thyroxine is depressed and thyrotropin (TSH) level is raised; the latter is only noted in primary hypothyroidism. An initial dose of thyroxine is 25 mg/day, increased in steps of 25 mg every week or two until a therapeutic level is reached. Estimation of free thyroxine should help with changes in dose. The usual dose of *l*-thyroxine is between 100 and 200 mg daily.

Goitre

Endemic goitres due to iodine deficiency may present as large multinodular tumours in some parts of the world. Retrosternal extension may cause pressure effects, such as dyspnoea and dysphagia and impaction in the thoracic inlet in labour is potentially lethal. It is important to exclude both hyper- and hypothyroidism. In most instances where the cause is iodine deficiency, increased thyroid activity makes the patient euthyroid. Iodine supplements are provided to compensate for fetal demands, especially in the first trimester of pregnancy, to prevent neurological cretinism which does not respond to treatment. When iodine deficiency occurs after the first trimester of pregnancy, the newborn suffers from hypothyroid cretinism and will respond provided the baby is treated promptly.

In developed countries where iodised salt is used, small euthyroid goitres may occur. Enlargements of these goitres may occur during pregnancy. They pose little difficulty to management except when doubt exists regarding thyroid malignancy. Ultrasonography, needle biopsy and a technetium ($^{99}Tc^{m}$) scan may help with diagnosis, but surgery may be indicated. When a pregnant woman has a simple goitre, small amounts of supplementary iodine in the form of iodised table salt are advised.

RHEUMATIC DISORDERS

Rheumatoid Arthritis

This chronic inflammatory disorder, affecting one or more joints, is more common in women.

Pregnancy has a beneficial effect on the disease, perhaps related to increased free cortisol levels, perhaps to changes in immune factors. Most patients develop recurrence of symptoms about 2 months after delivery, and almost all have an exacerbation within a few months.

The risk of spontaneous abortion, fetal growth restriction and perinatal mortality is no greater than in the general population.

Most patients with rheumatoid arthritis need only simple analgesics, usually non-steroidal anti-inflammatory agents such as aspirin and indomethacin, during pregnancy. These drugs are not responsible for congenital abnormalities but, as prostaglandin systhesis inhibitors, they tend to delay the onset of labour. Whether or not there is a small risk of premature closure of the ductus arteriosus and pulmonary hypertension in the newborn, if preterm delivery is affected, is debatable. Aspirin is irritant to the stomach and should always be crushed and taken with milk. If full doses are continued until the confinement, there is an increased risk of ultrasonically diagnosed intraventricular haemorrhage due to interference with fetal platelet function, particularly of preterm newborn, although there may be no untoward sequelae. Aspirin is best discontinued when delivery is anticipated within a few days. No special risks are documented with paracetamol.

Physicians are reluctant to treat rheumatoid arthritis with steroids in pregnancy, but there is no special risk provided supplements are given to cover surgical manoeuvres and labour.

Antiphospholipid Syndrome

This is an auto-immune condition. The most specific features are episodes of venous or arterial thrombosis, fetal loss (particularly 2nd or 3rd trimester fetal death), and auto-immune thrombocytopenia. There is a moderate to high increase in circulating antiphospholipid antibodies. The most readily available tests are for the lupus anticoagulant and IgG isotype of anticardiolipin antibodies, and a false positive serum test for syphilis should raise suspicion. Apart from fetal death, pregnancy-induced hypertension, utero-placental insufficiency and preterm birth are common.

Complications include vascular symptoms in almost any system. In particular, thrombosis, thrombocytopenia, haemolytic anaemia, livido reticularis, amaurosis fugax (transient ischaemic attacks affecting vision) and cerebrovascular stroke can occur.

Management of patients without relevant history or symptoms is with low dose aspirin. When there is a history of fetal loss, subcutaneous heparin 10,000–20,000 units/day in two or three divided doses, or subcutaneous low molecular weight heparin once daily, in addition to low dose aspirin, should be considered.

Systemic Lupus Erythematosus

Systemic lupus erythematosus is an auto-immune disease often associated with microvascular abnormalities. It usually affects women in the reproductive years and can present with a variety of manifestations, such as polyarthritis, myalgia, skin rash, alopecia, pleurisy, dyspnoea, pericarditis, proteinuria, anaemia, leucopenia and thrombocytopenia. The disease runs a fluctuating course. Detection of early stages by measurement of anti-DNA or anti-cardiolipin antibody and complement (C_3) levels has improved management of these patients.

Provided the disease is in remission, the outcome of pregnancy is generally good. This is where preconception counselling can be of major help. The effect of systemic lupus on pregnancy is an increased risk of spontaneous abortion, intra-uterine fetal death, premature labour, intra-uterine growth retardation and congenital heart block. Babies born to mothers with lupus nephritis and hypertension tend to be growth restricted, and the perinatal mortality rate is high. These patients should defer pregnancy until the disease is quiescent.

The effect of pregnancy on systemic lupus erythematosus is variable; there may be more exacerbations during pregnancy, in particular during the puerperium. Despite this, the maternal mortality and long-term prognosis are not affected. Anti-DNA antibodies are of little value for monitoring the disease during pregnancy; C_3 levels are more helpful in diagnosing exacerbation; symptomatology is the best guide.

The key to success in management is the free use of steroids when patients have been managed on other drugs; transfer to steroids before pregnancy (preferably not more than 10 mg/day of prednisolone) may be considered. When there has been a previous pregnancy loss taking other drugs, or the patient has been on steroids in the previous 2 years, transfer to steroids before or in early pregnancy is desirable. Patients taking steroids are not capable of the normal increased corticosteroid response to pregnancy, and prednisolone, 7 mg/day, should be regarded as a minimum replacement dose. Exacerbations are treated with increased doses, and if hypertension deteriorates beyond control with reasonable doses of hypotensive drugs, the dose of steroids is *increased.* Patients with a history of intrauterine growth retardation in a previous pregnancy should have low dose aspirin (75 mg/day) throughout pregnancy to minimise platelet aggregation. Labour is managed with parenteral hydrocortisone, continued for 24 hours after delivery. Puerperal exacerbation is common and may be prevented by increasing doses of prednisolone for a few weeks, followed by gradual reduction.

Patients with systemic lupus erythematosus should be tested for antiphospholipid antibodies, anticardiolipin and the lupus anticoagulant, preferably before they become pregnant. Those with elevated levels are at high risk for pregnancy loss, and need low dose aspirin and perhaps subcutaneous heparin. Patients with thrombotic variants of the disease need anticoagulation with subcutaneous heparin throughout pregnancy.

FURTHER READING

DeSwiet M., ed. (1995). *Medical Disorders in Obstetric Practice,* 2nd edn. Oxford: Blackwell Scientific.

Gleicher N., ed. (1992). *Principles of Medical Therapy in Pregnancy,* 2nd edn. New York and London: Plenum Press.

Hawkins D.F., ed. (1987). *Drugs and Pregnancy,* 2nd edn. Edinburgh: Churchill Livingstone.

Oakley C., ed. (1997). *Heart Disease in Pregnancy.* London: BMA Publishing Group.

11

Abnormalities of Pregnancy

HYPERTENSION

Hypertension in pregnancy can be classified as follows.

- Chronic hypertension, present before and continuing during pregnancy.
- Pre-eclampsia (PET) and eclampsia.
- PET superimposed on chronic hypertension.
- Transient hypertension without any other signs.

Chronic hypertension that does not change during pregnancy and which is controlled with medication is not usually a problem, unless there is superimposed pre-eclampsia which must be carefully watched for. The hypotensive therapy may be changed to methyldopa before or in early pregnancy as this is a good drug for the pregnant woman with a large therapeutic range. However unless the drug is an ACE inhibitor, the current therapy can be maintained.

Hypertension developing during pregnancy (>140/90 mmHg) in a previously normotensive woman is often accompanied by excessive fluid retention and less frequently by proteinuria. This triad of clinical signs is called pre-eclamptic toxaemia (PET). It must be differentiated from renal causes of hypertension, proteinuria and oedema, such as glomerular nephritis or renal abnormalities assoicated with other diseases such as the connective tissue disorders.

Pregnancy induced hypertension occurs in about 10% of pregnancies and is more common in women having their first pregnancy with a particular partner. The importance of prompt diagnosis and appropriate management lies in the prevention of rapidly worsening maternal hypertension with the subsequent risk of cerebral haemorrhage, eclamptic fits or placental separation as well as those of fetal hypoxia.

Factors Predisposing to Pregnancy Induced Hypertension

Genetic. A family history of pre-eclampsia or hypertension tends to increase the risk.

Primigravidae. It is at least twice as common in primigravidae as in multigravidae. A history of an early miscarriage may protect against the risk of PET, but pregnancy by a new partner increases the risk, suggesting that the disease has an immunological basis.

Social and economic. Pre-eclampsia is more likely to occur in poor and underprivileged women. Inappropriate diet may be a factor; failure to attend for antenatal care delays diagnosis and management. Women who smoke tend to have a lower incidence but, should pre-eclampsia develop, fetal outlook is worse.

Medical. Diabetes mellitus and chronic renal disease are predisposing diseases.

Obstetric. Pre-eclampsia is associated with hydatidiform mole, multiple pregnancy, hydramnios, and rhesus isoimmunisation.

Pathological Changes Occurring in Pregnancy Induced Hypertension

Vascular changes

Hypertension is caused by generalised arteriolar constriction with a normal cardiac output. A sudden rise of blood pressure may cause acute arterial damage with loss of vascular autoregulation, and the most common cause of maternal death from this condition is cerebral haemorrhage. Generalised arteriolar constriction also affects the vessels of the placental bed with a reduction of blood flow. Fibrin deposition in these vessels produces irreversible reductions. The consequences of chronically reduced placental blood flow are intrauterine growth retardation and placental infarction and sometimes abruption. Acute placental infarction may cause sudden hypertension as a result of thromboxane release, and fetal hypoxia if it is severe. Fetal hypoxia may also occur if the blood pressure is lowered by intravenous hypotensive drugs, too far and too fast, in response to the sudden increase in pressure.

Renal changes

Renal biopsies in patients with PET and proteinuria have shown a plethora of different varieties of pathological change. The most characteristic is oedema of the endothelial cells of the glomerular capillaries and fibrinoid necrosis in renal glomeruli and tubules. Renal tubular function is first impaired, causing a reduction of uric acid clearance, reflected by a rise in plasma creatinine or urea which indicates increasing renal impairment in the form of reduced glomerular filtration rate and subsequent reduction in urine output. Acute renal failure with tubular or cortical necrosis is more likely when placental abruption has occurred. Oedema is probably due to generalised changes in membrane function, but is associated with renal retention of both sodium and potassium and also to reduced plasma albumin. Although there is extravascular fluid retention, plasma volume is reduced and the haematocrit rises. Rare complications of fluid retention include ascites and pulmonary and laryngeal oedema.

Liver changes

These occur infrequently and only as a result of severe PET. Sometimes there is necrosis at the periphery of the lobule which may extend to involve the whole lobule. Occasionally, subcapsular haemorrhage is seen. Liver enzymes in the plasma are raised when there is liver impairment. Jaundice occurs rarely.

Coagulation changes

Disseminated intravascular coagulation (DIC) may occasionally occur in severe cases and tends to be worse if the liver is involved. Platelet count, fibrinogen, and factors V and VIII are reduced, with a rise in fibrin degradation products. Another hallmark of disseminated intravascular coagulopathy which places renal function at risk is the appearance of fragmented red cells in the peripheral circulation. Potential complications of clotting disturbances include haemorrhage and necrosis in the brain, kidneys, liver, adrenal and pituitary gland.

A combination of haemolysis, raised liver enzymes, and a low platelet count in a patient with rapidly worsening hypertension and proteinuria is called HELLP syndrome. This stands for Haemolysis, Elevated Liver enzymes, and Low Platelet count. Rapid delivery in these cases is essential if there is not to be DIC, renal failure or other pathology.

Possible Aetiology of Pregnancy Induced Hypertension

Numerous hypotheses have been put forward to account for this condition.

Abnormal vasospasm involving both uterine and renal circulations

The hypothesis that vasoconstrictor agents are released when there is excessive uterine distension was put forward to account for the fact that PET is more common in primigravid patients and those with multiple pregnancies. Renal ischaemia due to vasospasm allows the leakage of albumen through the tubules.

Coagulation abnormalities

Coagulation abnormalities have been said to account for the excessive fibrin deposition in the placenta and kidney which lead to placental infarction and glomerular damage characteristically seen in these cases. The increased fibrin deposition is accompanied by increased fibrinolytic activity and consequently there is an increase in circulating fibrin degradation products seen in cases of severe PIH. Placental damage leading to the liberation into the circulation of thromboplastic substances could cause generalised disseminated intravascular coagulation and consequently thrombocytopoenia, and a further rise in fibrin degradation products which are seen in severe PET.

Immunological aspects

The immunological barriers between mother and fetus that prevent rejection are not fully understood. Some inability of the mother to protect herself from the paternal antigens expressed in the conceptus has been suggested to explain the higher incidence of PET among first pregnancies and in cases of hydatidiform mole, as well as explaining the lower incidence of PET among antigenically similar couples. None of these theories provides an adequate explanation of its own. The likelihood is that the trophoblast plays a key role of some description and that there could be an interplay between immunological aspects, placental biochemistry and control of maternal blood pressure and coagulation factors.

Placental factors

What is the evidence for the placenta, and the trophoblast in particular, playing a key role in PET? (Fig. 11.1). Firstly, trophoblast cells invade the intima and media of maternal spiral arterioles in early pregnancy. This causes softening and loss of resistance in these vessels allowing for their expansion and so ensuring an adequate flow of maternal blood at low pressure into the intervillous space. The role of cell-cell adhesion molecules in facilitating or hindering this process may be important.

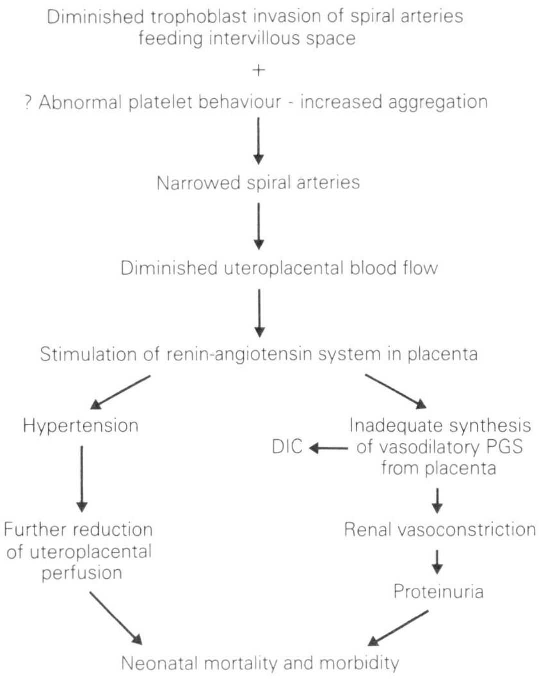

Fig. 11.1 *Possible aetiology of PET.*

A locally produced vasodilator to maintain the low flow and pressure state of the intervillous space should be of benefit. Candidates for this role are prostacyclin or nitric oxide. Nitric oxide synthase activity in the placental bed is reduced in cases of PET with increased vascular resistance in uterine vessels.

Secondly, the placenta produces renin and angiotensin and is able to carry out, in the same way as the kidney, all the enzymatic conversions within the renin-angiotenisn system (Fig. 11.2). The pregnant woman is refractory to angiotensin II infusions, which would cause hypertension in the non-pregnant woman. This suggests that some placental product modulates the pressor effects of angiotensin II. The kidney is also the site of the rennin-angiotensin pathway and the kallikrein-kinin pathway. The mother can influence the synthesis of these vasoactive compounds via estrogen and progesterone in early pregnancy.

The placenta and fetal membranes metabolise arachidonic acid to eicosanoids which are the products of the cyclooxygenase and the lipooxygenase enzyme systems (Fig. 11.3).

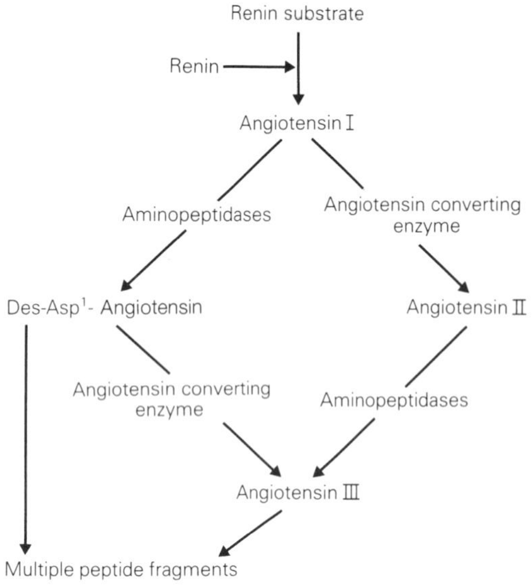

Fig. 11.2 *The renin-angiotensin system.*

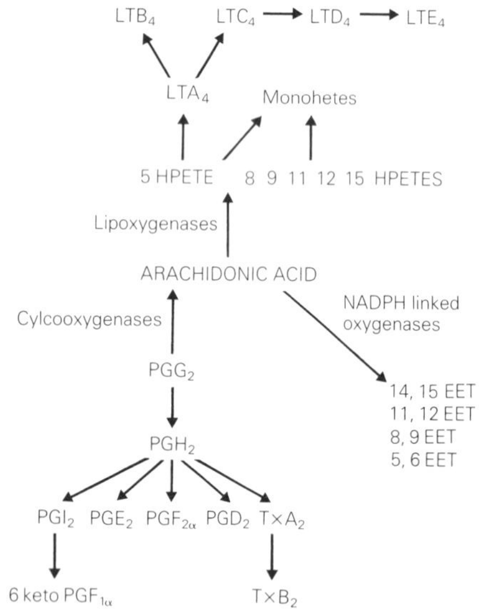

Fig. 11.3 *Metabolites of arachidonic acid with the cyclooxygenase and lipoxygenase enzyme pathways. PGG_2, PGH_2 = endoperoxides; PGI_2 = prostacyclin; TXA_2, TXB_2 = thromboxane A_2, B_2: HPETE = hydroperoxyeicosatetraeonic acid; LTA_4, B_4, C_4, D_4, E_4 = leukotriene A_4, B_4, C_4, E_4; ETT = epoxyeicosatrienoic acid.*

Prostacyclin is a very potent vasodilator and inhibitor of platelet aggregation, while thromboxane A2 has the opposite effect. The placenta has platelet anti-aggregatory activity which could be due to ADPase or prostacyclin. In cases of PET, there is a reduction in synthesis of prostacyclin as determined by low levels of urinary metabolites, reduced levels of 6-oxo-$PGF_1\alpha$ in amniotic fluid and the reduced conversion of C14 arachidonic acid to prostacyclin by the umbilical cord. Increased platelet aggregation leading to fibrin deposition and placental infarction would increase local thromboxane production both from platelets and from damaged placental tissue. A local imbalance in these two cyclooxygenase products could then ensue and be important in altering the biochemical balance necessary for maintaining a normal blood pressure.

The roles of lipoxygenase products in reproductive physiology are unknown, but their production in relatively large amounts by placental tissue and fetal membranes from early in pregnancy suggest that they are of importance. Leukotrienes and monohydroxy fatty acids have both contractile effects on smooth muscle and increase capillary permeability. This could therefore cause vasospasm and an increase in extravascular, and the corresponding reduction in intravascular, fluid volume seen in severe PET. Deficiencies of essential fatty acids have been demonstrated in PET which favour increased synthesis of lipoxygenase products which, in turn, will inhibit prostacyclin synthesis. Lipoxygenase products may affect the maternal immune response as leukotriene B_4 (LTB_4) induces active suppressor T cells which down regulate the maternal immune response. An abnormal interplay between the maternal immunological system, alterations of arachidonic acid metabolism and other biochemical factors responsible for control of maternal and fetal vascular homeostasis may be some of the reasons for PET.

Other possible factors in the aetiology of PET are the raised levels of ELAM1, which is an inducible cell adhesion molecule for neutrophils, and increased lipid peroxides causing endothelial damage. The levels of antioxidants which protect against endothelial cell damage may also be important, although the evidence for this is equivocal at present.

Abnormal coagulation factors, expressed in severe cases of PET as disseminated intravascular coagulation, are probably of a secondary nature as a result of placental infarction. These include raised levels of fibrin degradation products and reduced platelet count. There are some suggestions that increases in coagulation factors such as factor VIII may precede the onset of the hypertension.

Diagnosis

Pre-eclampsia is considered when the blood pressure taken in a sitting position reaches 140/90 mmHg in a previously normotensive woman. The upper limits of normal are between 130/80 and 135/85 mmHg. PET very rarely occurs before the 20th week of pregnancy except in the case of hydatidiform mole. Usually hypertension is the first sign, but it may be preceded by a sudden retention of fluid manifest by clinically obvious oedema of legs, hands and face or by a sudden weight gain of two or more kilos within a week.

The proteinuria is largely albumen and represents renal ischaemia causing leakage of protein through the glomeruli and tubules. It is usually between 0.5 and 3 g per day. It is a sign of a more severe form of PET, as renal pathology often reflects the placental pathology. The perinatal mortality rate in these cases is several times higher than in PET without proteinuria. Fulminating PET presents with hypertension, proteinuria, headache, hyperreflexia, irritability and sometimes epigastric pain due to distension of the liver capsule or, rarely, subcapsular haemorrhage.

Management

Management is determined by the need to minimise the possible harmful effects to mother and fetus. Perinatal mortality in severe PET with proteinuria is increased tenfold. However, this may be partly due to obstetricians' reluctance to perform an elective delivery sufficiently early. Recent experience of delivery between 28 and 32 weeks in cases of severe PET suggest that the perinatal mortality in these cases can be substantially reduced if the fetus is delivered before significant hypoxia *in utero* can exert its harmful effects.

If severe PET occurs suddenly around 26 weeks, with blood pressures of greater than 150/100 mmHg and with proteinuria, the patient must be admitted to hospital immediately and preferably to a centre with neonatal intensive care facilities. Intravenous hypotensive therapy using hydralazine and an anticonvulsant such as diazepam or chlormethiazole given i.v. is commenced. Methyldopa may be used in addition, for its longer term action.

Fetal weight and liquor volume together with as extensive an assessment of fetal state as possible are carried out ultrasonically. Cardiotocagraphy is performed twice daily to detect the earliest onset of fetal hypoxia. Renal function is determined by urine output, specific gravity of urine, total protein in grams per 24 hours, plasma creatinine urea and uric acid levels. Fibrin degradation products and platelet count should be carried out. Delivery will be indicated if (1) hypertension is difficult to control without the use of more than one hypotensive drug; (2) there is evidence of rapidly worsening renal function; (3) fetal growth stops; and (4) there is evidence of fetal hypoxia. If delivery is anticipated between 28 and 32 weeks, it is necessary to administer corticosteroids to the mother in the form of dexamethasone 12 mg i.m. on two consecutive days, the course finishing at least 24 hours before delivery if possible. This therapy reduces the incidence of respiratory distress syndrome and intraventricular haemorrhage in the low birth weight, preterm baby. The mode of delivery depends on the degree of control of maternal blood pressure and whether or not there is fetal distress. Caesarean section will be the preferred mode of delivery in the majority of cases of severe PET to minimise the risks of fetal hypoxia and maternal hypertension.

Moderate (150/100–160/110 mmHg) or mild (less than 150/100 mmHg) cases of PET will require hospitalisation, bed rest and therapy to maintain the blood pressure around 140/90 mmHg, and to improve placental blood flow. Hypotensive drugs suitable for use in pregnancy are described in Chapter 10. It is undesirable to reduce maternal blood pressure excessively, as this will reduce placental perfusion and cause fetal hypoxia. Anticonvulsant therapy is not usually needed unless the blood pressure exceeds 150/100 mmHg or there are signs of increased irritability, visual disturbance, severe headache or epigastric pain. Fetal monitoring should be by ultrasound scan every 2 weeks to assess fetal growth and liquor volume and by daily or twice daily fetal cardiotocography and fetal movement charts. Severe fetal growth retardation is unusual, but milder degrees (10th–3rd centile) are not uncommon. The timing of delivery depends on blood pressure control and fetal well-being. Renal function is not usually significantly impaired in these cases. Delivery will usually be vaginally unless there is fetal distress.

Management in labour

The principles of management in labour and delivery are (1) adequate control of both systolic and diastolic blood pressure, (2) the use of anticonvulsants if required, (3) adequate analgesia, and (4) delivery by forceps or caesarean section. Continuous fetal monitoring is mandatory. Epidural analgesia is an effective way of providing analgesia and reducing the blood pressure, but coagulation must be normal for it to be used. The use of an anticonvulsant prior to induction of general anaesthesia is desirable.

Management of eclampsia

Eclampsia occurs when a woman with severe pre-eclampsia starts to have convulsions. This constitutes a major emergency as the patient can rapidly suffer from any of the following:

1. Cerebral haemorrhage due to sudden further elevation in her blood pressure.
2. Acute asphyxia due to convulsions or obstruction of her airway by the tongue or inhalation of vomit.
3. Severe fetal hypoxia as a result of the above or from concealed accidental haemorrhage.

If the patient is not in hospital, immediate treatment is directed at reducing the blood pressure rapidly, ensuring an airway, and giving anticonvulsant drugs and then transferring to a major obstetric unit after stabilisation. Thereafter, delivery of the fetus should take place as soon as possible. A number of therapeutic regimens are used for this emergency. Diazepam, magnesium sulphate and chlormethiazone are used as anticonvulsants and should be given intravenously. Hypotensive therapy also needs to be given intravenously, the most commonly used drugs being probably hydralazine, although magnesium sulphate has some hypotensive effects. The drugs must be given in combination; a commonly used effective combination is 10 mg of hydralazine of and 10 mg of diazepam of given intravenously, in a period of 30 minutes. However, recent trials have shown that magnesium sulphate has given the best results.

Delivery of the baby should be by caesarean section once the blood pressure and fits are controlled and provided it is still alive.

Fluid overload should be avoided. Urine output during the first 24 hours after an eclamptic fit may be reduced to less than 500 ml, particularly if there has been a Caesarean section carried out. This is not a cause for concern but, if urine output continues at less than 500 ml into the second 24 hours, an osmotic diuretic such as mannitol is indicated.

Prophylaxis

On the grounds that enhanced platelet aggregation plays a key role in the pathogenesis of PET, drugs that suppress this may be of benefit if commenced early in pregnancy and before significant placental or renal damage has taken place. Aspirin in low doses blocks the cyclooxygenase enzyme in platelets by acetylation and, as they cannot synthesise new enzyme, they can no longer produce thromboxane A_2 during their lifetime in the circulation. Higher doses of aspirin partially block prostacyclin synthesis by vascular endothelium. Dipyridamole inhibits platelet aggregation and may also be helpful. Recent studies suggest that low dose aspirin (75 mg per day) from early pregnancy has been beneficial in pregnancies where excessive placental and vascular thromboxane production might be harmful. The possible beneficial effects of new thromboxane synthetase inhibitors require evaluation.

INTRAUTERINE GROWTH RETARDATION (IUGR)

Aetiology

Either the fetus is intrinisically small and, if so, it is often abnormal, or the growth retardation develops at a later stage of pregnancy. The reason for the latter is a reduced flow of maternal blood into the intervillous space and reduced fetal blood flow. When the ratio of the head to abdominal circumference remains constant, growth retardation is defined as being symmetrical.

Asymmetrical growth retardation is diagnosed when there is a progressive change in this ratio. Increase in the growth rate of the abdomen is markedly reduced compared with that of the head as a consequence of loss of body fat and liver glycogen.

Asymmetrical intrauterine growth retardation may be associated with severe PET or severe essential hypertension and is slightly more common in older women and in those who are very active or stressed throughout pregnancy. However, in about one-third of cases there is no obvious associated factor. A reduced blood flow through the uteroplacental circulation, either by fibrin deposition in the cases with severe PET or vasospasm in the other instances, leads to the reduced growth.

The pathological appearances of IUGR are a small infarcted placenta with evidence of fibrin deposition around the villi. The fetus will be relatively long and thin with little subcutaneous fat, an increased head to abdominal circumference ratio and an absence of vernix. Its weight will be below the 3rd, 5th or 10th centile for gestational age depending on the definition used.

The invasion of trophoblast cells during early pregnancy and again at about 20 weeks of gestation into the media of spiral arterioles, making them soft and dilated, seems to be important in allowing an adequate flow of maternal blood at low pressure into the intervillous space. Platelet aggregation and subsequent fibrin deposition and reduced blood flow through the fetal placental circulation are well-documented in cases of IUGR. The possibility that there is a deficiency of locally produced prostaglandins has been suggested, but the evidence is not conclusive. Recent evidence linking severe IUGR, leading to mid-trimester fetal death and abortion, with the presence in the circulation of anticardiolipin antibodies is of considerable interest. These antibodies are thought to act by preventing the liberation of arachidonic acid from cell membranes and so, by reducing substrate availability, altering the quantity, and possibly range, of arachidonic acid metabolites produced. These antibodies are found in patients with a variety of connective tissue disorders, particularly those with thrombotic complications. They are present in women with recurrent abortions of the type described, but without evidence of connective tissue disorders, although some of these women may go on to develop these later in life.

Diagnosis

Clinical awareness of the problem and regular palpation of the uterus, preferably by the same individual, are of vital importance. Failure of maternal weight gain or increase in abdominal girth are not of signficant prognostic value. A less than expected pubic symphysis to uterine fundal height may be of value. Ultrasound carried out at 18 to 20 weeks to confirm gestation and to exclude fetal abnormalities is important. The subsequent diagnosis of fetal growth retardation is best made by ultrasound scan and an accurate assessment of duration of pregnancy is vital in making the diagnosis. Important measurements are the biparietal diameter, head circumference, abdominal circumference, femur length and an assessment of liquor volume. In the symmetrically growth retarded fetus that has no congenital abnormalities, the pathology will have started early in pregnancy and be severe. All the measurements will have a similar relationship to each other. In the asymmetrically growth retarded fetus, the limb length will be appropriate for gestational age, while the circumference of the head will be reduced less than that of the circumference of the abdomen, thereby increasing the ratio between them. In both instances, there will usually be reduction in liquor volume. Blood flow in the arcuate arteries, in the umbilical vessels and in the fetal aorta can be demonstrated using Doppler ultrasound. An alteration in these measurements precedes fetal hypoxia and may be an indication for delivery.

Treatment

At present there is no treatment apart from bed rest, which seems to increase the uterine blood flow and improve fetal growth in mild cases. In more severe cases, with or without severe PET, bed rest alone does not usually improve fetal growth. On the grounds that there is an enhancement of coagulation mechanism and fibrin deposition in the placental circulation, various combinations of dipyrimadole and heparin have been tried with some evidence of success. Low dose aspirin therapy (75 mg or less per day) which inhibits platelet thromboxane A2 synthesis and so diminishes platelet aggregation has also yielded some success, but both possible therapies need testing in large scale trials. However, the problems of setting up these trials in an appropriate manner are formidable. If there are anticardiolipin antibodies present in a significant titre, immunosuppression using prednisolone in doses of up to 40–50 mg per day may be beneficial either with or without azothioprine and some form of antithrombotic therapy. In these cases, low dose aspirin combined with low molecular weight heparin has been shown to be beneficial. Daily fetal cardiotocography is necessary to warn of the early onset of fetal hypoxia, any signs of which indicate delivery without delay by the most appropriate method if growth retardation is mild. When growth retardation is moderate or severe, delivery should be considered at an appropriate gestation, even in the presence of normal fetal heart traces so as to avoid the neonatal problems of a compromised low birth weight baby. If the fetal weight, estimated by ultrasound is less than 1.5 kg, delivery should probably be by lower segment caesarean section. Otherwise, if there is no fetal distress, a vaginal delivery can be considered, but with careful monitoring during labour.

The growth retarded baby is particularly vulnerable to hypoglycaemia and hypothermia. Blood sugar and calcium estimations should be carried out at birth and repeated during the first 24–48 hours. Temperature control and adequate oxygenation either by head box adminstration or mechanical ventilation is important. Intravenous glucose may be necessary.

ANTEPARTUM HAEMORRHAGE

Placenta praevia

This is defined as a placenta situated wholly or partially in the lower uterine segment. Its significance is that when the lower uterine segment is taken up and the cervix is effacing either before or during labour, placental separation, and thus inevitable haemorrhage, will occur. The aetiology of placenta praevia is not known, but it can be recurrent and is said to be more common in multiple pregnancies because of a larger placenta. Its presence is determined at the site of implantation by defective decidual reaction allowing the placental site to extend. Traditionally, placenta praevia has been graded 1–4 as follows (Fig. 11.4).

Grade 1: placental edge in lower uterine segment.

Grade 2: placental edge reaches internal cervical os.

Grade 3: placental edge covers internal cervical os.

Grade 4: complete placenta central over the internal cervial os.

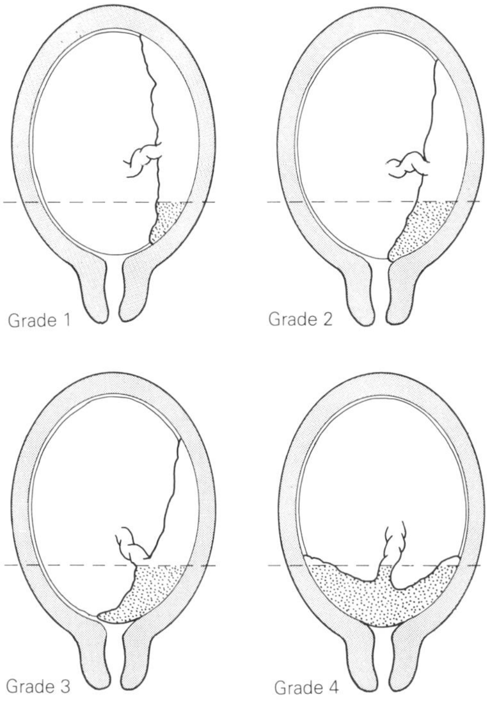

Fig. 11.4 *Grades 1–4 of placenta praevia.*

In practice, it is difficult to be so specific and, indeed, cases of grade 1 placenta praevia may never be diagnosed. A division into major and minor degrees of placenta praevia is a practical one, the major degrees being grades 3 and 4, where delivery by caesarean section is mandatory, while a minor degree of placenta praevia would encompass grades 1 and 2 in which vaginal delivery may or may not be possible, depending on the circumstances.

Presentation

Placenta praevia presents during the antenatal period with a relatively small, painless antepartum haemorrhage sometimes associated with intercourse, or with an unstable fetal lie. Occasionally, there are no warning signs until there is a brisk haemorrhage during labour. Bleeding from the lower genital tract should be excluded by a speculum examination using a Sims speculum to avoid stretching the vault and lower uterine segment.

Diagnosis

Diagnosis is nowadays by ultrasound, which is extremely accurate at localising the placenta and in determining its position relative to the internal cervical os. There is no place for other forms of imaging to localise the placenta.

Management

Admission to hospital during the last trimester of pregnancy is considered necessary because of the unpredictability and sometimes catastrophic nature of the haemorrhage. Cross-matched blood must be available at all times. As there is not a large area of placental separation, fetal growth is not usually impaired and pregnancy in the absence of severe haemorrhage may safely continue until 37–38 weeks. Delivery is usually considered at this time because of the increasing likelihood of the onset of labour with inevitable bleeding. A minor degree of placenta praevia, particularly if the placenta is on the anterior uterine wall, warrants assessment for possible vaginal delivery. An examination under anaesthesia in theatre prepared for immediate lower segment caesarean section will be carried out, followed by either rupture of the membranes and i.v. oxytocin to induce labour, or lower segment caesarean section, depending on the circumstances. For a major degree of placenta praevia, elective caesarean section is mandatory.

Accidental Haemorrhage (Abruptio Placentae)

This can be either revealed, concealed (retroplacental) or both together.

Revealed

This form of haemorrhage implies a variable degree of separation of the placenta with the blood tracking behind it to the vagina. Bleeding is usually painless and the volume of blood lost probably reflects the extent of placental separation. Admission to hospital is necessary, and a diagnosis is made by exclusion of other causes of bleeding from the lower genital tract. A Sim's speculum examination should be carried out, but not a bimanual vaginal examination. Placenta praevia is excluded by ultrasound examination at which time a blood clot behind the placenta may be seen.

Management. If bleeding is not repeated and has been slight, the fetal prognosis is good and so the mother can be discharged after a few days. If there has been no further bleeding, the pregnancy can be allowed to continue to 38 or 40 weeks, with a careful watch kept on fetal growth. If bleeding is persistent or repeated, however slight, then there will be increasing areas of placental separation and diminishing placental reserve. Fetal monitoring involving daily fetal cardiotocography and twice weekly ultrasound scans to determine fetal growth is essential. The volume, persistence, or recurrences of the haemorrhage, together with the state of the fetus, will determine the timing of delivery, usually at or before 38 weeks. If the fetus is uncompromised, or unless the bleeding is very heavy, delivery should be vaginally.

Concealed haemorrhage

Blood loss from a concealed antepartum haemorrhage is all retained retroplacentally or is extravasated into the myometrium. Revealed and concealed blood loss can occur from different parts of the placenta, these cases being called mixed antepartum haemorrhage. The aetiology is not clear, but concealed antepartum haemorrhage is more common in women with severe hypertension when the increased pressure of the blood entering the intervillous space could be of importance. Other associations are with multiparity. Physical forces such as those of an external cephalic version, or after rapid reduction in size of a previously overdistended uterus, can lead to shearing between the placenta and its uterine attachment. Folate deficiency has been suggested as a factor in causing a possible inadequacy of vascular development. Occasionally, abruptio placentae can recur in successive pregnancies.

Diagnosis. The main symptom of concealed antepartum haemorrhage is uterine pain and tenderness, usually of sudden onset and sometimes getting progressively worse as the area of placental separation increases. In mixed cases, the above will occur together with overt vaginal bleeding. Retroplacental clot can be seen ultrasonically. In severe cases, there will be evidence of shock, namely peripheral vasoconstriction, hypertension and sometimes, paradoxically, a normal or slow pulse rate. Shock is due to the pain and to the blood loss. There can be up to 2 litres of blood lost quickly in retroplacental clot and extravasated into the myometrium. In these cases, the uterus is larger than expected, hard and tender. Fetal heart sounds may be absent or, if present, difficult to hear.

Management. In cases where only a very small abruption is diagnosed or where there is doubt about the diagnosis, expectant management in hospital is appropriate. Blood should be cross-matched as a larger haemorrhage may occur unexpectedly. Daily fetal monitoring should be carried out. If there are recurrent small concealed antepartum haemorrhages, delivery is the best option, as sooner or later there will be a large one, with potentially serious fetal and maternal consequences. In moderate or severe cases, delivery as soon as possible is appropriate, as further extension of the haemorrhage may be fatal to the fetus and dangerous to the mother. Shock must be treated promptly with i.v. blood, or plasma if blood is unavailable. Transfusion should be as rapid as possible to retain normal jugular venous pressure measured by a central venous pressure catheter. Blood loss, particularly in cases of concealed antepartum haemorrhage, is usually underestimated and prolonged hypovolaemia and hypotension will increase fibrinolysis. Disseminated intravascular coagulation can occur due to release of placental thromboplastins into the circulation leading to hypofibrinogenaemia. The clotting time needs quick assessment while awaiting laboratory investigations which comprise measurement of fibrinogen, fibrin degradation products and platelet count. Treatment with i.v. fibrinogen and fresh platelets may be needed but, if blood transfusion is prompt and adequate, the coagulation abnormalities are rare. Urinary output may be impaired, so this must be watched carefully, usually by means of an indwelling catheter. Prompt correction of hypotension and hypovolaemia will reduce the risks of renal problems. The mode of delivery depends on the circumstances, such as fetal viability, maternal blood pressure, extent of haemorrhage and cervical dilatation. Labour can be quick in such cases, as there are a lot of prostaglandins released from the damaged uterine and placental tissue initiating uterine contractions, but this is a risky approach as there are real dangers of intrauterine death. For most cases with a definite diagnosis, caesarean section is the best method of delivery.

Vasa Praevia

Rarely, antepartum haemorrhage may be slight and consist of fetal blood from rupture of a placental vessel overlying the internal os. This may happen at artificial rupture of the membranes. The umbilical cord may be inserted at the edge of the placenta. If the bleeding is recurrent or severe, the fetus may die from haemorrhage or suffer the effects of prolonged anaemia. Abnormal fetal heart traces, such as marked decelerations or fetal tachycardia, may suggest this type of haemorrhage. The diagnosis is confirmed by carrying out a Kleihauer test to differentiate maternal and fetal red blood cells within the blood lost.

HYDATIDIFORM MOLE

In this abnormal pregnancy, there is no fetus, but only an overgrowth of placental tissue with hydatidiform vesicular changes.

Hydatidiform degeneration of the chorionic villi can occur involving the stroma and blood vessels. The degenerate villi are swollen, due to stromal oedema. They become avascular and the epithelium is thickened over their surface. The chorionic epithelium of some vesicles proliferates. Very occasionally, hydatidiform degeneration can occur in a normal placenta and is found more commonly in abortions. When the whole conceptus is involved, it becomes a hydatidiform mole. Depending on the state of the proliferative epithelium, moles can be benign or malignant (choriocarcinoma). There is an intermediate stage of invasive, but histologically non-malignant mole, which involves the myometrium, but does not metastasise. Hydatidiform mole is uncommon in Europe, the incidence being about 0.1%, but in Southeast Asia the incidence can be as high as 1%.

Diagnosis

Hydatidiform mole is suspected if the uterus is large for dates, fetal movements are not felt, there is severe hyperemesis, pregnancy induced hypertension occurs before 20–24 weeks, or there is persistent slight bleeding during the first half of pregnancy. Diagnosis is by ultrasound scan when the appearances are very characteristic. Serum ßHCG levels may be excessively raised by at least one order of magnitude.

Management

Expulsion of the mole can be induced medically using either intravenous oxytocin or intravaginal or intrauterine prostaglandins. Suction curettage to complete the emptying of the uterus may be needed, but extra care must be taken to avoid perforation and haemorrhage due to uterine softening and atony.

Histological assessment of the tissue is essential. Serum or urinary βHCG estimations are carried out every 3 months for a period of 2 years to ensure complete removal of chorionic tissue and to check against a recurrence in the form of choriocarcinoma. Pregnancy should be avoided during this time. Choriocarcinoma can follow any form of pregnancy. It is a rapidly metastasising tumour, which can present with irregular vaginal bleeding (uterine tumour) or haemoptysis or other pulmonary symptoms (pulmonary secondaries). Diagnosis is by measuring elevated βHCG levels, histological confirmation from curettage or by characteristic cannonball appearances of the pulmonary metastases on chest X-ray. Late metastases can occur in any relatively vascular organ. Treatment is often successful if started early, with rapid elimination of the tumour using methotrexate and folinic acid, or other related cytotoxic agents. Long-term follow-up using urinary βHCG estimations is essential.

HYDRAMNIOS

This is defined as a significant excess of liquor amnii (greater than 1.5 litres). The exact causes are unknown, but there may be an increased production of liquor from the membranes or there may be a reduction in its passage through the fetus or both. It can occur in either an acute or chronic form — the latter being the more common. Hydramnios is often found in association with congenital abnormalities in which the fetus cannot swallow, such as anencephaly, oesophageal atresia or severe muscular disorders. It is associated with diabetes and multiple pregnancy, often uniovular, in which case it may be acute. It can occur without any abnormality being detected.

Diagnosis

Diagnosis is made on clinical palpation when the uterus is tense and distended. Fetal parts are hard to feel, and a fluid thrill is present. Ultrasound examination will confirm this. The presence of fetal abnormalities should always be considered in cases of acute or chronic hydramnios. A thorough ultrasound examination of the fetus is very important.

Management

Premature labour due to uterine distension may occur and require treatment with drugs which inhibit myometrial contractions (tocolytic drugs). Amniocentesis to reduce pressure and relieve symptoms is not successful, as the fluid rapidly refills and the procedure may stimulate labour. Bed rest helps the discomfort, but this alone is rarely a cause for preterm delivery. Usually the patient will go into spontaneous labour or labour is induced. If the latter, liquor volume should be reduced slowly to reduce the chances of shearing off the placenta and causing an abruptio placentae. After delivery, immediate examination of the baby for possible congenital abnormalities such as oesophageal atresia is very important.

MULTIPLE PREGNANCY

Multiple pregnancy may occur:

1. By the division of an ovum fertilised by one sperm, which then divides at the two-cell stage into two separate cell bodies. Chromatin is common, so twins will be identical.

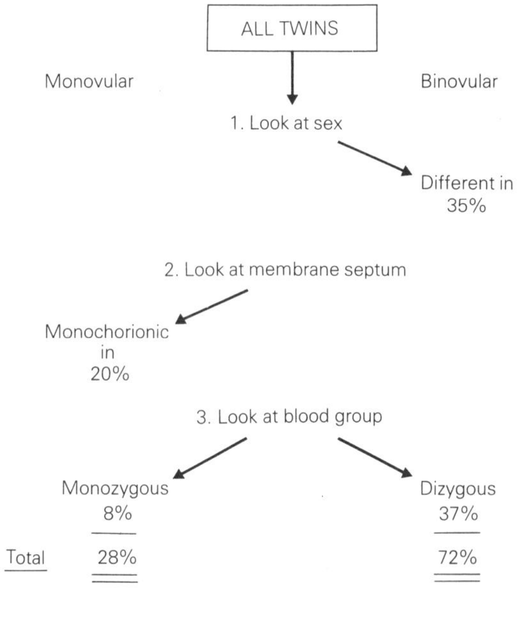

Fig. 11.5 *Determining types of twins.*

2. By more than one egg being fertilised by more than one sperm. There is a familial tendency for this to happen. Although they may be of the same sex, these twins will not be identical.

Multiple pregnancies with more than two babies may be a combination of multiple fertilisation and division at the two-cell stage. The incidence of twins in Europe is 1 in 80, triplets 1 in 8000 and quadruplets 1 in 500,000. Multiple pregnancies are more common in some countries such as in Africa. Induction of ovulation using clomiphene or gonadotrophins leads to a higher incidence of multiple pregnancies. The same is true of *in vitro* fertilisation when often three or more embryos, fertlised *in vitro,* are replaced into the uterus to improve the chances of a successful pregnancy (see Chapter 34). Determination of whether twins are identical or not is difficult. Figure 11.5 depicts a logical scheme for such determination.

Diagnosis

The diagnosis of multiple pregnancy is suspected when the uterus is thought to be larger than expected for the gestational period. Ultrasound scan is usually reliable at determining multiple pregnancies and the advent of routine scans at 18–20 weeks has detected most of these. There is no role for X-rays in the diagnosis of multiple pregnancy.

Associated problems

1. *Increased uterine size* and increased venous pressure lead to problems such as varicose veins of the legs and vulva, haemorrhoids and oedema of the legs.
2. *Anaemia* is more common due to the haemopoietic requirements of more than one baby. Iron and folic acid supplements are necessary.
3. *Congenital abnormalities* and *hydramnios* are more common and more often associated with uniovular twins.
4. *PET* is more common, but the reasons are not yet known. However, some fetal and/or placental factor may be involved.
5. *Intrauterine growth retardation* is another possible complication of multiple pregnancy. This may be equal in both babies due to inadequate uteroplacental circulation. On the other hand, there may be increased growth of one at the expense of the other twin, which is due to anastamosis of their placental circulations. The larger twin will be hypervolaemic and polycythaemic which may result in heart failure. The growth retarded twin will be correspondingly anaemic, also leading to heart failure. Regular ultrasound scans are needed to detect this problem and to deliver the babies before it becomes severe.
6. *Preterm labour* is the most important potential complication of multiple pregnancy. Most women with multiple pregnancy will go into spontaneous labour before 38 weeks and a number do so considerably earlier. Prophylactic bed rest or small doses of oral tocolytics do not seem to be reliable in preventing this. In threatened preterm labour, i.v. β sympathomimetic drugs, such as ritodrine, terbutaline or salbutomol are usually effective for some time. However, once the membranes have ruptured, delivery is usually imminent and effective for some time. For all these reasons more frequent antenatal care is necessary.

Mode of delivery

Vaginal delivery is appropriate in most cases of twins, unless they present by the breech between 26 and 34 weeks' gestation, or unless there is a malpresentation with the first twin, when caesarean section may give a better fetal outcome. Three or more babies are usually delivered by caesarean section as the risks of malpresentation and obstruction to delivery increase, as do the risks of hypoxia from placental separation or cord compression during prolonged vaginal delivery. The conduct of labour until delivery of the first baby is the same as for a single fetus. After the delivery of the first baby, the lie of the second is checked and, if longitudinal, the membranes are ruptured. Intravenous oxytocin may be needed to expedite delivery of the second twin. If the lie is not longitudinal, an external cephalic version should be carried out before rupturing the membranes and using intravenous oxytocin. Postpartum haemorrhage due to uterine hypotonia is a potential problem, so continuation of intravenous oxytocin for some hours after delivery is advisable.

Fetal abnormalities

Congenital abnormalities are either genetic or environmental in origin. Major congenital abnormalities occur in about 1.5% of live births and account for a large part of neonatal mortality and morbidity. About one-half of perinatal mortality is currently due to congenital abnormalities: chromosomal disorders account for the majority of congenital abnormalities and disorders of chromosomal number in the autosomal structure account for the majority of these. They account for about three-quarters of chromosomal abnormalities and include trisomy 21, and those of the sex chromosome such as XYY; XXY; XXX; mosaics of these and XO. Disorders of autosomal structure account for about one-quarter of chromosomal abnormalities and include translocation (balanced or unbalanced) or deletion of chromosomes.

Single gene disorders include the autosomal dominant conditions such as polycystic renal disease, achondroplasia, Huntingdon's chorea, polydactyly or the autosomal recessive conditions such as cystic fibrosis and β thalassaemia or other inborn errors of metabolism.

Examples of sex linked (X) recessive conditions are muscular dystrophy, mental retardation, haemophilia and Christmas disease and, of course, the most common, red/green colour blindness.

Environmental causes of congenital abnormalities include abnormal hormonal environment, infections, radiation, drugs or biochemical abnormalities induced by the diet. There are definitive examples of (1) hormones, such as testosterone or progestogens, causing virilisation of a female fetus; (2) of infections such as rubella and treponema, causing a variety of structural defects in the fetus; (3) radiation in high doses (50 rads) causing an increased incidence of a number of congenital abnormalities; (4) drugs such as warfarin causing a variety of fetal abnormalities.

There is no evidence that dietary deficiencies of certain vitamins or essential fatty acids cause congenital abnormalities, although it has been suggested that folic acid and vitamin supplements given from conception reduce the incidence of neural tube defects. Currently folic acid 400 ug daily is advised for all pregnant women during the first 13 weeks of pregnancy. Should there be a history of neural tube defect then the dose should be increased to 5 mg daily. Cause and effects are very difficult to prove and, unless there are large numbers of similar defects resulting from a common agent, the evidence will always be anecdotal.

The potential teratogen has to be involved at the critical time of organ development; for example, active rubella infection at 6–10 weeks of pregnancy may result in eye or heart abnormalities, while at 16 weeks it is very unlikely to have any effect. Finally, the potential teratogen such as a drug may not act directly, but through an intermediate, metabolic step which could vary from person to person.

Rhesus isoimmunisation

Of the six main genes involved in the rhesus group, three are dominant and three recessive. These are C, D, E and c, d, e, respectively. A rhesus negative person must, therefore, be homozygous (c, d, e/c, d, e), while heterozygocity leads to being rhesus positive with D being present in any genetic combination. Fetal red cells can enter the maternal circulation at the time of abortion, during pregnancy or delivery, or during the third stage. These antigenic rhesus positive fetal cells may sensitise the mother so that, when there is a further similar stimulus in a subsequent pregnancy, anti-D antibodies will be produced. These cross the placenta causing fetal haemolysis and an increased fetal excretion of bilirubin into the liquor.

Diagnosis

All women have their rhesus and antibody status assessed at booking. A positive antibody titre indicates isoimmunisation, but it is not an accurate guide to the extent to which the fetus is affected. The reason for this is that the placental transfer of antibody from mother to fetus is variable. If the antibody titre is significant (1 in 16 or greater), then the severity of the condition is assessed by estimating the bilirubin content of the liquor collected by amniocentesis at 20 weeks. The higher the liquor content of bilirubin, the more severely the fetus is affected. The amniocentesis is repeated in 2 weeks and the two results plotted on charts prepared to determine the severity of timing of intervention (Fig. 11.6). If greater accuracy in diagnosis is needed, particularly in severe cases, then sampling of fetal blood from the umbilical cord can be performed in a fetal medicine centre. In moderate or severe cases, the fetus will be

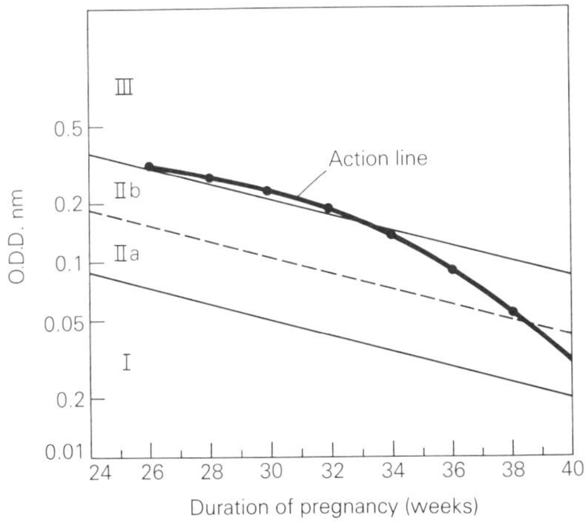

Fig. 11.6 *Optical density difference (O.D.D.) of liquor measured at 450 nm. Zone I = very mildly affected or unaffected fetus; Zone II (a & b) = moderately affected fetus; Zone III = severely affected fetus. When plot of O.D.D. reaches the action line, either intrauterine transfusion or delivery of fetus is required.*

anaemic and if severe and prolonged, cardiac failure will occur leading to peripheral oedema (hydrops fetalis). This can be seen on ultrasound and is a late sign of severe disease indicating a bad prognosis for the fetus. Serial ultrasound scans may also be helpful in assessing the severity of the condition. Moderately affected cases warrant assessment by amniocentesis or by haemoglobin estimation on cord blood, followed by delivery at the appropriate gestation. In mildly affected cases, invasive procedures may not be necessary and delivery could be as late as 38 weeks. Moderately affected cases will be delivered usually between 34 and 38 weeks, either by caesarean section or vaginally, depending on individual circumstances. Severely affected babies, if diagnosed before 28 weeks, will require intrauterine transfusion to prevent severe anaemia and its sequelae. Direct i.v. transfusion into the umbilical/placental vessels under ultrasound control is appropriate. This is repeated until the fetus is mature enough to be delivered and withstand the subsequent neonatal exchange transfusions, probably at 32 weeks, although delivery may need to be as early as 30 weeks if intrauterine transfusion is proving difficult. Management in the neonatal period depends on the age of the baby. Phototherapy would commence if the bilirubin levels were 50–60 μmol/l within the first 24 hours of life. After 48 hours of age, treatment in the form of phototherapy or exchange transfusion is needed if the level reaches 150–350 μmol/l depending on the gestational age at delivery.

Prevention

The injection of anti-D gamma globulin (IgG) to all rhesus negative women after abortions and to those with rhesus positive babies within 48 hours of delivery will destroy the fetal Rh positive cells in the maternal circulation and prevent sensitisation. The administration of anti-D gamma globulin during pregnancy has been shown to have some benefit in reducing the risk of immunisation. Many units now give anti-D prophylactically to primigravid women at 28 and 34 weeks.

FURTHER READING

Creasy R.K., Resnik R., eds. (1994). *Maternal-Fetal Medicine,* 3rd edn. Philadephia: Saunders.

Editorial (1986). Aspirin and pre-eclampsia. *Lancet* **i**: 18–20.

Kierse M.J.N.C. (1984). The small baby. In *Clinics in Obstetrics and Gynaecology,* Vol. II, No. 2. Howie P., Patel N. (eds). pp. 415–36. London: Saunders.

12

Physiology, Mechanisms and Management of Normal Labour

PHYSIOLOGY OF THE UTERUS AND CERVIX

The human uterus is a muscular organ adapted to support the growth of the fetus during pregnancy and then to expel it when the fetus is mature. It is approximately pear-shaped and consists of two main parts, the body (or corpus) and the cervix (see Fig. 2.1. p. 10). The body is mostly composed of smooth muscle, comprising up to 90% of the upper segment. The lower segment contains a diminishing proportion of muscle, so that when it merges into the cervix, muscle fibres make up only 10% of the tissue. The remainder is made up of connective tissue with a large admixture of elastic fibres.

The uterus is covered with a layer of peritoneum (the serosa) and lined with a mucosa, the endometrium. The endometrium contains large numbers of glycogen secreting glands that serve to nourish the developing embryo before the development of the placenta.

The blood supply of the uterus is essentially from the uterine and ovarian arteries, derived from the internal iliac arteries and the aorta respectively. They feed a plexus in the myometrium from which a series of arcuate arteries pass up into the endometrium. These short, straight vessels pass through the basal endometrium and give rise to the spiral arteries which, in pregnancy, open into the maternal portion of the placenta (the intervillous space).

Like the smooth muscle of the bowel, uterine muscle is spontaneously contractile. A biopsy specimen, removed and suspended in a physiological solution, will contract every 2–5 minutes without being stimulated. This spontaneous activity can be suppressed by hormones, notably progesterone and β_2 agonists, It is thought that a major function of the secretion of progesterone in the luteal phase of the menstrual cycle is to suppress uterine activity and prevent the expulsion of a developing blastocyst. Once implantation has taken place, progesterone production is taken over by the placenta. Initially, chorionic villi cover the developing embryo, but by 6 weeks they begin to atrophy, except at the site of the developing placenta. As the conceptus and uterus enlarge, the area of the endometrium increases more rapidly than that of the placenta, and uterine muscle at a distance begins to escape from progesterone suppression. Thus, at between 20 and 24 weeks' gestation, spontaneous uterine contractility starts to re-assert itself. At first, contractions are limited to single groups of fibres and produce only small rises in intrauterine pressure ('A' waves). However, as pregnancy progresses, oestrogen levels rise, resulting in the formation of 'gap junctions' between adjacent myometrial cells. These junctions provide low resistance pathways for the conduction of electrical activity from cell to cell and thus promote propagation and synchronisation of uterine activity. When large areas of muscle begin to contract in an organised fashion, they are able to raise intrauterine pressure to levels approaching those seen during menstruation and labour, ranging from 4 to 12 kPa (30–90 mmHg). These are termed 'B' waves, which are commonly known as the 'uterine contractions' of labour. Because of the greater concentration of muscle fibres at the fundus, uterine contractions tend to start there and then sweep down the uterus towards the cervix. This is termed 'fundal dominance' and may be physiologically important in the stretching of the lower segment and the dilatation of the cervix during labour. There is some evidence that the insertion of the fallopian tube into the uterus is a common site for the origin of contractions and it is sometimes called the 'cornual pacemaker'.

The 'B' waves that occur during pregnancy are painless, because the cervix is not being dilated. Nevertheless, they slowly stretch the lower segment of the uterus, which becomes elongated and thinned. In the third trimester, it balloons out during contractions, eventually allowing the descent of the presenting part into the pelvis. The contractions may also play a part in changing the consistency of the cervix prior to the onset of labour. Painless contractions occurring before the onset of labour are clinically termed 'Braxton-Hicks', after a 19th century obstetrician.

The uterine cervix is predominantly composed of collagen and connective tissue with only a little muscle. In the non-pregnant state, the cervix has a firm consistency likened to that of the end of the nose. It usually acts effectively to retain the developing gestation sac within the uterus throughout pregnancy. However, during pregnancy there is a softening process which eventually allows the cervix to stretch and permit delivery of the fetus, following which it reforms once again. How this remarkable feat is achieved is poorly understood, but it is thought to involve changes in the ground substance, particularly the breakdown of collagen by proteolytic enzymes and alterations in the relative amounts of the glycosaminoglycans, which normally bind the collagen fibrils together. There is also an increase in water content mediated by hyaluronic acid. It is thought that these changes are produced partly by alterations in oestrogen level and partly by other hormones such as prostaglandins. Prostaglandin E_2 is produced in increasing amounts by the amnion, chorion and decidua immediately prior to and during labour. It is known that disturbance of the membranes by vaginal examination ('sweeping the membranes') in late pregnancy produces considerable transient local prostaglandin release, and that this can precipitate the onset of labour. Relaxin, a hormone produced by the ovary, may also play a part in the cervical softening process known clinically as 'ripening'.

PHYSIOLOGY OF LABOUR

Onset of Labour

The mechanism of the onset of labour in the human is complex and, as yet, incompletely defined. Such evidence as we have points to fetal maturity being a major controlling factor, rather than, for example, parturition being triggered simply by the fetus reaching a particular size. The difficulty lies in discovering which particular fetal signal or signals interact with the mother to start labour. In some species, such as the sheep, the fetal hypothalamic-pituitary-adrenal axis, in conjunction with the placenta, is clearly in control of the onset of parturition. A sharp increase in fetal cortisol acts on the placenta to reduce progesterone secretion, augment oestrogen production and, perhaps, to increase prostaglandin production. However, a sharp rise in fetal cortisol associated with the onset of labour has not been demonstrated in the human, and attempts to induce labour with cortisol have not been successful.

On the other hand, prostaglandins (notably PGE_2) are much more strongly associated with the onset of labour in the human than in many other animal species. Both maternal and fetal production of oxytocin from the posterior pituitary are also involved. Although secretion rates do not alter, the concentration of oxytocin receptors in the uterus increases several hundred fold during pregnancy, so the uterus responds more to a static concentration of circulating oxytocin. Stimulation of the oxytocin receptor causes the release of prostaglandins both from the fetal membranes and uterine decidua. Effective blocking of labour can therefore be achieved with both prostaglandin synthase inhibitors, such as indomethacin and oxytocin receptor antagonists, such as atosiban.

Contractions can also be suppressed by administration of β_2 receptor stimulants such as salbutamol and ritodrine. This causes a rise in cyclic GMP within the cell, and uterine muscle relaxation. Adrenaline has a similar effect, and this may be why excessive maternal anxiety is associated with dysfunctional labour. Randomised controlled trials have shown that the presence of a supportive partner for the woman in labour is associated with better progress and outcome in labour.

Labour is divided into the first, second and third stages. The first stage begins with the onset of labour and ends when the cervix is fully dilated. The onset of labour is not an acute event, but a steadily accelerating process, which probably starts with the Braxton-Hicks contractions. Under their influence, the cervix 'ripens', becoming steadily softer and shorter (the latter is termed 'effacement'). Ripening normally becomes clinically apparent at about 36 weeks' gestation in the primigravida and even earlier in the multigravida, although the length of gestation is not affected by parity. Over the same period, uterine contractions become more frequent and regular, and may also become stronger. Eventually, the cervix begins to dilate progressively. This is the central event defining the onset of labour. The complete regularisation of contractions into the normal labour pattern frequently accompanies the onset of progressive dilatation, but may also precede it by a few hours or, less commonly, even days. Occasionally, the cervix may start to dilate before regular contractions are properly established. Rupture of the amniotic membranes before the onset of contractions (pre-labour rupture of the membranes, PROM) is quite common, occurring in 10–15% of all pregnancies, although contractions begin within 24 hours in over 80% of such cases. It is clear from this, that it is often impossible to define a precise time for the onset of labour. The clinical aspects of the diagnosis of labour will be dealt with in more detail later in this chapter (p. 159).

FIRST STAGE

The first stage of labour is divided into two main phases, the latent phase and the active phase (Fig. 12.1). The latent phase is that period when the cervix is exposed to regular uterine contractions, but is still softening and effacing. Cervical dilatation proceeds slowly, and does not normally reach more than 2–3 cm in this phase, which may last up to 12 hours or occasionally even longer. Once the cervix reaches 3 cm dilatation, full effacement and softening have usually occurred. At this point, the rate of cervical dilatation begins to increase (acceleration phase). From 4 to 9 cm, the cervix goes through the most rapid rate of dilatation (active phase), after which there is sometimes a deceleration phase. The mean rate of cervical dilatation over the whole of the active phase depends on the parity, with women in their first labour dilating at a mean rate of about 1 cm per hour and parous women at about 1.5 cm per hour. This reflects differences in the compliance of the cervix and pelvic soft tissues. The maximum rate of dilatation may be considerably more than 1–1.5 cm/hour.

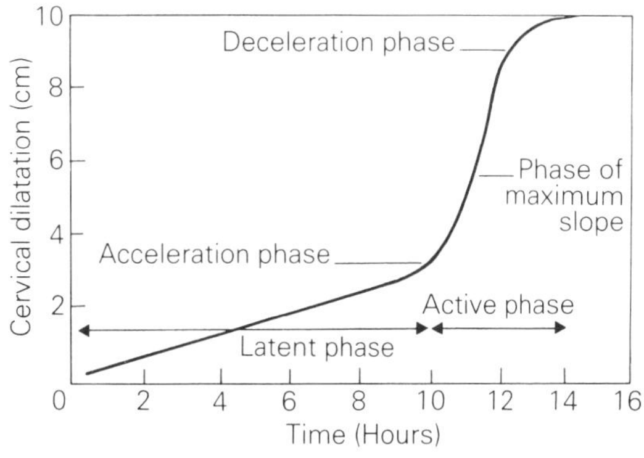

Fig. 12.1 *Latent and active phases of labour.*

Effect of Contractions on Fetal and Placental Blood Flow and on Oxygenation of the Fetus

The rise in intrauterine pressure during a contraction has no direct effect on the fetal circulation. This is because the whole of the fetal compartment is within the uterus, and thus changes in pressure occur equally at all points. The difference between fetal arterial and venous pressures is therefore unchanged and flow is unaltered. The best analogy here is with a diver in a compression chamber whose circulation continues happily despite being exposed to three or more atmospheric pressures. The only exception to this is when there is direct pressure on a structure; for example cerebral blood flow may be reduced by direct head compression, or umbilical flow may be reduced by direct pressure on the cord if it is prolapsed alongside the head, or wrapped tightly round the neck. In general, the fetus is protected from these effects by the surrounding liquor which, like all fluids, is virtually incompressible. Direct pressure effects are, therefore, most likely during the late first stage, as the fetus moves down through the pelvis, and following rupture of the membranes. Rupture of the membranes usually releases only a small proportion of the amniotic fluid volume, as the head normally blocks the lower segment like a plug, preventing the escape of the majority of the liquor.

In contrast, the rise in intrauterine pressure during a contraction has a major effect on the circulation through the maternal side of the placenta. This is because the arterial pressure supplying the intervillous space is derived from the maternal circulation outside the uterus, and is therefore not increased by the same amount as the intrauterine pressure during a contraction. Between contractions, intrauterine pressure normally exceeds intra-abdominal pressure by about 1–2 kPa (7.5–15 mmHg). This is known as the 'baseline' or 'resting' tone. Arterial inflow pressure in the spiral arteries is usually about 4–6 kPa, being reduced and evened out by the unique structure of these arteries. Thus a pressure of about 3 kPa provides a steady blood flow through the intervillous space. Too high a pressure or flow rate would tend to dislodge the placenta. The first event to occur during a contraction is that the rising intramyometrial pressure cuts off the low pressure venous drainage of the intervillous space. The arterial inflow continues, and the maternal pool of blood increases by up to 500 ml, as demonstrated using ultrasound, trapping a large reservoir of oxygenated blood in the placenta. When the intrauterine pressure rises to 4 kPa or more, the arterial inflow is arrested, and the maternal part of the placenta now becomes a closed system. The fetal circulation continues, and oxygen is extracted from the reservoir of maternal blood. Even so, the oxygen supply to the fetus declines steadily with time as the maternal blood becomes exhausted (Fig. 12.2). This decline continues until the intrauterine pressure once again falls below 4 kPa and fresh maternal blood can enter the placenta. It then takes some time for the oxygen-depleted blood to be washed out of the intervillous space, and thus the oxygen supply to the fetus is not restored until about a minute or so after the contraction has worn off. The reduction in fetal oxygen supply resulting from contractions can be demonstrated using transcutaneous oxygen monitoring, and the resulting increase in anaerobic metabolism produces a small, but measurable, decline in fetal pH during labour. These regular episodes

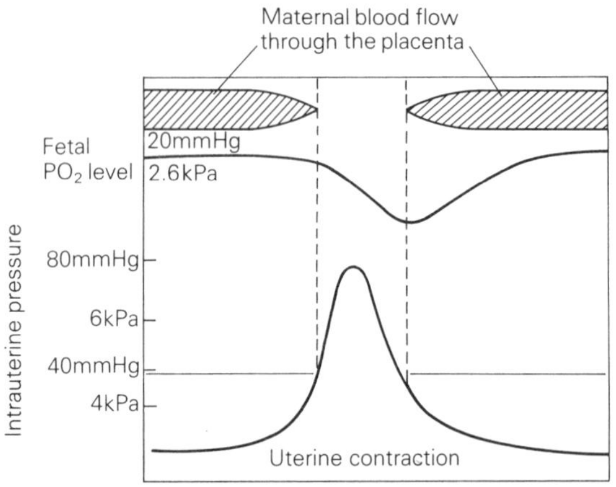

Fig. 12.2 *Effect of uterine contraction on fetal PO_2 level.*

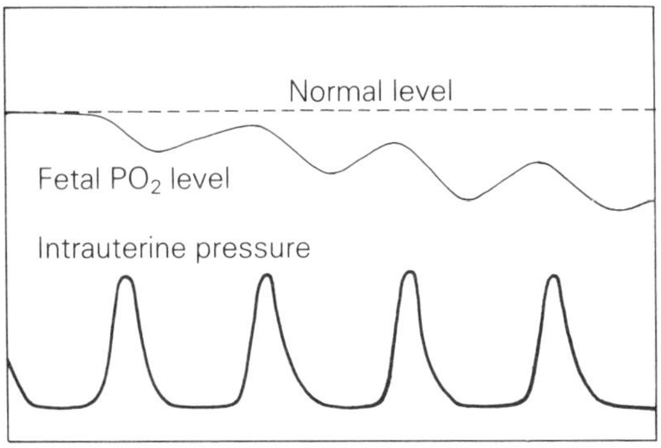

Fig. 12.3 *The effect of excessive frequency of contractions upon fetal oxygenation.*

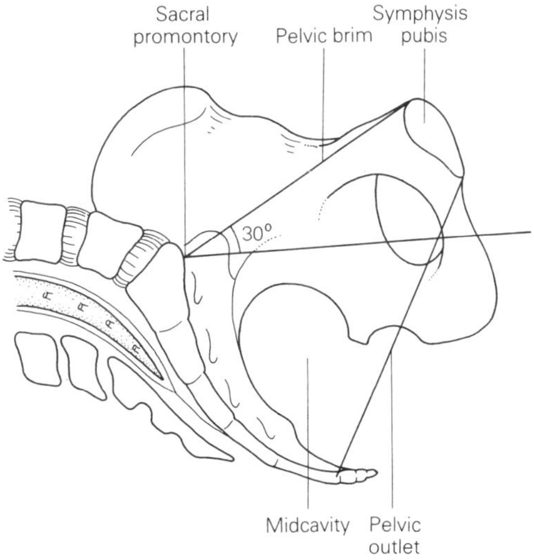

Fig. 12.4 *Lateral view of pelvis in a woman lying supine.*

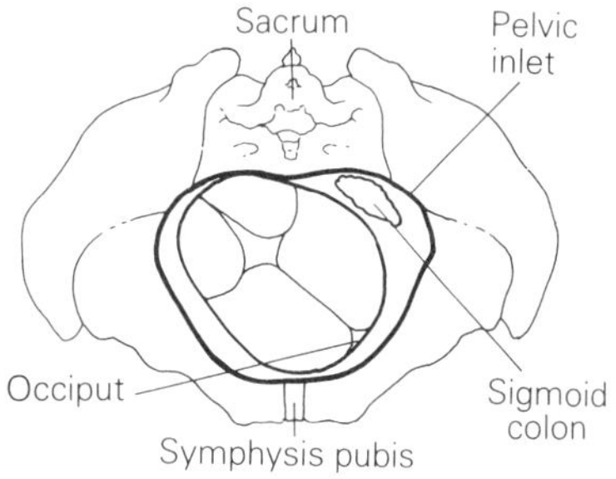

Fig. 12.5 *Relationship between the shape of the fetal head and the shape of the pelvic inlet.*

of relative hypoxia explain why labour is a stress for all fetuses, and are a particular problem for fetuses without much metabolic reserve (e.g. growth restricted) or with poor placental function (e.g. after placental abruption). They also explain why an adequate interval between contractions is vital to the well-being of the fetus in labour, being literally a 'breathing space', and why excessively frequent contractions (defined as more than one every 2–3 min) are very dangerous (Fig. 12.3).

MECHANISMS OF LABOUR

First Stage

Engagement is defined as the descent of the presenting part of the fetus (the head in over 95% of cases) into the cavity of the pelvis. The head is said to be engaged when its widest diameter has passed through the brim. Two important points should be noted. Firstly, the brim is at an angle of 30' to the horizontal in the supine woman (Fig. 12.4). Thus the direction of engagement is backwards towards the mother's sacrum rather than down towards her feet. Secondly, the pelvic brim is normally heart-shaped, as shown in Fig. 12.5, with its widest diameter in the transverse. The shape of the fetal head is such that the best fit is obtained in the oblique occipito-anterior (OA) position, and the majority of fetuses present in this way. The left occipito-anterior position is the most common, possibly because the presence of the sigmoid colon on the left side of the sacrum takes up some of the available space in the other diagonal. It is thought that the fetus selects its position simply by moving about until it settles in the position of 'best fit', rather as one would complete a jigsaw puzzle with one's eyes closed. This hypothesis is supported by the high rate of malpresentation in disorders which limit fetal movement such as fetal abnormality, or oligohydramnios; or reduce the pressure pushing the fetus down into the pelvis as in polyhydramnios. Engagement can occur as early as 36 weeks in the nullipara, although, in most parous women and many nulliparae, it only occurs during the process of labour. In the African pelvis, where the brim is often almost horizontal in the supine woman, engagement may not occur until the second stage.

Once the fetal head has entered the midcavity of the pelvis, it is free to rotate in any direction. At this point, the shoulders encounter the brim. The baby will then move around until the shoulders find the position in which they will best fit into the brim, which is when they are transverse. Because the shoulders have their widest diameter at right angles to the widest diameter of the fetal head, the head is forced to take up a position in the anteroposterior plane (Fig. 12.6). This rotation of the head from the transverse to the OA plane is known as internal rotation. It is most likely to be occipito-anterior, because the shortest distance between the occiput and the neck is down the back of the baby's head, which fits neatly behind the pubic bone, the shortest side of the pelvis. Similarly, the long sloping part of the fetal head from the occiput down over the face fits best into the curve of the sacrum (Fig. 12.7). As the fetus continues to be pushed down by regular uterine contractions, it becomes 'compacted' by flexion of the trunk and neck, so that the vertex now becomes the presenting part, rather than the top of the head. The presenting diameter accordingly becomes the suboccipito-bregmatic rather than the occipito-frontal.

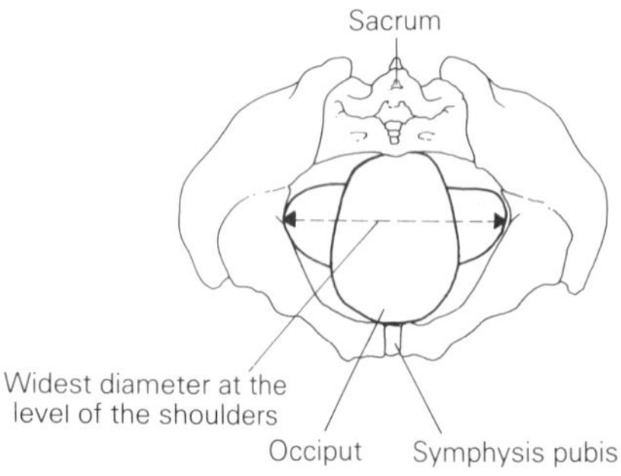

Fig. 12.6 *Positioon of head and shoulders when the head is in the midcavity and the shoulders are in the brim.*

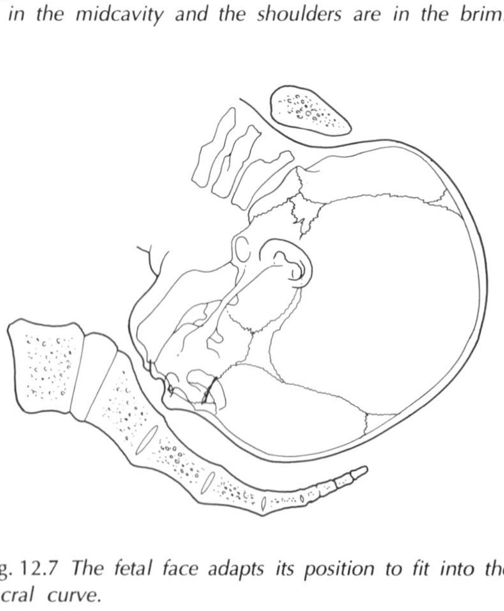

Fig. 12.7 *The fetal face adapts its position to fit into the sacral curve.*

As the fetus is pushed even further down, its head passes round the curve of the birth canal, extending its neck as it goes. Because of the process of internal rotation, it is in the correct position to pass through the outlet of the pelvis, whose widest diameter is in the OA plane. As the head emerges from the outlet, the shoulders enter the midcavity. They now have to rotate into the OA plane in order to negotiate the outlet. As they move round, the head naturally has to follow. This is known as external rotation. The anterior shoulder is normally the first to deliver, slipping under the symphysis pubis. The posterior shoulder is then born, followed easily by the rest of the body.

The corkscrew motion of the human fetus during delivery is often difficult for students to understand, but the most important point to remember is that the widest diameter of the fetal head is from front to back, while the widest diameter of the shoulders is from side to side. For the pelvis to allow delivery without being unduly wide, with consequential locomotional instability of the pelvis, it is necessary for the inlet and outlet to be separated by the length of the head, from vertex to shoulders, to be oval in shape, and to have their widest diameters at right angles to one another. This means that the head can be negotiating the outlet at the same time that the shoulders are passing through the brim, without twisting the fetus's neck into an impossible position. It is also appropriate for the widest transverse diameter to be at the brim, above the hip joints, rather than at the outlet, where the available transverse diameter is limited by the presence of the legs.

Second Stage

The second stage begins with full dilatation of the cervix, which is traditionally taken to be at 10 cm although, of course, the true dimension will vary with the size of the fetus. It ends with the delivery of the baby. The median duration of the second stage is 50 minutes in first labours and 20 minutes in second and subsequent labours.

Third Stage

The third stage of labour is from delivery of the baby to delivery of the placenta. The duration of the spontaneous third stage is about 20–60 minutes; the widely practised active management reduces this to about 5 minutes. Once the fetus has been born, the uterus continues not only to contract, but also to retract. Retraction is a process whereby, following a contraction, the muscle fibres do not return to their previous length, but become progressively shorter. As a result, the internal surface of the uterus is greatly reduced, shearing off the attachment of the placenta. Bleeding is controlled by the fact that the uterine muscle fibres are arranged in a criss-cross fashion around the perforating vessels supplying the placental bed. The retraction of the muscle fibres compresses the lumina of these vessels, the fibres thus acting as 'living ligatures'. Once the placenta is completely separated, it is squeezed out of the uterus by the continuing retraction of the upper segment. This process is often aided by maternal bearing down.

DIAGNOSIS AND MANAGEMENT OF FIRST STAGE LABOUR

Diagnosis of Onset of Labour

The primary signal that labour is occurring is progressive dilatation of the cervix in response to uterine contractions. There are three clinical signs, which are all related in some degree to this phenomenon.

A show

This is the passage of the plug of mucus that normally helps to seal the cervix during pregnancy against the ingress of infection. It falls out as the cervix begins to dilate, and may sometimes be mixed with a few streaks of blood, more blood than this should always be considered potentially abnormal. However, because cervical ripening occurs from about 36 weeks onwards in nulliparae and even earlier in parous women, the passage of a 'show' often precedes active labour by many hours, and sometimes days. The diagnosis of labour should, therefore, never be made on the basis of a show alone.

Regular painful contractions

As previously mentioned, coordinated uterine activity can be demonstrated from about 24 weeks' gestation onwards. Normally, however, contractions only become painful once the cervix starts to dilate. The onset of regular, painful contractions is, therefore, an important indirect indicator that cervical dilatation is taking place. However, because women's pain thresholds vary, and the onset of labour is often not abrupt but can take place over several days, irrevocable clinical actions such as artificial rupture of the membranes should not be undertaken without evidence of appropriate cervical dilatation obtained by vaginal examination.

Spontaneous rupture of the membranes (SROM)

In about 10% of pregnancies, SROM is the first sign that labour is starting. Contractions and progressive cervical dilatation will follow within 24 hours in 80% of cases. In the remaining 20%, there is a small risk of amniotic fluid infection occurring, usually with organisms derived from the vaginal flora. Group B streptococcus is particularly dangerous as it can affect the fetus, causing intrauterine pneumonia and even septicaemia. For this reason, most obstetric units have a policy that labour should be augmented with oxytocics, if contractions do not commence within a specified time (often 24 hours). An urgent vaginal examination is sometimes recommended to exclude cord prolapse with SROM, however, in the absence of malpresentation, this is extremely rare and can effectively be excluded by a normal cardiotocograph (CTG) tracing. In most cases, if membranes are intact at the onset of labour, they will rupture spontaneously as labour progresses. Some obstetric units have a policy of routine artificial rupture of membranes (ARM) at 4 cm dilatation. This has the advantage that meconium staining of the liquor can be detected, and a direct electrode can be applied to the fetus for CTG monitoring. It also promotes contractions in labours, where these are not yet fully established. Against this, many women feel ARM to be an unwarranted intrusion upon the normal progress of labour. Each case must, therefore, be dealt with on its merits.

Management

As explained above, the only irrefutable evidence that labour is established is progressive cervical dilatation. In all other cases, the diagnosis must be considered carefully before irrevocable action, such as ARM, is undertaken to avoid inappropriate induction of labour. The following procedures should help to clarify the situation where there is doubt.

Spontaneous rupture of membranes

A speculum examination, usually with a Cuscoe's speculum, is important to confirm that SROM has actually occurred. Often the diagnosis is clear, and copious liquor containing white specks of vernix can be seen flowing through the cervix. Sometimes, however, the history is equivocal and, on examination, only a little or even no fluid is seen in the vagina. Asking the woman to cough may produce a spurt of liquor from the cervix. Sometimes, nitrazine sticks ('amnistix') are used to test the pH of the vagina. At the normal vaginal pH of <5, the indicator is yellow, but it turns blue-green when the pH rises above 6.5. Because the pH of liquor is above 7, if the sticks turn black, it suggests the presence of liquor in the vagina. However, bacterial vaginosis is also associated with a raised pH, and contamination with maternal urine can also produce this colour change. In doubtful cases, where there are no epidemiological risk factors for infection, and the cervix is unfavourable, it may be better to take a high vaginal swab (HVS) to check for the presence of potentially pathogenic organisms, such as group B streptococci, and do nothing further if these are not found, rather than intervene with oxytocics and risk a failed induction of labour.

Contractions with an unfavourable cervix

The favourability of the cervix is normally described using the Bishop score (Table 12.1), published by E.H. Bishop in 1964 and devised by him to predict the outcome of induced labour. If the score is less than 4, 40% of induced labours in nulliparae will end in caesarean section for prolonged labour. In general, if the membranes are intact, it is unwise to intervene in labour if the Bishop score is less than 7. This applies even if the woman appears distressed with her contractions, since subsequent measurement of intrauterine pressure often shows that these women have weak contractions with a low pain threshold. It is better to assess the condition of the fetus carefully with CTG and to provide emotional support, and sometimes analgesia,

Table 12.1
Bishop Score

Cervix	0	1	2	3
Dilatation	0	1–2	3–4	5–6
Consistency	Firm	Medium	Soft	–
Canal lengths (cm)	>2	1–2	0.5–1	<0.5
Position	Posterior	Mid	Anterior	–
Station	–3	–2	–1.0	+1+2

to the mother. The active phase of labour normally starts at a Bishop score of 11, with the cervix 4 cm or more dilated and, if associated with contractions, it is then safe to diagnose labour.

Monitoring of labour progress

In current practice, a partogram is almost invariably used to monitor the progress of labour. This is a chart on which all the observations made in labour are recorded, its focal point being a graphical representation of the rate of cervical dilatation. Prior to 1970, it was common for labours to continue for many hours before recognition that adequate progress of cervical dilatation was not being made. Labours sometimes lasted several days with all the attendant risks of infection, progressive fetal asphyxia and maternal exhaustion. The pioneering work of Philpott in Zimbabwe, Studd in England, and O'Driscoll in Eire led to the concept of the 'active management of labour'. This philosophy involves regular monitoring of labour progress, allowing early intervention by oxytocin infusion or caesarean section, as appropriate, to prevent unduly prolonged labour. Current evidence suggests that failure of the Bishop score to improve by at least one point per hour in the latent phase, or of the cervix to dilate by at least 1 cm every hour in parous women or 1 cm every two hours in nulliparae should be considered abnormal, and augmentation of labour by oxytocin infusion should be considered. Randomised controlled trials have shown that such a policy reduces the duration of labour, which many women prefer. A reduced duration of labour also makes it easier to offer one-to-one care, which reduces the incidence of interventions and operative delivery. However, the use of syntocinon *per se* has no effect on the mode of delivery.

Augmentation of labour

The basic terminology of the description of uterine contractions is shown in Fig. 12.8. Mean values for the various parameters are shown in Table 12.2 as are the values below which it is generally agreed that slow progress is likely and oxytocin augmentation is warranted. Oxytocin is a potentially dangerous drug in that an overdose can cause prolonged and excessively frequent contractions, which will

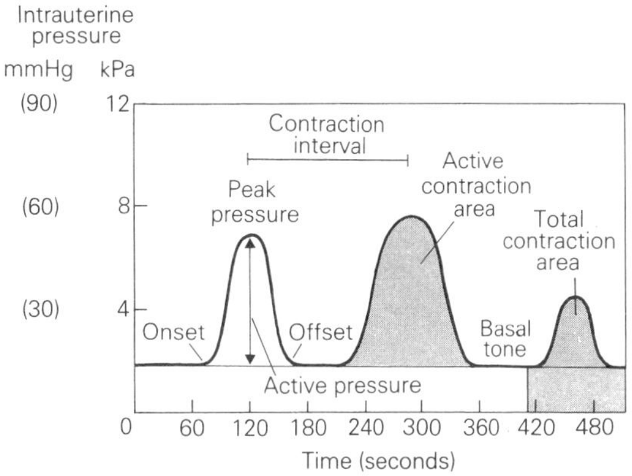

Fig. 12.8 *Terminology used when describing uterine contractions. Active pressure = peak pressure minus basal tone; active contraction area = area under contraction curve, but above basal tone; uterine activity integral (UAI) = active contraction area measured over a period of 15 min; kPa (kilo Pascal) = S.I. unit of pressure (13.3 kPa = 100 mmHg); kPa (kilo Pascal seconds) = S.I. unit of UAI (i.e. units of pressure x time).*

Table 12.2
Normal Values for Uterine Contractions

Measurement	Mean values (SD)	Lower limit below which augmentation with oxytocin is indicated
Frequency	3 per 10 min (1)	1.5 per 10 min
Active pressure	5 kPa (1.3)	3 kPa
	40 mmHg (10)	25 mmHg
Montevideo units	140 (65)	90
kPas/15 min	1100 (333)	700

asphyxiate the fetus. In the parous woman, excessive contractions may cause the uterus to rupture. Oxytocin is structurally related to ADH, and having an antidiuretic action, it can cause water retention. In association with excessive i.v. fluid administration, fits due to water intoxication can occur. Many workers have also reported an increase in neonatal jaundice when large amounts of oxytocin have been used. Ideally, therefore, the need for and the response to oxytocin stimulation should be monitored using an intrauterine catheter, in the same way that a hypotensive drug is monitored by measuring the blood pressure. However, due to lack of equipment and staff trained in its use, most obstetric units cannot do this. They must, therefore, rely on careful clinical monitoring of contractions and on observation of fetal condition, preferably by continuous fetal heart rate monitoring. Clinical monitoring of contractions can be difficult; for example if the woman is obese, and studies show that observers' impressions of the intensity of contractions are often related more to the parturient's reaction to labour than to the true intrauterine pressure. Clinical monitoring, therefore, depends heavily on measuring contraction frequency and, unfortunately, this is poorly related to overall uterine activity. The major factor in determining the rate of cervical dilatation is the active pressure of contractions. Nevertheless, prevention of excessively frequent contractions, defined as more than four in 10 minutes, is an important safeguard for fetal oxygenation. Intravenous oxytocin infusion is normally commenced at a rate of 1–2 mU/min, and increased every 15–30 minutes until adequate uterine activity is achieved. It is unusual for more than 8 mU/min to be required, and once normal contractions are established, the infusion rate can often be considerably reduced or even discontinued. Oral and vaginal prostaglandin administration for the augmentation of labour have been investigated but appear to be more unpredictable in their efficacy. They do have the advantage of allowing the patient to be ambulant.

Maternal condition should be monitored carefully during labour, with measurement of pulse rate, blood pressure and temperature every hour and more often if abnormal. Urine output and fluid intake should also be charted.

MANAGEMENT OF SECOND STAGE LABOUR

Longitudinal studies of fetal acid-base status are all agreed that there is a slow decline in fetal pH in the first stage of labour, due to the mild hypoxia produced by contractions. This continues unchanged once full dilatation has occurred, but accelerates once maternal bearing down commences. Very prolonged second stages can therefore asphyxiate even the healthy fetus. Thus, the practice grew up that if the second stage of labour, diagnosed from full dilatation, lasted longer than 30 minutes in a parous woman, or 60 minutes in a first birth, delivery should be expedited. These values represent the 90th centiles of normal spontaneous second stage labour.

However, these limits need to be modified when epidural anaesthesia is being used. Without analgesia, the woman usually becomes aware that the fetal head has descended onto the perineum, because she feels it stretching and contractions increase in intensity which is referred to as 'transition'. With epidural anaesthesia, the woman is not aware of this. Regular vaginal examinations therefore have to be performed to detect full dilatation. This can result in the diagnosis of the second stage before the head has descended and well before it would be reasonable to expect the mother to bear down. Secondly, the use of continuous fetal heart rate monitoring has enabled the birth attendant to be more objective about the diagnosis of 'fetal distress'. Thus, in the presence of epidural anaesthesia, the second stage can be allowed to continue so long as there is no sign of fetal asphyxia, and descent of the head continues. However, the duration of bearing down should not normally exceed one hour.

If it becomes evident that progress has stopped, or the mother becomes exhausted, a thorough search for the cause should be made. One or more of the following causes should be sought:

1. An overfull bladder or, rarely, rectum.
2. Malposition of fetus — commonly occipito-posterior or transverse or even, rarely, a malpresentation.
3. Too small a pelvis or a contracted outlet with a narrow subpubic angle and prominent ischial spines.
4. Inability of mother to push effectively. The use of epidural anaesthesia has increased the forceps rate in many units where it is used. In most cases of prolonged or arrested second stage labour, vacuum extraction or forceps delivery offer a suitable solution: caesarean section may be necessary if there is significant disproportion or fetal asphyxia. Operative delivery is covered in detail in Chapter 13.

MANAGEMENT OF THIRD STAGE LABOUR

If allowed to occur spontaneously, the placenta takes about 10–60 minutes to deliver. During this process, there is blood loss from the uterus, before the 'living ligatures' are fully effective. In about 10% of cases, this will exceed 500 ml and be by definition a 'primary postpartum haemorrhage' (PPH) which is loss of >500 ml of blood within 24 hours of delivery. The use of 'syntometrine' (0.5 mg ergometrine and 5 iu syntocinon given I/M or I/V with the delivery of the anterior shoulder or head of the fetus) produces a rapid and prolonged tonic contraction of the uterus, and reduces the incidence of PPH and therefore the need for blood transfusion by about 50%. However, this contraction can trap the placenta in the uterus, requiring 'manual removal'. The practice of 'active management' has, therefore been developed whereby the placenta is withdrawn by careful traction on the cord as soon as separation is evident. Suprapubic pressure is used to minimise the risk of inversion of the uterus. Such 'active management' is the usual practice in most developed countries.

Complications of the Third Stage

Retained placenta

This may occur if the placenta is morbidly adherent to the uterus, or if the cord is pulled off due to excessive traction. The management plan that should be followed is:

1. Set up an i.v. infusion if one is not already in place.
2. Take blood and arrange for 2 units to be cross-matched.
3. Call an anaesthetist.

Do *not* attempt to remove the placenta until the anaesthetist has arrived and the blood is ready, as such an attempt may precipitate a severe haemorrhage. If bleeding is excessive, it can usually be controlled by an i.v. infusion of oxytocin (10 i.u. per litre at 30 drops per minute). When everything has been prepared, the operator should 'scrub up' and clean the perineum. The bladder should be catheterised and a gentle vaginal examination performed, as in many cases the placenta will have separated spontaneously and be lying in the vagina, in which case it can be delivered without further ado. If not, the woman is then given an anaesthetic. If an epidural is already in place, it can be topped up to give complete anaesthesia. The cervix is then dilated manually with the hand in a funnel shape and the placenta sheared off with the fingers, grasped and withdrawn.

Postpartum haemorrhage

This is described in Chapter 14.

LABOUR AND THE FETUS

The fetus is adapted in many ways to the relative hypoxia of the intrauterine environment. For example, the dissociation curve of fetal haemoglobin is shifted to the left compared with adult haemoglobin, which allows the effective delivery of oxygen at partial pressures much lower than in the adult. This is necessary because the fetus obtains its oxygen via its mother, rather than directly from the atmosphere, and operates at an arterial pO_2 of 3–4 kPa rather than the normal adult value of 12–14 kPa. This shift results in the preferential transfer of oxygen from the maternal blood to fetal blood across the placental interface and also means that significant amounts of oxygen are held in reserve in fetal haemoglobin even when the pO_2 falls as low as 1–1.5 kPa. The low pO_2 at which the fetus lives has many important secondary effects. For example, it maintains the patency of the ductus arteriosus, which acts like a shunt allowing blood to bypass the lungs, which are not yet functional. It is also thought to maintain a high level of cerebral endorphins ('endogenous morphines'), a phenomenon also seen in severely hypoxic adults. A powerful action of endorphins is the suppression of breathing reflexes, an action also seen with 'synthetic endorphins' such as pethidine. The fetus does make some breathing movements *in utero*, which are important in the proper development of the lungs, but these are sporadic and interspersed with long periods of apnoea. In labour, the further reduction of pO_2 produced by uterine contractions effectively abolishes regular fetal respiratory movement, replacing it with intermittent gasping. This gasping is important at delivery, since the rapid rise in pO_2 produced by gasping and expansion of the lungs switches off the production of endorphins and allows the establishment of regular respiration. Endorphins may also play a part in regulating the cerebral state of the fetus. Ultrasound study of fetal heart rate and activity patterns, coupled with EEG recordings during labour, suggest that the fetus spends less than 5% of its time in a state which in the adult we would term 'awake'. Most of its time is, therefore, spent in various forms of 'sleep'. In view of the very limited environmental stimulation available to the fetus, this would seem an appropriate adaptation. Initially, there is no differentiation within the sleep state, but from about 30–32 weeks' gestation upwards, periods of 'quiet sleep' become distinguishable from periods of 'active sleep'. In quiet sleep, fetal activity is at a minimum. In active sleep, there is considerable fetal movement, usually associated with increased heart rate variability and accelerations in fetal heart rate. 'Rapid eyeball movements' that are associated with dreaming in the adult, can also be demonstrated. Fetal breathing movements are also more in evidence. Active and quiet sleep alternate at intervals of between 20 and 40 minutes and the transition between them is often abrupt. These alternating periods continue during labour and appreciating them is vital to the clinical interpretation of CTG traces.

Fetal Monitoring in Labour

In order to understand the analysis of fetal heart rate (FHR) patterns, it is necessary to appreciate how they are produced, using a cardiotocograph machine. In such a machine, signals representing cardiac action, either electrical (the 'R' wave of cardiac depolarisation) or more commonly ultrasound (Doppler signals representing cardiac movement) are used to measure the duration of the cardiac cycle. This measurement is correctly expressed in milliseconds. However, clinical measurement of heart rate has traditionally been by counting the number of beats in a given interval, usually one minute. In order to convert the measurement of cardiac cycle length into a figure readily understood by clinical personnel, it has become customary to programme the CTG machine to divide the measurement in milliseconds into 60,000 (one minute), thus obtaining the rate which would be counted if that interval continued unchanged for the next minute. For example, a beat-to-beat interval (one cardiac cycle) of 500 ms is equivalent to a heart rate of 120 beats per minute (bpm); one of 333.3 ms is approximately equivalent to 180 bpm, etc. In practice, of course, the fetal heart rate does not beat with such regularity, there normally being a variation of

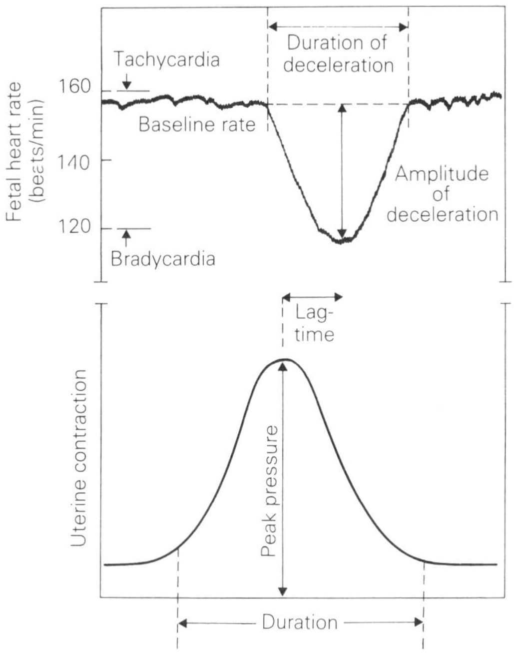

Fig. 12.9 *Terms used in the study of continuous records of FHR.*

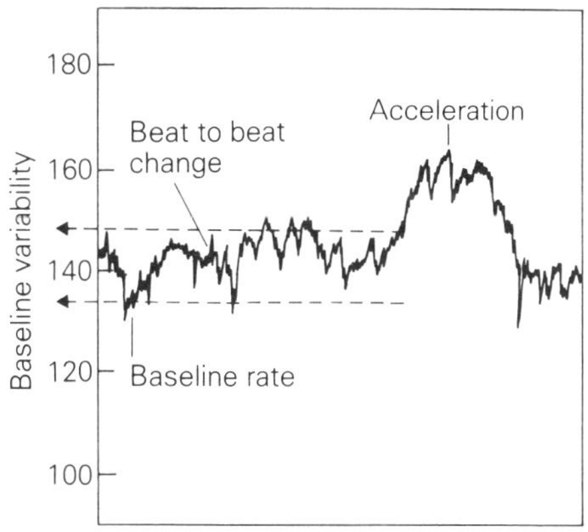

Fig. 12.10 *Beat-to-beat variation and baseline variabilituy.*

0.4–1.2 bpm between beats, this being defined as the beat-to-beat variation. The significance of beat-to-beat variation has been studied for many years, but at present its clinical implication is obscure. Because of this, the normal CTG machine uses a chart recording system, which is not designed to demonstrate beat-to-beat variation, but rather the more gross fluctuations in rate known as baseline variability, accelerations and decelerations. The chart recorder is by convention operated at a paper speed of 1 (UK) or 3 (USA) cm per minute. The terminology used in normal CTG analysis is shown in Fig. 12.9.

Baseline rate

This is the lowest rate to which the fetal heart rate consistently returns. The average baseline rate during labour is about 135 bpm, with two standard deviations of $\pm$ 25 bpm. Accordingly, FIGO (Federation International Gynecologie et Obstetrique) guidelines give the normal range as between 110 bpm and 150 bpm. A rate slower than this is called bradycardia and a faster rate is called tachycardia. Confusingly, the traditional British range of normality is 120–160 bpm. In practice, the higher or lower that the rate is beyond the FIGO limits, the more concerned one should be. A rise during labour, for example from 120 bpm to 150 bpm, should also be considered as suspicious as it may indicate the release of catecholamines in the fetus consequent upon accumulating hypoxic stress.

Baseline variability

This consists of oscillations in rate which normally range between 5 and 15 bpm (Fig. 12.10). There are usually about 2–5 oscillations per minute. They reflect the fine adjustments of heart rate produced by the autonomic nervous system in response to fluctuations in the fetal environment.

Accelerations

Accelerations are increases in rate of more than 15 bpm which last for more than 15 seconds. They are often associated with fetal movement, as both occur mostly in active sleep.

Decelerations

Decelerations are decreases in rate of more than 15 bpm for more than 15 seconds. There are two main types of deceleration:

Reflex decelerations are neurologically mediated via the vagus nerve. They are most often produced by head or cord compression. Head compression raises intracranial pressure. This activates the baroceptor mechanisms, which normally control intracranial pressure by regulating the pressure of the blood supply; blood pressure is, therefore, reduced via a vagally mediated bradycardia. Cord compression cuts off 25% of the fetal peripheral circulation producing a dramatic rise in peripheral resistance. Blood pressure rises as a consequence, and stretch receptors in the aorta act via the vagus nerve to produce bradycardia, limiting the rise in pressure. Both head and cord compression normally occur only during contractions. The resulting decelerations, therefore, occur synchronously with the contraction, with the nadir of the deceleration being at the peak of the contraction.

Hypoxic decelerations usually occur only if the pO_2 in fetal arterial blood falls below 1–1.8 kPa. At these levels, lactate produced in the myocardium has a direct effect to reduce FHR. The pattern of reduction in rate follows the pO_2 level, usually reaching a nadir at, or after, the end of a contraction (see Fig. 12.3). These decelerations are therefore delayed, or late, with respect to the contraction.

Techniques of monitoring the fetal heart rate

External FHR monitoring uses ultrasound (approximately 2.5 MHz) which is beamed from a piezo-electric transmitter towards the fetal heart. The movement of the heart alters the frequency of the reflected sound (Doppler effect), which is detected via a piezoelectric receiver. The transmitter and one or more receivers are usually combined in a single transducer. Air, which transmits ultrasound poorly, is excluded from the transducer-skin interface by a coupling medium, usually arachis oil or a proprietary gel but water can be used for short term monitoring. The Doppler signal, which reflects fetal heart activity, is used to trigger a rate meter and the rate is recorded continuously on a chart recorder. The signal is rather diffuse and, therefore, difficult to time, and so most CTG machines use various technical 'tricks', such as autocorrelation, to produce an interpretable trace. However, it should be noted that this produces a recording which is different in detail from a simultaneous trace produced using the R wave of the fetal ECG as a trigger for the rate meter. The fetal ECG can be detected from two electrodes placed on the mother's abdomen, but the signal strength is often poor and heavily contaminated with the maternal ECG and EMG noise. In labour, therefore, it is usually derived from an electrode placed directly onto the presenting part of the fetus, whose voltage is compared with an electrode in the maternal vagina. This technique usually produces a very clear and easily interpreted tracing, and, unlike ultrasound, recording is relatively insensitive to disturbance by maternal or fetal movement. The major disadvantage of using a direct electrode for electronic fetal heart rate monitoring (EFHRM) is that it requires the membranes to be ruptured. However, there are no proven deleterious effects of membrane rupture on the fetus other than an apparently innocuous increase in the incidence of synchronous decelerations due to head compression. In addition, ARM may speed desultory labour by encouraging contractions, and it also allows inspection of the liquor for the presence of meconium.

In normal, uncomplicated labour, modern technology using ultrasound is so good that it is nearly always used for fetal heart rate monitoring, especially as it is perceived as less invasive. However, the use of a fetal electrode should be considered if the tracing quality is poor.

Techniques of monitoring contractions

The easiest method of recording contractions is to use an external 'tocodynamometer' or strain gauge. However, this instrument can only record accurately the frequency of contractions; relative intensity is also registered, but the true intrauterine pressure (IUP) cannot be measured reliably per abdomen. Thus the technique is satisfactory if the contractions only need to be recorded as an aid to interpretation of the FHR trace. If the true IUP needs to be measured to investigate slow labour or to allow accurate control of an oxytocin infusion, then an intrauterine catheter must be used, which usually requires that the membranes be ruptured. Two types are available: an open-ended fluid-filled catheter connected to an external pressure transducer, and a closed catheter with a pressure transducer mounted on its tip, so that the transducer is inserted into the uterine cavity. The latter system is easier to use and less subject to artefact, but can be expensive if the sensitive transducers are damaged frequently by careless use. It can be seen from the above that for most routine monitoring, the external system of ultrasound FHR and tocodynamometer contraction recording is satisfactory but, in high risk cases, the more precise and reliable internal electrodes and transducers are preferable.

Normal traces. Figure 12.11 shows normal baseline rate, variability and reactivity and the absence of decelerations. If these criteria are fulfilled, the likelihood of a baby being born in poor condition with a 5-minute Apgar score <7 is less than 2%. A baseline rate between 100 and 110 bpm with no other abnormality can be considered normal, uncomplicated baseline bradycardia. Early decelerations of

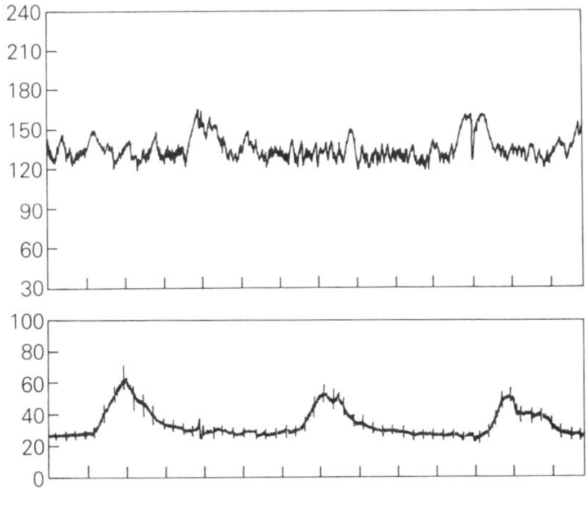

Fig. 12.11 *Normal trace.*

less than 40 bpm synchronous with uterine contractions but with no other abnormality can also be considered normal in advanced labour, but should be considered as suspicious in early labour as they may indicate cord compression. Larger decelerations with no late component, and normal baseline rate and variability, can also be considered normal in the second stage of labour, as they are often due to head compression during descent through the pelvis.

Suspicious traces. These are defined as such when one or two of the descriptive components of the CTG are abnormal. There are many permutations of the suspicious trace, and their implications are often different. However, some of the more commonly observed abnormalities are:

1. *Uncomplicated baseline tachycardia,* greater than 150 bpm with normal baseline variability and no decelerations, may be normal in some very preterm fetuses. This pattern is often associated with maternal pyrexia, which may be relatively harmless due to a hot room or interference with maternal sweating from epidural anaesthesia, but more seriously may be due to intrauterine infection. An uncomplicated baseline tachycardia may also represent the earliest sign of asphyxial stress and should, therefore, be investigated carefully.
2. *Uncomplicated loss of variability* may be physiological or due to drugs such as pethidine, diazepam or nitrous oxide (Fig. 12.12). However, it may be due to asphyxia and should, therefore, always be investigated if it persists for longer than 40 minutes.
3. *Uncomplicated variable decelerations* of >40 bpm with variable shape and timing most commonly reflect cord compression, usually due to cord entanglement around limb, body or neck, but occasionally indicate prolapse of the cord. They can also be produced by severe head compression. Acute problems with cord occlusion during delivery may occur. This pattern does not initially indicate asphyxia, but asphyxia may develop if the

cord compression interferes significantly with fetal circulation.

4. *Late decelerations* always indicate fetal hypoxia, but this may be relatively mild and temporary, and many normal fetuses can tolerate mild asphyxia for several hours without coming to serious harm. Nevertheless, when late decelerations are seen, attempts should always be made to identify the cause of the hypoxia and correct it. Common causes of reversible hypoxia are the supine position, uterine hyperstimulation with oxytocin and epidural hypotension. If late decelerations persist, further investigation is necessary (Fig. 12.13).

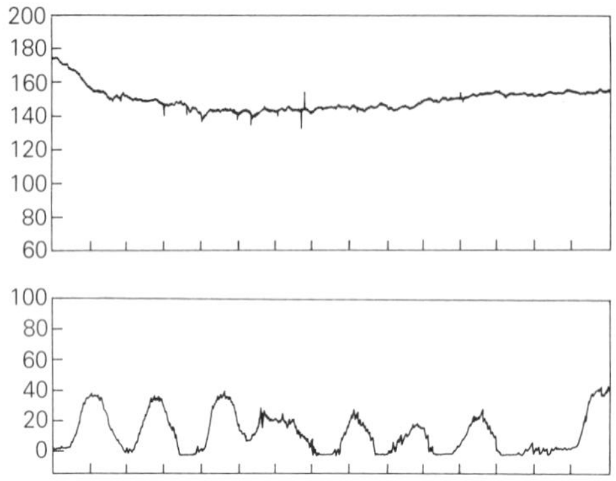

Fig. 12.12 *Uncomplicated loss of variability.*

Abnormal traces. At least three, and sometimes all, of the descriptive components of the CTG are abnormal. This is very serious and carries with it up to a 50% risk of fetal acidosis and a 20% risk of a 5-minute Apgar score <7. Such traces should be uncommon in

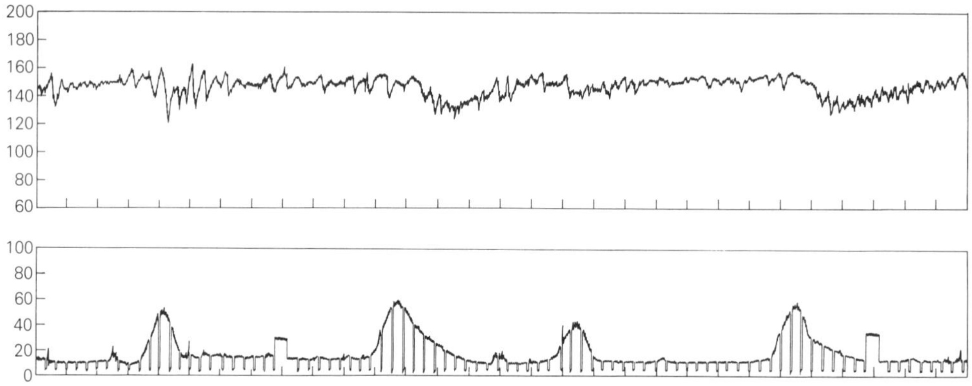

Fig. 12.13 *Late decelerations following epidural top-up.*

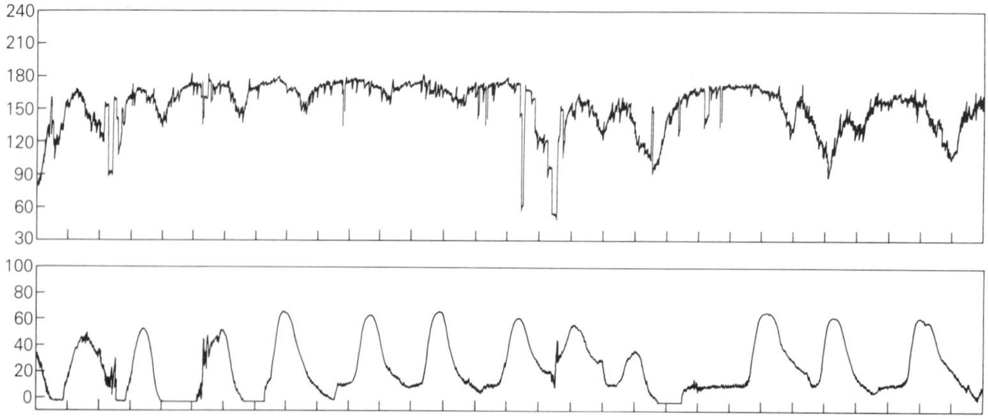

Fig. 12.14 *Abnormal trace showing non-reactive tachycardia with late decelerations.*

modern practice, since they usually progress from normal traces through one of the milder abnormalities described above. Corrective action to relieve the cause of the abnormality or to deliver the fetus should, therefore, usually prevent the appearance of a severely abnormal trace. The most common severely abnormal trace is a non-reactive tachycardia accompanied by late or variable decelerations (Fig 12.14). If there is also loss of variability, then the trace is likely to be preterminal and, even with prompt delivery, the risk of long-term neurological handicap is significant. It is followed by a fixed baseline bradycardia as the fetus actually dies.

Factors modifying the interpretation of the CTG

The predictive value of the CTG tracing taken alone is relatively low. For example, even using a short-term measure of neonatal outcome, such as a 1-minute Apgar score <7, only about 30% of fetuses with a suspicious trace will have an abnormal outcome, compared with about 10% if the trace is normal. Even if the CTG is severely abnormal, the predictive value only rises to about 50%. The predictive value of the CTG can, however, be improved if it is interpreted in conjunction with other indicators, such as meconium staining of the liquor, growth status of the baby, and pH of a fetal blood sample (FBS).

Meconium staining of the liquor. The passage of meconium by the fetus is a reflex response to stress which matures with age. Fetuses <34 weeks rarely pass meconium unless the bowel is directly irritated; for example, by infection with *Listeria monocytogenes.* On the other hand, one-third of fetuses of >42 weeks' gestational age will pass meconium in response to the normal stress of labour. It is, therefore, often a normal physiological event and, in the presence of a normal CTG, does not predict an abnormal neonatal outcome. However, excessive stress does increase the likelihood of meconium passage, and the combination of an abnormal CTG and meconium staining of the liquor, therefore, has an enhanced predictive value of about 40%.

Intrauterine growth restriction (IUGR). Many studies have shown that poorly grown fetuses are more susceptible to the effects of asphyxia than normally grown infants. The reasons for this are complex and not fully understood at the present time. Fortunately, a normal CTG in labour is just as predictive of normality in the growth restricted fetus as in the normally grown fetus. An abnormal trace, however, is almost twice as likely to be associated with an abnormal outcome in a growth restricted fetus compared with one that is normally grown. Moreover, the decline in pH in response to asphyxia is more rapid in the growth restricted infant. IUGR which is suspected on clinical, ultrasound or biochemical grounds before labour is, therefore, an important factor to be taken into account when interpreting the CTG trace.

Fetal blood sampling and pH measurement

CTG analysis is a screening technique, and cannot of itself quantify the effects of a stress on the fetus. If asphyxia is suspected, then the effects of this on the fetus should be quantified by taking a FBS for pH and, if possible, blood gas analysis. The scalp (or buttock in a breech presentation), is visualised via a metal tube called an amnioscope. The procedure cannot be performed if the cervix is less than 2 cm dilated. Ethyl chloride is sprayed on to cool the skin, following which a reactive hyperaemia occurs. This encourages the bleeding produced by piercing the skin with a 2 mm guarded blade mounted on a special holder. The blood is encouraged to form a discrete droplet by smearing the skin with silicone grease before the puncture is made, The blood is then drawn up into a preheparinised capillary tube, which is used to transfer the blood to a suitable blood gas/pH analyser.

The main objective of pH analysis of a FBS is to determine the degree of metabolic acidosis which has occurred as a result of asphyxial stress. Measurement of pCO_2 and base deficit helps to exclude the effects of transitory respiratory acidosis. If only pH measurement is available, then care should be taken not to take a FBS after an acute event when CO_2 is likely to be elevated.

The normal fetus has a pH between 7.30 and 7.45, a pO_2 between 3 and 4 kPa, a pCO_2 between 4 and 5 kPa and a base deficit less than 6 mmol/l. A pH between 7.25 and 7.30 suggests a stressed fetus, but is not dangerous in the short term. A pH between 7.15 and 7.25 is definitely abnormal, and operative delivery should be considered if spontaneous delivery is not imminent. A pH below 7.15 represents an emergency, and in association with an abnormal CTG trace is likely to be associated with asphyxia in greater than 50% of cases. A pH below 7.20 in the umbilical cord artery at birth carries a 10–15% risk of permanent neurological damage.

There is no doubt that use of CTG monitoring without a fetal blood sample results in an increase in the caesarean section rate, as operative delivery is undertaken in cases where the CTG is abnormal, but the outcome shows that the fetus was not, in fact, significantly asphyxiated. Even with the most abnormal CTG, a complicated baseline tachycardia, the likelihood of finding a significant metabolic acidosis on FBS is only about 50%. Unfortunately, FBS requires a level of equipment, staffing and expertise that is not available in many obstetric units even in the developed world. With women's increasing intolerance of long labours, and the risk of litigation in the event of a poor outcome, the caesarean section rate is now more than 20% in many UK maternity units. It is often perceived as easier and safer to perform a caesarean section, despite the significant but uncommon risks to the mother, than to perform a fetal blood sample, and consequently it is being performed less and less in current practice.

Risks Facing the Fetus in Labour

Asphyxia

The expression 'fetal distress' means simply a fetus thought to be in 'poor condition' and in need of delivery. Similarly, a baby in poor condition at birth is often said to be 'flat' i.e. in need of resuscitation. However, the causes of poor condition are many, for example, asphyxia, trauma, meconium aspiration, infection, and nuchal cord (cord around the neck). Asphyxia remains the most common single cause of distress. Originally meaning simply 'pulseless', from the Greek a-sphyxos, asphyxia is now defined more rigorously by the American College of Obstetrics and Gynecology as a combination of acidosis (pH<7.00), poor condition at birth, namely a five-minute Apgar score 3 or less, neonatal encephalopathy which presents usually as fits and poor feeding, and evidence of dysfunction of other fetal organs. The earliest manifestation of reduced oxygen supply to the fetus is hypoxaemia which, if prolonged, will eventually lead to metabolic acidosis as lactate from anaerobic respiration accumulates. If the interference with oxygenation is acute and severe, it is usually accompanied by hypercarbia, which produces respiratory acidosis. The fall in pH due to hypercarbia can be reversed rapidly if gas exchange is restored, unlike the more persistent metabolic acidosis. Chronic asphyxia can be caused by inadequate placental function and may, therefore, be associated with intrauterine growth restriction. This combination is doubly dangerous, because the growth restricted fetus's ability to cope with asphyxia is often severely compromised. Asphyxia can be caused by events such as placental abruption or cord prolapse, or by iatrogenic insults such as severe maternal hypotension secondary to epidural anaesthesia and the supine position, or uterine hyperstimulation with oxytocics.

Trauma

The most obvious form of trauma is that which can be inflicted upon the fetus during delivery. For example, during injudicious vaginal breech delivery, the fetus is at risk of trauma to the limbs, visceral trauma, particularly rupture of the liver, traction injury to the brachial plexus, and intracranial injury, such as tentorial tears and intraventricular haemorrhage. Intracranical injury can also occur as a result of forceps delivery, particularly rotational forceps. The risk of intracranial damage is potentiated if there is cerebral oedema secondary to asphyxia, because the brain is stiff and cannot cope normally with deforming forces. A less obvious form of trauma is due to severe and prolonged head compression; for example where there is cephalopelvic disproportion. This can be detected by assessing 'moulding' of the fetal head. If the sutures of the fetal skull are pressed closely together, there is said to be one '+' of moulding. If the sutures overlap, but can be reduced by finger pressure, the moulding is '++', and if it is irreducible, there is '+++' moulding. Prolonged severe head compression can lead to neonatal cerebral malfunction and should, therefore, be avoided. Moulding should not be confused with caput, which is simply oedema of the presenting part, and is much more common.

Meconium aspiration

The passage of meconium by the fetus in labour is not necessarily abnormal. However, when combined with gasping produced by asphyxia, it can lead to the inhalation of meconium with a resulting severe pneumonitis.

Infection

This is an uncommon, but potentially very serious, risk. It is associated with prolonged rupture of the membranes, and the presence of potentially pathogenic organisms in the vagina, such as group B streptococci. The risk is increased if an excessive number of vaginal examinations are performed. The baby may be born with pneumonia or even septicaemia. The mother may also become ill from endometritis or septicaemia. A pyrexia or fetal tachycardia should always alert the accoucheur to the possibility of infection, which should be investigated with appropriate cultures, and if necessary treated with a suitable antibiotic.

Inadequate ventilation at birth

Delivery normally induces reflex expansion of the chest, filling the lungs with air and causing a rapid rise in arterial pO_2. This, in turn, produces closure of the ductus arteriosus and the establishment of the adult pattern of circulation. This reflex may be inadequately developed, for example in the preterm fetus, or suppressed, for example by drugs such as narcotics or general anaesthetics. In severe asphyxia, the fetus may already have passed the point at which it is capable of responding to delivery by taking a breath. In all these circumstances, which are mostly predictable, the presence of a skilled paediatrician capable of intubation is vital.

CONTROL OF PAIN IN LABOUR

Although some women are lucky and have relatively little pain in labour, for many women it is the most painful experience of their lives. A lot can be done to prepare women beforehand and to give them confidence. Understanding the birth process is in itself helpful in removing the fear of the unknown, and all women should be encouraged to attend appropriate antenatal classes. Some women may also benefit from techniques such as psycho-prophylaxis, hypnosis and transcutaneous nerve stimulation (TENS). These all have the major advantage of being without significant side-effects. Their disadvantage is that they require considerable motivation and effort from all concerned over a fairly long period and are, therefore, seldom taken up by women in the poorer socioeconomic groups. They may also prove inadequate to deal with the pain, particularly if the labour is longer or more difficult than initially anticipated. There is, therefore, always likely to be a place for the pharmacological methods of pain relief. The simplest and oldest agents used for analgesia in labour are the narcotics. Pethidine, 50–150 mg, is most widely used in the UK. However, narcotics have been shown to be poor analgesics, and their effect is mainly to cause sedation and (sometimes) euphoria. Thus, women still feel pain, but care less about it. On the debit side, they frequently cause nausea and are, therefore, often given with an antiemetic such as metoclopramide. Some women find the psychic effects unpleasant, and some find the pain relief simply inadequate. The other main disadvantage is that when given within 1–4 hours of delivery, narcotics can suppress spontaneous neonatal respiration so that artificial ventilation is necessary, although this effect can be reversed rapidly with I.M. naloxone. The **inhalational anaesthetic agent,** nitrous oxide, can be used to supplement narcotics, or on its own. It is supplied as a 50/50 mixture with oxygen (Entonox) and is self-administered via a hand-held mask. It is not primarily an analgesic, but causes a feeling of detachment which many women find makes the pain more bearable. It is taken at the beginning of each contraction, and about four or five deep breaths are usually sufficient to provide the effect. It can be allowed to wear off between contractions as it takes effect very quickly. There are very few side-effects. **Pudendal nerve block** coupled with local anaesthetic infiltration of the perineum can provide reasonable anaesthesia for a non-rotational forceps delivery. However, it is not helpful in the first stage of labour and almost never provides sufficient pain relief for rotational forceps delivery.

Epidural Anaesthesia

A method of pain relief which has increased dramatically in popularity over the last 25 years is epidural anaesthesia. The basic anatomy of an epidural block is shown in Fig. 12.15. A plastic catheter is introduced into the epidural space and repeated injections of local anaesthetic can then be made. The aim is to stop transmission in the small pain fibres with, at the same time, minimal effect on the larger sensory and motor fibres. The development in the last ten years of so-called 'mobile' epidurals,

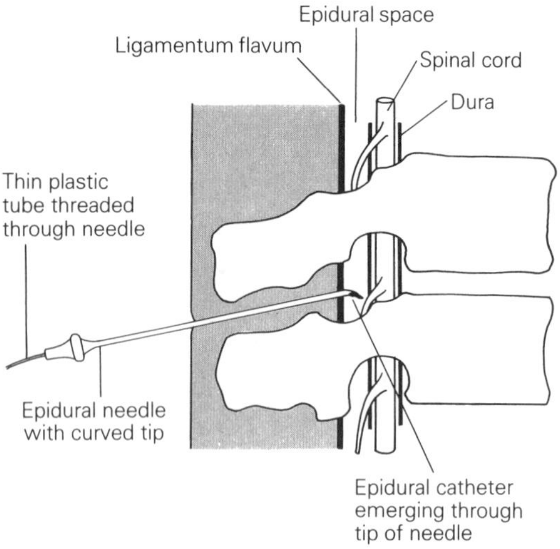

Fig. 12.15 *Principle of epidural catheter insertion.*

in which very low concentrations of marcaine are combined with opiates such as fentanil, has meant that numb, immobile legs are now much less common in women using epidural anaesthesia while over 80% of women experience complete relief of pain, with most of the remainder obtaining considerable benefit. This is why it is so popular; in many hospitals about 35% of women choose to have an epidural, and in some hospitals the figure is as high as 80%. There are, however, some potentially serious side-effects from epidurals, and these should always be borne in mind when they are used.

1. *Dural tap,* which is inadvertent penetration of the spinal canal. This occurs in up to 2% of cases, depending on the experience of the anaesthetist. Because a large gauge needle has to be used to pass the catheter, a considerable leak of cerebrospinal fluid may occur with reduction of pressure and subsequent severe headache if the patient is not lying flat. More seriously, if the puncture is not appreciated, direct injection of local anaesthetic into the subarachnoid space may occur, with resulting rapid anaesthesia of the whole spinal column, producing total paralysis and respiratory arrest.

It can be treated with artificial ventilation until the anaesthetic wears off; but deaths have occurred before the nature of the problem was appreciated.
2. *Hypotension.* Paralysis of the lumbar sympathetic outflow causes loss of vascular tone in the lower limbs with consequent blood pooling, reduction of venous return, and severe maternal hypotension. If this is exacerbated by caval compression from the supine position, death can result. Minor degrees of hypotension can produce severe reductions in uterine blood flow with consequent fetal hypoxia. Many of these problems can be prevented by infusion of 500–1000 ml of colloid solutions, such as Hartmann's, before the local anaesthetic is given. This technique is called 'preloading'. All women having an epidural must, therefore, have an i.v. line *in situ*.
3. *Increased incidence of forceps delivery.* The epidural interferes with normal sensation, and so bearing down efforts are often impaired. About 50% of nulliparae will require forceps delivery for this reason if they opt for an epidural; this figure can be reduced by allowing longer second stages, with careful monitoring. However, 85% of parous women will achieve a spontaneous delivery despite having an epidural.
4. *Interference with bladder function.* Loss of sensation means that women frequently have to be catheterised in labour. Normal bladder function can take 24 hours or even longer to return following delivery, and repeat catheterisations inevitably lead to an increased incidence of urinary tract infections.
5. *Long-term backache and paralysis.* Such complications can happen, but are extremely rare. Paralysis probably occurs in less than one in a million epidurals and when it does is probably due to the injection of the wrong material down the epidural catheter.

Absolute contraindications

1. Infection at or near the site of puncture.
2. Coagulopathy, for example in fulminating pre-eclampsia or abruptio placentae; or anticoagulant therapy. An epidural should not be placed if the platelet count is less than 80×10^9/l.

Relative contraindications

1. Actual or anticipated serious maternal haemorrhage with increased risk of sever hypotension.
2. Fetal hypoxia, which may be exacerbated disastrously if hypotension occurs.

It can be seen from the above that epidurals carry a significant medical risk; they should probably only be carried out when there is an anaesthetist and an obstetrician constantly available for the labour ward, and in a hospital with an intensive care unit.

Indications other than maternal request

Epidurals are useful in the management of twin labour, because the second twin may develop a malpresentation during the delivery of the first, which is uncorrectable except by internal podalic version which is inserting a hand into the uterus, grasping the feet of the baby and delivering it by breech extraction. An epidural eliminates the delay required to institute general anaesthesia and, if the version is unsuccessful, the surgeon can proceed directly to caesarean section. A similar advantage accrues to the use of epidurals in prolonged labour, or breech presentation, where a vaginal delivery may have to be abandoned at short notice and resort made to caesarean section. Epidurals also have many advantages for elective caesarean operations. They allow the mother and her partner to enjoy the birth of their baby, there is less risk of anaesthetic complications such as aspiration pneumonia and chest infections and no depression of fetal respiration. The mother must be tilted laterally to about 30° to prevent fetal hypoxia due to caval compression and inadequate placental perfusion during delivery.

FURTHER READING

1. Steer P., Flint C. (1999). ABC of labour care: Physiology and management of normal labour. *BMJ* **318**: 793–796.
2. Steer P. (1999). ABC of labour care: Assessment of mother and fetus in labour. *BMJ* **318**: 858–861.
3. Steer P.J., Danielian P.J. (1999). Fetal distress in labor. In: *High Risk Pregnancy — Management Options.* James D.K., Steer P.J., Weiner C.P., Gonik B. (eds). London: W.B. Saunders.

13

Abnormal Labour

Normal labour may be defined as the occurrence of regular uterine contractions with effacement and progressive dilatation of the cervix leading to spontaneous vaginal delivery of the baby between 37 and 42 completed weeks of gestation. Abnormal labour may be considered as all forms of labour which fall outside the limits of this definition thus providing a practical basis for discussing preterm labour, induction of labour, prolonged labour, operative delivery and malpresentations, each of which constitutes a form of abnormal labour.

INDUCTION OF LABOUR

Induction of labour is the initiation of uterine activity by an independent stimulus to achieve vaginal delivery of the fetus prior to the onset of spontaneous labour.

Since 1948, when the administration of oxytocin by i.v. infusion to induce uterine contractions became feasible, induction of labour has become a practical reality and a part of usual practice in every obstetric unit. At first, the availability of induction of labour was accepted enthusiastically by obstetricians with the genuine aim of reducing both maternal and perinatal mortality and morbidity. However, the last three decades have seen enormous swings in the frequency with which induction is used and this perhaps reflects that its use has not produced the dramatic improvement in perinatal mortality that was expected. Currently there is a downward trend in the frequency of induction of labour, but there remains a marked variation from one obstetric unit to another.

Indications

Indications for induction of labour may be obstetric or non-obstetric. A list of indications can never be complete, as obstetricians vary considerably in their views on acceptable reasons for induction of labour. Also, individual patients present differing circumstances which might make induction of labour appropriate or inappropriate.

Obstetric and medical conditions

Well-defined complications such as pre-eclampsia, hypertension in pregnancy, intra-uterine growth retardation, antepartum haemorrhage, multiple pregnancy, prolonged pregnancy, diabetes mellitus, rhesus isoimmuni-sation, gross congenital fetal abnormality and

Table 13.1
Indications for Induction of Labour

Indication for induction	Number (%)
Post-maturity	344 (41.8)
Pre-eclampsia/Hypertension	232 (28.2)
Static maternal weight/Weight loss at term	72 (8.8)
Previous caesarean section/Hysterotomy	46 (5.6)
Breech presentation	34 (4.0)
Antepartum haemorrhage	33 (4.0)
Placental insufficiency	25
Poor obstetric history	20
Diabetes/abnormal GTT	15
Spurious labour	23
Intrauterine death	10
Haemolytic disease	4
Congenital malformations	1
Multiple pregnancy	7
Others	34

fetal death *in utero* are generally accepted to warrant planned elective delivery. Table 13.1 lists the indications for induction of labour and their frequency in one obstetric unit. It is worth noting that not all of these indications would receive universal approval throughout the United Kingdom.

Relative indications

Individual patients will present differing features which are peculiar to themselves but which will influence a decision to deliver electively. Maternal age, poor obstetric history, previous infertility and a previous child suffering from the effects of traumatic childbirth or post-maturity are examples. Often a mother will have a combination of these factors and, although each factor on its own may constitute an insufficient reason for induction of labour, their cumulative effect cannot be ignored.

Social indications

On the whole, social convenience for both patient and obstetrician has not been generally accepted in the UK as an indication for the induction of labour. This was not the prevailing attitude in the United States, and since 1978, the Food and Drug Administration has required the pharmaceutical companies to include the following information with oxytocin supplied to hospitals:

Important Notice. Pitocin is not indicated for the elective induction of labour because available data and information are inadequate to define the benefits-to-risks considerations in the use of the drug's product. Elective induction of labour is defined as the initiation of labour in an individual with a term pregnancy who is free of medical indications for the initiation of labour.

The American College of Obstetricians and Gynaecologists (1982) recommended that induction of labour with oxytocin should be initiated only if required for the benefit of the mother or fetus.

There are occasional situations in which planned delivery may be necessary to provide the best level of care for a baby and/or mother. Such a planned delivery allows for the availability of anaesthetic, peadiatric and midwifery and nursing personnel and also intensive care facilities with laboratory back-up for investigations. These are usually more easily achieved if delivery occurs during the normal working day.

Despite the traditional, conservative approach to induction of labour outlined above, in recent years there has been increasing pressure from mothers for elective induction of labour and planned delivery with all the attendant benefits of convenience when it is successful. Planned delivery has become an important issue and is partly reflected by the current increase in elective caesarean section rates of 20% or more in many obstetric units.

Suitability for Induction of Labour

The approach to deciding if labour is to be induced should be as logical and rational as possible. The first question to be answered is 'should the pregnancy be interrupted before the onset of spontaneous labour?' If so, then the next questions are: 'what is the most appropriate mode of delivery, and if vaginal, what is the most appropriate method of induction?'. Although simplistic, such an approach at least lends itself to clarity of thought.

When the indication to induce labour is maternal, it must be certain that the process of labour will not place her at unnecessary risk. When fetal indications predominate, the ability of the fetus to cope with the physiological and mechanical stresses of labour and vaginal delivery must be assessed. Antenatal assessment of the fetus will include cardiotoco-graphy, fetal movement counts, estimation of fetal weight by head and abdominal circumference measurements by ultrasound scan, doppler assessment of blood flow patterns in fetal and utero-placental circulations, etc. Intrapartum continuous and intermittent fetal heart rate monitoring is usually employed to monitor fetal well-being after labour has been induced.

Once the decision has been made that labour should be induced and that vaginal delivery is reasonable, an assessment of the likelihood of induction of labour being successful is of value. Bishop devised a scoring system based on the findings at vaginal examination in relation to the state of the cervix and the level of the presenting part, and a modified version is shown in Table 12.1. Normal labour, as discussed in Chapter 12, is conveniently considered in two phases, namely prelabour, which is slow and time-consuming, and the active phase of labour, which is efficient and progressive. The Bishop score provides the clinician with information about the time required to complete the prelabour phase (Fig. 13.1) and the likelihood of success of the procedure to induce labour. The higher the score, the less time required for prelabour and the greater the likelihood of successful induction of labour. It is worthy of note, however, that this system describes a trend and even with a Bishop's score as low as 2, 80% of patients will still have a successful induction of labour (Fig. 13.2). Nevertheless, when the cervix is found to be totally unfavou-rable and/ or the presenting part is high, and the indication for delivery is fetal, the bstetrician may feel that delivery by elective caesarean section is more appropriate.

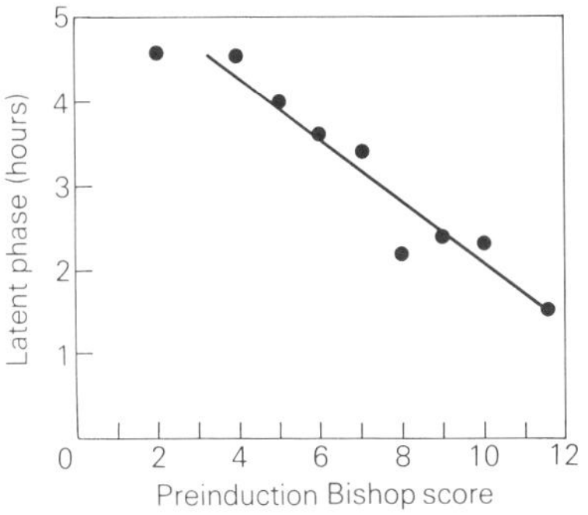

Fig. 13.1 *The longer 'latent phase' associated with a low preinduction Bishop score is an accurate indicator of the amount of prelabour which needs to be completed before active labour can proceed. (From data of Friedman et al. (1966). C.H. Hendricks (1983). Second thoughts on induction of labour. In* Progress in Obstetrics and Gynaecology, *Vol. 3. John Studd (ed). p. 104. London: Churchill Livingstone.)*

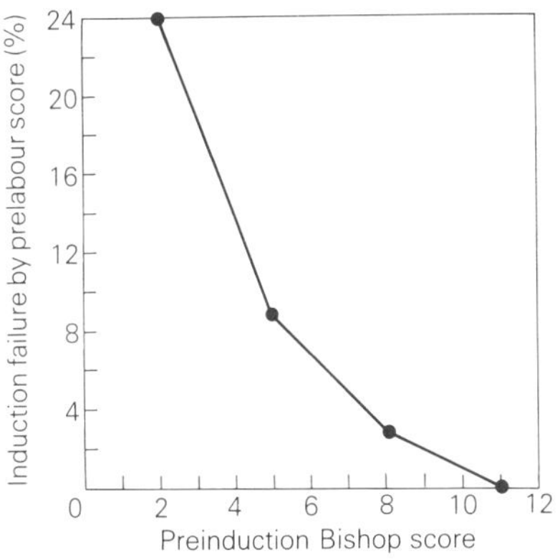

Fig. 13.2 *High preinduction Bishop score is a good predictor of successful induction. (From data of Friedman et al. (1966). C.H. Hendricks (1983). Second thoughts on induction of labour. In* Progress in Obstetrics and Gynaecology, *Vol. 3. John Studd (ed). p. 105. London: Churchill Livingstone.)*

Methods of Induction of Labour

Methods of induction of labour may be conveniently divided into surgical and medical categories. In practice, a combination of methods is often employed, but each will be considered separately for ease of reference.

Surgical

Traditionally, high and low amniotomy were the accepted methods of surgical induction of labour. The former has virtually disappeared from modern obstetric practice, but in the presence of a ripe cervix, both methods successfully induce labour in 80–90% of patients. In order to achieve artificial rupture of the membranes (ARM), the cervix must be 1–2 cm dilated and this, of course, improves the Bishop score for predictability of successful induction. Also, the membranes are routinely swept digitally from the lower uterine segment at the time of ARM and this will cause the local release of prostaglandins, thus enhancing the onset of uterine contractility. The membranes are ruptured by grasping them with a toothed forceps or using an amniohook to tear a small hole. Care must be taken not to traumatise the fetal presenting part. Liquor should be allowed to drain slowly. The fetal heart must be checked immediately following the procedure.

The true value of amniotomy is twofold. It sensitises the uterus to the action of syntocinon and allows more direct intrapartum surveillance of the fetus.

Medical

Syntocinon. Syntocinon is the commercially synthesised compound which is chemically similar to naturally occurring oxytocin.

When syntocinon became available, the methods of induction commonly employed were ARM alone or syntocinon alone with the membranes intact. While there was no doubt that uterine contractions occurred following syntocinon administration, the success rate of inducing labour was not as high as when the membranes had ruptured. Also with amniotomy alone, the rate of 90% successful induction of labour only occurred with up to a 48-hour delay and considerable risk of intrauterine infection. When amniotomy and syntocinon infusion were combined, 80–90% of patients were delivered within 12 hours. As a result, the modern practice of induction of labour combines these procedures, although there is variation among obstetricians in regard to the timing of syntocinon infusion relative to amniotomy and to the dose schedule used. Most dose regimens would commence syntocinon at the time of ARM or within 6 hours of the procedure.

The sensitivity of individual patients to syntocinon varies widely and the importance of titrating the dose administered against uterine response must be appreciated. Most regimens commence with a dose of 1 milliunit/ml which is doubled every 15–30 minutes until effective uterine contractions occur. Once active labour and cervical dilation have begun, the dose rate may be held constant or, more likely, reduced as the endogenous production of prostaglandins effectively maintains the labour. The majority of mothers whose labour is induced by this method can be expected to deliver within 12 hours of induction.

Side-effects of syntocinon infusion are rare. Water intoxication may occur with high dosage due to the anti-diuretic effect of syntocinon or when large volumes of fluid are used to administer a suitable dose of the drug. With awareness of this problem it should not occur. Syntocinon may cause haemolysis in the fetus and an increased incidence of neonatal jaundice after its use has been reported, but this is rarely serious.

Although the results of this method of induction of labour are satisfactory, there are certain drawbacks. The method remains unpopular with mothers. Some find the amniotomy painful, and dislike the restriction of movement imposed by the i.v. infusion. A minority of mothers show a poor response to this method of induction of labour. In particular, primigravidae with an unripe cervix at induction tend to have long painful labours, with fetal distress developing more often (Table 13.2).

Table 13.2

Details of Labour and Delivery of 125 Primigravidae Analysed by the State of the Cervix at the Time of Amniotomy

Cervical score	Number	Induction delivery intervals (hours) mean ± s.d.	Mode of delivery		
			Caesarean section	Forceps	Spontaneous
0–3	31	14.9	10	16	5
(unripe)		± 5.5	(32%)	(52%)	(16%)
4–7	69	8.9	3	38	28
(intermediate)		± 3.0	(4%)	(55%)	(41%)
8–11	25	6.4	0	11	14
(ripe)		± 2.2	(0%)	(44%)	(56%)

Prostaglandins. Although prostaglandin preparations were available for use in clinical practice for many years, their widespread use for induction of labour was slow to develop. This was mainly due to their side-effects after systemic administration. A single prostaglandin may have several actions throughout the body. Prostaglandin $F_{2\alpha}(PGF_{2\alpha})$ will stimulate the smooth muscle of the lungs, intestine and uterus. On absorption into the bloodstream, 90% of the drug is rapidly metabolised in the lungs and thus large doses are required to gain an effect on the uterus with a consequent increase of unwanted effects.

The production of an oral tablet of PGE_2 0.5 mg aroused interest and when used in conjunction with amniotomy in those with favourable Bishop scores (> 4), it has proved reasonably effective using doses of 0.5–1.5 mg hourly. The absence of an i.v. infusion is attractive, but the side-effects of nausea, vomiting and diarrhoea experienced are unpleasant.

Local administration of prostaglandin within the genital tract avoids these side-effects and PGE_2 vaginal tablets and gels are now commercially available. It is known that natural prostaglandins are involved in the process of cervical ripening and, when induction of labour is indicated and the cervix is unfavourable, administration of PGE_2 vaginally is of benefit. Not only will such treatment ripen the cervix, but labour will satisfactorily follow in up to 60% of patients. Even when the cervix is favourable, vaginal administration of prostaglandin may be preferred, thus deferring the need for an i.v. infusion and perhaps amniotomy. In multigravidae with a Bishop score of > 4, a single vaginal tablet, or gel, of PGE_2 and amniotomy 6 hours later achieves delivery in up to 90% of cases.

Choice of method for induction of labour varies amongst obstetricians and between hospital units. Variations also occur within a single unit depending on the clinical need (Table 13.3). As with syntocinon, patients vary in their sensitivity to prostaglandin. Prostaglandin and syntocinon should not be used concurrently as prostaglandins are known to sensitise the uterus to oxytocin. Excessive uterine activity may occur with hypertonus severe enough to endanger the fetus from asphyxia or the mother from uterine rupture.

Table 13.3
Method of Induction of Labour at St. Helier Hospital, Carshalton, 1999

	n(%)
Total induction	487
PGE_2 alone	43 (8.8)
PGE_2 + ARM	96 (19.7)
ARM +/− syntocinon	47 (9.7)
Syntocinon alone	53 (10.8)
PGE_2 + syntocinan sequentially	47 (10.9)
PGE_2 + ARM + syntocinon sequentially	104 (21.4)

Complications of Induction of Labour

The complications following induction of labour will be considered briefly.

Mode of delivery

It is generally accepted that there is a greater incidence of operative delivery following induced labour than spontaneous labour (Table 13.4) which will to some extent reflect the reasons for induction of labour.

Table 13.4
Complications of Spontaneous and Induced Labour. Peninsula Maternity Services, Cape Town

Nature of complication	Spontaneous labour-	induced labour
	%	%
Caesarean section	10.7	19.8
Forceps delivery	7.6	10.7
Failed induction or failure to progress in labour	0.9	4.6
Fetal distress	3.9	11.9
Prolapsed cord	0.3	0.6
Rupture of uterus	0.03	0.0
Total number of patients	9014	1022

(From V.K. Krutzen, H. Tannerberger, D.A. Davey (September 1977) *S. Afr. Med. J.* **52**(12): 482–485.)

Method of induction

Amniotomy. Prolapse of the cord is thought to occur in 0.5% of cases, which is very similar to the incidence following spontaneous rupture of the membranes. Rupture of the membranes above the presenting part, or hindwater amniotomy, can sometimes cause damage to a posteriorly situated placenta.

Syntocinon. Uterine hypertonus causing fetal asphyxia and water intoxication has already been discussed (p. 178).

Prostaglandins. When given i.v. or orally, diarrhoea, nausea and vomiting may occur. Uterine hypertonus may occur in occasional patients who are very sensitive to prostaglandins.

Failure of induction

Following amniotomy, there is a significant risk of intrauterine infection if delivery is delayed for more than 24 hours. Caesarean section must be considered then if vaginal delivery is not imminent.

Prematurity

Preterm infants may be delivered intentionally for obstetric reasons or in error due to incorrect assessment of gestational age. Such errors are avoided if confirmation of gestational age in early pregnancy by ultrasound scanning is performed.

Neonatal complications

Neonatal asphyxia may follow delivery of the at-risk fetus unable to cope with the stress provoked by a normal uterine contraction. Hypertonus provoked by uterine overstimulation will very rapidly produce fetal hypoxia.

Neonatal jaundice may be caused by the use of syntocinon in labour as a result of haemolysis. It is thought that the anti-diuretic effect of syntocinon influences the water content of the red cell in the neonate, altering its shape and promoting its destruction.

PROLONGED LABOUR

One of the most notable changes in obstetric practice over the last 25 years has been the reduced incidence of prolonged labour. The length of labour is now normally hours rather than days. The definition of prolonged labour varies from > 12 to > 24 hours. One large teaching hospital in Dublin has defined labour as being abnormal when its duration exceeds 12 hours. The dangers of prolonged labour are well appreciated and threaten both mother and baby. In brief they are intrauterine infection, fetal asphyxia, metabolic changes in the mother from dehydration and ketosis, and loss of morale which may have devastating effects on the mother's approach to future pregnancies. Dangers also occur as a result of a cause of prolonged labour, namely obstructed labour, and to cephalopelvic disproportion causing uterine rupture.

CAUSES OF PROLONGED LABOUR

The causes of prolonged labour are traditionally classified as:

Faults in the powers.
Faults in the passages.
Faults in the passenger.

The Powers: Inefficient Uterine Action

The function of uterine contractions is twofold: to dilate the cervix during the first stage of labour and to cause the presenting part of the fetus to descend to the pelvic floor during the second stage of labour. Uterine efficiency can be assessed by the time taken to achieve the delivery of the baby. The normal expectations may be depicted in graphic form by plotting the rates of dilatation of the cervix. Partograms which depict the progress of labour by cervical dilatation and descent of the presenting part are now generally accepted and are discussed in Chapter 12.

Once labour is established, the cervix should dilate by at least 1 cm per hour. Inefficiency of uterine action, or primary dysfunctional labour, occurs more often in primigravidae (26%) than multiparae (8%), and other causes of slow labour must be carefully considered in the latter.

During the first stage of labour, inefficient uterine action may present in one of two ways. Most commonly, the cervix dilates slowly right from the onset of labour. This, of course, assumes the initial diagnosis of labour has been correct. Less frequently, inefficient uterine action occurs late in the first stages of labour when the rate of cervical dilatation slows down after a normal start. This may reflect cephalopelvic disproportion and careful assessment is required.

During the second stage of labour, inefficient uterine action may occur when the presenting part fails to descend through the birth canal to the pelvic floor, following full dilatation. Again, careful assessment is required as the lack of progress may reflect cephalopelvic disproportion.

Treatment of inefficient uterine action

Amniotomy. When the membranes have remained intact, amniotomy alone will often improve uterine contractions. This improvement is probably mediated via the local release of prostaglandins.

Syntocinon. Syntocinon may be given by i.v. infusion in gradually increasing dosage until contractions are occurring regularly. In general, the diagnosis of cephalopelvic disproportion can only be justified in the presence of efficient uterine action. Care and regular assessment of the patient is required. The primigravid uterus virtually never ruptures, whereas the parous organ is more prone to rupture and so the use of syntocinon in multigravid women requires caution. Eighty per cent of primagravid and 90% of multiparous patients will respond to syntocinon.

The Passages: Cephalopelvic Disproportion

True contraction of the pelvis nowadays is very uncommon and reflects better nutrition in childhood years. Only very occasionally are congenital anomalies of spine or pelvis encountered and acquired defects, due to fractures, for example, only rarely affect pelvic capacity. The size of the baby is usually related to parental characteristics and small women tend to produce babies which are in proportion. Generalised fetal enlargement may be hereditary or acquired, such as in diabetes or rhesus isoimmunisation. Localised fetal deformity, such as hydrocephalus, usually proves an obstruction to vaginal delivery.

It is difficult to diagnose with certainty most cases of cephalopelvic disproportion in advance of labour. The labour is abnormal if there is poor dilation of the cervix during the first stage or failure of the head to descend during the second stage. Inefficient uterine action in the primigravid patient must be excluded or treated, otherwise a diagnosis of cephalopelvic disproportion is likely to be wrong. Efficiency of uterine action will often safely overcome minor degrees of cephalopelvic disproportion due to the ability of the fetal head to mould and the ability of the pelvic ligaments to stretch a little. When the cervical dilatation ceases and/or the head remains high in the presence of efficient uterine action, recourse to delivery by caesarean section is necessary. In the multigravid patient, abnormally slow labour is much more likely to reflect cephalopelvic disproportion and very careful assessment is required.

The Passenger: Occipitoposterior Position

It is well-known that when the fetal head adopts the occipitoposterior position, labour is likely to be prolonged. It is easily diagnosed by abdominal and vaginal examination. Labour may be abnormal in that cervical dilatation is slow or the head fails to descend and rotate. If rotation is incomplete, deep transverse arrest of the head may occur in the second stage of labour. Inefficient uterine action as the cause of poor labour may be excluded by the use of syntocinon during both the first and second stages of labour. If labour remains abnormal, then recourse to operative delivery is indicated.

Augmentation or acceleration of labour is often confused with induction of labour. The former is used to expedite a labour already commenced, whereas the latter is used to interrupt the pregnancy. Augmentation reduces the incidence of operative delivery, which is more prevalent for various reasons following the induction of labour.

OPERATIVE DELIVERY

The procedures involved in operative delivery are necessarily of a practical nature and, therefore, best learnt by seeing them performed. The student is encouraged to spend as much time as possible in the delivery suite to witness all forms of delivery. An understanding of the mechanisms of normal spontaneous, vaginal delivery is essential to comprehend the mechanics and rationale of forceps delivery.

Forceps Delivery

The idea of using instruments to expedite the delivery of the baby is approximately 400 years old. Modern forceps include a pelvic curve to the blades to allow easier introduction to the curved birth canal, a locking mechanism to join the blades together and a traction handle to allow the direction of pull to be applied in an efficacious manner. Slight differences of design and attendant gadgetry have led to the availability of a large number of different forceps, estimated by one source as being in excess of 600. However, we shall simply consider the essentials which allow a classification of three types:

1. Long-shanked forceps, e.g. Simpson, Neville-Barnes.
2. Short-shanked forceps, e.g. Wrigley.
3. Kielland or rotational forceps.

The constituent parts of the obstetric forceps and their types are illustrated in Fig. 13.3(a)–(c) The instrument consists of two blades, usually fenestrated to avoid excess weight, and held together when assembled by a simple locking mechanism akin to that of scissors. The blades are curved on the edge to fit the curve of the pelvis and on the flat to accommodate the baby's head.

Long-shanked forceps: (Fig. 13.3(a)). These were originally designed for application when

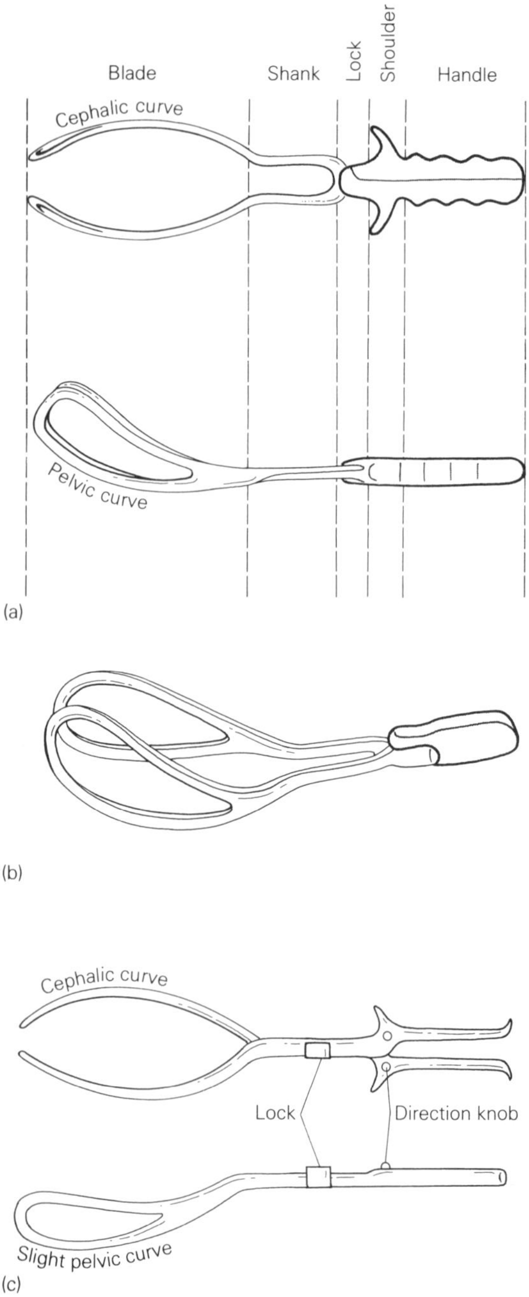

Fig. 13.3 *Types of forceps. (a) Simpson's; (b) Wrigley's; (c) Kielland's. (Adapted from Derek Llewellyn-Jones (1969).* Fundamentals of Obstetrics and Gynaecology, *Vol. 1, 'Obstetrics'. London: Faber and Faber.)*

the baby's head was still at the pelvic brim and unengaged and had a traction device to ensure that the direction of pull was applied in the axis of the birth canal. In modern obstetrics, 'high forceps' is not practised due to the unacceptably high risk of damage to both baby and mother. The forceps are now used for delivery when the head has descended at least to the midcavity of the pelvis and the fetal sagittal suture lies in the anteroposterior diameter of the pelvis. The instrument is also of great value in controlling the delivery of the aftercoming head in a breech delivery, and because of the length of the forceps, the operator's hands are well removed from the maternal perineum allowing the assistant ready access to clear the baby's mouth, nose and nasopharynx of liquor and mucus.

Short-shanked forceps: (Fig. 13.3(b)). These forceps are very light and used to deliver the baby's head when it has descended to the maternal perineum and vulval outlet. They can be applied relatively painlessly.

Kielland's forceps: (Fig. 13.3(c)). The use of these forceps remains controversial. Some would claim their only place in obstetrics is in the museum. All would agree their use should be treated with respect. Originally introduced to deliver the unengaged head, these forceps are now exclusively used when the head has descended at least to the midpelvis (the level of the ischial spines) and has remained in the transverse or posterior diameter of the mid or lower pelvis. The blades have minimal pelvic curve and, after application, the forceps are used to rotate the head so that the sagittal suture lies in the anteroposterior diameter of the pelvis in the occipitoanterior position. The locking mechanism allows the shanks of each blade to slip on each other, permitting the correction of asynclitism of the fetal head which arises due to lateral tilting.

Indications for forceps delivery

The indications for forceps delivery are:

Delay in the second stage of labour. It is traditional teaching that the second stage for a primigravid patient should last for no longer than 1 hour and for multigravida, 30 minutes. This timing has required reconsideration with the extensive use of epidural anaesthesia. Providing the fetal heart rate remains normal, it is reasonable to allow the second stage to continue for longer if epidural anaesthesia is being used and provided the labour continues to progress in the absence of maternal complications.

In general, however, the causes of delay in the second stage of labour are transverse arrest of the head in midcavity, persistence of an occipitoposterior postion of the head in midcavity, inadequacy of the uterine powers and minor degrees of cephalopelvic disproportion.

Maternal distress. Delivery of the baby may be indicated in the situation where the mother has become extremely distressed and is failing to cope with the second stage of labour. This is now an infrequent occurrence with better management during the first stage of labour and effective means of pain relief.

Associated maternal conditions. When the mother has associated conditions, such as preeclampsia, hypertension and cardiac disease, which may deteriorate if 'pushing' is prolonged during the second stage, forceps delivery may be performed as an elective procedure.

Fetal distress. If the baby is showing signs of distress during the second stage, delivery may be expedited by the use of forceps. The head should have descended to a level below the ischial spines.

Breech delivery. As the aftercoming head of the breech traverses the pelvic outlet and perineum, forceps may be used to control its delivery so that a sudden change in pressure is avoided as this may cause cerebral damage.

The indications for forceps delivery in a major UK hospital are shown in Table 13.5.

Table 13.5
Incidence and Indications for Forceps Delivery

	Number (%)
Number of cases	169
Incidence per cent	13.0
Indications:*	
Delayed second stage	92 (54%)
Fetal distress	90 (53%)
Eclampsia/Hypertension	0
O-P position/Deep transverse arrest	22 (13%)

*In some cases more than one indication were recorded.

Conditions necessary for forceps delivery

The following list of conditions are generally accepted as absolutely necessary to allow a forceps delivery:

Full dilatation of the cervix. Delivering the head through a non-fully dilated cervix may lead to extensive trauma of the cervix, vagina and lower uterine segment. Severe haemorrhage can result from such damage. A small, thin rim of remaining cervix may cause little trouble in the application of forceps by an experienced operator, but if the other factors permitting an easy delivery are absent, tissue damage is highly likely. The base of the broad ligament and uterine vessels may be involved and laparotomy may be required to control the resulting haemorrhage. The risks are, therefore, great and, if delivery prior to the full dilatation of the cervix is judged appropriate, use of the vacuum extractor is required.

Engagement of the fetal head. Engagement is considered to have occurred when the widest diameter of the presenting part has passed through pelvic brim. The application of forceps when the head is still high in the pelvis has no part in modern obstetric practice. Correct application of the forceps is extremely difficult to achieve in such circumstances and the non-dilatation of the soft tissue of the birth canal effect considerable resistance to the delivery. Damage to the baby and mother is extremely likely. Rarely, a high forceps delivery is justified in the multiparous patient when the cord prolapses or a second twin needs expeditious delivery in the absence of facilities for immediate caesarean section.

Cephalic presentation. Forceps can only be reliably applied to the fetal head and, in general, with vertex and face presentations.

Position of the fetal head. When the vertex presents, forceps may be applied with the occiput in an anterior, lateral or posterior position. The most common position by far in spontaneous vaginal delivery is occipitoanterior reflecting the optimal position of the head for delivery. Forceps delivery should mimic this as far as possible and occipitoposterior positions should generally be rotated to the anterior position. However, when the head is deep in the pelvis and close to the maternal perineum and in the occipitoposterior position, proceeding to delivery in this position may be more advantageous than exposure to the risks attendant with upward displacement and rotation of the fetal head. The vertex presentation in an occipitolateral position requires rotation to occipitoanterior. The rotation may be performed manually or with Kielland's forceps, both of which require skill and experience.

Rupture of the membranes. The membranes should be ruptured before application of the forceps blades.

Empty bladder. Ensuring that the bladder is empty is important for two reasons. Firstly, all the space within the pelvis is available for the fetal head when the bladder is empty and, secondly, it minimises the chances of bruising the bladder neck either by the forceps or the fetal head.

No cephalopelvic disproportion. The pelvis below the level of the fetal head must be adequate to allow vaginal delivery. The head should *never* be pulled past an obstruction. In these circumstances, delivery by caesarean section is required.

Adequate maternal analgesia. Instrumental delivery is an uncomfortable procedure for the mother and adequate anaesthesia or analgesia should be provided. This is commonly achieved by the use of epidural or spinal anaesthetics or a local pudendal block.

Complications following forceps delivery

The complications following delivery with forceps are as follows:

Fetal damage. Serious fetal damage caused by forceps can be avoided if the conditions required for forceps delivery outlined above are observed.

Immediately after delivery, the baby may have erythematous marks where the forceps blades have been applied. Occasionally, there may be slight bruising in these areas or to the lobe of an ear, but this is seldom serious.

A facial palsy may result from compression by the blades of the forceps on the facial nerve just as it runs in front of the baby's ear. While the paralysis may last a few days, it always recovers spontaneously and completely.

Intracranial haemorrhage in the baby may occur if the forceps are applied incorrectly or if excessive traction is used.

Maternal damage. Despite the use of episiotomy, further perineal and vaginal tears may occur, or the episiotomy extend. Occasionally, these tears may extend up to and through the anal sphincter.

Occasionally, the cervix may be torn, especially when it is not fully dilated at the time of application of the forceps. The cervix should be carefully checked after all rotational forceps deliveries.

After forceps delivery, there may be oedema in the proximal urethra/bladder neck region. This can cause acute retention of urine, but invariably settles with catheter drainage of the bladder.

Episiotomy

Episiotomy is virtually always performed before operative deliveries to prevent tearing of the perineum and vagina. It is also performed in other vaginal deliveries and is used in about 25–35% of cases. It involves incision by scissors of the perineal muscles and lower vagina at the end of the second stage of labour. It is usually made in a posterolateral direction following infiltration with plain local anaesthetic. Some operators favour a midline incision, although the risks of this incision extending posteriorly into the anal sphincters and rectum are greater.

The indications for episiotomy are:

1. To expedite delivery of the fetal head if there is fetal distress during the late second stage of labour.
2. To reduce trauma to the fetal head in cases of prematurity (< 34 weeks) and breech presentation.
3. To minimise risks of large perineal and vaginal tears if forceps are used, if the fetal head is very large or if the perineum is fibrotic and likely to tear during delivery.

The operation should never be performed without a clear indication that it is really necessary.

Repair of an episiotomy is not always easy. The vaginal incision should be repaired by a continuous suture. Interrupted sutures should be used to bring the perineal muscles together. The perineal skin should be closed with a subcuticular continuous suture of fine material. Vicryl is very suitable for all layers.

Post-operative pain is common because of the sensitivity of the perineum, the presence of oedema and chafing of the sutures while walking. Good surgical technique and a subcuticular skin suture will minimise discomfort, but perineal ice-packs and analgesics or occasionally ultrasound may be necessary for a few days.

During the late 1970s and early 80s midwifery and medical opinion suggested that perineal tears healed better and were less painful in the immediate puerperium. The rate of episiotomy fell significantly as a result. With time, clinical opinion has settled somewhere between the pro-episiotomists and those in favour of spontaneous tears and Table 13.6 reflects current practice, and demonstrates

Table 13.6

Perineal Damage During Childbirth For All Deliveries. St. Helier Hospital, Carshalton, 1999

Total Deliveries	3020	(%)
First degree laceration	360	(11.9)
Second degree laceration	730	(24.1)
Third degree laceration	31	(1.02)
Episiotomy	493	(16.3)

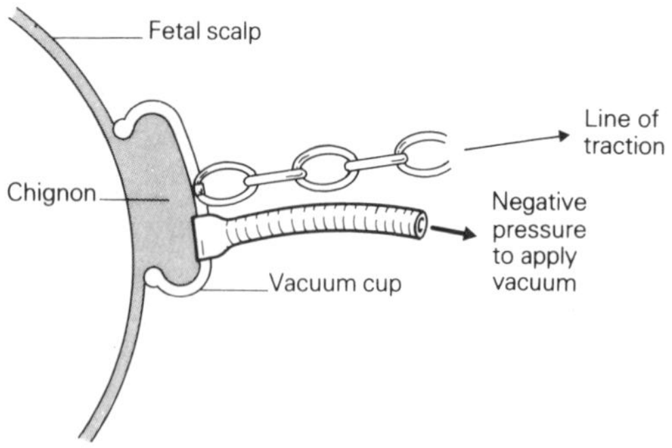

Fig. 13.5 *The application of the vacuum cup to the fetal scalp to permit traction. (Adapted from G. Chamberlain (1980). Forceps and vacuum extraction. In* Clinics in Obstetrics and Gynaecology. *I. MacGillivray (ed). London: Saunders.)*

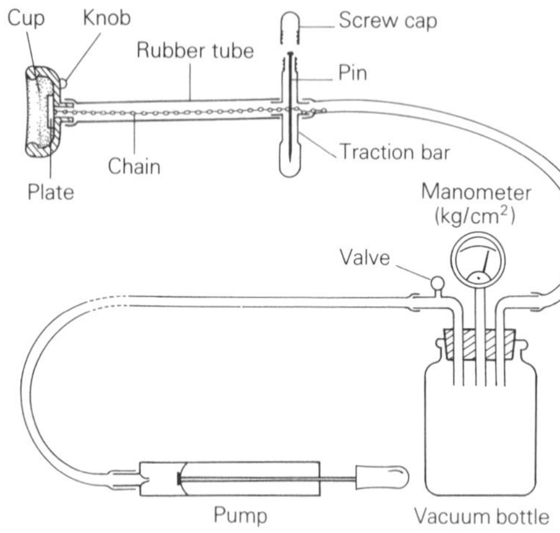

Fig. 13.4 *The vacuum extractor.*

the high incidence of perineal events with parturition.

Vacuum Extraction

Delivery of the baby by vacuum extraction is an old idea that only became a reality in obstetric practice in the early 1960s. The vacuum extractor is shown in Fig. 13.4. A metal or plastic/silastic cup is applied to the fetal scalp. When a vacuum is applied, the soft tissues of the scalp are sucked into the cavity of the cup forming a dome (chignon). Traction is then applied to the cup and, if excessive, causes detachment of the cup. (Figure 13.5), a feature considered to protect the baby from the effects or excessive traction.

Indications for vacuum extraction

1. During the first stage of labour

Slow progress in cervical dilatation. It has been claimed that vacuum extraction may be safely undertaken if the cervix is 5 cm or more dilated and the presenting part has descended to the midcavity of the pelvis. This is particularly true for the multiparous patient. There must be no cephalopelvic disproportion. Traction is applied intermittently to coincide with uterine contractions, bringing the head into contact with the undilated part of the cervix. Delivery can be effected safely within 20 minutes in the majority of cases.

When the level of the head lies above the ischial spines, there is a danger of trauma to the mother and fetus and a high incidence of failure to deliver. As with forceps delivery, a high vacuum extraction is to be avoided. An exception to this rule may be the delivery of the second twin. Where the tissues of the birth canal have already been dilated by the delivery of the first twin, application of the vacuum extractor to the head of the second twin, even if still high, may result in safe delivery.

Fetal distress in the first stage of labour. Controversy surrounds the use of the vacuum extractor in this situation. It is worth emphasising that the use of forceps and the vacuum extractor requires experience and skill. Once cervical dilatation has reached 7 cm, delivery can be effected quickly and safely using the ventouse (vacuum extractor). More often than not, delivery is achieved long before the time taken to organise a caesarean section. Here, more than ever, the experience of the operator is vital.

2. During the second stage of labour

The ventouse may be used as an alternative to forceps for delivery when the cervix is fully dilated and operative delivery indicated. Its use in such situations is popular in many European countries and has become increasingly popular in the UK. There is probably little to choose between the methods, given skilled operators. The vacuum extractor may be safer than rotational forceps when the head is occipitoposterior or transverse. Also, its use may produce less discomfort for the mother, avoiding the additional distension of the soft tissues and perineum incurred with forceps delivery.

Complications of vacuum extraction

The complications of vacuum extraction are described below.

Fetal. The chignon which remains after the removal of the cup from the fetal scalp looks formidable, but invariably settles quickly. There may be a circular area of bruising which dissipates within 3–4 days. When traction has been ill-directed or excessive, superficial scalp abrasions may occur. These heal rapidly and without treatment.

In approximately 1% of cases, cephalohaematoma occurs, which is not very different from the figure for all deliveries. As the haematoma resolves, neonatal jaundice may occur.

Maternal. Damage may occur to the cervix and walls of the vagina if they are inadvertently included during the application of the cup to the fetal scalp. Proper technique avoids this.

Very rarely, the cervix has been lacerated when the instrument is used during the first stage of labour. Such lacerations require suturing, but heal well.

Dilatation of the cervix using the vacuum extractor does not cause cervical incompetence.

Contraindications to the use of the vacuum extractor

The major contraindication to the use of the vacuum extractor is cephalopelvic disproportion. In this respect, the instrument offers greater safety than forceps in that, when excessive traction is applied, the cup detaches, thus protecting the baby's head.

In malpresentations, the vacuum extractor is used with caution. It may be of benefit in brow presentation, but has no place in the management of face presentation. In such a presentation, the vacuum would be applied over the eyes, causing severe damage.

Caesarean Section

Elective caesarean section is performed prior to the onset of labour and implies that vaginal delivery is containdicated. Emergency caesarean section is performed after the onset of labour and implies that safe vaginal delivery has become impossible.

Lower segment caesarean section describes the placement of the incision of the uterus in its lower segment, usually in a transverse direction, and is by far the most common procedure performed (Fig. 13.6). Classical caesarean section describes the placement of the incision of the uterus in the upper segment, invariably in a longitudinal direction.

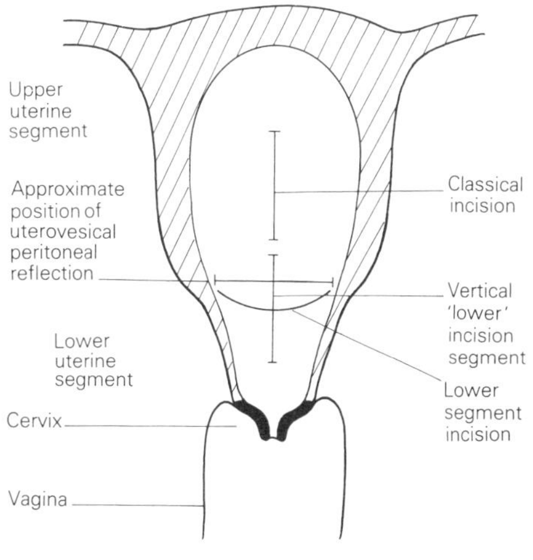

Fig. 13.6 *Uterine incisions for caesarean sections.*

Indications for elective caesarean section

It is virtually impossible to draw up a list of specific indications for elective caesarean section that would gain universal approval. The indications may be categorised in a general sense. These categories often combine fetal and maternal interests.

Cephalopelvic disproportion. Where there is an obvious discrepancy between the size of the baby and the birth canal, the risk of birth trauma may warrant delivery prior to the onset of labour.

Complications of pregnancy. This group includes conditions which cause placental insufficiency and render the infant incapable of withstanding the physiological stress of labour. Severe intrauterine growth retardation may warrant elective section solely in the interests of the fetus. Elective section in the presence of fulminating pre-eclampsia or severe abruptio placentae may combine both maternal and fetal interests.

Presentation of the fetus. A body of opinion firmly believes elective caesarean section is indicated in all breech presentations for fear of birth trauma. A greater proportion of obstetricians accept that a breech presentation combined with any other complication, such as hypertension, intrauterine growth retardation, prematurity (estimated fetal weight < 1.5 kg) or maternal diabetes, should not be allowed to deliver vaginally.

Obstruction to the descent of the presenting part. This group of indications includes cephalopelvic disproportion. The presence of placenta praevia, cervical fibroid or ovarian cyst may prevent the presenting part entering the pelvis. The occurrence of an unstable lie at term is accepted by many as an absolute indication for elective caesarean section.

Previous surgical incision of the uterus. In the past, previous hysterotomy or myomectomy were considered to be indications for elective caesarean section. However, views are now favouring a more conservative approach and these patients are usually allowed to deliver vaginally. Multiple myomectomy would be an indication for abdominal delivery.

Previous lower segment caesarean section for a non-recurring cause has generally been accepted as a poor reason for a repeat elective section. However, if two or more caesarean sections have been performed previously, the risks of the conservative approach must be considered carefully as the incidence of uterine rupture will be increased. Most obstetricians would recommend delivery by repeat elective caesarean section.

Poor obstetric history. Most obstetricians accept that there are circumstances in which previous reproductive/obstetric performance warrants elective caesarean section in a subsequent pregnancy. The would-be mother, particularly over 35 years of age, who has had several previous pregnancies ending in early or late spontaneous miscarriage, or the mother who has a handicapped child as a result of intrapartum asphyxia provide examples.

Delivery of the preterm infant. With the improvement in neonatal care, there has been a marked improvement in the outlook for the small, preterm infant. What risk these babies face, especially if presenting by the breech, in vaginal delivery poses a real dilemma for the obstetrician. There has been a marked increase in the use of elective caesarean section in these cases specifically to avoid fetal asphyxia and trauma (intracranial haemorrhage) during labour and delivery. Published figures are both confusing and contradictory, but it has been suggested on retrospective evidence that caesarean section is of value when the infant weighs between 1000 and 1499 g and presents by the breech. Caesarean section *per se* does not seem to benefit the preterm infant weighing 1000–1499 g whose presentation is cephalic.

Multiple Pregnancy. Triplets and quadruplets are rare events in obstetrics. However, most obstetricians accept that such multiple pregnancies are best delivered by elective caesarean section. With the increased use of *in vitro* fertilisation for infertility, there has been a rise in the incidence of such pregnancies. Elective caesarean section is now recommended for the delivery of mono-amniotic twin pregnancy which can be reliably diagnosed by ultrasound scanning.

Indications for emergency caesarean section

Fetal or maternal distress. Fetal distress in the first stage of labour may be severe enough to warrant prompt delivery. As outlined previously, delivery may be effected by use of the vacuum extractor if the cervix is nearly fully dilated, but the majority would advocate delivery by lower segment caesarean section.

Maternal distress during the first stage of labour is rarely, if ever, an indication for caesarean section due to the availability of adequate methods of providing analgesia.

Prolonged labour. As has been previously discussed, failure of labour to progress despite efficient uterine action may warrant delivery by caesarean section to reduce fetal and maternal risks.

Cephalopelvic disproportion/obstructed labour. This is an important diagnosis and may not be apparent until after labour has commenced. Caesarean section is indicated to avoid fetal injury and uterine rupture.

Type of caesarean section

The vast majority of caesarean sections performed in modern obstetric practice are of the lower segment variety. An incision so placed heals better, produces less risk to the integrity of the uterus in subsequent labour, is associated with less haemorrhage at the time of surgery and is less likely to cause intraperitoneal adhesions.

However, the use of the classsical procedure will never disappear entirely. Major degrees of placenta praevia may render the lower segment so vascular that an incision in the upper segment provides a safer option. An anterior wall fibroid in the lower segment may make access impossible. Compound presentation of the fetus, especially if the arm has prolapsed through the cervix into the vagina, or a transverse lie with the uterus contracted, may require an incision in the upper uterine segment to provide sufficient access to permit manipulation of the baby to enable delivery. These are rare occurrences, but deny any option in the type of procedure performed.

Complications of caesarean section

Maternal mortality. The risk of fatality following caesarean section is now less than 1 in 1000. The operation can, therefore, be considered as relatively safe. When the causes of death are scrutinized (Table 13.7), it can be appreciated

Table 13.7

Proportion of Maternal Deaths Connected with Caesarean Section. Classified According to Immediate Cause of Death

Cause of death	1967–1969 %	1970–1972 %	1973–1975 %	1976–1978 %
Haemorrhage	11.3	7.2	9.9	11.1
Pulmonary embolism	14.5	15.3	7.4	10.0
Sepsis and paralytic ileus	8.9	14.4	9.9	8.9
Hypertensive diseases of pregnancy	4.8	13.5	14.8	13.3
Anaesthesia	25.8	17.0	21.0	22.2
Other conditions (including associated diseases)	30.6	32.4	37.0	34.4

(From *Report on Confidential Enquiries into Maternal Deaths in England and Wales, 1976–1978*. London: HMSO.)

that hypertension, haemorrhage and pulmonary embolism increase the risks substantially. The administration of an emergency anaesthetic has significantly reduced as a major risk over the years.

Haemorrhage. Haemorrhage is the most common complication of the operation. The average blood loss is between 300 and 600 ml, mainly due to the large venous sinuses within the uterine muscle, which become even larger in the presence of placenta praevia. After delivery of the baby, the uterus naturally retracts and contracts, providing a very effective, mechanical means of controlling haemorrhage. Intravenous syntocinon (10u) is given as a bolus routinely after the delivery of the baby to aid this process and to overcome any relaxing effect the anaesthetic may have on uterine contraction.

Excessive haemorrhage is most often associated with extension of the uterine incision laterally causing damage to the uterine vessels. It can be avoided by using a curved incision, properly placed in the lower segment, and unhurried delivery of the head and shoulders. Suturing of this region is hazardous and requires extreme care to avoid damaging surrounding structures such as ureter and sigmoid colon.

Very rarely, haemorrhage is excessive and uncontrollable, but occasionally occurs with multiple fibroids, placenta praevia and uterine rupture. In these circumstances, internal iliac artery ligation or hysterectomy may offer the only hope of vascular control.

Bladder damage. Given proper surgical technique, this should occur only very rarely. In repeat caesarean section, the bladder is often very adherent to the lower uterine segment and requires careful, sharp dissection. When the bladder is damaged, recognition is essential as repair at the time of injury is usually straightfoward with good results.

Deep venous thrombosis/pulmonary embolism. Pregnancy causes increased coagulation potential, with increases in factors I, VII, VIII and X from approximately 14 weeks' gestation. This, associated with any circumstances which reduce venous bloodflow or damage the intima of the vessel wall, increases the potential for developing deep venous thrombosis and/or pulmonary embolism.

Many of the hazards are avoidable, such as prolonged labour, failure to correct dehydration and blood loss, misuse of lithotomy poles, failure to relieve calf pressure by ankle support at caesarean section and delay in mobilisation post-operatively. Early treatment of pelvic infection minimises the risk of pelvic vein thrombosis.

Post-operative ileus. Post-operative abdominal distension is common after caesarean section. The majority recover in 24–48 hours with simple measures such as intravenous fluids and aspiration of gastrointestinal contents.

Infection. As with any operative procedure, infection may occur within the pelvis or abdominal wound, but should occur in less than 4% of patients. Prophylactic antibiotics are now routinely prescribed at the time of the caesarean section.

MALPRESENTATIONS

These include breech presentations, face and brow presentations, transverse lie with possibly the arm or shoulder presenting and finally cord presentation.

Breech Presentation

The incidence is about 30% at 28–30 weeks' gestation and reduces to about 3% at term. The incidence of breech delivery varies between 2 and 3% depending on various factors such as the incidence of prematurity. The more common type of breech presentation is shown in Fig. 13.7. The hips are flexed, the buttocks and sacrum fill the lower uterine segment and cord prolapse is unlikely. The knees may be fully extended, splinting the body. The other form of breech presentation is when one or

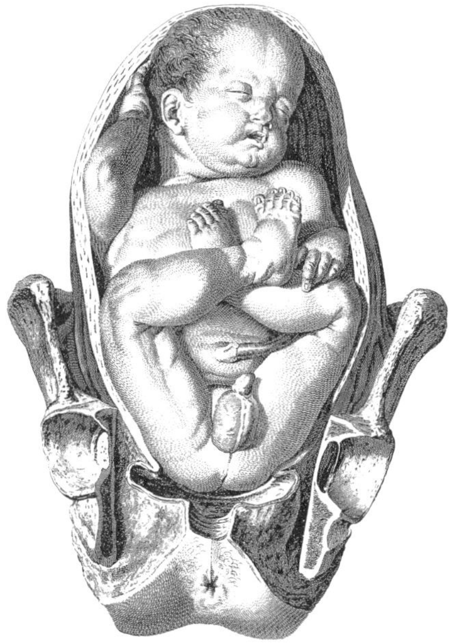

Fig. 13.7 *Common types of breech presentation. (From* William Smellie's Anatomical Tables. *Facsimile of 1754 edition published by University of Auckland, 1971.)*

both hips are extended with knees in varying degrees of flexion, consequently a knee or foot may present. The risk of cord prolapse in these cases is increased considerably.

External cephalic version

External cephalic version is when the baby is turned *in utero* from a breech presentation to a cephalic presentation by the manual application of external pressure on the uterus. Whether such manipulation reduces the incidence of breech delivery has been the subject of much debate. Traditionally it has been performed between 34 and 37 weeks' gestation. More recently, external cephalic version at or near term has attracted considerable interest, and results have demonstrated a significant reduction in non-cephalic births and caesarean section. The breech should be out of the pelvis and the uterus relaxed (tocolytics can be used) and no undue force should be exerted. The direction of rotation should be such as to encourage flexion of the fetus. The version may only be temporarily successful, it may cause placental separation, rupture of the membranes or, particularly if performed more than once, cord entanglement. It should only be attempted in singleton pregnancies and must not be carried out if there is: (1) a scar on the uterus, (2) hypertension, and (3) a history of antepartum haemorrhage.

Assessment of mode of delivery

Labour should only be allowed to proceed with a breech presentation if there is adequate room within the pelvis for easy passage of the aftercoming fetal head. There will be no time for moulding and while minor degrees of cephalopelvic disproportion can be dealt with naturally by moulding when the head presents, this can lead to disastrous fetal damage in breech presentation.

The pelvis can be assessed radiologically and clinically. An erect lateral film gives most information with a single X-ray and the details are given in Fig. 13.8. C.T. scanning has become more popular and offers similar information as an X-ray but with less exposure to radiation. Clinical pelvimetry is necessary to assess the pelvic outlet and, in particular, the width of the pelvis, the prominence of the ischial spines and the angle of the subpubic arch. If the pelvis is abnormal, with prominent ischial spines and a narrow subpubic angle, it suggests an android type or funnel-shaped pelvis. Breech

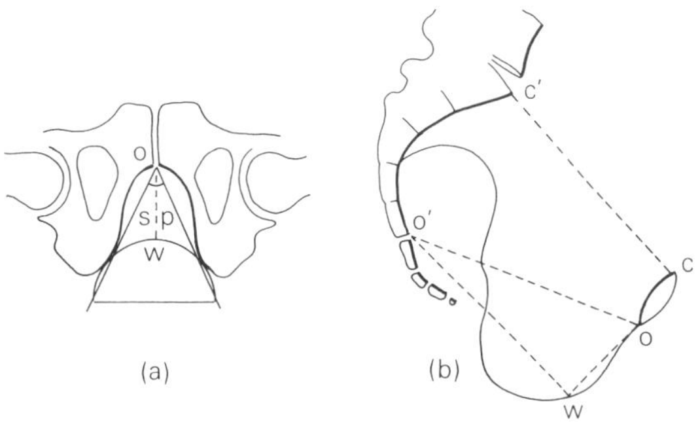

Fig. 13.8 *Radiograph of (a) outlet of pelvis, sp = subpubic angle; ow = waste space; (b) erect lateral view. cc' = shortest conjugate; ow = waste space between fetal head and subpublic arch; o'w = available antero-posterior diameter of pelvic outlet.*

delivery in those circumstances should only be considered if the fetus is preterm. Assessment of fetal size, including biparietal diameter and head and abdominal circumstances, should be made by ultrasound. A vaginal breech delivery in a primagravid patient should only be considered if the baby is not excessively large (< 3.5 kg) and the diameters of the pelvis are good. The anteroposterior diameter of the pelvic brim should be at least 11.5 cm and that of the pelvic outlet equally good.

Attitudes to breech delivery have changed considerably throughout the developed world during the last 15 years, with an increasing trend towards elective caesarean section, because of the increased fetal mortality and morbidity with breech delivery and a more litiginous general public and legal profession. Mothers are aware of the uncertainty surrounding breech delivery and will often request abdominal delivery.

The current practice in many developed countries is to allow vaginal breech delivery if the pelvis is obviously adequate and if there are no other abnormalities of pregnancy. Otherwise, lower segment caesarean section is the mode of delivery.

Management of labour in breech presentation

The membranes should be left intact for as long as possible, particularly if it is a footling presentation, as cord prolapse is more likely than when the presenting part fits snugly into the pelvis. Progress in labour in terms of descent of the presenting part and cervical dilatation should be steady, and if this is not the case in the presence of a frank breech, then serious consideration should be given to delivery by caesarean section before the second stage is reached. In breech presentation, the duration of the first stage of labour is usually longer than normal. The technical details of breech delivery are outside the scope of this book. However, some important principles for delivery of the frank breech should be known. These are:

1. Adequate relaxation and analgesia are essential to carry out the necessary manoeuvres — epidural anaesthesia is ideal.
2. The breech should be allowed to descend to the perineum before any intervention takes place.
3. An episiotomy should be performed.
4. The breech and legs should deliver spontaneously as far as possible before there is any assistance.
5. Once the legs are delivered, the umbilical cord is revealed and a loop pulled down to ensure that it is not too short to allow completion of the delivery.
6. The trunk is delivered either spontaneously or by gentle traction on the fetal pelvis. The shoulders are then rotated into the anteroposterior plane, the anterior arm is delivered by flexion and traction at the elbow followed by the posterior arm; any difficulty is probably due to extended arms. They are brought down by first getting the shoulders into the anteroposterior plane and then rotating the fetus with its back uppermost through 180°. This brings the previously posterior arm to behind the pubic symphysis and it is then delivered. Rotation back through 180° again with the back uppermost, allows delivery of the other arm (Lovset's manoeuvre).
7. Once the trunk, shoulders and arms are delivered, the body should be allowed to hang for a few seconds to encourage descent and flexion of the head.
8. Delivery of the head is by low cavity forceps or with manual control of flexion of the head (using Mauriceau-Smellie-Viet manoeuvre).

Face and Brow Presentations

These represent varying degrees of extension of the normally well flexed fetal head. Partial extension results in a brow presentation with the presenting diameter being the largest, namely the occipito-frontal. Obstruction during labour is vey likely and so delivery should be by caesarean section.

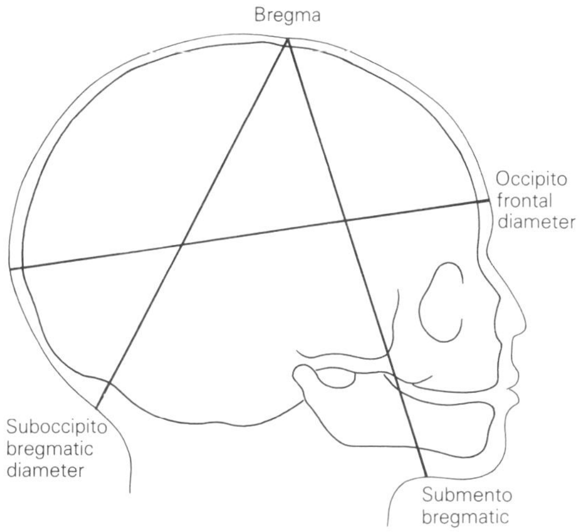

Fig. 13.9 *Fetal diameters presenting in face and brow presentations.*

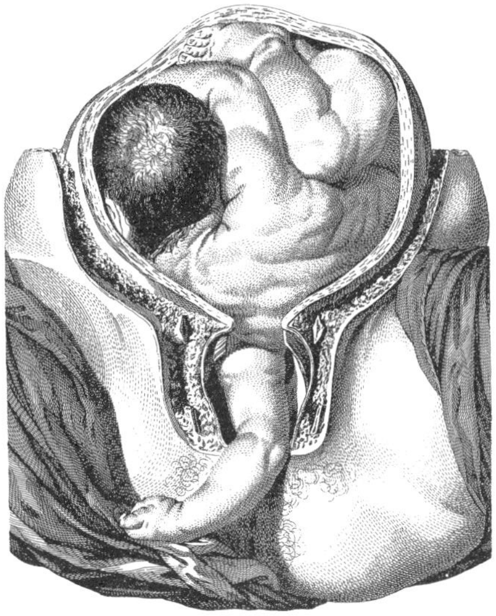

Fig. 13.10 *Transverse lie with arm descending through the cervix. (From* William Smellie's Anatomical Tables. *Facsimile of 1754 edition published by University of Auckland, 1971.)*

Full extension of the fetal head leads to the submento-bregmatic diameter being the presenting one and this approximates to the normal suboccipito-bregmatic diameter which presents when the head is well flexed (Fig. 13.9). Vaginal delivery is therefore possible, particularly if the chin is anterior (mentoanterior). If the presentation is mentoposterior, rotation to mentoanterior followed by a vaginal delivery may occur. If rotation fails, then the chin gets obstructed within the hollow of the sacrum and delivery by caesarean section is necessary.

Shoulder Presentation

This presentation may often lead to cord prolapse. It can occur if there is hydramnios, uterine abnormalities, minor degrees of placenta praevia or, spontaneously, in grand multiparae with uterine hypotonus.

If there is a transverse lie, an arm may descend through the cervix. Vaginal is therefore impossible as can be seen from Fig. 13.10. Delivery by caesarean section is necessary, otherwise the uterus may rupture.

Cord Presentation and Prolapse

Occasionally loops of cord will present behind intact membranes. Caesarean section is necessary to prevent cord prolapse when the membranes rupture. More often than not the cord will prolapse as a result of some other malpresentation, such as a footlong breech or transverse lie. Management of this obstetric emergency requires keeping the cord warm and moist by replacing it into the vagina, keeping pressure off it to prevent mechanical obstruction to the blood flow and to minimise its handling. Caesarean section should be carried out as soon as possible. Alterations in temperature and PO_2 cause chemical constriction of the cord vessels. Occasionally, if cord prolapse occurs when the cervix is fully dilated, immediate operative vaginal delivery may be appropriate.

PRETERM LABOUR

Definition

A baby born before 37 weeks' gestation (259 days from the first day of the last menstrual period) is classified by the World Health Organisation as preterm. A baby weighing less than 2.5 kg is classified as low birth weight and need not be premature.

In practice, in developed countries with good facilities, the outcome for babies born between 34 and 37 weeks is so good that prematurity only becomes a significant clinical problem at less than 34 weeks.

Preterm delivery is a major public health problem as with an incidence of 4–8% in developed countries, and much higher in underdeveloped countries, where it accounts for 75% of perinatal mortality and morbidity in the developed countries.

Mechanism of Labour

Labour be it preterm or term has a final common pathway, while the factors leading up to and initiating it will be different.

The myometrial intracellular events leading to contraction involves raised intracellular Ca++ which creates a calcium calmodulin complex which in turn activates myosin light chain kinase. This enzyme phosphorylates myosin leading to contraction of the cell.

The intracellular free Ca++ concentration is therefore of key importance. This is affected by calcium channels, gap junctions and compounds such as prostaglandins which release calcium bound to the sarcoplasmic reticulum and progesterone which increases intracellular binding of calcium.

Smooth muscle activity can be influenced not only by action potentials but by agonist/receptor stimulation. The link between the activated agonist/receptor complex and the effector system is in many cases G proteins. These affect adenyl cyclase and phospholipase C which in turn generate second messengers, that are involved in signal transduction across the plasma membrane. Second messengers include inositol triphosphate and diacylglycerol.

The fetal membranes produce prostaglandins (PGs), largely the amnion and deciduas. The chorion contains prostaglandin dehydrogenase for its metabolism. Factors that lead to inflammation in the membranes, principally in the decidua, will result in local PG release and myometrial contractions.

Preterm Labour

Elective preterm labour and delivery, often by caesarean section will be considered in Chapter 11. Here, we shall deal with spontaneous preterm labour of a normal weight for gestational age baby.

There are many associated factors linked to preterm labour and these can be grouped into obvious obstetrical factors and epidemiological and environmental factors.

Obstetrical factors

Such factors can be divided into 3 categories. The first is over-distention of the uterus which is thought, in the presence of high levels of oestrogen, to increase gap junction protein in the myometrial cell membrane. This facilitates Ca++ transfer between cells. Over-distension is due to multiple gestation or polyhydramnios which in turn may be due to fetal abnormalities.

The second is placental and membrane trauma which releases prostaglandins locally thus raising intracellular Ca++ concentration. This is clearly seen in cases of retroplacental haemorrhage, but also in other forms of antepartum haemorrhage.

The third is abnormalities of the uterus. Congenital abnormalities such as septate uterus lead to premature labour in up to 30% of cases. This is due to increased contractility of the uterus both before and during pregnancy but the reasons for this are not known.

Cervical incompetence can be congenital either due to absent or deficient tissue or to abnormal types of collagen. In all these, the sphincteric mechanism of the cervix is deficient, it opens up and allows exposure of th membranes and their premature rupture which is then followed by rapid spontaneous delivery.

Cervical trauma is also a cause and is acquired at D&C, cone biopsy, and childbirth. Cervical cerclage is effective in those cases where the diagnosis is correct, but the condition is overdiagnosed and its true value has been difficult to assess. The presence of foreign material in the vagina can increase the likelihood of infection, which in turn may cause the membranes to rupture and cause preterm delivery.

Epidemiological and environmental factors

Preterm birth has been associated with small stature (maternal height < 155 cm), low socio-economic status, high parity and low maternal age. These variables overlap considerably, and if short stature and low socio-economic status are combined, the preterm delivery rate is higher than for any single variable. When height and weight are considered together, height is not important if weight is appropriate, stressing the role of nutrition. Studies in New York and France have identified good nutrition as being important to reduce the incidence of preterm delivery.

Smoking during pregnancy is becoming uncommon but those that persist are usually of lower social class. However, the incidence of preterm labour is higher in smokers than non-smokers for each social class.

Previous reproductive history is not as helpful in predicting prematurity as would be thought. The incidence of preterm labour in subsequent pregnancies is not increased by previous spontaneous first trimester abortions. However, previous midtrimester spontaneous abortion or preterm delivery do increase the incidence of subsequent preterm labour. This is greater after two or more of such events. The risks of preterm delivery after induced abortion are low provided the cervix is not dilated to beyond 10 mm. The use of vaginal prostaglandin pessaries pre-operatively to soften the cervix and so reduce cervical trauma is recommended in primigravid women.

Other factors that are now recognised to be important are physical activity and stress. Excessive physical activity including prolonged standing at work have been shown to significantly associated with preterm labour. Reduction in these led to reduced incidence of prematurity in a study in France.

Stress causes an increase in corticosteroid production which is controlled by the hypothalamic hormone corticotrophin releasing hormone (CRH). This compound is also produced in increasing amounts by the placenta. It is kept inactive by being bound to a binding protein (CRHBP). There comes a time when the production of CRHBP is not enough to cope with the rising amounts of CRH which then become bioavailable.

This is normally at about the 37–38th week when the cervix starts to ripen. CRH has been shown to induce an inflammatory reaction in the fetal membranes resulting in cytokine and prostaglandin release. There are also CRH receptors in the myometrium with a high binding affinity. In women who are stressed, the levels of CRH are higher than normal and bioavailable CRH is present much earlier (Fig. 13.11).

Cause of Preterm Labour

The majority of cases of preterm labour have no obvious cause that fits into the categories described above and so were called idiopathic. However, recent research has cast some light on the aetiology of this large and important

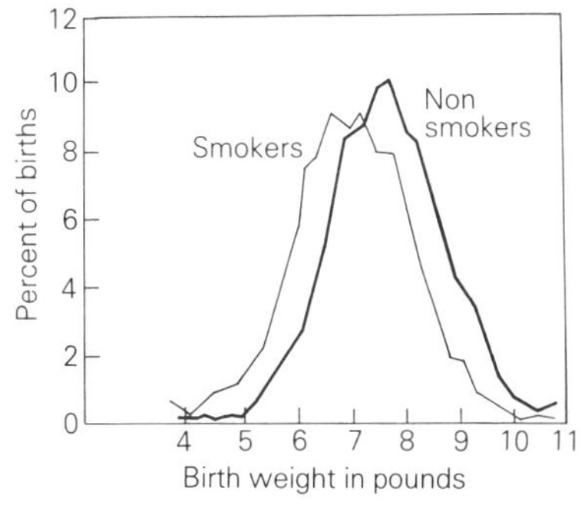

Fig. 13.11 *Distribution of birth weight by maternal smoking status. Smokers were those who consumed 20 or more cigarettes per day during pregnancy. (Adapted from E.J. Quilligan (1981). Pathological causes of preterm labour. In* Preterm Labour. *M. Elder and C.H. Hendricks (eds). p. 65. London: Butterworth.)*

group of cases. There are two categories that emerge. These are the early preterm labours from 16 to about 30 weeks (there is no logical reason to separate late spontaneous miscarriage with a live fetus from early preterm delivery), and those between 30 and 37 weeks.

There is a high incidence of infection among the earlier cases in the form of chorioamnionitis and neonatal and maternal morbidity, while in the latter group there is a very low incidence. This suggests that if infection is a factor, it will create the conditions for labour quite early in the pregnancy. If it is not a factor, then the mechanisms of normal labour are invoked but at an earlier gestation.

Early cases

Severe febrile illness such as pyleonephritis can cause preterm labour at any stage of pregnancy due to the presence of circulating endotoxins, which have been shown to stimulate an inflammatory response in fetal membranes.

However, the vast majority of so-called infections leading to preterm labour are either symptomless or have minimal symptoms.

Much stress was laid, during the 1980s, on identifying specific vaginal organisms that supposedly caused preterm labour. Predictably, many were implicated as the causative organism. While the presence of some organisms such as chlamydia trachomatis and ureaplasma urealyticum were more common than others, the important fact is that whatever the organism(s) it was probably causing a low grade inflammatory response in the fetal membranes, irrespective of the organism, which leads to the production of inflammatory cytokines such as interleukins1, 6 and 8, and TNFα. IL8 (neutrophil attracting factor) is thought to be the leucotactic agent leading to the infiltration of white cells into the cervix, and by their release of collagenase, cause it to ripen. The cytokines also stimulate prostaglandin production by the fetal membranes. The amnion and deciduas are the important sites, while the chorion contains PG dehydrogenase for its metabolism. Proximity of the decidua to the myometrium without an intervening metabolising tissue suggests that this is the major site of PG production for the onset of labour.

The most obvious inflammatory condition leading to preterm labour is bacterial vaginosis (BV). This is a condition characterised by a reduction or absence of lactobacilli in the vaginal flora plus overgrowth with organisms such as gardnerella vaginalis. The vaginal pH is raised to > 4.5 due to the lack of lactobacilli and so an important natural defence mechanism is lost. BV has been shown to be more common than normal in women having late miscarriages or early preterm labour and to be more common in African Americans in whom there is a much higher incidence of preterm delivery.

In most of these early cases, there will have been preterm premature rupture of the membranes (PPROM), histological or gross evidence of inflammation in the membranes and placenta (chorioamnionitis) and the fetus may or may not be infected.

Later cases

These are usually unassociated with infection. The incidence of PPROM is much lower and the usual onset is gradual, progressive contractions. Until we know the mechanism of normal labour, the cause of these contractions remains conjecture. Suffice to say that the mechanisms will be the same but the initiating factors or their timing will be different.

Factors such as stress acting through compounds such as CRH may bring forward physiological events. The role of receptors including progesterone and their availability and function in local tissues needs to be considered. So too do fetal signals such as the role of fetal cortisol, or PAF secreted from fetal lung, on maternal paracrine and endocrine function. This complex, multifactorial chain of events converts a situation of uterine quiescence in which progesterone and other relaxants such as nitric oxide probably have an important role, to one of contractility in which oxytocin, PGs and other compounds are involved.

In conclusion, while a lot of progress has been made in understanding early preterm labour, the complexity of the possible mechanisms outlined for later preterm labour mean that much more research will be necessary before the story can be fully told.

Prevention

This has been very poor as the incidence of preterm birth in the UK is 6% and it has not changed in the last 50 years. In the USA where the incidence is 7–8%, it is actually rising in the African American population.

Screening whole populations for markers of a disease is only of value if the marker is clear and with a high incidence, the screening is reliable and there is a definite remedy for the condition when found. None of these apply in the causation of preterm labour. Screening must therefore be restricted to those with a previous history so that there are clues as to what to look for. For example, in a patient with a history of one or more early pregnancy losses preceded by PPROM, then screening for vaginal organisms, BV, vaginal pH and treatment with the appropriate antibiotics and checking on cervical shortening or dilatation with serial ultrasound scans would be appropriate. Prophylactic cervical cerclage or waiting until there was definite ultrasound evidence of cervical change before cerclage would also be appropriate.

On the other hand, in someone with a history of a straightforward delivery at 34 weeks, enquiry into occupation, activity and stress and any appropriate remedy, would be needed.

In all cases of previous preterm labour, patients should be warned of the importance of noting and reporting early symptoms such as increased or altered vaginal dicharge, or an increase in uterine contractility. Staff in the obstetric unit must also be aware of the importance of these early signs and not dismiss them as normal until they have been properly assessed.

It is not easy to differentiate between vague abdominal pain from mild uterine contractions. An MSU should always be done as mild urinary tract infections present in this way. A specific swab from the upper vagina for onco-fetal fibronectin may also be helpful. Fibronectin is not normally present in cervical/vaginal secretions between 20 and 34 weeks of pregnancy. However, it is released into the cervical/vaginal secretions when there is breakdown of the decidual membrane interface. This can be due to physical separation if the cervix is ripening or from cell damage due to inflammation. A positive swab would therefore mean that preterm labour was likely and some positive action necessary. A positive fibronectin means that there is a 50% chance of delivery within 2 weeks. A negative result means that there is a 95% chance of the pregnancy continuing beyond 2 weeks.

While the final event of preterm labour appears to be sudden, the underlying process has probably been going on for days or weeks and attention to early signs can prevent labour from reaching the point of no return.

Management

Current management of preterm labour is simply trying to stop the process, when in many cases, it has become irreversible. If infection is the cause, prolonging pregnancy by even hours may not be in the baby's interests. Before using tocolysis, infection should be ruled out at least clinically.

Management depends on the intravenous infusion of drugs that will block some part of what is a complex pathway leading to myometrial contractions.

Beta-mimetic drugs have been widely used in Europe and elsewhere. They include ritodrine, terbutaline and salbutamol. Their efficacy and side-effects are similar. They act on adenylcyclase thereby reducing intracellular Ca^{++}. They have marked side-effects particularly tachycardia, cardiac arrythmias, myocardial ischaemia and tremor. Metabolic side-effects include hyperglycaemia which can go onto hyperinsulinaemia, hypoglycaemia and hypokalaemia. Pulmonary oedema can occur if the dose is high and it is given with too much fluid.

Magnesium sulphate is widely used in the US. Its action is to compete with calcium for access to the calcium channels and to competitively bind to calcium storage sites in the cell. Plasma magnesium levels are needed during administration to avoid the side-effects of respiratory depression and cardiac arrhythmias due to hyperkalaemia.

Atosiban, an oxytocin receptor antagonist has recently been licensed in Europe. It competes for oxytocin receptor sites and in trials has been shown to be as effective as beta-mimetics in delaying labour, but without the unpleasant and potentially dangerous side-effects. It should soon take over from the beta-mimetics as a safer and more pleasant drug to use.

As many cases of treatment for preterm labour are started late in the process, it is not surprising that they are not effective on a long term basis. They do however allow a delay of 48 hours in many cases which will allow for transfer to a tertiary referral unit and the administration of maternal corticosteroids.

There is no evidence that long term oral beta-mimetics or magnesium sulphate given prophylactically have any beneficial effect.

Maternal corticosteroids should be given to mothers if delivery is suspected between 24 and 34 weeks. In some units, this may be extended to 36 weeks. Betamethasone is usually given in two doses of 12 mg intramuscularly 24 hours apart. If dexamethasone is used, there are four doses of 6 mg given every 12 hours. These enhance surfactant production by the fetal lung and have been shown to reduce the severity of respiratory distress syndrome (RDS), thereby reducing the incidence of intraventricular haemorrhage and neonatal mortality. If preterm labour stops and delivery is no longer imminent, it is debatable as to whether to give weekly courses (as that is the duration of effectiveness of the course of steroids), or whether to wait and see what happens. Large doses of maternal corticosteroids have caused hippocampal atrophy in primates. At present, there are no clear guidelines on this issue.

Outcome

Prematurity accounts for about 50% of perinatal deaths and 75% of long term handicap. In the last 10 years, the numbers of very low birth weight babies that survive has increased considerably and between 50 and 75% of babies weighing less than 800 g now survive.

The proportion of these infants with severe handicap is probably constant and so there is an overall increase in the number of very low birth weight infants surviving with major handicap. Low birth weight is the single most important determinant of cerebral palsy.

What are the causes of brain damage?

Intraventricular haemorrhage

In preterm infants, the most common form of intracranial bleeding occurs in in the germinal matrix. This is a dense capillary network at the head of the caudate nucleus and bleeding occurring here will extend into the lateral ventricles. Half of these cases occur within the first 24 hours of life and are related to hypoxia and changes in cerebral blood flow brought about by ventilation. The incidence is strongly related to gestation being most common at 26 weeks and being much less by 34 weeks when the germinal matrix has largely involuted.

Perventricular Leukomalacia

This condition is due to anoxia affecting the same region of the brain and damaging the white matter. Oligodendrocytes are deprived of oxygen and glucose by the inability of the blood supply to respond to situations such as hypotension hypocarbia and hypoxia. There may be haemorrhage into these areas and subsequently cyst formation as the white matter atrophies. The condition is a major risk factor for spastic diplegic cerebral palsy.

Chronic lung disease with long term oxygen dependency is due to damage induced by ventilating pressures and high oxygen concentrations for long periods of time as well as the initial respiratory distress syndrome.

Visual and hearing impairment are other common types of handicap that the very premature baby is at risk of acquiring.

This paints a rather gloomy picture but it must be remembered that many, even very low birth weight babies are unaffected or have only minor problems. The obstetrician's role is to deliver the baby with no hypoxia or infection, so giving the small baby the best chance. The hypoxic or infected preterm infant has an uphill struggle from the very beginning.

FURTHER READING

Anderson A., Beard R., Brudenell M., Dunn P., eds. (1977). *Proceedings of the Fifth Study Group of the Royal College of Obstetricians and Gynaecologists.* London.

Beard R., Brudenell M., Dunn P., Fairweather D., eds. (1975). *Proceedings of the Third Study Group of the Royal College of Obstetricians and Gynaecologists.* London.

Beazley J.M., ed. (1975). Active management of labour. In *Clinics in Obstetrics and Gynaecology,* Vol. 2, No. 1. London: W.B. Saunders.

Elder M.G., Romero R., Harmont R., eds. (1997). *Preterm Labour.* New York: Churchill Livingstone.

MacGillivray I., ed. (1980). Operative obstetrics. In *Clinics in Obstetrics and Gynaecology,* Vol. 7, No. 3. London: W.B. Saunders.

Report on Confidential Enquiries into Maternal Deaths in the United Kingdom, 1994–1996. London: HMSO.

Hofmeyer G.J., Kulier R. (1999). *External Cephalic Version for Breeech Presentation at Term.* The Cochrane Library, Issue 4, Oxford.

14

Post-Partum Haemorrhage and Third Stage Problems

In a modern obstetric setting, it is easy to overlook the importance of the third stage of labour, the time from the delivery of the infant to the delivery of the placenta. The elation of delivering a baby can be swiftly followed by dangerous or even lethal maternal complications.

During the first and second stages of labour, the biological activity of the uterus is directed towards delivery of the baby. In the third stage of labour, the aim of the uterine activity changes towards stopping blood loss and delivering the placenta. Without this physiologica mechanism, mammalian reproduction would not have evolved. Uterine blood flow during pregnancy and labour is 600 ml/min, and so to avoid morbidity and mortality third stage haemostatic mechanisms have to begin rapidly after the infant is born. Several processes are involved in achieving these mechanisms; the most important by far is mechanical haemostasis via uterine contraction.

After the fetus is delivered, the uterine muscle both contracts and retracts (the muscle fibres get shorter and stay shorter). This process allows the placenta to be sheared off from the uterine wall. Once the placenta has been detached, it can be delivered. In addition, uterine contraction 'clamps off' bleeding blood vessels in the placental bed, limiting the amount of blood loss after delivery. The third stage is usually completed within 30 minutes, but often takes less than half this time.

MANAGEMENT OF THE THIRD STAGE AND PREVENTION OF HAEMORRHAGE

Active Management of the Third Stage

In the UK, nearly all women have the third stage of labour managed actively. The aim is to limit blood loss after delivery.

Active management consists of a triad of intervention:

(i) Early cord clamping
(ii) Controlled cord traction for removal of placenta
(iii) Oxytocic drugs.

The non-pharmacological interventions in active management, i.e. early cord clamping and controlled cord traction, have their origins shrouded in antiquity and have evolved over the centuries. Using oxytocic drugs is also not new, and this intervention has been widespread in the UK for most of the last century.

At the delivery of the anterior shoulder, an oxytocic drug is given via intramuscular injection. Oxytocic drugs stimulate contraction of uterine muscle. The most widely used drug is syntometrine, which is a combination of syntocinon (synthetic oxytocin) and ergometrine. The combination allows rapid-onset long-lasting contraction (Table 14.1).

The cord is clamped and cut quickly after delivery. After 'signs of separation' (lengthened cord, rising and contraction of fundus, small gush of blood vaginally) are observed,

Table 14.1

	Syntocinon	Ergometrine
Type of drug	Peptide hormone	Ergot alkaloid
Type of contractions	Rhythmic	Sustained
Time for onset of action	3 minutes	7 minutes
Duration of action	15–30 minutes	2–4 hours
Common side-effects	None	Headache Nausea and vomiting Hypertension

the left hand steadies the uterus while the right hand grasps the cord and the placenta is drawn out. The placenta and membranes must be checked for completeness after delivery.

Passive 'Natural' Management of the Third Stage

During antenatal classes, active management is discussed with pregnant women. In the UK, a small proportion (3%) of women opt out of active management, preferring to have 'natural' or 'passive' management of the third stage. No pharmacological treatment is given as the baby is delivered, and the cord is not clamped until its blood vessels have stopped pulsating. In theory, this allows the baby to maintain a higher blood volume after delivery, but it has never been proven to improve neonatal outcome. Instead of controlled cord traction, the woman is encouraged to use gravity to deliver her placenta. Women who choose passive management have to be told that there is a higher chance of both post-partum haemorrhage and retained placenta.

Measurement of Blood Loss

One of the most important aspects of third stage management is the monitoring of blood loss. Although this is notoriously difficult to do, after decades of experience, midwives in the UK have settled on using visual estimates, with less than 500 ml blood loss being considered as 'normal'. Blood loss estimation is essential in order to make a diagnosis of post-partum haemorrhage.

POST-PARTUM HAEMORRHAGE (PPH)

PPH is a life-threatening obstetric emergency. There are two types, primary and secondary.

Primary PPH

Primary PPH is defined as **estimated genital blood loss of more than 500 ml within the first 24 hours after delivery of the infant**. It is often seen within minutes. Primary PPH occurs in around 5% of all pregnancies. In developing countries, the facilities for treatment of primary PPH are scarce. The consequences are tragic: at least 200,000 deaths per year, or one-third of maternal deaths, are attributed to primary PPH. This highlights the value of using active management to prevent haemorrhage.

Causes of primary PPH

There are two main causes of primary PPH. **Inadequate uterine contraction**, often called uterine atony, occurs in around 75% of cases. As already described, contraction is needed to arrest bleeding. Risk factors are shown in Table 14.2.

Table 14.2
Inadequate Contraction — Risk Factors

Antenatal:-
Previous PPH
◊ Uterine overdistension (e.g. multiple pregnancy, big baby, polyhydramnios)
◊ Antepartum haemorrhage
- Placental abruption
  Blood trapped in the myometrium impairs contraction (Couvelaire uterus)
- Placenta previa
  Lower segment muscle cannot 'clamp off' bleeding efficiently

◊ High parity
◊ Uterine abnormalities (e.g. fibroids)

Intrapartum:-
◊ Long labour
◊ Operative delivery
◊ Retained placenta or placental fragments after delivery

Table 14.3
Trauma — Sites

External genitalia:-
◊ Episiotomy
◊ Vaginal tear
◊ Perineal tear (Risk factor: varicosities)
Cervix and uterus:-
◊ Cervical tear
◊ Uterine tear and uterine rupture (Risk factor: uterine scars, e.g. previous C-section or myomectomy)

Trauma to the genital tract accounts for most of the remainder (Table 14.3). There are also several rare causes, including pre-existing coagulopathy, uterine inversion, amniotic fluid embolism and abnormally adherent placenta (placenta accreta).

Consumptive coagulopathy

Regardless of the cause, rapid haemorrhage can be swiftly exacerbated by a consumptive coagulopathy. Haemostasis fails because the clotting factors have been used up. Identification and correction of this problem forms an important part of PPH management. It occurs in cases of severe PET or concealed accidental haemorrhage.

Diagnosing primary PPH

Significant haemorrhage is sometimes immediately obvious to the practitioner, especially if blood loss is rapid. However, it is more usual to diagnose PPH after estimating the blood loss. Blood volumes are difficult to measure after delivery, and in practice midwives/obstetricians make a visual estimate of both amount and rate of blood loss. It must be remembered that these visual estimates are sometimes underestimates.

In severe haemorrhage, apart from heavy bleeding there may be signs of hypovolaemic shock, including cold clammy peripheries and tachycardia. Hypotension is a late sign. Ideally the diagnosis and management plan should be implemented before shock ensues. However, bleeding can be much more insidious. For example, a litre of blood can be lost into a vaginal wall haematoma without being revealed. This emphasises the importance of monitoring the mother's condition after delivery.

Management of primary PPH

Primary PPH tests both the clinical skills of individual staff members and the efficiency of the obstetric unit as a whole. Women can rapidly go into shock and coma, and may exsanguinate within a matter of minutes. **The role of the first attending practitioner is to ensure that the resuscitation process has started and to get help.** Senior obstetric and anaesthetic involvement should be sought early, and many units make use of a 'major obstetric haemorrhage' protocol.

Resuscitation and initial measures. Women with PPH need particular emphasis on the circulation. Two size 18G i.v. cannulae are sited, and these are used to take blood samples for FBC, coagulation and cross-match (at least 4 units in the first instance).

While waiting for cross-matched blood, the patient can be given colloid (e.g. gelofusin) or ABO and Rh matched blood, depending on the haemodynamic status. As a last resort, O negative blood can be given. If the initial clotting tests are abnormal, the patient may require FFP, platelets and cryoprecipitate; this decision needs input from a senior haematologist. The woman should have direct pulse, blood pressure, urinary output and oxygen saturation monitoring. Consideration should be given towards monitoring central venous pressure and acid-base status.

PPH treatment is aimed at stopping bleeding. To start with, one or more further oxytocic agents is given, this time by the intravenous route to ensure rapid action. Suitable options include intravenous injection of ergometrine 0.5 mg, or syntocinon 40 units in 500 ml Hartmann's solution intravenous infusion. It is also helpful to rub up a contraction manually.

If the bleeding does not stop in response to these measures, causes other than, or additional to, inadequate contraction have to be considered before proceeding further, i.e. retained placenta or trauma.

Retained placenta. While this is going on, the placenta and membranes should be carefully checked. If they are either undelivered or incomplete (e.g. a missing cotyledon or succenturiate lobe), the uterus will not contract down and bleeding will continue. If the oxytocic agents fail to induce delivery of the remaining placental tissue, it should be manually removed.

Retained placenta may not always be accompanied by haemorrhage. Failure of the placenta to separate is associated with specific risk factors, including preterm labour, induced labour, grand multiparity and especially previous retained placenta.

Even in the absence of haemorrhage, the placenta should be manually removed if it has not delivered within 30 minutes. The longer one waits, the more likely it is that severe haemorrhage will ensue. Additional oxytocic agents are sometimes given before manual removal to encourage uterine contraction and placental separation. Manual removal is done in theatre under epidural or general anaesthesia. The placenta is gently lifted away from the uterine wall using the side of the hand. It is done under antibiotic cover.

Trauma. If the placenta and membranes are complete but haemorrhage does not respond to the oxytocic agents, the next step is to exclude trauma. Abdominal palpation of a 'contracted' uterus can be dangerously misleading — the only proof that an oxytocic drug has reversed inadequate contraction is if the haemorrhage stops. Trauma is diagnosed by examination under good anaesthesia to properly assess the uterus, cervix and vagina. Bleeding is stopped using sutures. Good illumination is essential, so this procedure should be done in theatre.

Persistent inadequate contraction. Once trauma has been excluded, inadequate contraction is again assumed. Repeated doses of carboprost (hemabate), a prostaglandin analogue, can be given by either intramuscular or intramyometrial injection to stimulate the uterus to contract. Recently, another prostaglandin analogue, misoprostol, has been given rectally to achieve a good therapeutic effect. Non-pharmacological methods are also useful, including bimanual compression.

Should all of this fail, more radical solutions may be needed to save the mother's life. The uterine or internal iliac arteries can be surgically ligated. A possible option is to embolise these vessels in the angiography suite. However, ultimately hysterectomy may be the only solution.

Secondary PPH

This is abnormal genital blood loss occurring at any time between 24 hours and 6 weeks after delivery. Fresh bleeding of any amount should not normally occur during this time. Secondary PPH is strongly linked to intrauterine infection, which in turn is usually, but not always, triggered by retained placental tissue or membranes. Although ultrasound scanning can sometimes show retained products, it is difficult to distinguish between these and collected blood, and the initial treatment is often to treat with broad-spectrum intravenous antibiotics. If the bleeding does not settle, the uterus can be gently explored under general anaesthesia. Retained products can be removed by suction curettage, but the post-partum uterus is very soft and uterine perforation is a danger.

RARE THIRD STAGE PROBLEMS

Placenta accreta is abnormal adherence of the placenta to the uterine wall. It is very rare, and is often associated with placenta previa. Placenta accreta is caused by a failure of the decidua to form properly. It often presents as difficulty in separating the placenta from the uterine wall during manual removal. If the operator does not recognise the problem, he or she can tear the sinuses and massive haemorrhage ensues. The traditional treatment is hysterectomy, but uterine artery ligation, curettage and oversewing of the placental site has also been shown to work.

Uterine inversion is also very rare. It can be complete or incomplete, depending on whether or not the fundus passes through the cervix. Traditionally the birth attendant has been blamed for pulling too hard on the cord while the placenta is attached, but in fact there are other risk factors including a fundal placental insertion, oxytocin augmentation and macrosomia. Inversion can result in rapid onset shock with or without haemorrhage, plus pain.

The treatment is to replace the uterus with placenta still attached manually as soon as possible. This is often not possible, as a 'constriction ring' forms around the cervix, so i.v. magnesium is given to relax the constriction, and replacement is done under general anaesthesia. An alternative is to seal off the introitus with one hand (or a silastic ventouse cap) while instilling saline in large volumes with the other into the vagina: hydrostatic pressure replaces the uterus. After the inversion is reversed, oxytocic drugs are given to prevent haemorrhage.

Amniotic fluid embolus is usually diagnosed after death, which occurs in 80% of cases. The fluid escapes from the sac into uterine veins, and causes an anaphylactoid reaction in the pulmonary circulation resulting in shock and DIC, collapse and dyspnoea. Treatment is general, resuscitative and supportive, including oxygen, circulatory support (dopamine, digoxin), and steroids.

FURTHER READING

James D., Steer P., Weiner C., Gonik B. (1999). *High Risk Obstetrics.* London: Saunders.

Department of Health (1998). *Confidential Enquiries Into Maternal Deaths (1996–1998).* London: HMSO.

15

Lactation and Puerperium

LACTATION

Breast-feeding confers important health benefits to both the mother and baby which deserve to be actively presented to young women. For the baby, protection against respiratory and gastrointestinal infections, reduced exposure to allergens early in life and a reduction in insulin-dependent diabetes are important. For the mother, breast-feeding is associated with a significant reduction in breast cancer, the most common cancer. It is also important to point out that breast-feeding does not increase the risk of post-menopausal osteoporosis. During pregnancy, growth of lobules and alveoli proceeds. Mammary growth during pregnancy is stimulated by oestrogen, human placental lactogen, progesterone, growth hormone and cortisol. The structure of the lactating breast is shown in Fig. 15.1.

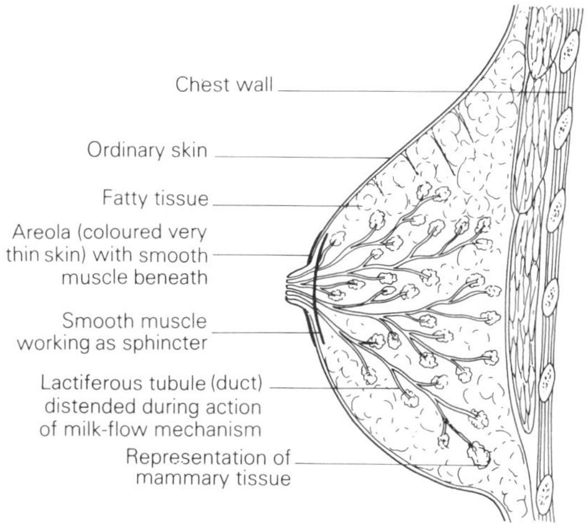

Fig. 15.1 *The structure of the lactating breast.*

Antenatal Assessment of the Breast

Although the nipple appears less protractile in some women, randomised trials have not shown that the success of breast-feeding is increased by the use of exercises or breast shields.

Milk Production

Milk is produced by the alveolar cells taking up precursors from the blood and synthesising the milk constituents, which are then passed into the lumen of the alveolus. This process is independent of neurological control, but is under endocrine control.

Prolactin

Prolactin is a polypeptide hormone produced in the anterior pituitary. Its amino acid sequence has some similarities to growth hormone. Human placental lactogen (HPL) is secreted throughout pregnancy by the placenta, but the high levels of oestrogen and progesterone block the lactogenic effect. After birth, the levels of oestrogen and progesterone fall. This removes the block and allows a full secretory response. With the delivery of the placenta, HPL levels fall. If the mother does not breast feed, serum prolactin remains at around 10 ng/ml but, in mothers who breast feed, prolactin levels rise to 20–50 ng/ml. The sucking stimulus brings a rapid rise to about 1000 ng/ml.

The pathway for prolactin secretion is from two origins. One is from the frontal cerebral cortex and the other is the sensory innervation of the nipple. Both inputs go to the anterior hypothalamus close to the third ventricle. From

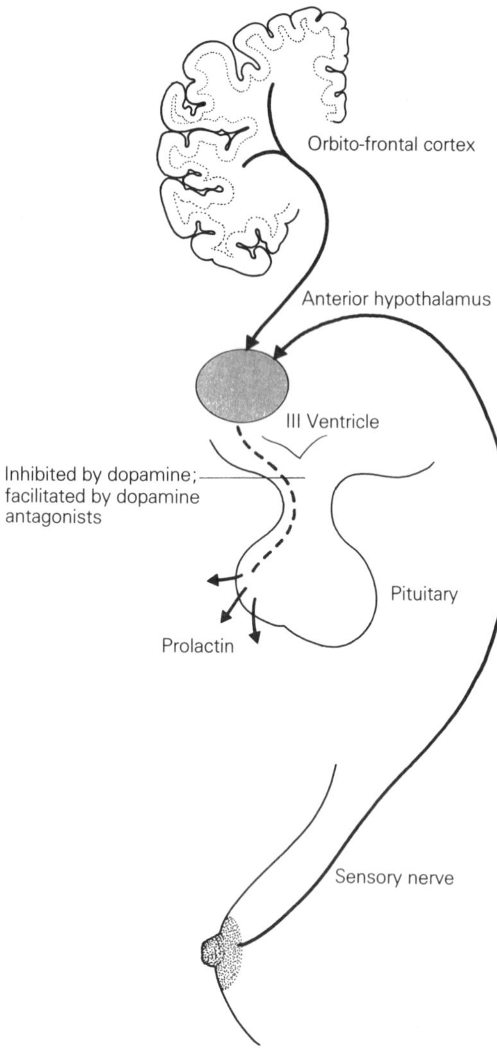

Fig. 15.2 *Necessity of prolaction secretion for the initiation and maintenance of lactation.*

there, neurotransmitters are conveyed to the anterior pituitary by the hypophyseal portal system (Fig. 15.2).

Prolactin secretion is inhibited by the neurotransmitter — *dopamine.* L-dopa inhibits lactation in this way. Bromocriptine, a dopamine agonist, is a more powerful inhibitor of lactation and can be used therapeutically in doses of 2.5–5.0 mg daily to mothers who do not wish to breast feed. Oestrogens can also be given to inhibit lactation as they block the effect of prolactin. Secretion of prolactin can be increased by the administration of hypothalamic thyrotrophin-releasing hormone (TRH). Dopamine antagonist drugs such as the phenothiazines stimulate prolactin, and this has been used to increase milk production in mothers who cannot supply all their baby's needs. Chlorpromazine, metoclopramide, domperidone and sulpiride have all been used in this way.

Milk Removal

Milk, when produced, is stored in the alveoli, ducts and cisterns of the breast. The milk in the larger ducts and sinuses is available to the baby sucking. Milk is transported from the alveoli by the contraction of myoepithelial cells which envelop the alveoli. Contraction is stimulated by oxytocin from the posterior pituitary gland in response to the stimulus of the baby sucking on the breast. This sudden availability of milk is known as the 'milk ejection', 'draught' or 'let down' reflex. The reflex can also be stimulated by the sight and sound of the baby and by gentle touch on the breast. This pathway is from the sensory nerve endings in the nipple to the spinothalamic tract, then the paraventricular nuclei from which neurosecretory axons run to the posterior pituitary. The reflex takes less than a minute from stimulation.

Oxytocin is released in repeated bursts and produces pressure waves of over 15 mmHg in the ducts of the breast. These changes occur in both breasts while the baby is sucking from only one. Thus some milk usually drips from the opposite breast even when no sucking is applied.

Continued breast-feeding may result in amenorrhoea and thus provides some degree of contraception, particularly when suckling is frequent. Once night feeding is reduced or stops, ovarian follicular function commences, and ultimately so does ovulation.

Contraception is advisable during lactation.

Composition of Breast Milk

Table 15.1 shows the composition of mature human milk compared to cow's milk. The

Table 15.1
Composition of Milk

	Mature breast milk	Preterm breast milk	Cow's milk
Protein	1.0	1.9	3.3 g/dl
Fat	3.8	3.5	3.7 g/dl
Carbohydrate	7.0	7.1	4.8 g/dl
Sodium	15	32	58 mg/dl
Calcium	33	30	125 mg/dl
Phosphorus	15	15	96 mg/dl
Energy	67	67	66 kcal/dl

(From T.E. Oppe, 1974. *Present Day Practice of Infant Feeding.* DHSS Report on Health and Social Subjects. London: HMSO.)

protein content of cow's milk is higher and much of the protein content is casein which tends to form large curds in the stomach. The sodium and phosphate content of cow's milk is much higher than human milk. The carbohydrate content of cow's milk is lower and the fat content varies according to the breed of cow. The composition of mature human milk is ideal for human babies' growth. The high sodium content of cow's milk may result in a baby becoming dangerously hypernatraemic if fluid loss from diarrhoea or fever occurs. The high phosphate content may give excessive plasma phosphate levels with reciprocal hypocalcaemia and convulsions.

Preterm babies, especially those born before 32 weeks, have different requirements from full-term babies and need larger amounts of sodium, calcium and phosphate. Breast milk from mothers who deliver preterm has a different composition from mature breast milk, having significantly higher protein and sodium levels, but no change in phosphate content. Human milk has a number of important *protective substances* of which the most important is IgA globulin fraction. During the first few days, the initial milk, known as colostrum, is particularly rich in IgA. Lactoferrin is a protein which binds iron in the lumen of the intestine and makes in unavailable for bacterial growth, while intestinal absorption can continue. Lysozyme is a non-specific antibacterial protein. White blood cells are present in breast milk and may also have a protective effect in the body. Cow's milk and artificial formulae have no protective effect on human babies.

Cow's milk protein allergy

This is a cause of some cases of failure to thrive, infantile eczema and perhaps colic. While allergy to human milk is much less common, it is still possible for a baby to react to very small amounts of antigen's (cow's milk, egg, etc.) from the mother's diet which have passed into the breast milk.

Nutritional Requirements

All the requirements of a full-term baby are supplied by breast milk if the volume of feed is approximately 150 ml/kg/day. Sufficient protein, calories, electrolytes, minerals, trace elements and essential fatty acids are provided.

No supplementation is needed until the baby is at least four months of age when solid foods such as rice cereal and puréed apple may be given for variety and to space out the meals, but are not nutritionally essential.

The only nutritional supplement which is advisable is vitamin K. This is essential for the synthesis of coagulation factors. If no Vitamin K is given at birth, a small but definite number of breast-fed infants become deficient and develop a clinical bleeding disorder within a few days (early haemorrhagic disease of the newborn) or after several weeks (late haemorrhagic disease of the newborn). This haemorrhage can be intracranial and fatal. In most countries, intramuscular vitamin K 1 mg is given after birth to all infants and is very effective in preventing such bleeding. Three oral doses of vitamin K is an alternative.

If the mother's diet is grossly deficient, then the breast milk may be reduced in volume rather than protein and calorie content. Vitamin D and vitamin B_{12} may be deficient in breast milk if the mother's diet is severely reduced in these nutrients.

Techniques of Breast-Feeding

The mother should be in a comfortable position. She can be sitting upright or lying down. If she is sitting up, it may help to lean forward slightly. The breast should be quite free of the brassiere. The baby can be held in one arm (left arm for left breast, right arm for right breast) with the arm supporting the neck and head and holding his mouth and nose level with the nipple.

If the mother is lying down, the baby can be laid on his side parallel to her trunk. The breast can then be moved so that the nipple is level with the baby's mouth.

The baby can be put to the breast within minutes of delivery. The release of oxytocin may be helpful in contracting the uterus. Subsequently, the baby can be put to the breast for a few minutes every three hours or more frequently if there is demand. There will be small volumes of colostrum released in the first two days, but by the 3rd or 4th day the volume of milk increases.

The baby obtains milk by:

1. The milking action of the baby's jaw and tongue.
2. Suction with each swallow.
3. The milk ejection reflex.

The nipple should go right to the back of the mouth so that the areola comes between the jaws and milk is obtained by compression of the ducts under the areola. This milking action of the jaws and tongue is the most important mechanism, because it obtains milk and also stimulates oxytocin secretion. With the milk ejection reflex, the rate of flow from the breast may be 30 ml or more per minute early in a feed. The position of the baby's head may have to be adjusted, close to the breast with the chin against the skin and the head slightly extended.

Problems of Lactation

Some common problems are:

1. **The nipple is not far enough into the mouth.** The milk ducts are not compressed and there is inadequate stimulation of the milk ejection reflex.
2. **The mother is afraid or anxious.** If the baby feed for a short time and then stops, feel the breast. If the breast is empty, it is soft. If the milk ejection reflex has not been stimulated, the breast will feel full. If there is insufficient milk production, extra feeding may stimulate prolactin secretion. Helping the mother to relax mentally and physically, and maintenance of the fluid intake, will help with breast-feeding.

   Dopamine antagonists, such as metoclopramide, have been shown to increase milk production, but emotional support, explanation and encouragement are probably more helpful. Oxytocin does not increase milk production but helps milk ejection, and when given sublingually (100 units) or nasally (40 units), increases the volume of milk per feed.
3. **Fighting the breast** is the term used to describe the baby turning his head away from the nipple, crying, arching his back and pushing with his fists. This upsetting behaviour is usually due to difficulty with breathing, the upper lip riding up and covering the nostrils. This is more likely to happen if the nipple protracts poorly.
4. **Engorgement** is a painful accumulation of milk which may occur on the 3rd or 4th day. By the 3rd day, milk production may exceed the baby's capacity and the milk ejection reflex may not be working satisfactorily. If the pressure within the breast rises, obstruction to the lymphatic drainage may occur, causing oedema. The lax tissues beneath the areola may swell and harden, thus making it more difficult for the baby to take the areola into his mouth. Engorgement should be prevented by the baby emptying the breast at each feed. The treatment for engorgement is to give analgesia and empty the breast using a pump. Manual expression is not easy for many mothers to learn and a hand or electric pump will empty the breast more efficiently.
5. **Acute intramammary mastitis.** This condition occurs when an excessively distended

set of alveoli leak milk into the surrounding tissues. An inflammatory reaction occurs with local swelling, tenderness, redness and a fever. Early emptying of the breast by pump may resolve the problem. If the condition has established itself over two days, milk suppression, analgesia, local application of warmth and antistaphylococcal antibiotic cover will be necessary.

If not controlled early, secondary invasion with staphylococci may lead to a breast abscess, with segmental redness and oedema.

Suppression of Lactation

Suppression of lactation after it has commenced is seldom necessary, but it may be required if the nipples become very cracked and sore, a breast abscess develops or there is bleeding from the nipple. A dopamine agonist inhibiting prolactin secretion such as bromocriptine is the most effective treatment and it is used in doses of 2.5 mg b.d. for up to two weeks. The use of large doses of oestrogens is no longer acceptable because of side-effects, including an increased risk of venous thromboembolism. Preventing lactation from starting may often be achieved by avoiding emptying the breast, using firm supports, analgesics if required, and fluid restriction for two to three days. If this conservative approach is unsuccessful bromocriptine is again recommended.

Breast-Feeding Small-For-Gestational-Age Babies

Babies below the 10th centile for birth weight may have low stores of carbohydrate and fat. There is a need for a substantial nutritional intake in the first 48 hours to prevent hypoglycaemia. Milk production may be much less than the 80–100 ml/kg/day that the baby requires, especially if the mother is primiparous. Hypoglycaemic convulsions at 24–48 hours may permanently damage the baby. Thus extra effort is required to help mothers with such babies and blood glucose must be monitored every 4–6 hours.

Breast-Feeding and Preterm Babies

Babies born before 35 weeks' gestation are not usually able to breast feed for themselves. Tube feeding is required either by the use of an indwelling nasogastric tube, indwelling orogastric tube or intermittent orogastric tube (gavage). Mother's milk can still be given by using an electric or hand pump to express the milk which can either be given fresh or may be frozen to be thawed and given later. Boiling breast milk (to kill any bacteria) destroys all the protective substances and milk lipase. If decontamination, for example of milk donated by other mothers is considered necessary, pasteurisation at 62°C for 30 minutes should provide adequate sterilisation while preserving most of the protective substances. Mother's milk is even more important for small and preterm infants than it is for full-term infants. Gastric emptying is better with breast milk than with cow's milk formula and this is important in reducing the need for intravenous nutrition which has a significant risk of septicaemia. The potentially fatal condition, necrotising enterocolitis is six to nine times more common in preterm babies fed formula than in those fed breast milk.

Drugs and Breast-Feeding

Many drugs may enter breast milk and so be ingested by the infant. However, the significance of this to the infant depends on the nature of the drug, degree of protein binding and the quantity in which it is transferred. Protein-bound drug is not transferred. Transfer to breast milk usually takes place by diffusion. Drugs that ionise and have a basic pH diffuse more readily than acidic ions, as the pH of milk is weakly acid compared to that of maternal plasma, which is weakly alkaline. Some drugs are actively transported into breast milk. Drugs with large molecular size do not, as a rule, pass into breast milk. These include heparin and insulin. Some maternal drugs which may have harmful effects on the breast-fed baby sufficient to contraindicate breast-feeding are shown in Table 15.2.

Table 15.2
Maternal Drugs which Contraindicate Breast-Feeding

Methotrexate
Cyclophosphamide
Iodine and radioiodine
Amiodarone
Lithium
Thiouracil
Phenindione
High dose benzodiazepines

It is an unfortunate consequence of the free market that pharmaceutical companies are not compelled by the regulatory authorities to document transfer of maternal drugs into milk and the pharmacological consequences for the infant. Many companies do not carry out the necessary research and avoid responsibility by advising against lactation when the drug is being taken when there is insufficient basis for avoiding breast-feeding. The appropriate attitude is that the benefits of breast-feeding are so well documented and important that medication should only be prescribed for lactating women if it is really necessary.

Fortunately, most commonly used drugs for bacterial infections, cardiovascular and psychiatric conditions can safely be combined with breast-feeding.

PUERPERIUM

Puerperium is derived from the Latin puerperus meaning childbirth. It refers to the period of time from the end of the third stage of labour until most of the changes of pregnancy have reverted to normal, usually six weeks. Some of these changes such as involution of the uterus are obvious and occur rapidly, while others, such as the reversion to normal of the urinary tract, are much more gradual and less obvious.

UTERINE INVOLUTION AND OTHER CHANGES

The uterus reduces in weight from about 1 kg at term to about 50–100 g in the non-pregnant state. Contractions occurring after delivery and throughout the puerperium are stimulated by oxytocin. These are particularly strong and sometimes painful during breast stimulation, i.e. suckling. Muscle fibres remain constant in number, but are reduced in size, losing intracellular constituents in the form of amino acids which are excreted. The puerperal woman is, therefore, initially in negative nitrogen balance. Fibrous tissue undergoes hyaline degeneration. Veins thrombose and undergo hyaline degeneration, while arteries have their lumen occluded by subendothelial swelling. Withdrawal of progesterone leads to autolysis and shedding of the decidua. The placental site is obliterated by the following processes: (a) vascular constriction and occlusion causing haemostasis; (b) ischaemic necrosis; (c) hyalinisation; and (d) autolysis. The endometrium regenerates from the basal layers (decidua basalis) and by growing in from the margins of the placental site.

Lochia

These consist of the autolytic products of the degenerating decidua from the placenta site. Until haemostasis is complete, blood is present in the lochia and so they are red for the first two or three days of the puerperium. Blood is replaced by serous exudates, while leukocytes, mucus, vaginal epithelial cells and non-pathogenic saprophytic bacteria appear in increasing amounts. The lochia are, therefore, brown from Days 3–6 approximately as the number of red cells decline and, thereafter, become cream coloured. Passage outwards of the lochia and their alkalinity protect against ascending uterine infection. Vaginal douches, therefore, should not be used.

Cardiovascular Changes

The increased blood volume and cardiac output that occur during pregnancy revert to normal during the first few days of the puerperium, a diuresis frequently being obvious. Coagulation factors VII, IX and X are all raised during pregnancy, and there is a further rise during the first few days of the puerperium before a gradual return to non-pregnant levels. There is an increase in venous tone and gradual reduction in varicose veins commonly found in pregnancy. However, they will persist for some time into the puerperium. Increased coagulation factors and increased platelet adhesiveness found post-operatively mean that the puerperal woman who has undergone an operative delivery is at risk for venous thromboembolism. Adequate hydration, prevention of anaemia, good surgical technique and, above all, early and active mobilisation reduce the risk of deep vein thrombasis to one that is very small (two per thousand deliveries). Superficial thrombophlebitis is more common, but less serious as subsequent embolism is very rare. Treatment of anaemia in the puerperium is usually by oral iron. Folic acid will be needed if there is a macrocytic anaemia. If oral iron is poorly tolerated, then consideration should be given to using i.m. iron sorbitol, or citric acid complex. Deep venous thrombosis must be treated promptly with anticoagulants, namely i.v. heparin for 48 hours, while oral anticoagulation with warfarin is being established.

Alimentary Tract

Constipation is common during the puerperium because of reduced food intake, perineal pain due to episiotomy and/or haemorrhoids, lax abdominal muscles and intestinal atony persisting from pregnancy. Treatment is by increasing fluids, bulk in the diet and use of a bulk laxative (bran, agar) if necessary.

Urinary Tract

The increased glomerular filtration rate, ureteric hypertrophy and dilatation of renal calyces, pelvis and upper ureter which occur during pregnancy, revert gradually to normal. An intravenous urogram (IVU) should not be performed within three months of childbirth, as residual effects of pregnancy such as ureteric dilatation will make interpretation difficult. Mild trauma to the bladder neck causing oedema may occur during delivery and this, together with bladder atony and perineal pain, may lead to urinary retention during the first few days of the puerperium. Intermittent catheterisation as necessary is the correct management. Indwelling catheters and use of parasympathomimetic drugs should be avoided, because of the increased risk of vesico-ureteric reflux and so infection. Urinary tract infection is more common during the puerperium for the reasons already stated. Awareness of the potential problem, prompt diagnosis and treatment with appropriate antibiotics will prevent the more serious complication of chronic pyelonephritis.

Puerperal Pyrexia

The common causes of puerperal pyrexia are uterine infection, urinary tract infection, breast engorgement (with or without infection), and pelvic or lower limb deep vein thrombosis.

Normally, the flow of lochia prevents ascending infection from the vagina to the uterus. However, the presence of pieces of placenta or blood clot within the uterus can encourage the growth of bacteria, leading to infection. A subinvoluted tender uterus with offensive lochia are diagnostic, and treatment is by emptying of the uterus and antibiotics.

Ascending urinary tract infections may occur in the puerperium as a result of diminished local resistance secondary to trauma and urinary stasis. Stasis allows bacteria a longer incubation time and interferes with the host's natural defence mechanism such as phagocytosis or destruction of bacterial cell walls by leukocytic lysozymes. Diagnosis is by the symptoms and from culture, and treatment is by the appropriate oral antibiotic.

Deep vein thrombosis can occur in the puerperium, particularly after an operative delivery, due to tissue damage and/or infection in the presence of increased coagulability of the blood which is a feature of pregnancy and the early puerperium. Deep vein thrombosis in the pelvic veins may only present by a mild fluctuating pyrexia and pelvic tenderness. Deep vein thrombosis in the lower limbs need not be associated with infection and presents with pain, swelling and localised tenderness in the calf and a positive Homan's sign. Diagnosis can be made using Doppler ultrasound or venogram. Treatment should be with anti-coagulants and antibiotics if necessary.

IMMUNISATION

Rubella vaccine should be given to all non-immune mothers during the puerperium. The immunity induced may be impaired if a blood transfusion is given during the puerperium. It is important that efficient contraception is used during the subsequent three months. Anti-D γ-globulin should be given to all rhesus negative women delivering rhesus positive babies. Anti-D must be given within 72 hours of delivery and preferably sooner if iso-immunisation is to be avoided. If the Kliehauer count indicates a greater than normal transfer of fetal cells into the maternal circulation, a double dose of immunoglobulin should be given.

POSTPARTUM CONTRACEPTION

Lactating women do not ovulate until the frequency of suckling starts to diminish, particularly when night feeds are cut out or spaced to 4–6 hourly intervals. Hormonal contraception such as progestogen-only pills, progestogens given by injection, implant or intrauterine device are suitable as they do not affect milk production. The combined pill may reduce milk volume. All hormonal methods should be avoided during the first few weeks of lactation, as trace amounts of the steroid will reach the infant and theoretically may affect its future sexual behaviour. For the non-lactating woman, any form of hormonal contraceptive that is appropriate can be initiated soon after delivery. Insertion of intrauterine devices in the immediate postpartum period is best avoided as the incidence of expulsion or removal for bleeding is higher than when the device is inserted six weeks after delivery.

STERILISATION

Sterilisation is quite often performed during the puerperium for convenience. The failure rate is increased twofold due to a greater chance of recanalisation of the tubes. It should also be remembered that the first week of life is the most dangerous and an unexpected neonatal death following sterilisation may cause the decision to be bitterly regretted.

Diaphragms should not be fitted until involution of the genital tract is complete.

PSYCHOLOGICAL CHANGES

Postnatal depression is discussed in Chapter 16.

FURTHER READING

Bowes W.A., ed. (1980). The puerperium. In *Clinical Obstetrics and Gynaecology*, pp. 971–1142. Hagerstrom: Harper & Row.

Gunther M. (1973). *Infant Feeding*. Harmondsworth: Penguin.

Hartmann P.E. (1986). The breast and breast feeding. In *Scientific Foundations of Obstetrics and Gynaecology*, 3rd edn. Phillip E., Barnes J., Newton M. (eds). pp. 286–296. London: Heinemann Medical.

Oppe T.E. (1974). *Present Day Practice of Infant Feeding*. DHSS Report on Health and Social Subjects. London: HMSO.

The Cochrane Library. Update Software. Oxford 2000: Issue 2.

16

Psychological Aspects of Reproduction

INTRODUCTION

Professor Lord Winston introduces his book "Making Babies" with the statement

> "The most important thing that nearly all of us do is to bring a child into this world".

We also know that when someone experiences a pregnancy loss, either in real terms or of the "hoped for" child, we struggle to know what to say or do to help that person. We feel uncomfortable as witnesses to their suffering.

In this chapter we will look at the emotions people experience in pregnancy, in the loss of a pregnancy and in trying to achieve pregnancy through artificial reproductive techniques. By understanding the complexity of these feelings, we can begin to understand the needs of such people when things go wrong.

Most people wanting to start a family plan the timing best suited for them, take the necessary steps to conceive and hope that nine months later they will give birth to a child. When this does not happen people become worried, but their concern is normally tempered by the belief that medicine has advanced sufficiently in our society to allow for thorough diagnostic assessments and hopefully action to "put things right". People feel secure in the belief that they have control.

"Everybody has the right to have a child" seems to be an irrefutable assumption and expectation in our society. If reality indicates otherwise the resulting devastation can lead to major emotional, social and psychological difficulties not only for the individual and couple, but also in their interactions with others.

By contrast, there are those who find themselves involuntarily pregnant, and having not planned for a child, are faced with the difficult decision about what to do. Enormous implications can arise in choosing termination particularly if the woman should subsequently be unable to conceive.

Much of what is known about how people cope with trying for a child, experiencing disappointments and enduring treatment can be understood in the context of Bereavement Theory of which four authors are mentioned here. Kubler-Ross in her work with the terminally ill, Murray Parkes in his work with the widowed, Bowlby in his studies of attachment and loss, particularly with children, and Engel, who saw the process of mourning as similar to the process of healing in his work "Is grief a disease?"

Models of bereavement are helpful in understanding people's reactions to reproduction because studies of pregnancy, pregnancy loss, termination and infertility all note that how people cope with their desire for children follows a similar pattern to how people cope with a major loss or death. Pregnancy, or the desire for children, is recognised as one the major goals or yearnings of people in adult life and therefore the analogy of the loss of the child that might never be born gives a powerful allusion to death, as is the realisation that there are life events over which we have no control.

Bereavement theory provides a highly respected and valued tool in understanding the natural responses to grief and loss and is therefore useful in understanding the feelings witnessed in Reproductive Medicine. However the "stages of grief", as they are commonly referred to in the literature, should not be taken to imply a smooth progression from one set of feelings to the next. The process of grieving is not so simple. Rather the stages represent a range of feelings, which are likely to exist and provide a framework for understanding the process by which people find they might move. Sometimes they move back and forth between or within stages, all the while hopefully moving towards a positive future.

Bereavement theory denotes four stages of grief — Shock and Disbelief, Denial, Growing Awareness, and finally, Acceptance — all part of a normal reaction to profound grief and loss.

Shock and Disbelief

When a person is first diagnosed, they are faced with a sense that life has lost its meaning. Shock can take the physical form of pain or numbness, or consist of complete apathy, withdrawal or anger. Numbness can act as a defence so people can go on and cope with the immediate issues in their lives.

Denial

This comes when news is unwelcome or unexpected and can be a powerful tool in protecting the person from the enormity of their situation.

Growing Awareness

For the person tackling crises in their life, there will be a strong force within trying to find answers, going over things that have happened to find explanations, this can lead to depression as slowly the person comes to a realisation of the huge change ahead.

Acceptance

Infertile couples must grieve their inability to become pregnant, and experience parenthood. Since there is no visible death, others may not understand their anger, depression, and sense of emptiness. Accepting these reactions as normal will be a comfort to those who feel alone in their struggle.

Trying to talk, especially with the partner can help to evaluate what is important — marriage, work, interests, without imagining they need to take the place of wanting a child, these are important elements in the process of moving on.

Couples should be encouraged to seek support from friends. A counsellor or support group might help in understanding the feelings, a first step to finding new ways of coping.

The next section will look at ways in which a person adjusts and copes with pregnancy and situations that arise following natural conception. This will be followed by circumstances where things subsequently go wrong. Then the psychological processes a person might struggle with when pregnancy seems unattainable. After discussion about infertility or subfertility a more detailed discussion is given of the often-traumatic emotional and psychological implications of infertility treatments including a look at the implication of Egg and Sperm Donation.

Finally, there is a section on how people survive these experiences.

PREGNANCY

In Bryant Higgins Book "Infertility New Choices New Dilemma" Higgins speaks for many men and women when he says

> "Perhaps like most men, I always assumed I should eventually have children. It would be a natural part of marriage, a natural part of life". (p. 15)

When a couple decide they want to start a family, it is known that for the majority of normally fertile women having sex with a normally fertile partner, a pregnancy will be achieved within the first twelve months of trying.

Society's commitment to family life means that throughout a woman's pregnancy, she will be closely monitored and have the support of a range of services from the GP to the hospital and other complementary services in the community.

Few parents feel fully prepared for the major event that is about to take place. Most struggle with fears about their adequacy as parents and their ability to adapt to the rigours of parenthood. But for most couples by the time they enter the second half of the pregnancy, they are actively engaged with ways to accommodate the child. By this stage, the baby is often already considered part of the family and may even have a name.

Depression After Birth

However thrilled with a new baby there is often a degree of "let down" when the drama of the birth is over. A sudden bout of weepiness around day three or four is common. Feelings of exhaustion and of being unable to cope as the realisation of taking full charge of the baby are also common.

There are physical causes for this such as hormonal upheavals, the body does not settle down until at least six weeks after the birth. Practical causes are numerous too. Possible post-birth discomfort from stitches, the necessity of caring for the newborn at night. Emotions can run riot. A new baby is a total and long-lasting responsibility, which means rethinking one's image and a change in relationship with the partner. Practical assistance and emotional support together with accepting one's feelings as normal and transient are vital.

However if tears and fears still beset the woman by the time of the first postnatal check-up, she might be suffering from postnatal depression. She should be urged to speak to the doctor who can offer help and guidance.

Postnatal Depression

Postnatal depression is generaly held to affect between 10–15% of all new mothers. It can manifest itself in many different ways with some symptoms harder to detect than others. Some women can be virtually disabled by it, unable to care for themselves or their baby. Others have symptoms not so overwhelming, and manage to hide how they are feeling from family and friends. Recovery time varies greatly from several weeks or months.

The main features of postnatal depression are lethargy, tearfulness, anxiety, guilt, irratibility, confusion, disturbed sleep, excessive exhausion, difficulties making decisions, low self-esteem, no enjoyment in motherhood, loss of libido, hostility or indifference to people she normally loves, shame at being unable to be happy. Symptoms will differ according to the level of support a woman has. Although all new mothers may identify some of these features, a depressed mother feels little joy and delight in the baby, or in motherhood and her negative feelings predominate.

The causes of postnatal depression are not certain, but help is available, usually from the local front line health professionals in the form of counselling, support and medication. Medication can cover a range of options from hormone treatment to antidepressant drugs. Specialist referral is reserved only for those women who show severe symptoms.

One or two in every 1000 women will experience pueral psychosis — a severe and often dramatic mental breakdown after childbirth. Symptoms associated with this condition can include hallucinations, excessive energy, the developement of obsessions about germs or tidiness. The condition can be treated with medication followed by or combined with admission to hospital. Recovery time is usually quite short.

PROBLEMS IN PREGNANCY

When things go wrong in a pregnancy, support is not always readily available. In fact, our society seems ill equipped to cope beyond the minimal medical intervention required. Yet it is often among those who can only dream of a healthy pregnancy where an understanding of the psychological aspects of reproduction are most clearly needed.

In the following, some of the situations where normal pregnancy can spontaneously go wrong will be described and then situations where the couple might choose or have to consider termination.

Miscarriage

Miscarriage is a very common event occurring in one in three pregnancies in this country. Neuberg says:

> "To experience miscarriage can be a waking nightmare. At one moment, there you are, happy and buoyed up with hope, expectation and joy in the new life you are growing. The next moment you are bleeding... told you are loosing your baby, given a D & C, and then sent home". (in Neuberg "Infertility Tests, Treatments and Options" p. 183)

After a miscarriage, the society we live in can often appear very cruel. You are told, and its meant to console you that — "it's Nature's way of getting rid of something that's wrong". However, in the initial stages after miscarriage it is much more likely that the woman will have feelings of "Why me?", a sense of failure, of profound loss. The grief for the loss of one's child is very real, and it is right for the couple to mourn for the child that will not be born and for whom there is no parting ritual, no coffin and no goodbyes.

The psychological wounds after miscarriage can remain for a long while, with the person experiencing huge oscillations from one moment a feeling of healing and resigned acceptance, "at least I know I can get pregnant" to suddenly feeling despair, depression and aloneness.

What is essential for the eventual well-being of the couple is to be able to talk, although not all couples find themselves able to do this. Many couples or women in particular report that they are expected to "get on" with life and say that their feelings were never really understood.

Often the man feels excluded from events. Perhaps because in our culture we tend to regard fatherhood as beginning at birth rather than conception. As a result, men are seen as not so intensively affected by miscarriage, or other pregnancy losses they are involved in, and they tend to keep whatever reactions they have to these events to themselves, often in deference to their female partners feelings.

Ectopic Pregnancy

This form of pregnancy occurs when an embryo implants itself outside the womb usually in one of the fallopian tubes. It is a potentially dangerous and life-threatening condition because the tube may rupture as the fetus grows. If the woman has already had a positive pregnancy test, then to discover that the baby is growing in the wrong place will be devastating.

The recovery from an ectopic pregnancy can be as difficult and fraught as from miscarriage. Added to which a woman can feel her body has been violated. A precious part of her reproductive system has gone and with it a reduction in the chances of conceiving naturally. Some couples struggle to regain a healthy physical relationship when surgery has been necessary.

The way to negotiate this difficult period is by talking together, or with close family or friends. Many couples find it difficult to help each other in this way. Men in particular find it difficult to express their feelings and suffer a sense of helplessness because they want to "make things right" for their partner. Both partners might end up finding it more acceptable to say nothing. However, it cannot be emphasised strongly enough that talking about the loss is an important way to accept what has happened and to heal.

If grief seems overwhelming, clinical depression may be indicated. Indicators that include a person feeling they cannot function even some of the time, or when grief shows no sign of easing, or a person feels stuck or totally unable to cope with day-to-day life, is unable to sleep or eat, in these circumstances it will be helpful to seek guidance or medication from the doctor.

Termination

Abortion is a difficult choice for many women emotionally, morally and spiritually. Although every abortion like every pregnancy has an individual context and a particular personal meaning, those who choose abortion will be all too aware of society's view.

Some may wish to deny their grief over the loss of their offspring because it is "inappropriate". They may imagine that because, according to pro-choice supporters, abortion is a simple common medical procedure it will have few if any profound consequences. At the other extreme, there will be those who struggle with intense feelings of shame about their decision, often influenced by the extremist pro-life view that abortion is to be equated with murder.

The experience of a late-term genetic abortion can carry an even greater nightmarish quality at once terrifyingly real but also utterly incomprehensible, for example when prenatal diagnostic testing reveals genetic abnormalities in the baby. The woman may be required to undergo labour and delivery. She may face a decision as to whether she sees the child. There may or may not be a burial, or funeral service and no sympathy cards.

Perinatal Loss

When a baby is stillborn or dies in the first week of life, the situation is fraught with difficulty. The idea of death before birth is almost too cruel to fathom. The reality of the loss is unquestionable — there is a full-term baby delivered, a body which most parents are encouraged to view, and normally a funeral service.

The death of a child is one of the most difficult losses a person will ever face. It is also known that sudden death is particularly difficult to come to terms with. Perinatal loss has both these characteristics. My own work with couples has confirmed what is known from the literature, that such traumatic loss can take many years for a couple to absorb or even be able to talk about.

Although the figures for stillbirth or early death in absolute terms are low, they are twice as high among babies produced by assisted conception than in the general population. IVF babies tend to have more problems at birth, and stillbirth maybe slightly more common. This trend is not due to IVF itself but because women who conceive through IVF are more likely to be in the "high risk group".

Apart from stillbirth or perinatal loss, one overriding feature of all the situations of loss outlined so far, is the fact that couples have few if any rituals to call upon to acknowledge the death of their child or hoped for child. There is no special place where a person can go to continue to quietly grieve. As time goes on there becomes less support and the opportunity to speak about what has happened diminishes. Yet comments like "cheer up you should be getting over it by now" are unkind, thoughtless and not conducive to healing.

Infertility

In England today, one couple in six who hope to have a child will have difficulty conceiving. For one in ten couples the cause of infertility will be a male factor, which is difficult to treat. Many cases of infertility are due to a combination of problems in both partners.

The fact that many women are waiting to a later age before trying for a child is likely to be a factor in the increase in numbers of couples remaining childless. This is because of the fall in women's fertility after the age of 30.

The causes of infertility are discussed in detail elsewhere in this book. It is helpful, however, to state the most common causes since diagnoses in these cases almost always leads to patients being encouraged to consider treatment, and with the hope of treatment, we see the major psychological consequences of infertility clearly demonstrated.

There are four common causes of infertility: — initial problems, ovulatory failure, a sperm dysfunction, and unexplained infertility.

Each of these conditions can be tackled with programmes of assisted conception. A couple can be offered *in vitro* fertilisation with its associated hurdles, one in three chance of achieving pregnancy, and 25% chance of actually "taking home a baby". Couples can be offered intracytolplasmic sperm injection (ICSI) or associated techniques, all highly invasive, emotionally charged options for those with poor sperm. Or they may be offered donor insemination, with significant implications for the couple and child. For all these options, couples find themselves thrust into an emotional experience well beyond anything they may have faced before. Compounded by the fact that offering treatment of whatever type does not guarantee pregnancy or the birth of a child. Treatment only offers the ***hope*** of success and this is almost always the single most difficult aspect for a couple to manage.

Before discussion of how specific treatments give rise to psychological problems, we should be aware of how any couple trying to conceive, yet remaining unsuccessful is likely to proceed.

Waiting For a Diagnosis

The process a couple goes through to arrive at a clinic where diagnosis is made, and a treatment plan offered, can be long and fraught with anxieties. Each month will hold its own hopes followed, on bleeding, by enormous disappointment. There is likely to be daily monitoring of temperature and ovulation charts, with timed coitus, so that the spontaneity and joy of intercourse is removed. Each month holds the possibility that others might announce news of pregnancy. Seeing pregnant people in the street can be painful. Couples often describe themselves as feeling "excluded from a club". Many couples say they are no longer able to continue normal living as they withdraw from any possible contact with children. Requests to join in family celebrations, birthdays, etc. all become times that bring acute pain and despair.

After the couple's GP has agreed to refer to a specialist, there is usually a delay waiting for the referral appointment. The specialist will then typically request various tests before a diagnosis is made. This means more waiting. A picture emerges of a couple clearly anxious, fearful and concerned to hear "The News". Finally, at the consultation when the diagnosis and possible course of action is given, many couples say they would have liked more time with the doctor. For them, this appointment is the culmination of a long and difficult journey and there will be great investment in hoping for a positive outcome. Often, not all that is said is clearly remembered or understood.

Counselling

Begins, and often before a diagnosis is reached, clinicians have found counselling to be of great benefit to both partners. Counselling is a rather general term, that in this case covers the need for a couple to explore concerns about subfertility and later medical investigations or subsequent treatment.

The Human Fertilisation and Embryology Act (HFEA) 1990 requires all licensed centres to provide counselling where treatment is offered. The HFEA suggests the following four categories of counselling be made available: information, implications, support and therapeutic counselling. When clinics offer counselling, the couple are given the opportunity to ensure they have all the necessary information about treatment and any implications, are offered support through what may be a very difficult time, particularly after an unsuccessful treatment or when treatment is finally to be discontinued. Finally, therapeutic counselling should "concentrate(s) on healing, especially in helping the couple adjust to hard circumstances... some people may need it, if only occasionally, for some years".

IN VITRO FERTILISATION (IVF)

Treatment for Ovulatory Failure

A patient who has ovulatory problems has the possibility of achieving a pregnancy with the use of stimulatory hormone treatment. Only IVF treatment is mentioned here, although intrauterine insemination (IUI), a less invasive procedure, has a similar emotional impact on patients.

IVF treatment requires an ability to manage a complicated procedure with what patients describe as "many hurdles". Each hurdle passed brings a sense of achievement, another marker along the road to a hoped for child. Couples must manage their feelings, which in tandem with hormonal drugs taken to stimulate the woman's ovaries, can make for a very turbulent time. Daily injections, frequent visits to the hospital, waiting for results of blood tests and scans, together with coping with possible side-effects from the drugs such as irritability, hot flushes etc. all make for a difficult time. A woman can feel very isolated yet despite fears, will want to be positive. Embryo transfer is a particularly difficult time for couples who then wait for two weeks for the pregnancy test.

For couples tackling this traumatic regime, we know that the outcome in terms of the couple's mental well-being will more speedily be restored if the sense of hope during treatment is tempered with a reality that they should be under no illusions about the outcome. But as Robert Winston says in his book "Infertility: A Sympathetic Approach":

> "The worst risks of *in vitro* fertilisation are emotional and psychological".

Number of Treatments

The number of times IVF is attempted will depend on a range of factors. National Health Service treatment is normally restricted to a few specified attempts and for these couples, the pressure during treatment can be immense. Conversely, there is often a sense of relief that "at least we tried" and couples do move on, albeit slowly, the experience of treatment leading to resigned acceptance.

For those couples paying for treatment, some clinics allow repeated cycles of IVF, assuming previous cycle results have been favourable. We know that for couples to benefit and achieve a full recovery after continued unsuccessful treatment the question of, how many times they try IVF, should be within their own control. Most clinics will look at age, response to drugs, quality of embryos before advising on the likelihood of a success. But should pregnancy continue to evade, it is important for the long-term well-being of the couple, that their autonomy be acknowledged and the decision to stop treatment be made by them. When a couple is encouraged to make their own decision, they are more likely to feel resolved in their own minds if they can say to themselves "we did everything *we* could".

When IVF is not successful, couples face an even greater test of their relationship than during the treatment and some couples do separate because of the strain of childlessness, particularly when one or other of them perceive that one partner still has the chance for a child in another relationship.

Multiple Births

One of the recognised outcomes of hormone treatment used in the management of infertility is multiple pregnancy. By 1996, the last year for which records are available, the multiple birth rate had remained consistently at between 25–30% over the previous six years. Many couples are overjoyed to discover a multiple birth but it is important that couples are mindful of the risks involved.

Notwithstanding the initial euphoria of success when multiple pregnancy follows a history of infertility, it can mean massive confusion for the couple, as the implications of the pregnancy become real. Some couples seek counselling at this stage but feel embarrassed to admit to feelings of ambivalence about their new status.

Occasionally, issues concerning embryo reduction will be discussed. The clearest case for reduction would be on the grounds of substantial risk of a premature baby being born with such severe physical and mental abnormalities as to be seriously handicapped. The Multiple Birth Foundation gives written as well as personal advise.

> "Inevitably would-be parents can only do their best when new but sad choices prove inescapable".

When a multiple pregnancy is indicated, the woman is likely to find herself tiring, and particularly in the case of triplets, might have to be admitted to hospital for rest. Complications such as high blood pressure and premature labour are common. Multiple births are likely to have a higher mortality rate than singletons. Babies are often born by caesarean section and below normal birth weight. They might require care in special baby units. Premature delivery also carries a risk of having a brain damaged child.

Once the pregnancy has ended and the children born are well, a couple face a whole new set of circumstances to test their individual strengths and that of their relationship. If there are other children in the family, the psychological impact of multiple birth will also resonate for them.

Sperm Donation

There are a number of circumstances where a couple will have to consider the use of donated sperm. The major reason would be if the man had a poor sperm count or problem with sperm motility, although other indicators might be a hereditary condition, or blood matching incompatibilitiy. The only circumstance looked at here will be the more common one of low sperm count or poor motility and where donation is by an anonymous donor.

When a man is found to have impaired sperm or sperm function, not only is it a shock but one that leaves a man feeling inadequate, calling into question his masculinity and virility. This can trigger problems with sexual performance, and intimacy which can elude a couple at a time when it is most needed. The issue of a man's fertility is a taboo subject in our society and is not a matter easily aired by either partner between themselves, let alone beyond the privacy of their relationship.

Bereavement theory can help to explain the process by which the couple gradually adjust to the new situation. The man will not only be grieving the loss of his masculinity, he also has to face the fact that he cannot procreate children of his own. One man quoted in Snowdens Book "The Gift of a Child" says:

> "What depressed me most... was this idea that at this point my genetic channel stops".

Men can and do feel enormously distressed and profoundly guilty at being infertile. They have to live with the loss and can, albeit illogically, feel deeply ashamed. Frequently, the sense of failure will spill over into other areas of a man's life.

However, if a couple are to tackle their desire for a child then they will need to talk, and if necessary be helped by speaking with a counsellor or sympathetic doctor. There is also a self-help group in this country, the Donor Conception Network set up by couples that have undergone sperm donation.

If a man is to come to terms with his infertility, the couple must be able to acknowledge the finality of the situation. Once the couple accept the fact that they are not going to be able to have a child in the usual way, they can begin to come to a new decision about future plans and work out what would be the best course of action for them. Having treatment through sperm donation does not resolve the finality of "genetic death", but it does allow the man to nurture a child, one conceived with his partner's genetic material, and for many couples, this is the key factor in the decision to proceed with donation.

All couples who decide on donor treatment are required by law, under provisions set out by the Human Fertilisation and Embryology Act 1990, to have a counselling session and subsequently to sign consent forms that they understand the implications of what they are doing. Aside from the potential ethical, religious and emotional issues associated with donor treatment there are also legal implications in the use of anonymous donor sperm, most crucially in the area of confidentiality and anonymity and the question of the child's right to know of his or her origins. Treatment cannot proceed without the written consent of both partners; the husband or partner must consent in writing to become the legal father of any child born as the result of treatment.

The law requires that non-identifying facts about the donor be registered (such as hair colour, build and nationality). The donor may wish, but is not required, to add a list of his hobbies/interests and occupation. From the age of 18 (or 16 if they plan to marry) the child has the legal right of access to non-identifying information from the HFEA Register.

For parents with children conceived in this way, a major issue is whether or not to tell their children or others.

The HFEA is currently considering whether the donor's identity should be disclosed. This is in response to pressure from groups concerned about the child's right to know about their origins. If the law governing donor treatment changes in the future, then the retrospective identity disclosure could be instituted if Parliament passed legislation.

Some couples diagnosed with a sperm problem are offered the opportunity for treatments such as intracytoplasmic sperm injection (ICSI), microsurgical epididymal sperm aspiration (MESA), sub-zonal insemination (SUZI), the mechanics of which are discussed elsewhere in this book.

From the psychological point of view, these techniques have meant the possibility of using the man's sperm, which when isolated and injected into the eggs of his partner's, and should embryos be successfully developed, gives the couple the possibility of their own genetic offspring, in the same way as in IVF. There has been success with treatment but when not successful it can create enormous dilemmas for couples, as each partner must be reconciled as to when or why to stop.

Egg Donation

In the case of egg donation, couples proceed with donation either from a known or anonymous donor. The law concerning registration of the origins of children born from these treatments is the same as for sperm donation. With egg donation, it is the woman who has the task of coming to terms with the loss of her ability to procreate her genetic material. It does seem that women are more accepting of the idea of social rather than genetic mothering.

It is too early to know how children born of donor treatments will fare in the future, as legislation about their right of access to non-identifying information does not come into effect until 2008.

Unexplained Infertility

When a couple has undergone all available tests, it may be that nothing sufficiently abnormal can be found to explain the difficulty in conceiving. The lack of an explanation can be extremely frustrating as people feel it would be easier to cope if there was something definite wrong.

Couples report that the major struggle for them is in not being able to put a finger on the cause, and as reported from many counselling sessions with people who have "unexplained infertility", couples are quick to realise that without an explanation their guilt at not being able to conceive becomes a minefield for fantasies about what could be going wrong. On the other hand when no cause has been found there is always the prospect that a pregnancy might happen one day.

When couples remain unsuccessful and have no clear cause they can blame, it can be almost impossible to "give up" hope and move on with life.

FACING CHILDLESSNESS

There is an implicit belief in our culture that it is not psychologically healthy to dwell on one's sorrows. To dwell on the past, we believe, will slow us down, encumber us and stop us achieving our goals. However, it does not encumber us to look back on our losses, but actually frees us to move forward on our lives. To be endlessly pre-occupied with our sorrows can be a way of avoiding the difficulties of the present but for the most part any fear of getting stuck if we look back too long is, as Kluger-Bell says:

> "wildly out of proportion to the danger that looking back actually poses".

The real danger comes if we never look back at all. Facing loss directly allows for the "letting go" of the past and to genuinely move on. For this reason, public ceremonies such as funerals and memorial services, including for the "hoped for child" who was never born have a place in helping people. Making grief public and thereby important makes it more bearable.

It is not possible to have a reproductive crisis which results in stillbirth, ectopic pregnancy, abortion, premature menopause, destruction of frozen embryos, secondary infertility, sperm problems and lack of success with treatment and not have feelings that need to be expressed. The way in which any particular event can affect a person's life will vary from person to person, just as the personal significance of any loss varies. What is clear is that the impact of the loss will depend on the kinds of hopes, dreams and fantasies wrapped around that child.

We all need recognition by other people of the things that happen to us in our lives, to help us make sense of them and bear them more easily. This is especially true of the traumas, setbacks and losses we suffer. Finding a place where a person can speak freely about their loss, where a person can be heard and understood, is critical. This place can be a support group, among sympathetic friends or family, or in the presence of a counsellor, therapist, doctor or spiritual leader.

Grieving takes time, and for carers it is not easy to witness distress nor to watch and feel helpless to provide any significant assistance. However the grieving person can, if allowed to process their loss, eventually be able to appreciate the riches of life again. None of the things a person might choose is a solution to losing a pregnancy and the regret will never go, but a time will come as Bryant says when:

> "Those of us who have not finally succeeded in having children will seek a mode of life that is creative and rewarding in other ways".

It would be impossible for a person to forget that they are childless. But a day does arrive when it is not uppermost and at this point the "coming to terms" will have arrived.

FURTHER READING

Professor Robert Winston (1999). *The IVF Revolution: The Definitive Guide to Assisted Reproduction Techniques.* Vermilion.

Robert, Elizabeth S. (1993). *The Gift of a Child.* Exeter University Press.

Anna F. (1997). *The Infertility Companion: A User's Guide to Tests, Technology and Therapies.* Thorsons.

William Worden, J. (1998). *Grief Counselling and Grief Therapy.* Tavistock Publications.

Kim K.-B. (1998). *Unspeakable Losses: Understanding the Experience of Pregnancy Loss, Miscarriage, and Abortion.* W. W. Norton.

Elizabeth B., Ronald H. (1995). *Infertility New Choices, New Dilemmas.* Penguin.

Virginia I., Sarah B. (1995). *The Subfertility Handbook.* Sheldon Press.

17

Adaptation to Extrauterine Life

In the womb, the fetus receives a continuous supply of oxygen and nutrients from the placenta. Removal of waste products also occurs via the placenta. Within minutes of delivery, the newborn baby has to change from continuous dependence upon the placenta to independant control of its entire metabolism. The newborn baby has to utilise pulmonary gas exchange, commence intermittent orogastric feeding with intestinal digestion and eliminate its own waste products.

In this chapter, the normal processes of adaptation will be described. Failure to adapt normally to extrauterine life leads to many serious problems for the baby and death may result.

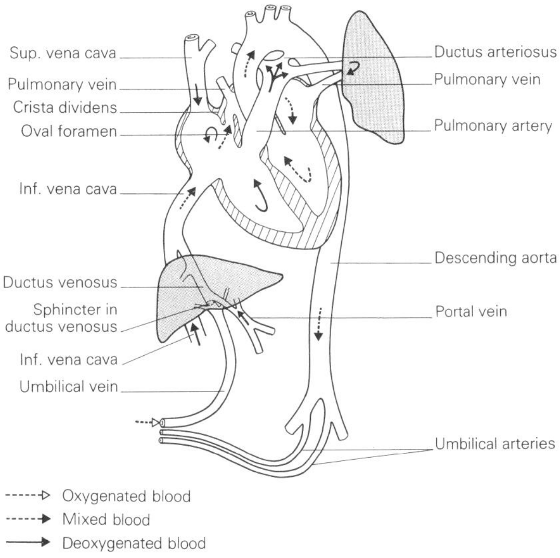

Fig. 17.1 *Plan of the human circulation before birth. Arrows indicate the direction of blood flow.*

FETAL CIRCULATION

The circulation of blood in the fetus differs from the mature infant's circulation as the fetus is dependant upon the placenta. The fetal circulation is shown in Fig. 17.1. Oxygenated blood from the placenta returns to the fetus via the umbilical vein, bypasses the liver via the ductus venosus and enters the right atrium. The right atrial pressure is higher than the left atrial pressure in fetal life and this keeps the foramen ovale open. Oxygenated blood flowing via the inferior vena cava into the left atrium is channelled through the patent foramen ovale into the right atrium. From there the oxygenated blood crosses the mitral valve, enters the left ventricle and is pumped via the ascending aorta to the brain and other organs.

The deoxygenated blood from the brain flows down the jugular veins and superior vena cava to the right atrium. Some mixing with the oxygenated blood flowing up from the umbilical vein occurs in the right atrium, but most of the deoxygenated blood flows through the tricuspid valve into the right ventricle from where it is pumped to the pulmonary artery. The fetal pulmonary circulation is tightly vasoconstricted thus generating a high vascular resistance and a pulmonary artery pressure that is slightly higher than aortic pressure. This is in contrast to postnatal life when aortic pressure is normally considerably higher than the pulmonary artery pressure. As a result of the high pulmonary vascular resistance, only 10% of the blood flowing along the pulmonary artery perfuses the lungs, 90% flowing through the ductus arteriosus into the descending aorta.

Fetal arterial Po_2 is approximately 4 kPa and Pco_2 6 kPa. To help the fetus to transport oxygen around the body in the presence of relatively low Po_2, the haemoglobin concentration is raised to 16–22 g/dl and consists of fetal haemoglobin (HbF). HbF has a higher affinity for oxygen than adult haemoglobin and can thus take up more oxygen in the placenta at a relatively low Po_2.

FETAL LUNG DEVELOPMENT

By 26 weeks' gestation, the respiratory bronchioles and a rich supply of capillaries have developed. From this time, the alveoli are developing as clusters of thin-walled saccules lined by flattened epithelium (type I pneumonocytes). Type II pneumonocytes are also present at this gestation (Fig. 17.2) and contain surfactant (Fig. 17.3). Surfactant is a phospholipid-lipoprotein complex that lowers the surface tension in the fluid film which lines the alveoli. This facilitates expansion of the lung during inspiration. The terminal bronchioles of babies born at 28 weeks are very small and have a strong tendency to collapse in expiration. This collapse on expiration is prevented by the surfactant molecules being forced to take up an almost crystalline structure as they are pushed closer together as the alveoli get smaller in expiration. The type II pneumocytes of the preterm infant produce little surfactant and thus the lungs of the preterm infant are hard to inflate and tend to collapse on expiration.

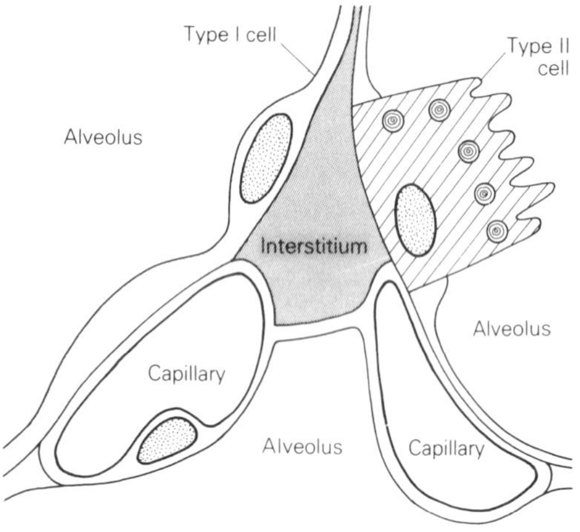

Fig. 17.2 *An alveolus with type I and type II pneumocytes.*

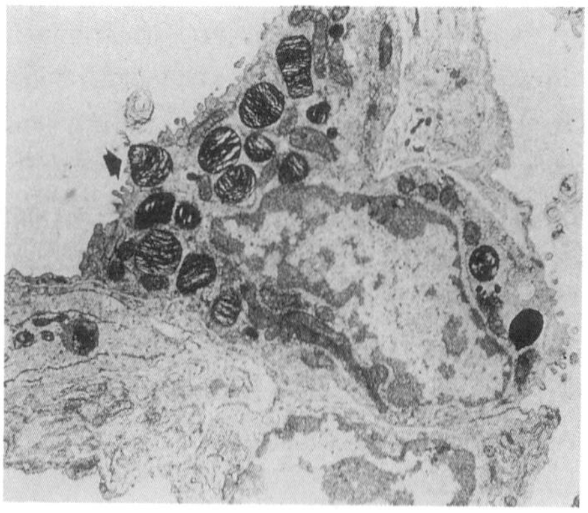

Fig. 17.3 *Electron micrograph of a type II pneumocyte showing the lamellated osmiophilic bodies which are thought to contain surfactant.*

During fetal life, the lungs are filled with fluid secreted by the lungs themselves. During labour, adrenaline is secreted by the fetal adrenal medulla. This inhibits the secretion of lung liquid and stimulates the absorption of lung liquid by the pulmonary lymphatics. Some of the fetal lung fluid is also physically forced out of the thorax of the fetus by compression during each contraction.

The First Breath

Why does a baby cry vigorously after delivery having breathed quietly and regularly for months *in utero*? Sudden loss of weightlessness and compression, exposure to cold and physical squeezing followed by release are the most likely stimuli to initiate breathing. After birth, the chemoreceptor control of respiration is changed, Pao_2 normally being maintained around 10 kPa and Pco_2 around 5.3 kPa. The first breath in a full-term baby is about 30 ml and requires a negative intrathoracic pressure of -40 to -100 cm H_2O. Very soon functional residual capacity is established and a negative pressure of only a few cm H_2O is required for each tidal volume.

CIRCULATORY CHANGES AFTER BIRTH

The umbilical vessels constrict in response to thromboxane released by natural stimuli such as animals chewing at the cord of their offspring or to cold, drying and increased oxygen tension. Filling the lungs with air produces a fall in pulmonary artery pressure and a large increase in pulmonary blood flow. Thus ventilation and perfusion of the lungs increase in parallel and *the pulmonary circulation converts from high resistance low flow to low resistance high flow.*

The tying of the umbilical cord removes a low resistance circuit from the fetal arterial

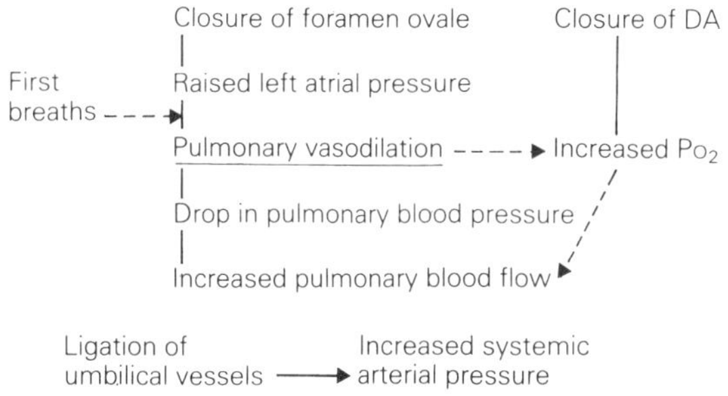

Fig. 17.4 *Key changes in the transition from fetal to neonatal circulation.*

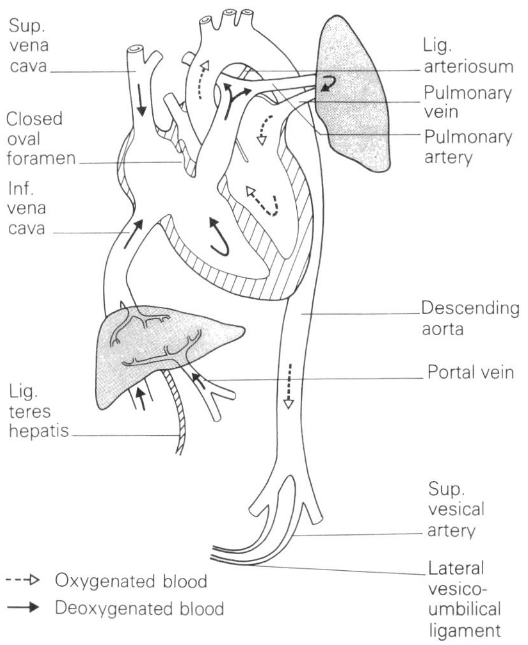

Fig. 17.5 *Plan of the human circulation after birth. Note the changes occurring as a result of the beginning of respiration and the interruption of the placental blood flow.*

circulation. The systemic arterial pressure then rises above that of the pulmonary artery, resulting in reversal of the flow through the ductus arteriosus.

As the pulmonary blood flow increases, blood returning to the left atrium increases and the left atrial pressure rises above that of the right atrium. When this happens, there is no more right-to-left shunt between the atria, and the foramen ovale closes as a simple flap.

As the arterial Po_2 rises, the ductus arteriosus constricts. The ductus venosus constricts soon after umbilical flow ceases (Fig. 17.4). The neonatal circulation is shown in Fig. 17.5.

DISORDERS OF CARDIOPULMONARY ADAPTATION

Respiratory Distress Syndrome (RDS)

Respiratory distress syndrome (RDS) is the condition affecting the lungs of preterm infants deficient in surfactant. Lacking the surface-tension-lowering phospholipid, the alveolar saccules and terminal bronchioles are difficult to inflate and the alveoli tend to collapse in expiration and remain collapsed. Worsening hypoxia occurs as more and more alveoli are not ventilated and the work of breathing increases as the lungs become stiffer. Clinically, the baby develops increasing tachypnoea, grunting, subcostal and sternal recession, nasal flare and cyanosis. As the baby fatigues, respiratory and metabolic acidosis increase.

Chest X-ray shows a diffuse granular pattern throughout both lungs, "the ground glass appearance" of RDS. As the lungs are underinflated with collapsed alveoli, they do not contain air. The bronchi, which do contain air, may be seen as black outlines against the hazy light grey lung fields, the "air bronchogram".

Treatment of RDS within a neonatal intensive care unit consists of monitoring arterial blood gases and giving increased concentrations of inspired O_2 to maintain an adequate Pao_2 (7–10 kPa). Continuous positive airway pressure (CPAP) applied usually by the nose helps to maintain lung volume, improves oxygenation

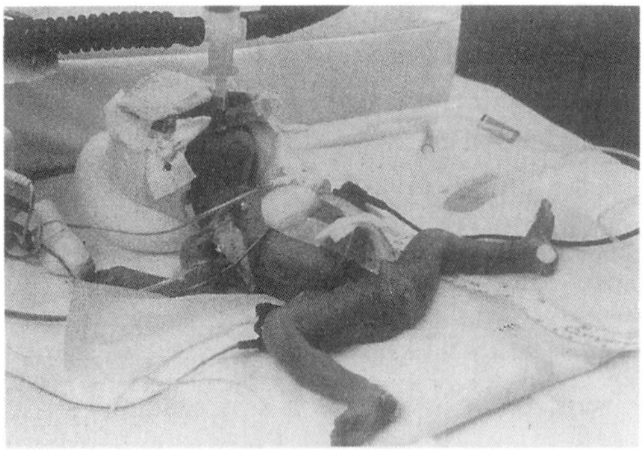

Fig. 17.6 *A 26-week gestation infant connected to a ventilator.*

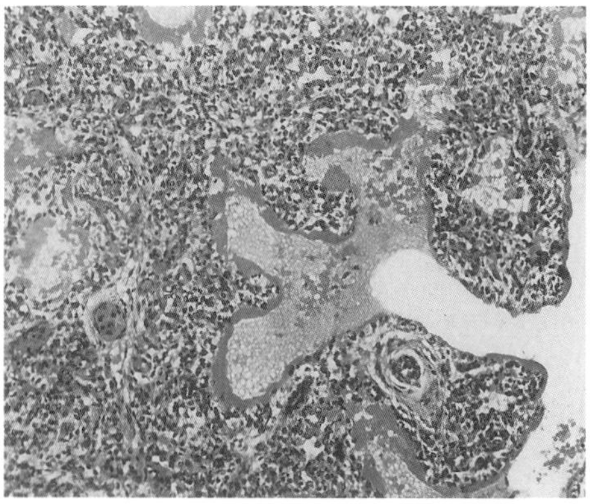

Fig. 17.7 *Section of lung from an infant of 29 weeks' gestation who died with respiratory distress syndrome at 30 hours of age. There is a dilated bronchiole with several branches containing red cells and proteinaceous material and lined with thick layers of amorphous hyaline membrane. The surrounding cellular tissue comprises the collapsed air spaces. Haematoxylin and Eosin stain. Magnification x90.*

and reduces apnoea. Mechanical ventilation with positive-end-expiratory pressure is needed for persistent hypoxaemia, respiratory acidosis and prolonged apnoea (Fig. 17.6). Surfactant may be extracted from the lungs of pigs or cows or made synthetically. Instillation of surfactant into the lungs of the ventilated newborn preterm infant with RDS is now routine. This results in a rapid improvement in the condition of the lungs by reducing the surface tension within the lung so allowing inflation of the lung and also helping to prevent collapse in expiration. In randomised trials, natural surfactant has reduced mortality by 40% when given prophylactically to infants with gestation under 30 weeks.

At autopsy, the lungs of a preterm infant with RDS are very poorly expanded and histologically, there is a pink hyaline membrane lining the alveoli and terminal bronchioles (Fig. 17.7). Hyaline membrane disease (HMD) is used as a synonym for respiratory distress syndrome, but strictly, it is a pathological diagnosis.

Advances in obstetrics and neonatal medicine have decreased the severity and frequency of RDS but deaths still occur from complications such as pneumothorax and cerebral intraventricular haemorrhage. Asphyxia damages the type II pneumocytes and increases the risk of RDS. Thus careful monitoring with operative delivery to avoid asphyxia reduces the chances of RDS in preterm infants. The risk increases as gestational age shortens and is greater in male than female infants. Experiments with pregnant ewes have shown that giving ACTH or glucocorticoids induces earlier production of surfactant. Subsequent studies have shown that 24 hours of maternal treatment with a glucocorticoid such as betamethazone has a maturing effect on surfactant production if the infant is delivered before 34 weeks' gestation. In randomised trials, antenatal corticosteroids have reduced mortality, RDS and severe cerebral intraventricular haemorrhage in preterm infants.

Retained Fetal Lung Fluid or Transient Tachypnoea of the Newborn (TTN)

Retained fetal lung fluid affects babies at all gestational ages including term and is more common following elective caesarean section, when the fetus has not experienced any thoracic squeezing or adrenaline secretion to expel lung liquid. The newborn infant shows the clinical signs of respiratory distress: tachypnoea, grunting, subcostal and sternal recession nasal flare and cyanosis. Hypoxaemia is frequent, but is easily relieved by a moderate increase in inspired oxygen almost always without the need for mechanical ventilation. X-rays of the chest typically show well inflated lungs, hence dark lung fields, but lung fluid may be seen in the horizontal fissure of the right lung and in the lymphatic drainage of the lung as perihilar streaks. This condition is also known as transient tachypnoea of the newborn (TTN) and may resolve within 24 hours, occasionally taking 48–72 hours.

Intrapartum Asphyxia

If the fetus is asphyxiated by significant hypoxia from obstetric complications, such as prolapsed cord or placental abruption, metabolic acidosis from accumulation of lactic acid occurs. Systemic vasoconstriction may result in blood being shifted from the baby's side of the fetal circulation to the placenta. After delivery, there may be systemic hypovolaemia as a result.

The hypoxic fetus may pass meconium into the amniotic fluid and, if severely distressed, may gasp, thus inhaling meconium into the airways. Meconium aspiration is most common in postmature babies and the respiratory problem may be severe. The particles of meconium exert a chemical irritant effect inactivating surfactant and setting up pulmonary inflammation. The meconium particles also have a ball-valve effect so that inspiration may be obstructed much less than expiration resulting in trapping of air and overdistension of the lung. Air leaks in the mediastinum and pleural space are common complications.

If intrapartum asphyxia persists before delivery, worsening acidosis, bradycardia and hypotension will subject all the baby's vital organs to hypoxia and ischaemia. This includes the brain, kidneys, intestines and heart. Treatment is emergency delivery and resuscitation to restore oxygenation and improve perfusion. For the baby who is limp, has a bradycardia and is apnoeic, endotracheal intubation and manual ventilation are the most effective means of oxygenation. If severe bradycardia (< 60 beats per minute) persists, external cardiac massage should be started at 120/min. If the heart rate remains < 60 bpm adrenaline should be given into the heart through a cannula sited via the umbilical vein. The Apgar score is the universally acknowledged system of marking a baby's state at birth and its response to resuscitation (Table 17.1). An Apgar score of 5 or less necessitates active resuscitation. If the score is still 6 or less after 5 minutes, the response to treatment has not been good. If the baby takes more than 10 minutes to establish respiration, then the effects of hypoxia on the brain (hypoxic-ischaemic encephalopathy or HIE) are likely to be clinically significant. The processes by which brain cells die continue to operate for hours and days after oxygenation and circulation have been restored. HIE involves visible changes in the tone and reflexes of the baby with the most severe infants losing brain stem responses and respiration. Convulsions are common. The basal ganglia, thalamus and brain stem are especially vulnerable. Infants with severe HIE either die or survive with cerebral palsy and varying degrees of cognitive disability and epilepsy. Several post-hypoxic-ischaemic

Table 17.1
Agpar Score

Clinical feature	0	1	2
Heart rate	Absent	< 100	> 100
Respiration	Absent	Gasping or irregular	Regular or crying lustily
Muscle tone	Limp	Diminished or no movements	Normal with active movements
Response to pharyngeal suction	Nil	Grimace	Cough
Colour of trunk	White	Blue	Pink

interventions have been shown to reduce brain damage in newborn animals and the most promising treatment, mild hypothermia, is now undergoing clinical trials.

Persistent Pulmonary Hypertension (Persistent Fetal Circulation)

Following severe asphyxia and in severe respiratory distress syndrome, hypoxaemia and acidosis may stimulate pulmonary vasoconstriction. This results in pulmonary hypertension, reduced pulmonary blood flow and reduced pulmonary venous return to the left atrium. The reduced left atrial pressure results in right-to-left shunting through the foramen ovale. Thus deoxygenated blood shunts into the systemic circulation further worsening the hypoxaemia. The pulmonary hypertension may additionally cause pulmonary-to-systemic shunting through the ductus arteriosus which opens as a response to hypoxaemia. Thus, a vicious circle of hypoxaemia stimulating further hypoxaemia characterises persistent pulmonary hypertension and results in failure to establish the normal neonatal circulation. Treatment involves mechanical ventilation with high concentrations of inspired oxygen, restoring the blood volume, correcting any acidosis and using pulmonary vasodilator drugs such as inhaled nitric oxide gas or prostacyclin.

Patent Ductus Arteriosus (PDA)

Normally, the ductus arteriosus constricts within hours of birth. If the baby is very preterm (less than 32 weeks), this is often delayed for days or weeks. Usually the systemic arterial pressure is higher than the pulmonary arterial pressure after birth, and this causes blood to shunt left-to-right, i.e. aorta to pulmonary artery.

If the ductus arteriosus is patent, this can cause serious problems to very preterm infants because:

1. Pulmonary blood flow may be increased to the levels where the lungs are 'wetter' and stiffer. Thus more effort is required to breathe. Babies below 1500 g may become fatigued and apnoeic.
2. A large fraction of the left ventricular output is wasted in that it does not perfuse the systemic circulation. Thus the left ventricle has to increase its output substantially to keep up with the demand. Hypotension and cardiac failure may result. The failure to adequately perfuse the brain of the preterm infant in the first few days of life may result in severe cerebral intraventricular haemorrhage. Poor perfusion to the gut of a preterm infant may result in bowel ischaemia and necrosis (due to necrotising enerocolitis: see below).

The frequency of PDA can be minimised in babies under 32 weeks by avoiding excessive fluid intake, hypoxaemia and anaemia. If a PDA causes a clinically significant shunt with symptoms and signs, indomethacin, which inhibits the production of vasodilatory protaglandins is effective in closing most PDAs. If a troublesome shunt persists, then surgical ligation of PDA can be safely carried out even in tiny infants.

Pulmonary Hypoplasia

Normal lung growth and development requires fetal breathing movements with adequate space in the chest, adequate amniotic fluid to breathe and good muscle power. The lungs may fail to

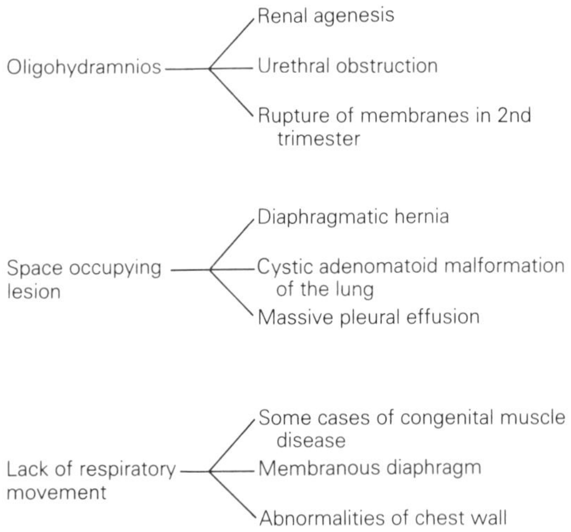

Fig. 17.8 *Causes of pulmonary hypoplasia.*

grow and develop if there is deficiency of amniotic fluid, a mass occupying space in the chest, or if severe neurological abnormalities inhibit respiratory movements (Fig. 17.8).

Clinically, pulmonary hypoplasia presents as severe respiratory difficulty which responds poorly to endotracheal intubation and ventilation, and tension pneumothorax is a common terminal event.

NUTRITION

The fetus receives a continuous supply of glucose, amino acids, electrolytes, mineral and essential fatty acids via the umbilical vein. The fat intake is relatively small, most of the calories being supplied by glucose. Subcutaneous fat, which is white adipose tissue, is laid down in the fetus from 26 weeks' gestation, most of the triglyceride being synthesised from glucose.

After delivery, the baby changes from a continuous high carbohydrate diet to an intermittent high fat diet. Fetal blood glucose is normally slightly lower than maternal blood glucose. After birth, there is a fall in blood glucose during the first few hours, but this stabilises above 2.6 mmol/l after about 4 hours of age when milk feeding has started and the infant switches its metabolism to use energy substrates apart from glucose.

The neonatal brain uses 50% of the total consumption of oxygen and calories. At birth, the carbohydrate store (glycogen) is only sufficient for about 12 hours in a full-term infant. However, glycerol derived from the breakdown of fat in adipose tissue can be converted to glucose in the liver. By studying arteriovenous differences, it has been possible to show that the neonatal brain may take up not only glucose, but also acetoacetate and β-hydroxybutyrate which are formed in the liver from fatty acids. Free fatty acids lactate, pyruvate and glycerol are not utilised directly by the brain. After birth, free fatty acid levels rise and double by 12 hours. Vital organs, such as the heart, can utilise free fatty acids and within hours of birth the respiratory quotient falls from 1.0 to 0.7, indicating a switch from carbohydrate to fat utilisation.

Digestion

Carbohydrate in breast milk is in the form of *lactose*. This is hydrolysed by lactase on the brush border of the intestinal mucosa to glucose and galactose. This enzyme is present even in very preterm infants. Lactase deficiency may occur as a result of injury or infection in the small intestine. Profuse watery diarrhoea results.

Protein Digestion

Pancreatic peptidases such as trypsin, chymotrypsin and elastase are present even in very preterm infants. Further digestion occurs by proteases on the brush border. There is evidence that some animal species can absorb intact proteins in the neonatal period. It is not clear how important this process is in humans, but absorption of immunoglobulins from breast milk may give some protection, and absorption of antigens (in cow's milk, egg and wheat) may stimulate allergic responses. Over 80% of babies with *cystic fibrosis* have a deficiency of pancreatic enzymes because of obstruction of pancreatic ducts. Trypsin is normally detectable in neonatal stools. Absence of trypsin from stools, or an excessive level of trypsin in blood, is suggestive of cystic fibrosis.

Fat Digestion

Triglycerides are hydrolysed by pancreatic lipase into monoglycerides and fatty acids. Bile salts facilitate the absorption of monoglycerides and fatty acids. Breast milk contains a lipase which is activated by bile salts in the duodenum. Boiling breast milk to sterilise it, destroys the lipase and thereby reduces fat absorption.

Necrotising Enterocolitis

Apart from congenital abnormalities of the gut, such as atresias at various levels, the most serious gastrointestinal disorder in the neonatal period is necrotising enterocolitis (NEC). This condition occurs mainly in small, sick infants. The pathogenesis involves: (a) an injury to the integrity of the intestinal mucosa, usually hypoxic-ischaemic, from respiratory failure, cardiac failure, PDA, shock, catheters in the arteries or veins supplying the gut, (b) the availability of substrate for bacterial growth, and (c) invasion of the wall of the gut by gas-forming anaerobic bacteria. The ileum and jejunum are most commonly affected.

Clinically, there is abdominal distention, bile-stained vomiting, and bloody diarrhoea. If infarction of the intestine or perforation with peritonitis occurs, there is considerable mortality. Most at risk are babies in neonatal intensive care units with severe respiratory distress syndrome, severe congenital heart disease, extreme prematurity, or those infants requiring exchange transfusion.

Fluid and Electrolyte Balance

The main function of the fetal kidney appears to be as a source of amniotic fluid. In renal agenesis, there is extreme oligohydramnios and severe pulmonary hypoplasia (Potter's syndrome). After birth, there is normally obligatory loss of water which gives a 5–10% weight loss in the first four days. This is partly due to continued excretion of water and sodium despite a small intake.

At birth, glomerular filtration rate and renal blood flow are both about one-third of that expected and gradually increase with age. Renal tubular function is also immature in that sodium excretion is limited and the maximum concentration is 700–800 mOsm/k, whereas an older child can excrete urine with osmolality of 1200–1400 mOsm/k. Apart from regulation of fluid and electrolyte balance, another important renal function is the elimination of drugs. Aminoglycoside antibiotics, such as gentamicin, are entirely cleared in the urine and elimination is significantly slower in the first week of postnatal life than later. To avoid potentially toxic accumulation of these drugs, the doses need to be less frequent than in older children.

In preterm babies, especially those below 32 weeks, all aspects of renal function are less mature than at term. Not only is sodium excretion limited, but the GFR is lower. There is also a relatively high plasma aldosterone level.

The skin of the preterm infant is particularly thin but cornifies rapidly over the first two weeks of life. As a result, huge amounts of water may be lost from the premature infant by diffusion through the skin and evaporation in the first few days of life. In fact, the amount of fluid lost solely through the skin of a very premature infant in the first few days of life may be more than twice the urine output. This predisposes the infant to rapid dehydration and hypernatraemia. Transepidermal water loss may be reduced by nursing the preterm infant in 80% humidity and by applying barrier creams to the skin to prevent evaporation.

Thus the care of sick and small infants involves very careful calculation of changes and requirements of fluid and electrolytes because of the limited ability of the newborn to maintain correct balance.

BILIRUBIN

Bilirubin is formed by the breakdown of haem from old red blood cells. In fetal life, this is removed by the placenta and accumulation only takes place in the fetus if there is extremely severe haemolysis as in rhesus incompatibility. After birth, the neonatal liver has to remove bilirubin. Bilirubin is initially released from the reticulo-endothelial cells as unconjugated bilirubin. This is more fat-soluble than water-soluble and cannot be excreted effectively by the kidneys. Plasma albumin has a considerable capacity to bind bilirubin and only a small fraction is actually unbound in plasma. Unconjugated bilirubin is taken up by specific receptors in the liver and by a series of steps is conjugated to bilirubin glucuronide. This is more water-soluble and is normally excreted in the bile. The process of conjugation frequently

Table 17.2
Causes of Neonatal Unconjugated Hyperbilirubinaemia

Haemolysis	Rhesus, ABO and other blood group incompatibility Red cell defects, e.g. spherocytosis enzyme defects Bruising, e.g. cephalhaematoma
Short gestation	
Breast milk jaundice	
Infection	
Dehydration	
Hypothyroidism	

fails to keep up with need in the first week after birth, and unconjugated bilirubin accumulates without there being any disease present (Table 17.2). This 'physiological jaundice' occurs in about one-third of all normal full-term babies and is usually fading by ten days of age.

High plasma levels of unconjugated bilirubin in plasma are potentially harmful because the binding capacity of albumin may become saturated by bilirubin. Thus free bilirubin may enter the brain and damage the basal ganglia and VIII nerve nuclei. This pattern of brain damage (kernicterus) gives choreo-athetoid cerebral palsy and sensori-neural deafness.

Some breast fed infants remain mildly, but definitely, jaundiced for several weeks with unconjugated bilirubin. They thrive well and investigation reveals no other pathology. This is breast milk jaundice and is thought to be due to unknown substances inhibiting the pathways that influence glucuronidation. It is not necessary to stop breast-feeding.

In well full-term infants, plasma levels of bilirubin up to 340 μmol/l and slightly higher are considered safe, but the shorter the gestation and the more ill the baby, the lower is the threshold for kernicterus. A plasma bilirubin over 200 μmol/l in a sick infant below 1500 g carries a significant risk of sensori-neural deafness. Thus all newborn infants must be scrutinised daily for jaundice in the first week and investigated if jaundice is marked.

Phototherapy with white or blue light is usually effective in controlling hyperbilirubinaemia by photo-isomerisation of the bilirubin molecule such that it becomes water soluble and excretable. However, exchange transfusion is still necessary in severe haemolytic disease and in very-low-birth-weight babies.

TEMPERATURE REGULATION

At birth, the baby emerges from a perfectly centrally heated environment to be exposed to cold stress. Cooling by several degrees may occur within minutes if the wet neonate in the delivery room is not dried off, wrapped up and placed in a warm cot or against the mother's body. Cold stress can be a serious threat to newborns, especially preterm infants, and has been shown to increase mortality.

Children and adults may increase heat production by shivering, but newborns are unable to do this. Their principal source of heat production is from brown adipose tissue. These cells contain many fat vacuoles and numerous large mitochondria in the cytoplasm. In contrast, subcutaneous or white fat has a single fat vacuole with relatively few mitochondria. This metabolically active brown fat has a rich blood supply and is distributed around the main arteries, and has been called 'oil-fired central heating'. The cells can take up glucose, glycerol and fatty acids from the circulation, to be stored as triglyceride. Heat production is controlled by the sympathetic nervous system. When the temperature drops, sympathetic nerve endings release noradrenaline which activates the brown adipose cell, via cyclic adenosine monophosphate (cyclic AMP), to oxidise fatty acids. This oxidation is uncoupled from the generation of ATP and heat is produced which can be carried by the circulating blood to the rest of the body. A full-term infant may increase metabolic rate from 6 ml of oxygen/kg/min to a maximum of 15 ml oxygen/kg/min. Thus hypoxia, hypothermia and hypoglycaemia are interrelated. Hypothermia increases the need for oxygen to fuel brown adipose tissue. Hypoxia and hypoglycaemia impair the ability of brown fat to respond by burning more fuel.

The lower the birth weight, the higher is the surface area to weight ratio and thus the greater is the surface for heat loss by convection, radiation and evaporation. In addition, small-for-gestational-age babies often have a relatively large head for the rest of the body, and thus have high metabolic requirements.

Sick and small babies who require intensive care procedures are most conveniently nursed under a radiant heater which can be servo-controlled to maintain the baby's skin temperature at 37°C. The side of the abdomen or buttock is a good site for an 'average' skin temperature. The use of such radiant heaters increases the evaporation of water from the newborn skin and this is further increased in the more immature baby. However, the effects of this can be reduced by putting a thin layer of plastic sheeting over the baby between procedures and the increased water loss can be compensated by carefully increasing fluid intake.

Very-low-birth-weight infants who do not require frequent procedures are most conveniently nursed in a closed incubator in which the air temperature can be carefully controlled. The environmental temperatures for thermal neutrality (i.e. minimum metabolic requirement) have been determined, i.e. a 1000 g baby on the first day may require a temperature of 36°C.

Larger babies (over 1500 g) can be adequately maintained if well wrapped in a cot in a warm room (24°C or 75°F). In many countries, the best place is in bed with the mother and being held naked against the mother's skin between the breasts has been successfully used for very-low-birth-weight infants in Colombia.

Neurological Adaptation to Extrauterine Life

A full-term baby is able to open the eyes and fix visually on a face within minutes of birth. This is best demonstrated if the baby is wrapped up well, held upright or inclined and if the lighting is slightly subdued. He or she will also orientate to sound and show a number of postural reactions and neonatal responses. Neck flexion is usually slightly stronger than neck extension. Leg and arm recoil are brisk. The Moro and grasp reflexes are present. Within the first week, visual preference for a striped pattern to a grey background can be demonstrated and the baby becomes able to distinguish the smell of his mother's breast from that of other mothers.

The main threats to the neonatal brain are:

1. *Hypoxic-ischaemic encephalopathy resulting from intrapartum asphyxia.*
2. Respiratory distress syndrome and asphyxia in preterm infants resulting in *haemorrhage in and around the cerebral ventricles* (Fig. 17.9).

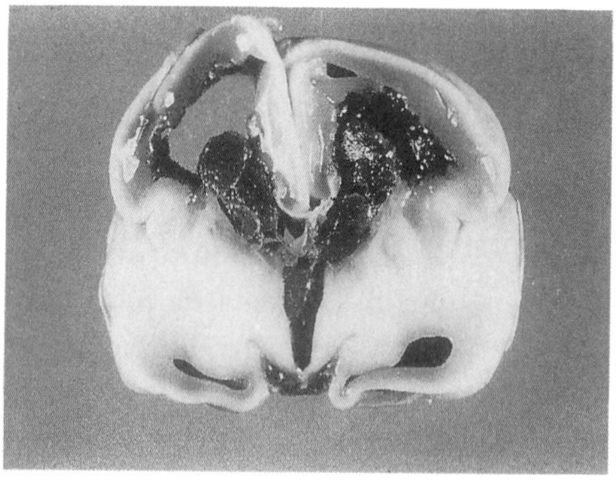

Fig. 17.9 *A coronal section of a preterm brain at autopsy. Massive intraventricular haemorrhage with ventricular dilatation.*

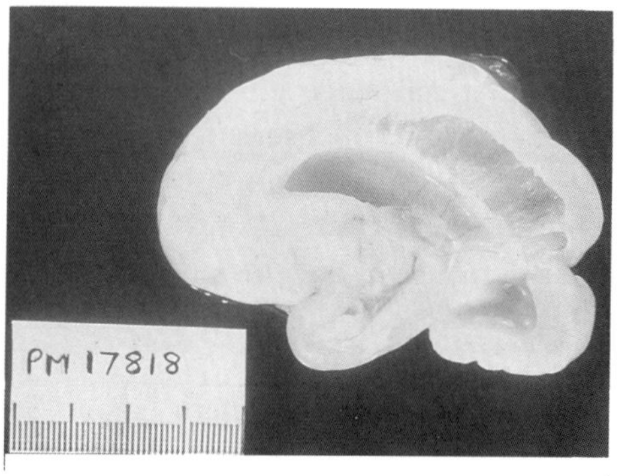

Fig. 17.10 *A parasagittal section of a preterm brain at autopsy. Massive cyst formation adjacent to the ventricle indicates periventricular leukomalacia.*

3. Underperfusion and inflammation giving *periventrincular leukomalacia* in preterm infants (Fig. 17.10).
4. *Hypoglycaemia.*
5. *Meningitis.*

The potential problems of adaptation to extrauterine life are usually successfully overcome by full-term infants. The more premature the baby, the more numerous are the potential problems.

FURTHER READING

Davis J.A., Dobbing J. eds. (1981). *Scientific Foundations of Paediatrics.* London: Heinemann Medical.

Rennie J., Roberton N.R.C. (1998). *A Manual of Neonatal Intensive Care.* London: Arnold.

Wigglesworth J. (1984). *Perinatal Pathology.* Philadelphia: W.B. Saunders.

18

Abnormal Menstruation

Period problems are the most common reason for women to request a gynaecological referral and hence are extremely prevalent in routine gynaecology clinics. The undergraduate should, therefore, have a good basic grasp of the common problems and the typical treatments. Areas to be covered in this chapter are:

Dysmenorrhoea
Menstrual irregularity
Inter-menstrual bleeding (IMB)
Post-coital bleeding (PCB)
Menorrhagia
Dysfunctional uterine bleeding (DUB)
Secondary amenorrhoea.

DYSMENORRHOEA

Primary or Spasmodic Dysmenorrhoea

This term means literally difficult monthly flow. More than half of all women suffer discomfort and pain at the time of menstruation. The majority have a normal uterus and no pelvic pathology. The risk of dysmenorrhoea is up to 6 times greater in smokers compared with non-smokers. Following pregnancy and child birth there are commonly fewer complaints of pain.

What causes the pain? Women who suffer from primary or spasmodic dysmenorrhoes have increased uterine activity during menstruation — the myometrium is actively contracting with pressures up to 120 mmHg. Blood flow to the endometrium is less when the contractions occur and the aetiology of the pain is largely ischaemic. Prostaglandins mediate uterine contractility and may themselves increase the sensation of pain by their inflammatory nature. The aetiology is related to excessive prostaglandin production and release from the endometrium, as the levels of particularly $PGF_{2\alpha}$ in endometrium, menstrual and peripheral blood are significantly higher in women with primary dysmenorrhoea. Ovulatory cycles are more painful than anovulatory cycles because the endometrium is thicker and synthesises and releases more prostaglandins.

Cramping lower abdominal pains starting just before or with the menses are characteristic. There are often associated gastrointestinal symptoms such as nausea, vomiting and frequent loose bowel motions at the time of the worst pain. These symptoms as well as vaso dilatation are due to increased circulating prostaglandin levels. $PGF_{2\alpha}$ is responsible largely for the increased gastrointestinal motility and PGE_2 for the vasodilatation.

Pelvic exmination is normal except during the period when the uterus is tender.

Treatment of Primary Dysmenorrhoea

Firstly reassurance is important. Many women feel that there must be something wrong with them which is usually not the case, and they do not realise how common the condition is. Abolishing ovulation so that the endometrium becomes atrophic, usually achieved by prescribing the combined pill is often appropriate. Sufferers are often between 18 and 30 and so in many cases the pill is acceptable for contraceptive purposes as well.

Non-steroidal anti-inflammatory drugs (NSAIDs) which inhibit prostaglandin synthesis are also appropriate remedies. These include indomethacin, mefenamic acid, brufen and naproxen. They are more efficacious if taken a few hours before menses and symptoms start if this can be predicted. Combination of NSAIDs and the pill may be needed in severe cases.

Calcium channel blockers such as nifedipine which relax smooth muscle have been found to be effective.

Secondary or Congestive Dysmenorrhoea

Secondary dysmenorrhoea is pain which starts before the onset of menses, often many days beforehand. It may be relieved by the onset of menstrual flow or it may continue throughout and even after the period. There is always some form of pelvic pathology present and accounting for the symptoms. There may also be superadded spasmodic dysmenorrhoea. This form of dysmenorrhoea occurs usually in the older patient who complains of the symptoms described above.

The most common causes are pelvic inflammatory disease, endometriosis, adenomyosis and fibroids. Irritable or inflammatory bowel disease can also have menstrual exacerbations.

Diagnostic hysteroscopy or laparoscopy is often needed and treatment is that of the underlying cause. Suppressing menstruation in the case of endometriosis or suspected adenomyosis may help. NSAIDs may be partially helpful. Surgery may be required in the more severe cases.

MENSTRUAL IRREGULARITY

What is a 'normal' cycle interval (the number of days between the first day of one period and the next)? Although one might anticipate a figure of 28 days, long term studies on normally cycling women have confirmed that anything between 21 and 35 days can be considered normal, with relatively few women having an exact 28-day cycle. Even when there is a 'typical' cycle interval, then a fluctuation of several days either side is commonplace. Various potential causes of menstrual irregularity are given in Table 18.1.

Table 18.1
Causes of Menstrual Irregularity

Pregnancy related	Ongoing pregnancy — complicated by bleeding Retained products — following miscarriage Ectopic pregnancy — either acute or chronic
Anovulation	More frequent around menarche or before the menopause Disorder or disease of the hypothalmus or pituitary Polycystic ovarian syndrome Thyroid dysfunction

It is important to enquire about contraceptive practice in sexually active women to ascertain whether they could potentially have a complication of pregnancy causing their problem. Also the contraceptive method itself can have an effect, the progesterone only pill and a recently inserted mirena will frequently result in irregular bleeding.

The diagnosis of polycystic ovarain syndrome is made by ultrasound and/or the finding of a raised follicular phase luteinising hormone (LH) to follicle stimulating hormone (FSH) ratio (greater than 3 to 1) and possibly an elevated serum testosterone. Hypothalamic, pituitary and thyroid gland abnormalities are also screened for by the relevant serological tests.

It is common to have predominantly anovulatory cycles for the initial couple of years after menarche and prior to the menopause. In association with this, there is variability in cycle interval of an underlying physiological basis.

Treatment may involve simple reassurance or the inducing of regular endometrial shedding with progestogens alone or in combination with oestrogens with the combined oral contraceptive pill. Where there is a desire for pregnancy, then ovulation induction may be appropriate.

INTER-MENSTRUAL BLEEDING (IMB)

This is bleeding which occurs outside of the menstrual periods. This should not be confused

Table 18.2
Potential Causes of IMB

Physiological	Ovulation Stress/illness Foreign bodies e.g. intrauterine device
Endometrial	Polyps Endometritis Endometrial hyperplasia Endometrial cancer
Hormonal	Anovulation Thyroid dysfunction

Table 18.3
Causes of Post-Coital Bleeding

Local disease	Urethral polyp/prolapse/caruncle Vulval problems Vaginal lesions (rare)
Genital tract infections	e.g. Chlamydia
Cervical	Ectropian Cervicitis Cervical polyp Cervical cancer

with the normal (often described as brown) light loss the day preceding a period or on the last day or two of menstruation. Causes of IMB are summarised in Table 18.2.

IMB can be a worrying symptom, although the majority of cases have a benign underlying cause. At the time of ovulation there is a transitory drop in oestrogen levels which in some women is sufficient to provoke endometrial bleeding. IMB associated with stress of illness is frequently self-limiting. Any foreign body with the cavity, the most common of which is a contraceptive device can be associated with IMB and resolved by its removal (if a suitable alternative contraceptive can be offered). An endometrial polyp can be avulsed at the time of hysteroscopy and cure associated IMB. Particularly in the woman over 40, the possibility of endometrial hyperplasia or malignancy should be kept in mind and excluded. Such pathology may be of relevance in a younger woman who is markedly obese, and therefore who has an adipose source of oestrogen and/or in women with a history of prolonged anovulation where there has been infrequent or absent progesterone endometrial exposure.

POST-COITAL BLEEDING (PCB)

With this complaint, the relatively uncommon but important cause of cancer of the cervix should always be ruled out. Any other part of the lower genital tract can be traumatised at the time of intercourse and therefore bleed. Treatment of infection can cure PCB. Occasionally, cervical cautery is used to encourage overgrowth of glandular epithelium on the ectocervix with squamous cells.

MENORRHAGIA

Menorrhagia is clinically the complaint of excessively heavy periods, usually with associated episodes of flooding (uncontrollable flow, soiling clothing and bed linen) and sometimes passing clots of blood. It is objectively defined as a loss of 80 ml or more per period. Other than for the purposes of research, blood loss is rarely measured which is a pity, for it has been repeatedly shown that the perception of 'heavy periods' is frequently grossly inaccurate. Around half those women complaining of heavy periods will have an actual blood loss within the normal range, an average of 35 to 45 ml.

Investigations of Heavy Periods

Anaemia is more frequent in woman who lose in excess 80 ml per period and therefore a full blood count (which will also assess other blood constituents such as platelets) is a useful first step. In the presence of other suggestive symptoms and cycle irregularity, thyroid function studies may be of value as correction of the over- or under-active thyroid can result in resolution of menstrual problems. In the young girl with menarchal onset severe menorrhagia, formal haematological investigation may be warranted, as in up to 30% this may be the first presentation of an inherited bleeding disorder.

Around half the women with heavy loss have an entirely normal examination. Ultrasound is a useful adjunct to examine the uterus for other pathology that may be causing the heavy periods, such as sizeable endometrial polyps or fibroids which indent and enlarge the uterine cavity. Rarely a forgotten intrauterine device may be seen. There is no good data that endometriosis or chronic pelvic inflammatory disease is a cause of menorrhagia. Underlying endometrial pathology such as hyperplasia or even malignancy should be excluded in women over 40. Examination of the cavity and biopsy should be optimally combined with visualisation at hysteroscopy.

Table 18.4
Medical Treatment of Menorrhagia

Drug	Average reduction in blood loss	When taken	Comments	Potential adverse effects
NSAIDs	20–45%	With menses	Also helps dysmenorrhoea. Has no effect on cycle regularity.	Dizziness, dyspepsia, bronchospasm.
Tranexamic acid	50%	With menses	No help with dysmenorrhoea or cycle regularity.	Gastrointestinal upset. Rarely a disturbance of colour vision.
Luteal phase progestogens	20% to a 20% increase in blood loss!	From day 19 to 26 of the cycle	Increased cycle predictability and enables postponement of menstruation. Not recommended — a poorly effective treatment for reducing loss.	Pre-menstrual type symptoms, weight gain, bloating. Dysmenorrhoea.
Extended dose progestogens	30% in ovulatory women, 60% in anovulatory women	For three weeks out of four	Increased cycle predictability and enables postponement of menstruation.	See above for luteal phase.
Combined oral contraceptive pill	50%	For three weeks out of four	Increased cycle predictability. Reduction in dysmenorrhoea. Excellent contraceptive efficacy.	Nausea, headaches, breast tenderness, hypertension, thrombosis.
Danazol (200 mg daily dose)	60 plus %	Continuous daily for 3 months	Helps pre-menstrual syndrome and sore breasts. Androgenic side effects may limit usefulness. Contraception required.	Weight gain, acne, greasy hair and spots. Muscle cramps, rash, headaches.
Gonadotrophin -releasing analogues	Majority have complete amenorrhoea	Monthly injection or frequent nasal spray	Useful for pre-operative fibroid shrinkage and/or enabling the haemoglobin to rise. Limited to 6 months because of deleterious effect on bone mass.	Menopausal symptoms of hot flushes, sweats, vaginal dryness.
Mirena	80% reduction at 6 months, > 90% reduction 12 months following insertion	Intrauterine system, fitted as one-off normally as an outpatient	Effective for at least 5 years. Excellent reversible contraceptive effect. Need counselling to ensure amenorrhoea an acceptable outcome.	Potential initial 3 to 6 months of protracted irregular bleeding and spotting.

Treatment of Menorrhagia

Reassurance is important, that heavy periods are common and that there is only rarely a sinister underlying cause may be all that is required. Initially, medical therapy is usually instituted before resorting to surgery if this fails. A wide variety of preparations are available and outlined in Table 18.4.

Costs

The pill, NSAIDs and the mirena are the more economic preparations for long term administration, but counselling as to the anticipated bleeding pattern to include the acceptability or otherwise of amenorrhoea will influence how happy the patient is with a mirena. It is an expensive device (around £100) to fit for a matter of a few weeks.

There are potentially problems with medical treatment in that they do not always reduce bleeding sufficiently, need to be taken long term, are associated with adverse effects.

Non-Medical Treatments

For women who have completed their family, more permanent means of reducing blood loss are attractive. A hysterectomy is successful means of achieving amenorrhoea, but in recent years newer less invasive techniques are gaining popularity.

Local Endometrial Techniques

Endometrial biopsy has already been mentioned in relation to diagnosing pathology, but does not have any therapeutic effect on blood loss. Local pathology such as a polyp or the electrical resection and removal of fibroid(s) which indent the cavity may reduce blood loss, yet preserve fertility.

Endometrial destruction can be achieved by a variety of techniques, such as heat, surgical resection and laser vaporisation. The advantages of such techniques are that they avoid major surgery, often being capable of being performed on an outpatient or day case basis. The uterus is left intact, together with the nerve and blood supply. Amenorrhoea however cannot be guaranteed with any of these techniques, but most women experience at least a reduction in flow. There is a strong regenerative potential within the endometrium, which is more likely in the younger woman and therefore, the closer the woman is to menopausal age, the less likely she is to express dissatisfaction with these local techniques and pursue hysterectomy. Contraception is still required as although the cavity is scarred, islands of endometrium may persist and permit implantation. Progestogen opposition to the oestrogen component is needed when HRT is prescribed.

Hysterectomy

In the early 1990s it was established that 60% of women referred with 'menorrhagia' alone or in combination with other symptoms have hysterectomy within 5 years. By 55 years of age, around 1 in 5 women have had their uterus surgically removed. The vast majority of these women having their uterus removed for benign gynaecological disease. Whereas in the past the menopause gave relief from bleeding, many women take HRT, if only briefly, encouraging a hysterectomy operation in the perimenopausal age group. The operation, which can be conducted laparoscopically, vaginally or abdominally has a high satisfaction rate, around 85% of women went ahead six months after the surgery. If the cervix is retained, then continued cervical smears are necessary. Prophylactic oopherectomy is discussed in the over 40 age group as a potential means of preventing the future development of ovarian cancer.

DYSFUNCTIONAL UTERINE BLEEDING (DUB)

The term DUB is frequently used, but a definition of exactly what is meant is often lacking, it is most helpfully attributed to 'Abnormal bleeding (heavy, prolonged or frequent) after the exclusion pelvic pathology, pregnancy, and medical disease'. It is really a diagnosis of exclusion and often there is confusion between clinicians as to what exactly is meant by this term. On the whole therefore, it is often best to simply describe the symptoms, rather than use this 'shorthand'. Such as a woman complaining of excessively heavy and frequent periods with a normal examination and ultrasound. That way the complaint(s) and potentially associated abnormality on clinical examination are specifically outlined.

Similarly, such terms as 'polymenorrhagia' or 'metropathica haemorrhagica' are seen in textbooks in chapters related to abnormal menstruation. Again there can be confusion as to what precisely is meant by these terms and again therefore, in this author's opinion, it is best to stick to simple descriptive terms of actually what it is the patient is complaining of and what is considered to be an underlying abnormality.

SECONDARY AMENORRHOEA

This is described in detail in Chapter 3 and a summary is given here.

Secondary amenorrhoea is defined as the absence of periods for 6 months in someone who has previously menstruated. The causes of primary amenorrhoea (never having had a period at all) are usually different and not covered in this chapter. There are a variety of causes which are most easily grouped into the controlling mechanisms for menstruation, which are outlined in Table 18.5.

Table 18.5
Potential Causes of Secondary Amenorrhoea

Physiological	Pregnancy Lactation
'Higher' brain centres	Eating disorders Stress Significant illness
Hypothalamus	Tumour Functional
Pituitary	Tumour Surgery Radiotherapy Infarction (Sheehan's syndrome) rare Prolactin producing adenoma
Ovarian	Surgery Radiotherapy Chemotherapy Autoimmune disease Premature ovarian failure 'Resistant' ovarian syndrome Polycystic ovarian syndrome (PCOS)
Uterine pathology	Asherman's (Intra-uterine adhesions) Tuberculosis Chemical inflammation
Endocrine disease	Thyroid over- or under-activity Diabetes mellitus Cushing's disease Addison's disease
Drugs **Drugs which elevate prolactin**	Depo-provera Phenothiazines Haloperidol Cimetidine Reserpine Methyldopa Metoclopramide

Management of Secondary Amenorrhoea

This will obviously depend upon the cause, which may be elucidated by taking a thorough history; to include the past gynaecological history, recent pregnancy or the possibility of this condition. Enquiries should be made about weight changes, eating disorders and stress. Specific enquiries should be made about any drugs they may be taking, the presence of galactorrhoea (milky discharge from the breasts) which may be present in patients with an elevated prolactin or the presence of menopausal symptoms. Examination should look for acne and hirsuitism, the body mass index calculated, and for stigmata of endocrine or generalised disease.

First line investigations may include a pregnancy test, follicle stimulating hormone (FSH) level and prolactin level.

SUGGESTED FURTHER READING

Most larger textbooks have comprehensive chapters on the topic.

A readable and informative short book is "Menstrual problems for the MRCOG" by Lumsden, Norman and Critchley, published by RCOG Press. Editor: Peter Milton.

19

Vaginitis and Pelvic Inflammatory Disease

VAGINITIS

Physiology

The squamous epithelium of the vagina and vulva is thin and undifferentiated in the child and the post-menopausal woman because of the lack of oestrogen. Oestrogens cause a thickening of the epithelium and differentiation into the well recognised, basal, intermediate and superficial cell layers, characteristic of the reproductive years. The percentage of flattened superficial cells with a high nuclear-cytoplasmic ratio indicates the degree of oestrogenic activity. Progesterone causes a decrease of the number of superficial cells, while the intermediate cells increase (Fig. 19.1).

The vaginal epithelial cells contain much glycogen. The formation of glycogen, abundant within the superficial cells, is another oestrogenic effect, thus providing a dense protective epithelium. Glycogen is easily fermented or broken down to produce lactic acid and, therefore, increases the acidity of the vagina, which is toxic to many pathogenic organisms and saprophytes. The healthy vagina of the woman of reproductive age contains lactobacilli and acidogenic corynbacteria. Fungi, which would otherwise grow, are restricted by this acid pH (pH 3.5–4.1). The acidity of the vagina can be changed by other factors: drugs, intercourse and cervical erosions. The columnar cells of the endocervix produce an alkaline cervical mucus, so if there is an excess of these, as in any ectropion or large cervical erosion, then the vaginal pH will rise. Intercourse provokes an increase in the vaginal pH as the vaginal lubricant secreted by the vaginal epithelium increases the pH to 6 or 7 as will the seminal fluid. This pH will persist for hours after intercourse. Frequent intercourse causes the vagina to be alkaline, toxic to the lactobacilli and corynbacteria, but suitable for pathogens.

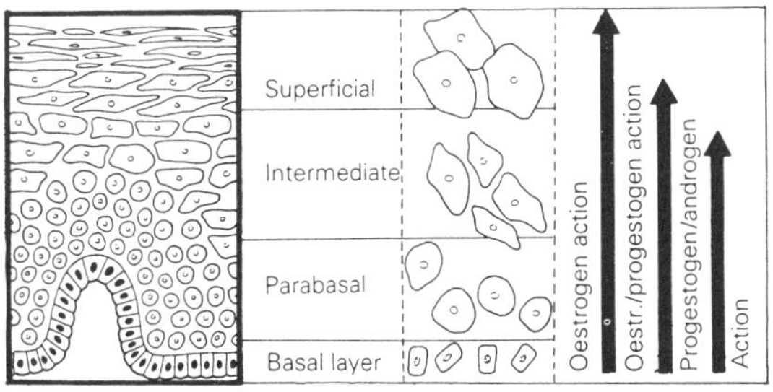

Fig. 19.1 *Vaginal epithelium.*

Descriptions of vaginal infections with *Candida albicans, Trichomonas vaginalis, Neisseria gonorrhoea, Chlamydia trachomatis, Herpes genitalis and bacterial vaginosis* follows.

Vaginitis in children is uncommon. It may be due to trichomonal or other pathogenic organisms acquired by non-sexual contact in the home, or secondary to an intravaginal foreign body.

Candida albicans (C. albicans)

Candida albicans is the most virulent of the *Candida* species of yeast. It possesses hyphae, pseudohyphae and spores, which are recognised easily on a wet preparation slide. The hyphae and buds of the fungus are seen clearly when 10% potassium hydroxide (KOH) solution, which lyses epithelial cells, inflammatory leucocytes and debris, is added to the wet preparation slide. When blastospores predominate, it is a pathogenic and saprophytic infection. *C. albicans* is a low grade opportunitistic organism and is often present in the vagina without causing clinical symptoms or signs. An overgrowth commonly occurs in pregnancy, diabetes, long-term corticosteroid and immunosuppressive therapy as well as treatment with broad spectrum antibiotics. The widespread use of antibiotics and the fashion of nylon knickers, tights and jeans, which produce a warm moist culture medium for *Candida*, has contributed to the recent dramatic rise in the incidence of candidal vaginal infections. Indiscriminate antibiotic treatment of similar infections has also contributed to this increased incidence.

Symptoms and signs

Candidal vaginitis causes vulval and vaginal itch and irritation which varies from woman to woman. There is an intense vulval pruritis, exacerbated at night by moisture causing a thick discharge likened to 'curdled milk'. Sometimes symptoms do not correlate with the signs. Whilst some women with pronounced symptoms may have little to be seen on examination, others have more obvious infection and are not disturbed by their symptoms. Erythema of the labia minora is an unusual presentation. A blood sugar should be performed when glycosuria and a candidal infection is encountered in the young child or post-menopausal woman. Any patient complaining of dysuria should be examined for vaginal discharge.

Diagnosis

A wet preparation is crucial, and as previously mentioned hyphae and spores are identified easily if a drop of 10% KOH is added. A vaginal swab must be taken in determination of the vaginal pH using narrow pH range paper and this can also be taken in the gynaecology clinic. Normal vaginal pH is < 4.5. If the pH is in the range of between 4.0 and 4.5, then *Candida* can be suspected. Candidal infections can occur at all pH values but the majority occur within the normal pH.

Treatment

Polyene anti-fungal drugs such as nystatin are effective. These cause increased permeability of the fungal membrane and leakage of cellular components. They can be applied by cream or pessary. Creams are more effective than pessaries, because the cream is evenly spread across the vaginal membrane, but patient compliance is poor. Imidazole derivatives such as clotrimazole, miconazole and econazole are also effective in the form of a one dose oral pessary, which dissolves after three days. These are not associated with any serious adverse reactions but they are more expensive than topical treatments. Recalcitrant candidal infections do occur which seem resistant to treatment and longer courses of oral treatment and monthly courses of imidazole pessaries may be required. There may also be women with symptoms which are highly suggestive of candidiasis but who probably have an allergy to detergents used in washing powders or soaps, or a rubber allergy in condoms. There may be concurrent infections with other organisms, such as bacterial vaginosis.

Systemic ketaconazole in a single dose is effective in resistant cases where there may be gastrointestinal involvement. It should be used with care, as cases of hepatotoxicity have been described.

The male partner of any woman with a fungal vaginitis requires treatment. Men can carry the fungus and are often symptomless, thereby re-infecting the woman. Treatment is by using antifungal cream applied to the glans penis and prepuce twice daily for 5–7 days.

Trichomonas vaginalis (T. vaginalis)

Trichomonas (T) vaginalis infection is the second most common vaginal infection (Fig. 19.2).

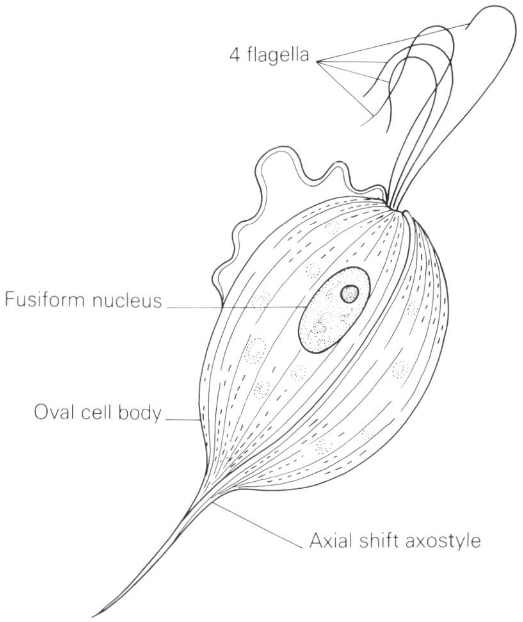

Fig. 19.2 *Trichomonas Vaginalis.*

It is caused by a flagellated protozoan which inhabits female and male paraurethral glands from whence it can autoinfect susceptible vaginae. *T. vaginalis* has been known to survive for up to 25 hours in chlorinated swimming pools, but usually is sexually transferred when an inoculum is transported in the buffered alkaline medium of semen.

Symptoms and signs

Patients complain of a profuse discharge with pruritis, which is less severe than a candidal pruritis. Up to 50% of women will be asymptomatic. *Trichomonas vaginalis* commonly co-exists with bacterial vaginosis because *Trichomonas vaginalis* alters the vaginal flora creating an anaerobic environment. On examination, the vagina will be reddened and inflamed. The discharge is classically described as 'greenish, effervescent and frothy' but this is, in fact, rarely seen. Indeed a frothy vaginal discharge is more likely to be casued by *Gardnerella vaginalis.* This trichomonal discharge is usually a grey-white opaque colour with an occasional bubble with a pH between 5 and 7. *Trichomonas* is rarely found in a discharge with a low pH. Occasionally the classic 'strawberry' appearance of the vagina and cervix is seen.

Diagnosis

T. vaginalis can be easily seen on a wet prep and examined under the microscope. It has a characteristic swirling movement under the microscope where the flagella seem to move independently from the oval body. Colposcopy shows the characteristic Y-shaped blood vessels on the cervix. Some trichomonal infections will also be diagnosed by cervical cytology, although it is not absolute. Trichomonas diagnosed on cervical smears may be confused with inflammatory cells or cell fragments and so the sensitivity of diagnosis is relatively inaccurate.

Treatment

Metronidazole, 200 mg tds for 7 days is the specific treatment for *T. vaginalis.* This organism is sexually transmitted, so the partner must also be treated. The drug is contraindicated in early pregnancy and when breast-feeding. It is also associated with nausea which is aggravated by alcohol.

Genital Herpes

Herpes is caused by herpes simplex virus II (HSV II), although HSV I is increasingly found in vaginal herpes, because of oral sexual habits. Vaginal herpes is often asymptomatic, but primary vulval herpes is a distressing and painful condition.

Symptoms and signs

Primary herpes causes malaise, low grade fever, inguinal lymphadenopathy and thin watery discharge. Single herpetic vesicles appear or coalesce to form clusters, which then ulcerate. The intense pain of primary herpetic urethritis sometimes causes urinary retention. A latent infection follows the primary infection when this virus inhabits the sacral ganglia, but it re-appears periodically causing mild recurrent infection.

Diagnosis

This is difficult, although culture is preferred to high antibody titres which reflect pre-existing latent infection.

Treatment

Oral acyclovir is the preferred treatment of choice. However, this will only ameliorate the condition and will not be a cure. Oral acyclovir may reduce the shedding of virus particles in recurrent episodes, and topical treatment will speed up the healing of vesicles.

Genital Warts

Condylomata acuminata result from infection with human papovavirus (HPV) and are sexually transmitted. They are extremely infectious, infecting 65% of the patients' consorts. Invasive cervical cancers are associated with human papovavirus (HPV) types 16 and 18, while cervical dysplasia which is associated with types 6 and 11 rarely progress to malignancy.

Treatment

The application of 25% podophyllin cream twice weekly has been the traditional treatment, but this can be awkward and causes local ulceration. Treatment with electrocautery, cryocautery or laser coagulation is effective.

Bacterial Vaginosis

Bacterial vaginosis disturbs the normal vaginal flora, and hence, the high vaginal pH. It is now the most common cause of vaginal discharge in the United Kingdom, especially in genito-urinary clinics. Lactobacilli are normally the predominant organism in the vagina and these are reduced and replaced by a number of organisms, including *Gardnerella*, *Mobiluncus*, urea plasma, bacteroides and other anaerobes. Bacterial vaginosis presents with a white/grey fishy smelling discharge. The pH of the vagina ranges between 4.5–7.0. The cause is unknown but it may be related to the rise in vaginal pH following exposure to alkaline semen during unprotected intercourse. There has been confusion about the classification of *Gardnerella*. This gram negative bacillus was previously known as *Haemophilus vaginalis* and may occur in 33% of asymptomatic patients and approximately 98% of patients with non-specific symptomatic vaginitis. Concurrent infection with other organisms, especially *Trichomonas vaginalis* is common. Furthermore episodes of candidal vaginitis may be followed by a bacterial vaginosis in women who have had recurrent bacterial vaginosis as a reflection of active bacilli in the vagina. Patients with bacterial vaginosis should be advised to avoid douching and the use of soaps, bubble baths and gels as these may alter the vaginal pH and also eradicate lactobacilli. Women who have recurrent bacterial vaginosis may benefit from a once-monthly course of metronidizole for 7 days after menstruation.

Symptoms and signs

Bacterial vaginosis causes a thin, watery and opaque vaginal discharge with a disagreeable smell, especially after intercourse. This smell is accentuated when a drop of 10% KOH is added to the wet preparation slide. Clue cells are seen on wet preparation. These are granular vaginal, epithelial cells with an irregular outline which have huge numbers of *G. vaginalis* bacilli attached to the surface. They can be seen on Papanicolaou smears. Over 90% of women with a vaginal discharge and a vaginal pH of 5–7 or greater will have either *T. vaginalis or G. vaginalis* vaginitis. Culture of this organism is difficult, which accounts for the confusion about its pathogenicity.

Treatment

Metronidazole 200 mg 8-hourly for patient and consort for 7 days is effective. Clindamycin vaginal cream (2%) applied in a 5 g dose every night for 7 nights is also effective, but is expensive.

Neisseria gonorrhoeae (*N. gonorrhoea*)

This is a sexually transmitted vaginal infection caused by this gram negative intracellular diplococcus. It may infect the cervix, urethra and rectum and is easily transmitted by direct sexual contact. It is highly infectious as there is a 90% chance of infection from a single exposure. The majority of women are asymptomatic and examination may be normal. However, the endocervix may be infected causing salpingitis or pelvic inflammatory disease. Swabs should be taken from these sites in all cases of suspected gonorrhoea.

Syjmptoms and signs

Some patients, however, may complain of painful vulval oedema several days after sexual transmission, caused by an inflammation of the vulval mucous membranes, inflamed Skene's ducts and congested Bartholin's glands, which are found in the vestibule and fourchette, respectively. Both may form an extremely painful and tender Skene's or Bartholin's abscess. Surgical drainage under general anaesthesia is required and Bartholin's abscesses are traditionally marsupialised. This means excising the skin over the abscess and suturing it back in four segments, so that the abscess cavity is opened up completely. Healing is by granulation and re-epithelialisation. Antibiotic treatment alone encourages a chronic infection.

Diagnosis

Gram stains should be prepared in outpatients. Swabs for culture must be taken from the cervix, urethra and peri-rectal areas, and if possible, around Skene's and Bartholin's glands. These should be plated immediately or kept in Stuart's medium for 24–28 hours. it is important to remember that concurrent infection with other organisms, particularly *C. trachomatis*, *T. vaginalis* and genital warts, is common with gonococcal infection and syphilis must not be forgotten.

Treatment of Neisseria gonorrhoea

Procaine penicillin 2.4 mg i.m. into each buttock is compulsory with 1 g of oral probenicid to delay excretion of penicillin. Oral treatment in the form of ampicillin/amoxycillin 2–3 g plus 1 g of probenicid can also be given. An oral quinolone antibiotic, ciprofloxacin 250 mg, may be given as an alternative. Gonorrhoea diagnosed in a gynaecology clinic should be referred to a genito-urinary clinic. A second endocervical swab should be taken for culture within 24 hours of diagnosis and it is also important that her sexual partner is screened and appropriately treated.

Chlamydia Trachomatis

Chlamydia trachomatis is now the most predominant sexually transmitted disease in the UK. Its prevalence rates vary but according to the population studied, in genito-urinary clinics the incidence is approximately 5–15%, and in young women presenting for termination, the incidence may be up to 8%. It may also occur in up to 12% of women attending their general practitioners for regular smear tests. Women with vaginal *C. trachomatis* infections may have non-specific symptoms, such as vaginal discharge, lower abdominal pain or urinary frequency. The clinical findings are often normal.

Diagnosis

Chlamydia trachomatis is difficult to culture. There are a number of diagnostic tests available but some of these are expensive and not readily available. These include enzyme immunoassay (EIA) or direct immunofluorescence (DFA) performed on a sample from the endocervix. Methods of detection are based on molecular biological techniques, such as polymerase chain reaction (PCR), which was developed to test endocervical swabs. Ligase chain reaction (LCR) has been demonstrated to have a high sensitivity, particularly of urine specimens. Current evidence suggests that the most effective and acceptable method of diagnosing *C. trachomatis* is by a DNA amplification technique on first-void urine specimens. These tests are more sensitive and specific than ELISA techniques.

Treatments

Treatments are with tetracyclines or microlide antibiotics. The standard treatment is doxycycline 100 mg twice daily for 7 days. Compliance may be poor because of gastric irritation and erythromycin may also be used. Treatment with azalide macrolide antibiotics, such as azithromycin in a single 1 g oral dose is known to be effective but is expensive.

Psychological Vaginitis

Some women are more bothered than others with vaginal discharge and vaginitis. Discharge varies in all women. There can be an underlying fear of having something seriously wrong or a suspicion of having an underlying sexually transmitted disease. These patients should be thoroughly investigated and treated with the utmost discretion before making this diagnosis.

PELVIC INFLAMMATORY DISEASE

Introduction

The terminology of pelvic infection is confusing and there is no recent definition suitable to cover all causes. The term 'pelvic inflammatory disease (PID)' is increasingly used and is synonymous with salpingitis and pelvic sepsis. Microbial invasion of the female upper genital tract may result in PID. The acronym ESP (Endometritis–Salpingitis–Peritonitis) is commonly used in the United States. It can be defined as a microbial inflammatory process involving the endocervix, endometrium and tubal epithelium with subsequent inflammation of the parametrium and spill of tubal exudate into the peritoneal cavity. It is usually associated with ascending genital infection in sexually active women of childbearing age. It is a common disease and is often silent. Pelvic inflammatory disease, if left untreated, can result in the possible tragic sequelae of ectopic pregnancy, infertility, chronic pelvic pain, perihepatitis, let alone subsequent remorse and depression in the patient years later.

Epidemiology

The promiscuity of the permissive society provoked a dramatic increase in this condition in the 1960s and 70s. There was a decline in the 1990s attributed to greater awareness and more restrained sexual attitudes.

Aetiology

The causes are listed in Table 19.1.

N. gonorrhoea

N. gonorrhoea remains a major cause of PID throughout the world. It causes a bilateral

Table 19.1
Causes of Pelvic Sepsis

1 PRIMARY PELVIC SEPSIS (Ascending genital infection)	
Exogenous agents	**Iatrogenic**
Sexually transmitted:	
N. gonorrhoea	D & C
C. trachomatis	Termination of pregnancy
Mycoplasma hominis	Hysterosalpingogram
U. urealyticum	Insertion of IUCD
Viruses	Post-operative
Endogenous agents	
Bacteroides	
Peptococcus	
Anaerobic streptococci	
E. coli	
Actinomyces	
2 SECONDARY PELVIC SEPSIS	
Pelvic peritonitis	
Mycobacterium tuberculosis (bloodborne)	

endosalpingitis leading to destruction of ciliated endothelial cells within the fallopian tube. These specialised cells are necessary for sperm and ovum transport. Moderate infection causes pyosalpinx formation and sever infection, tubo-ovarian abscess with formation of adhesions. A resolved pyosalpinx forms a hydrosalpinx causing permanent occlusion of the fimbrial ostia.

Chlamydia trachomatis

Chlamydia trachomatis (C. trachomatis) is another major cause of pelvic infection. The chlamydiae were formerly classified as rickettsia, being very small, immobile, spherical or rodlike parasitic organisms, which resemble bacteria but which, like viruses, cannot reproduce outside the cells of their hosts. They have a complicated life cycle and the infectious particle, the elementary body, is small and metabolically inactive. It has a rigid, hard envelope and is similar, to gram negative organisms. It is taken into the host cell by phagocytosis, re-organising to form, within 12 hours, the reticulate body, which is intracellular and metabolically active. This reticulate body divides repeatedly by binary fusion, so that within 20 hours, the cytoplasm of the host cell contains many reticulate bodies. These eventually re-organise into inclusions — namely the elementary bodies. Latency, or the persistence of the organism in an inapparent infection is characteristic of chlamydial infections. They may prove difficult to isolate or observe in chronic infections and persist in the genital tract as subclinical salpingitis which is re-activated when host resistance is low. They may cause a considerable degree of permanent fallopian tubal endothelial cell destruction despite appearing to be such a mild infection. *C. trachomatis* is difficult to culture, but the recent development of monoclonal anti-chlamydial antibody techniques and DNA amplification techniques and offers a more rapid and reliable diagnosis.

Ureaplasma urealyticum

Mycoplasma was first isolated from a Bartholin's abscess in 1937. A tiny mycoplasma was later described — hence *T. mycoplasma,* now known as *Ureaplasma urealyticum.* This is a very small sexually transmitted organism which is difficult to isolate and is responsible for less than 10% of cases of PID. *C. trachomatis and U. urealuyticum* are both sensitive to tetracyclines. Iatrogenic causes of PID are listed in Table 19.1.

Intrauterine devices

The intrauterine device is not a direct cause of PID, but can facilitate ascending infection by sexually transmitted organisms via the threads. However, recent studies suggest there is a low risk of PID associated with the intrauterine device. This pelvic infection is strongly related to the insertion process and the background risk of sexually transmitted disease. Pelvic infection rarely occurs three weeks after insertion. Therefore the previous opinion that intrauterine contraception should not be offered as a first choice contraceptive to young nulliparous women who are having a stable monogamous relationship is no longer relevant.

Other causes

Severe pelvic infection commonly follows illegal abortion. PID commonly occurs after therapeutic abortion and is related to the high incidence of *C. trachomatis* and bacterial vaginosis amongst those young girls seeking termination. In fact, screening for *C. trachomatis* and bacterial vaginosis has been recommended. This is often impractical so empirical prophylactic treatment is offered to all women having a termination. Postoperative pelvic infection can occur and prophylactic antibiotics are commonly given to hysterectomy patients. Hysterosalpingograms are an unusual cause of pelvic infection, but this procedure can cause a recrudescence of chronic PID. The endogenous agents causing pelvic infection are listed in Table 19.1. These are of low pathogenicity and some may be classified as secondary invaders. PID is known to be polymicrobial and these agents (especially anaerobes) cause a superimposed infection after tissue destruction, initially caused by a sexually transmitted organism. Bacteroides and actinomycetes may be found in tubo-ovarian abscesses. Anaerobic streptococci are a common cause of ascending puerperal pelvic infection. Today, a bloodborne secondary pelvic infection by *Mycobacterium tuberculosis* causing an obliterative endosal-pingitis is rare in the UK, but it is a possible cause of infertility in immigrants.

Diagnosis

The classic criteria for diagnosis are listed in Table 19.2. Unfortunately, these signs and symptoms may be based on unconfirmed observations. The clinical diagnosis may only be correct in 65% of women with laparoscopically verified PID.

The differential diagnosis includes appendicitis, endometriosis, ectopic pregnancy and bleeding or ruptured ovarian cysts. Fever may be present in only 30% of cases of PID. Chlamydial salpingitis is a mild insidious relapsing condition with few signs, so liberal use of these classic criteria are set out in Table 19.3 and liberal use of the laparoscope is recommended, especially where there is any doubt of the diagnosis. All patients with suspected PID, not responding to adequate and appropriate therapy, should be laparos-coped. The liver should be routinely examined at every diagnostic laparoscopy for 'violin-string' adhesions typical of the Curtis-Fitzhugh syndrome. This is a result of chlamydial hepatic and perihepatic infection, which may follow pelvic chlamydial infection.

Table 19.2
Classic Clinical Criteria for Diagnosis of Pelvic Sepsis

1. Lower abnormal pain
2. Purulent endocervical discharge
3. Cervical excitation tenderness
4. Adnexal tenderness
5. Fever
6. Leucocytosis

Treatment

Before commencing treatment, any *in situ* intrauterine contraceptive device (IUCD) should be removed.

Mild pelvic inflammatory disease

Mild pelvic inflammatory disease does not require admission to hospital — patients have localised symptoms, do not feel very ill and can go about their daily activities. Antibiotic therapy for clinically diagnosed PID should be effective against *C. trachomatis*, *N. gonorrhoeae* and the anaerobes characterising bacterial vaginosis. The Royal College of Obstetricians and Gynaecologists (RCOG) study group recommend an oral regimen of oflaxacin 400 mg twice daily plus clindamycin 450 mg four times daily or metronidazole 500 mg orally twice daily,

Table 19.3
Referral Criteria for the Diagnosis of Pelvic Sepsis

1. Abdominal tenderness with or without rebound tenderness	All three necessary for diagnosis
2. Cervical excitation tenderness	
3. Adnexal tenderness	

Plus one or more of the following:

1. Positive endocervical swab showing Gram negative intracellular diplicocci
2. Temperature of 38°C or greater
3. Leucocytosis of 10,000 or greater
4. Purulent material (with WBC present) from peritoneal cavity
5. Pelvic abscess or inflammatory mass demonstrated on ultrasound

all for 14 days. Sexual partners should be traced and treated. The RCOG study group also advise a properly organised local mechanism for this important task of contacting these partners.

Moderate to severe pelvic inflammatory disease

Patients are admitted to hospital for bed rest, as they usually feel unwell, some with pyrexia and all with marked pelvic and lower abdominal pain and tenderness. Laparoscopy is performed where possible and especially if the diagnosis is doubtful, or the pain persists for more than 24 hours. After appropriate tests for *C. trachomatis* and *N. gonorrhoeae*, a standard antibiotic regimen against those organisms most likely to be implicated in PID commenced. The RCOG study group recommends the following treatment — Cefoxitin 2 g intravenously (i.v.) 6-hourly, plus doxycycline 100 mg orally 12-hourly continued for a minimum of 48 hours after the patient demonstrates substantial clinical improvement, followed by doxycycline 100 mg orally twice up to a total of 14 days; or clindamycin 900 mg i.v. 8-hourly, plus gentamycin 2 mg/kg as i.v. or as an intramuscular (i.m.) loading dose, then 1.5 mg/kg 8-hourly, again for a minimum of 48 hours, followed by doxycycline 100 mg orally twice daily or clindamycin 450 mg orally four times daily, all for 14 days. Oral metronidazole 500 mg twice daily for up to 14 days may also be considered. Laparoscopy is not essential, particularly if a large tubo-ovarian abscess is suspected. However, if an ectopic pregnancy or torted ovarian cyst is included in the differential diagnosis, then a laparoscopy should be performed, sooner rather than later! Treatment remains conservative and laparotomy is not advised unless a tubo-ovarian abscess ruptures, or requires draining. Peritoneal lavage and oophorectomy, not hysterectomy, can then be life-saving.

Tubo-ovarian and pelvic abscesses

Large tubo-ovarian abscesses are an unusual event in the UK but relatively common in the US and Africa. Again, treatment is conservative and overlaps with the medical treatment of severe sexually transmitted pelvic sepsis unless (1) clinical signs fail to show response to clinical management within 24 hours; (2) generalised peritonitis persists beyond a 24-hour period, or (3) if there is no reduction in size of pelvic mass within 28 hours.

Pelvic clearance is not recommended and only the adnexal mass is removed. Hysterectomy is not advised, but may be reluctantly considered in severe puerperal infection.

Posterior colpotomy, or piercing the pouch of Douglas through the apex of the posterior vaginal wall to drain a tubo-ovarian abscess, is contentious as it may not resolve all cases. However, it can easily be performed when there is a large fluctuant mass bulging into the posterior vaginal fornix.

Sequelae

It has been estimated that one episode of PID causes a 13% incidence of infertility; two episodes cause a 35% incidence and three episodes a rate of 78%. The exact incidence of ectopic pregnancy following PID is uncertain, but is thought to be high. Reconstructive tubal microsurgery of hydrosalpinges offers a 20% chance of a successful pregnancy, but is less if extensive deciliation has occurred. Microsurgical correction of cornual disease offers approximately a 50% chance of successful pregnancy. There is, however, approximately a 10% risk of subsequent ectopic pregnancy. The degree of residual tubal damage often means that surgical correction is impossible, and that *in vitro* fertilisation offers the only hope of a successful pregnancy. The patient with chronic lower abdominal pain resulting from previous pelvic sepsis is well known to all medical practitioners, and pelvic clearance may not be the panacea. Early diagnosis, prompt treatment and adequate follow-up are necessary to prevent these tragic sequelae.

20

HIV in Obstetrics and Gynaecology

BACKGROUND

HIV Infection: Epidemiology

Throughout the world, over 33.6 million people are estimated to be infected with HIV, of whom 95% live in developing countries. Approximately 46% of infected adults are women, but differences in routes of transmission give rise to substantial regional variation; in sub-Saharan Africa, where heterosexual transmission predominates, women represent over half of all adult infections. In Western Europe and the USA, where transmission is more common among male homosexuals and intravenous drug users (IVDU), around 20% of HIV-infected adults are women. However, the rate of heterosexual transmission is rising in the developed world, and women are likely to represent an increasing proportion of HIV-positive adults in these countries.

HIV Infection: Transmission

HIV is a retrovirus containing reverse transcriptase. This enzyme allows the virus to transcribe its RNA genome into DNA, which then integrates into the host cell's DNA. There are two strains of HIV — types 1 and 2; HIV-2 is less pathogenic than HIV-1 and is relatively rare outside West Africa. As HIV is a highly variable virus, HIV-1 has been further classified into groups M and O; the M group has a number of subtypes, known as clades. HIV infects cells expressing both a chemokine co-receptor (mainly CCR5 or CXCR4) and a CD4 molecule. Such target cells include T-lymphocytes, macrophages and dendritic cells.

Table 20.1
HIV Transmission: Routes of Infection and Risk

Mother-to-child transmission (no intervention)	1:4
Needlstick injury	1:300
Receptive anal intercourse	1:300–1000
Male to female vaginal intercourse	1:500–1000
Female to male vaginal intercourse	1:1000–3000

The different routes of transmission and their associated risk of HIV infection are shown in Table 20.1. Individuals with high levels of circulating free virus (high plasma HIV viral load) are most at risk of transmitting HIV through any route. Genital infections and ulceration increase the risk of both transmitting HIV and acquiring HIV through sexual intercourse.

HIV Infection: Natural History

Seroconversion occurs 2–6 weeks after infection. At this time the plasma viral load is high, and individuals may experience a glandular fever-type illness (acute seroconversion). Seroconversion is followed by a prolonged clinical latency phase; during this time viral replication continues but is controlled by host immune responses. The number of CD4-positive T lymphocytes (CD4 count) gradually falls, resulting in impaired immune function. This ultimately leads to the opportunistic infections and malignancies characteristic of AIDS. During this last phase, the plasma viral load increases and the associated decline in CD4 count accelerates.

HIV Infection: Progression

The rate of disease progression varies between individuals; without treatment, the median time from infection to AIDS is approximately 10 years. However, the recent introduction of highly active antiretroviral therapy (HAART) is dramatically reducing the rate of disease progression and improving survival.

Diagnosis of HIV

The standard means of diagnosing adult HIV infection is by detection of HIV-specific antibodies in the blood, using the enzyme-linked immunosorbant assay (ELISA). A positive ELISA result is then confirmed by Western Blot, whereby selected viral proteins are bound by HIV-specific antibody, which can then be visualised. The HIV antibody test is 99.9% specific and sensitive when performed 12 weeks or more after primary infection. This is because it may take up to 12 weeks for an individual to develop a full antibody response. During this period, individuals may test antibody negative. However, due to the associated high plasma viral load, they are likely to be particularly infectious at this time. Although plasma viral load, determined by polymerase chain reaction (PCR), is generally used for monitoring the progression of HIV infection, it may also be used to diagnose primary HIV infection, within the initial period. PCR is also used in the diagnosis of HIV in infancy (see below).

Management of Women with HIV Infection

Highly active antiretroviral therapy

Patients with HIV are monitored by regular clinical assessments, plasma CD4 counts (reflecting the degree of immunosuppression) and plasma viral load measurements (indicating the rate of viral replication). Indications for treatment of HIV infection depend on these three parameters; treatment should be considered for any patient with a viral load of greater than 30,000 copies/ml and/or a CD4 count less than $350 \times 10^6/l$. Three classes of antire-troviral drug are currently used; nucleoside analogues (NA) and non-nucleoside reverse transcriptase inhibitors (NNRTIs) prevent viral replication by blocking the reverse transcriptase enzyme used by HIV to transcribe RNA into DNA, while protease inhibitors (PIs) block the protease enzyme, resulting in the production of non-infectious virions. The current standard of care is to initiate treatment with at least three antiretroviral drugs. These potent combinations of drugs are often referred to as highly active antiretroviral therapy (HAART). Patients should consider that such therapy will be lifelong. Consistent adherence to HAART minimises the risk of viral resistance, which is the principal cause of treatment failure.

Prophylaxis for opportunistic infections

Pneumocystis cariniii pneumonia (PCP) is the most common opportunistic infection in those with HIV disease. Indications for prophylaxis include severe immunosuppression (determined by clinical assessment and/or CD4 count less than $200 \times 10^6/l$), or a past history of PCP. The first-line regimen is oral co-trimoxazole, 960 mg three times weekly, and alternatives include oral dapsone, 50 mg daily, or inhaled nebulised pentamidine, 300 mg monthly.

OBSTETRICS

Prevalence of HIV in Pregnant Women

The prevalence of HIV infection in pregnant women varies widely within the UK (Table 20.2),

Table 20.2
Prevalence of HIV Infection in Women Giving Birth

Inner London	33.9
Outer London	13.3
Rest of England and Wales	1.4
Scotland	2.3

the highest prevalence being in inner London, where 33.9 women per 10,000 who gave birth in 1998 were HIV positive, the highest annual number ever reported. These data are taken from the unlinked anonymous HIV seroprevalence screening programme, which was set up in 1990 to assess the spread of HIV infection, whether diagnosed or not, in accessible sentinel groups of the adult population. The number of HIV positive pregnant women giving birth is surveyed by infant dried blood spot testing; although the blood sample is taken from the baby, it is actually giving information about the HIV status of the mother, as all babies (whether HIV infected or not) born to HIV positive mothers will test HIV antibody positive because of the presence of maternal antibody. The proportion of HIV positive pregnant women whose infection is diagnosed prior to delivery is estimated by correlating unlinked anonymous data with confidential reports of HIV positive pregnancies made to the Royal College of Obstetricians and Gynaecologists (RCOG). Compared to the USA and other European countries, the UK has been slow to implement a policy of universal antenatal HIV testing, and in 1997 over 70% of maternal HIV infections remained undiagnosed at the time of delivery, despite overwhelming evidence that most cases of mother-to-child transmission of HIV could be prevented. In 1999, new national guidelines were announced, which stated that all pregnant women throughout the UK should be offered and recommended a HIV test as an integral part of their antenatal care, with the national objective of achieving an 80% reduction in mother-to-child transmission of HIV by 2002.

Effect of Pregnancy on HIV

For pregnant women with severe immunosuppression, who are not taking appropriate antiretroviral therapy, there is evidence that pregnancy may accelerate the progression of HIV infection. However, for pregnant women with early HIV infection and those receiving effective HAART, pregnancy does not appear to accelerate HIV progression.

Effect of HIV on Pregnancy

Evidence from developing countries suggests that HIV positive women with severe immunosuppression have an increased risk of adverse pregnancy outcomes, including fetal loss, intrauterine growth retardation, preterm birth and low birth weight. In developed countries maternal HIV infection has been associated with an increased risk of first trimester miscarriage, but for pregnant women with early HIV infection and those receiving effective HAART the course of pregnancy appears to be otherwise unaffected. HIV positive women are not at increased risk of congenital abnormalities.

Preventing Mother-to-Child Transmission of HIV

The risk factors for mother-to-child transmission of HIV are listed in Table 20.3. Although transmission has been reported in the first trimester, infection prior to the third trimester is rare, and the vast majority of transmissions occur during late pregnancy, at delivery and postnatally through breast feeding. The best predictor of mother-to-child transmission is high maternal plasma viral load, with low CD4 count and clinically advanced HIV disease being important related risk factors. Obstetric factors include prolonged membrane rupture, chorioamnionitis and events or procedures involving fetal exposure to maternal blood. Bacterial vaginosis and other cervico-vaginal infections also increase the risk of transmission.

Table 20.3
Risk Factors for Mother-to-Child Transmission of HIV

- Maternal plasma viral load
- Clinically advanced HIV disease
- CD4 count $< 200 \times 10^6$/l
- Breast feeding
- Prolonged rupture of the membranes
- Chorioamnionitis
- Preterm birth
- Bacterial vaginosis
- Vaginal delivery

There are thought to be two mechanisms by which mother-to-child transmission may occur; firstly, as a result of oro-mucosal exposure, through direct contact between the baby and infected blood and secretions within the genital tract. Alternatively, it may occur when microtransfusions of maternal blood enter the fetal circulation as a result of uterine contractions during labour and/or the presence of areas of placental rupture. Although both mechanisms probably play a significant role in vertical transmission, there is increasing evidence to support the relative importance of the former hypothesis. Firstly, the longer the duration of membrane rupture, the greater the risk of vertical transmission. Secondly, at twin deliveries, the first-born twin has twice the risk of HIV infection compared with the second twin if both are delivered vaginally.

Antiretroviral therapy

Antiretroviral therapy reduces mother-to-child transmission both by reducing maternal plasma viral load, and by direct pre-exposure and post-exposure prophylaxis of the fetus and/or neonate. Women who do not require antiretroviral therapy for their own health should receive oral zidovudine monotherapy from the third trimester, intravenously during labour and postnatally to the infant for the first three weeks of life. The evidence for this 'three-part' zidovudine regimen is from a landmark study of HIV positive pregnant women, known as ACTG 076, where in the absence of breast feeding, a three-part zidovudine regimen was associated with a 67% reduction in vertical transmission.

Women who require treatment of their HIV infection should be treated with HAART in a similar way to non-pregnant individuals, and where possible their HAART regimen should include zidovudine, as this is the only antiretroviral drug with proof of efficacy in reducing vertical transmission. There are very limited data on the safety of most antiretroviral drugs in pregnancy, and it is usually possible to defer initiation of HAART until after completion of the first trimester. As well as improving the health of the mother, increasing numbers of observational studies are reporting little or no transmission in pregnant women taking HAART regimens, even where the baby is delivered vaginally.

Caesarean section

Evidence from a European randomised controlled trial and a meta-analysis of 15 prospective studies have demonstrated that elective Caesarean section performed prior to labour and where the membranes are intact reduces the risk of mother-to-child transmission of HIV by at least 50%. In non-breast feeding women receiving 3-part zidovudine prophylaxis who are delivered in this way, the risk of transmission is around 2%.

The technique of 'bloodless' Caesarean section has been proposed to further reduce the risk of transmission. In order to deliver the baby through an almost bloodless field, the wound edges of the lower uterine segment incision are sealed using a disposable staple gun. Although this technique has not been evaluated in a randomised controlled trial, it is biologically plausible that minimising the

Table 20.4

Intervention	*Vertical transmission risk*
None	20–30%
No breast feeding	14–15%
Zidovudine prophylaxis and no breast feeding	5%
Zidovudine prophylaxis, no breast feeding and elective Caesarean section	~ 2%
Highly active antiretroviral therapy +/– elective Caesarean section	< 2%

exposure of the fetus to maternal blood will further reduce mother-to-child transmission.

Postnatal Intervention

A meta-analysis of 5 prospective studies of mother-to-child transmission of HIV in Europe suggests an additional 14% (95% CI 7–22%) risk of transmitting HIV if a mother breast feeds rather than formula feeds. All HIV positive women who have access to safe bottle-feeding should continue to avoid breast-feeding (Table 20.4).

Management of the HIV Positive Pregnant Woman

The principles of managing HIV positive pregnant women are shown in Table 20.5.

Antenatal care

The antenatal care of HIV positive women should involve a midwife, an obstetrician, a HIV physician and a paediatrician. Interventions to reduce the risk of mother-to-child transmission should be discussed, a screen for sexually transmitted infections (STIs) performed on at least one occasion during pregnancy, and a cervical smear taken (if one has not been performed within the last year). A HIV physician should review the patient at regular intervals during the pregnancy, and plasma viral load measurements and CD4 counts should be performed every 4 to 6 weeks.

Intrapartum care

A decision about mode of delivery should be made antenatally, and clear instructions should be written in the case records (see Table 20.5).

Postpartum care

Women delivered by Caesarean section should be monitored for complications in the usual way. All HIV positive women should be given support and advice regarding formula feeding. Mothers taking oral zidovudine prophylaxis should discontinue therapy after the delivery, but those taking HAART should continue their treatment.

Table 20.5
Guidelines for the Management of HIV Positive Women During Pregnancy and Postpartum

Antepartum Avoid: • Cervical cerclage • Chorionic villus sampling • Amniocentesis • Placental biopsy • External cephalic version	Advise: • Zidovudine monotherapy from third trimester or • Highly active antiretroviral therapy, to include zidovudine
Intrapartum Avoid: • Fetal blood sampling • Fetal scalp electrodes • Amniotomy • Episiotomy • Forceps • Ventouse	Advise: • Intravenous zidovudine to start one hour before start of elective Caesarean section or at onset of labour, to continue until cord is clamped • Early cleansing and drying of baby • lective Caesarean section at 38 weeks gestation or • Planned, carefully monitored vaginal delivery
Postpartum Avoid: • Breast-feeding	Advise: • Oral zidovudine to the infant for first 3 weeks of life • Oral co-trimoxazole from 3 weeks to 6 months of age • Follow-up by paediatrician for at least 18 months

Care of the infant

Oral zidovudine should be administered to the infant for the first 3 weeks of life. Co-trimoxazole should be started thereafter until 6 months of age. Avoiding concurrent zidovudine and co-trimoxazole therapy reduces the risk of bone-marrow toxicity, as both these drugs are associated with bone-marrow suppression. Maternal antibodies cross the placenta and are detectable in the vast majority of neonates born to HIV positive mothers. PCR is used to diagnose infant infection, and tests are carried out at birth, then at 3 weeks, 2 months and 6 months of age. In the absence of breast feeding, over 90% of infants testing negative at 3 weeks and 99% testing negative at 6 months of age will be uninfected. The definitive test is the HIV antibody test; a negative result at 18 months confirms that the child is uninfected.

GYNAECOLOGY

Safe Sex

The male latex condom used together with a water-based lubricant throughout sexual intercourse provides very effective protection against sexual transmission of HIV and other STIs, and they should be recommended to all couples where one individual is HIV positive and the other is HIV negative. They should also be recommended to couples where both partners are HIV positive, to prevent an individual acquiring other strains of HIV which may increase the speed of HIV disease progression.

Sexually Transmitted Infections (STIs)

Throughout the world, most women acquire their HIV infection through sexual intercourse and are therefore more likely to be co-infected with other sexually transmitted pathogens. A screen for STIs should be included as part of the initial assessment of women diagnosed HIV positive. All STIs should be treated effectively, and where possible partners should be screened and treated in the usual way. The presentation of uncomplicated STIs is unaffected by HIV infection *per se*. However, HIV-related immunosuppression is associated with recurrent candidiasis, genital warts and severe infectious vulval ulceration, all of which may be resistant to treatment. Syphilis infection is more likely to be associated with unusual serological responses, and treatment failure is more common.

The incidence of pelvic inflammatory disease (PID) is probably no greater in HIV positive women. However, HIV positive women are more commonly found to have lower white cell counts at presentation, and the frequency of tubo-ovarian masses is increased. There is no difference in the microbiology of PID in women with or without HIV infection.

Contraception

The male latex condom is associated with a pregnancy rate of 12% across all age groups, and many couples who do not wish to conceive choose additional methods of contraception. The progestogen-only pill, parenteral progestogen-only contraception (such as Depo-provera) and sterilisation have similar indications and contraindications in HIV negative and positive women. However, the efficacy of the combined oral contraceptive pill is reduced by some antiretroviral drugs, notably certain PIs (ritonavir and nelfinavir) and NNRTIs (nevirapine and efavirenz), which reduce the bioavailablility of synthetic oestrogens as a result of hepatic enzyme induction. Women taking these drugs should be advised to use alternative methods of contraception.

In the past, the intrauterine contraceptive device (IUCD) was considered to be an unacceptable choice of contraception for HIV positive women, principally because of concerns of an increased risk of pelvic infection and increased menstrual flow. However, recent evidence suggests that complications associated with IUCD use are no greater in appropriately selected HIV positive women compared with their HIV negative counterparts. The levonorgestrel intrauterine system (IUS) is becoming a more popular choice of contraception in HIV positive women because of the decreased risk of pelvic infection, high efficacy and reduced menstrual flow.

Cervical intraepithelial neoplasia

There is a strong association between HIV infection and detectable papillomavirus (HPV) infection, and this association increases with progressive immunosuppression. Young HIV positive women have a two-fold increased risk of cervical intraepithelial neoplasia (CIN) and a 1.7-fold increased risk of cervical cancer compared to their HIV negative counterparts. There is also evidence that in HIV positive women, CIN progresses more rapidly and is less responsive to treatment.

For these reasons, HIV positive women with CD4 counts greater than $500 \times 10^6/l$ are recommended to have annual cervical smears with or without colposcopy. CIN 1 abnormalities in HIV positive women should probably be treated because of the increased risk of rapid progression to CIN III. All women, irrespective of HIV infection should have CIN II and III lesions treated by large loop excision of the transformation zone (LLETZ). More frequent follow-up is necessary for HIV positive women, because of their increased risk of recurrent dysplasia.

Menstrual Abnormalities

A high prevalence of menstrual disorders (menorrhagia, oligomenorrhoea and amenorrhoea) and premature menopause has been described in HIV positive women, but controlled studies have failed to demonstrate any clinically significant direct effect of HIV or HIV-related immunosuppression. However, co-existent substance misuse and weight loss associated with advanced HIV disease may cause amenorrhoea.

Menstrual abnormalities in HIV positive women should be managed in a similar way to HIV negative women.

Planning Pregnancy

Life-expectancy for people with HIV infection has improved significantly over recent years and increasingly, couples where one or both individuals are HIV positive are deciding to have children. All HIV positive women should be encouraged to plan their pregnancies, and they should be given the opportunity to discuss their concerns. Antiretroviral medication known to be teratogenic, such as efavirenz, should be avoided in women of childbearing age. Women planning pregnancy who continue to require prophylaxis against opportunistic infections should not discontinue their prophylaxis. Again, maintaining the woman's health must be given priority. Couples discordant for HIV infection require special consideration.

HIV positive woman, HIV negative man

The peri-ovulation phase of the woman's menstrual cycle where conception is most likely should be determined by the use of an ovulation detector kit or temperature chart, and during this time artificial insemination using the partner's sperm may be carried out at home.

HIV negative woman, HIV positive man

For discordant couple where the man is HIV positive, intrauterine insemination using 'washed semen' may be carried out in order to reduce the risk of HIV transmission to the woman.

Infertility

Increasingly, couples where one or both individuals are HIV-positive are requesting investigations and treatment for infertility. Cases should be assessed individually, with the involvement of local ethics committees.

CONCLUSIONS

Highly active antiretroviral therapy has had a great impact on life expectancy for those diagnosed HIV positive, and HIV infection has become a chronic treatable disease, akin to insulin-dependent diabetes. Increasing numbers of HIV positive women are becoming pregnant while taking HAART, and the safety of anti-retroviral drugs in pregnancy is an area of concern that requires continued surveillance. For HIV positive pregnant women in developed countries, antiretroviral therapy, formula feeding and delivery by elective Caesarean section, have reduced the risk of vertical transmission to below 2%. It is now widely believed that in these countries, mother-to-child transmission of HIV can be virtually eradicated. Implementation of the government guidelines, that all pregnant women throughout the UK should be offered and recommended a HIV test as an integral part of their antenatal care, will bring us much closer to this goal.

FURTHER READING

Smith J.R., Low-Beer N., Barron B.A. (in press). *HIV in Obstetrics and Gynaecology.* Oxford, UK: Health Press.

Connor E.M., Sperling R.S., Gelber R. *et al.* (1994). Reduction of maternal-infant transmission of human immunodeficiency virus type 1 with zidovudine treatment. Pediatric AIDS Clinical Trials Group Protocol 076 Study Group. *N. Engl. J. Med.* **331**: 1173–1180.

21

Ectopic Pregnancy

DEFINITION

An ectopic pregnancy is a pregnancy that has occurred *outside* the uterine cavity.

SITES OF ECTOPIC PREGNANCIES

The most common site for an ectopic pregnancy is in the ampullary portion of the tube. This is closely followed by the isthmic portion, interstitual or intramural portion, fimbrial portion, and then lastly, areas outside the fallopian tube such as the ovary or even bowel.

AETIOLOGY

There are several pre-disposing factors that increase the instance of ectopic pregnancy. Not surprisingly, most of these centre around the fallopian tube, although in many cases, the exact aetiology is unknown.

Pelvic Infection

Any history of past pelvic or abdominal infection, such as pelvic inflammatory disease or appendicitis, significantly increases the chance of a pregnancy being ectopic. Most infections in the pelvis will affect the tube is some way. This may be overtly such as peritubular adhesions and even distal tubal blockages, or covertly, particularly in the case of chlamydial infections which affect the microcilia inside the fallopian tube, so that the tubal function and tubal transport is impaired. Whatever the way the tube is damaged, this will significantly increase the chance that the fertilised egg does not pass down the fallopian tube into the uterine cavity where it would normally implant around Day 5, but more likely get "stuck" inside the fallopian tube and start to implant there.

Iatrogenic Tubal Damage

Females who have had previous sterilisation procedures on their fallopian tubes have a very low chance of falling pregnant (ses chapter on sterilisation and its reversal), but if they do fall pregnant, they have a higher proportion of tubal ectopics. This is thought to be because of the impairment of the tubal transport mechanism which does not allow easy passage of the fertilised egg into the uterine cavity.

Any other surgical procedure performed on the fallopian tube ranging from tubal microsurgery to correcting an anatomical problem, through to previous ectopic pregnancies that have been treated conservatively, will also increase the proportion of tubal pregnancies in those that subsequently fall pregnant.

There is an increased incidence among patients who have had a previous termination of pregnancy, irrespective of the gestation or reason for the termination. Indeed the more terminations that the patient has had, the higher the incidence of subsequent ectopic pregnancy. This is likely to be due to either the operative procedure itself and the associated post-operative infection rate, or because patients who have had multiple terminations of pregnancy also have a higher associated risk for sexually transmitted disease and pelvic inflammatory disease.

Other Pre-Disposing Factors

Salpingitis isthmica nodosa (SIN)

This is a disease of the proximal portion of the tube whose aetiology is unknown. It is not thought to be infective. SIN can either cause a total proximal block or, in the case of ectopic pregnancies, an area of fibrosis in the proximal portion which appears to cause an increased incidence of ectopic pregnancies. The reason for this is not known but it is thought to relate to the constriction of this proximal portion due to the fibrosis which may allow the small spermatazoa through to fertilise the egg in the ampulla but not the much larger fertilised egg back into the uterine cavity.

Intrauterine contraceptive devices (IUCDs)

Although the instance of pregnancies in patients with IUCDs is low, the proportion of these pregnancies that happen to be ectopic is higher than in patients who do not have an IUCD. This may be due to the presence of the IUCD in the uterine cavity which would prevent implantation but would not prevent conception taking place in the tube. A past history of IUCD usage is also a risk factor that predisposes to ectopic pregnancy. This is most likely to be due to the associated increased incidence of pelvic infection in users of IUCDs.

Fertility treatment

Any patient who is undergoing fertility treatment ranging from ovulation induction to intrauterine insemination (IUI) or *in vitro* fertilisation (IVF) has an increased incidence of ectopics. The reasons for this range from the hormonal manipulation affecting the tubal function to the associated increased incidence of tubal damage in these patients. It surprises a lot of patients that even with IVF where the embryo is replaced directly into the uterine cavity, that they still have a significant chance of any resulting pregnancy being ectopic. This is due to embryo transmigration, where the embryos that are put back into the uterine cavity, move into a tube due to the contractions of the uterus. Any patient undergoing an IVF cycle should therefore be warned that this does *not* exclude the chance of an ectopic pregnancy.

SYMPTOMS

Many patients who have ectopic pregnancies may initially have no symptoms at all. The only sign that is present in nearly all of these patients is that of a missed or delayed period.

The most common symptoms are: abnormal vaginal bleeding and abdominal pain. If an ectopic has ruptured, then the presentation can be that of an acute abdomen and cardiovascular collapse with hypotension and tachycardia.

DIAGNOSIS

With the advent of sensitive home pregnancy tests which detect the beta subunit of HCG, then most patients know that they are pregnant within one week of a missed period. Any patient presenting with the above signs or symptoms should always have the pregnancy test confirmed by the medical or nursing staff and a transvaginal ultrasound arranged. The only case whether this would not be appropriate would be in the acute presentation of the cardiovascularly shocked patient. If the pregnancy test is positive, then blood should be taken for quantative HCG as well as a transvaginal ultrasound arranged. Because of the higher frequency of the transvaginal probe and the closer proximity of the probe to the affected region, the acuity of these pictures are much better than with the use of a transabdominal probe. A transabdominal probe is also much more affected by obesity and often requires a full bladder to get an adequate picture of the pelvis. Pregnancy testing and ultrasound scanning, are the two most essential tools in the diagnosis of ectopic pregnancy.

There is a golden rule that if the pregnancy test is positive and an intrauterine pregnancy cannot be seen on ultrasound, then the patient has got an ectopic pregnancy until proven otherwise. Although a certain proportion of patients with these two findings may have had a complete miscarriage, or even be in the stages of a very early intrauterine pregnancy, they have to be treated with the utmost caution until an ectopic pregnancy has been disproven. If a patient has a positive pregnancy test and an empty uterus on ultrasound, then they must be admitted to hospital, bloods taken for full blood count and group & save, a large bore intravenous cannula inserted and observed regularly for further signs and symptoms. If the patient has significant signs with abdominal pain, particularly with rebound and/or guarding, then a laparoscopy should be arranged as soon as is safely possible. Laparoscopy is the standard in diagnosing ectopic pregnancy. During laparoscopy, both tubes should be thoroughly inspected as well as the rest of the pelvis if an obvious ectopic is not seen in one of the tubes. Free blood in the pelvis is a worrying sign and even if both tubes appear normal, then a thorough pelvic and even abdominal survey should be undertaken until the ectopic is found or one convincingly excluded. The uterus should not be instrumented until an ectopic has been found just in case it is a very early intrauterine pregnancy which would be adversely affected.

If the patient is relatively asymptomatic, then a laparoscopy does not need to be arranged as an emergency. Indeed, with the growing knowledge that a lot of these ectopic pregnancies will be tubal abortions and not proceed to rupture, then sometimes a more conservative approach can be adopted. If the patient is asymptomatic, then a further quantative beta HCG is arranged two days after the first and a further transvaginal scan performed. The beta HCG level would normally double within two days if it is a healthy intrauterine pregnancy but the rate of increase is often lower with an ectopic pregnancy. With the levels of beta HCG greater than 2000 iu/l, one would normally expect to see an intrauterine pregnancy.

TREATMENT

The treatment of ectopic pregnancies can be sub-divided into expectant management, medical treatment and surgical treatment.

Expectant Management

As previously noted, a significant portion of these ectopic pregnancies in the fallopian tube will not result in continuing growth and rupture, but indeed become tubal abortions. Expectant management should only be performed on the patients who are cardiovascularly stable, asymptomatic and where there is rapid access to surgical facilities as well as laboratory facilities where the results of the quantative beta HCG are received the same day. If the patients remains asymptomatic, then they can generally be released from hospital when there has been a significant reduction in the levels of beta HCG. Even when the levels are falling, there is still a very small chance that the ectopic can rupture and the patient should be advised of this and advised to return to hospital if they get any sudden onset of pain.

Medical

Although many agents have been used to treat ectopics medically, the one that has got the most data regarding efficacy and safety is methotrexate. This is normally given as either a single dose of 50 mg/m^2 intramuscularly, or some clinicians repeat this two days later. This is normally used for ectopics that are asymptomatic but the HCG is still rising, albeit slowly. Some authorities believe that the cases where methotrexate has its best effects are ones that were tubal abortions and would have resolved themselves in any case.

Surgical

Until ten years ago, the vast majority of surgery for ectopics was by open procedures at laparotomy. The ectopic was diagnosed laparoscopically but for therapeutic purposes the patients then had a laparotomy, normally through a pfannensteil incision, and the tube removed. If the ectopic has not ruptured, then the tube can be treated in a conservative fashion with a linear salpingostomy performed. This is a linear incision normally performed with needle point diathermy on the border opposite the mesentery of the fallopian tube. The incision is made over the area of greatest distention where the ectopic has implanted. The ectopic is then shelled out, any bleeding areas coagulated with the diathermy, the pelvis thoroughly washed out and the abdomen closed in the usual way.

A conservative approach to an ectopic pregnancy is normally performed if the tube is otherwise relatively healthy and this is the first ectopic in that tube. If the tube is diseased in other portions of it, or, this was an ectopic pregnancy resulting from an IVF pregnancy, then most authorities would advocate salpingectomy as opposed to salpingostomy.

Laparoscopic Techniques

Over the last ten years, surgeons have tried to treat ectopic pregnancies in a less invasive surgical form. These are centred around laparoscopic or keyhole surgical techniques. The three main treatment options with the laparoscopic techniques are direct injection with a chemotherapeutic agent, salpingectomy and linear salpingotomy.

Direct injection

Several agents have been used ranging from potasium chloride, 50% dextrose and methotrexate. Again, the most successful one of these has been methotrexate in a dose of 50 mg in 2 ml injected directly into the area of the gestational sac. Side-effects are minimal and resolution rates excellent. There are cases though where you get persistent trophoblastic tissue which will either necessitate removal by further surgical techniques or systemic methotrexate which has more side-effects.

Salpingectomy

A salpingectomy can be performed laparoscopically either using special 'lassoo' type sutures if it is in the ampullary portion or, the tube can be removed with bipolar diathermy along the mesenteric border and then cut away after coagulation has been performed. The tube containing the ectopic can either be removed piecemeal or placed in a specially designed bag inserted down one of the secondary trocars and taken out complete. This latter method is preferred as it reduces the risk of seeding of the trophoblastic tissue around the pelvis or at the incisional site.

After all conservatively or medically treated ectopics, then the patient should be followed up with quantative beta HCG. As long as the patient remains asymptomatic, the first one of these should be within 7 to 10 days after the operative procedure and should generally reduce down to below 50. If it is still above 50, then a repeat sample several days later should show the continuing trend. If the trend is increasing, then the likelihood of persistent trophoblastic tissue is high and further treatment will be required. As previously noted, this can either be systemic methotrexate or by further surgical procedure, depending on the initial technique used.

SUMMARY

Ectopic pregnancies are common and still result in fatalities every year in the United Kingdom. With increasing awareness amongst the general population and more sophisticated diagnostic tests, both the mortality and morbidity should continue to decrease. More conservative approaches to ectopic pregnancies are now being used, but they do require a high level of skill and more specialised facilities. If surgery is required, then the more minimally invasive techniques are preferential as they allow for a speedy recovery to return.

Note: Every female patient, of reproductive age, attending casualty should have a pregnancy test performed. If it is positive, then an ectopic pregnancy should be suspected until it is ruled out by further investigation.

FURTHER READING

RCOG Guidelines on Ectopic Pregnancy (1999).

Margara and Trew (1997). Ectopic pregnancy, In *Gynaecology*, 2nd edn. Churchill Livingstone.

22

Benign Disorders of the Uterus

UTERINE FIBROIDS

Fibroids or leiomyomata are the most common tumours not only of the female genital tract, but also in the human body. Approximately 20% of all women are thought to have them and the majority are silent and symptomless. They can be single or multiple, varying from the size of a pea to that of a football. The aetiology of these benign smooth muscle tumours is unknown but oestrogen is thought to play some part. They are more common in black women, and also in nulliparous women. Symptoms are caused by increasing size and often occur around 30 years of age. They regress after the menopause and, like the uterus, undergo atrophy.

Classification

This is shown in Fig. 22.1. Fibroids are divided into three groups — subserous, when they project from the peritoneal surface of the uterus; mural, when they are within the wall of the uterus; and submucous, when they project into the uterine cavity. They can develop long stalks and occasionally pedunculated submucous fibroids may be seen protruding through the cervix and even the introitus. Fibroids are characteristically firm but may be soft due to hyaline or cystic degeneration, or rock hard due to calcification. When cut across, fibroids are seen to be contained in a false capsule of compressed uterine muscle and are thus easily enucleated. Red degeneration or infarction especially of pedunculated fibroids commonly occurs in pregnancy. Fibroids rarely become infected and sarcomatous change is unusual (< 1%).

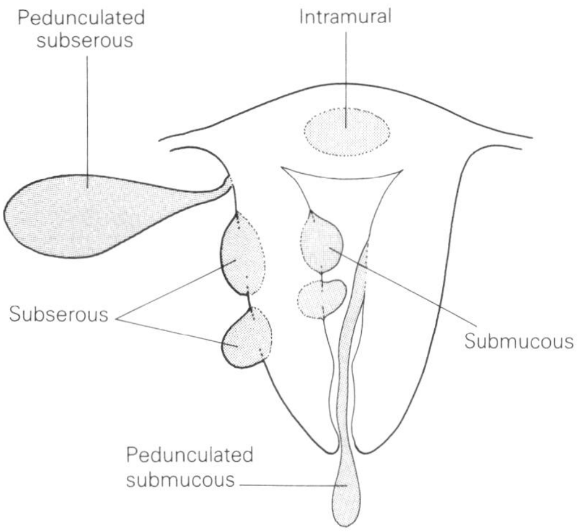

Fig. 22.1 *Types of uterine fibroids.*

Clinical

Fibroids are often silent and symptomless even when they grow to a considerable size. They are discovered at vaginal or abdominal examination or the patient may notice a gradual increase in girth. Symptoms produced by fibroids are summarised in Table 22.1. Pressure effects on surrounding organs, such as constipation, is unusual, but the retroverted impacted fibroid uterus may cause acute urinary retention or occasionally urinary frequency. The increased size and vascularity of the uterus may cause menorrhagia, especially if these are submucous fibroids protruding through the cervix, presenting as intermenstrual or postcoital bleeding which may be heavy. Fibroids do not cause infertility, rather prolonged infertility is associated with the development of fibroids. Submucous cornual fibroids may occlude the proximal part of the fallopian tubes, but this

Table 22.1
Symptoms of Fibroids

Pressure effects	Urinary frequency Retention of urine Backache Constipation
Bleeding	Menorrhagia (enlarged uterine cavity) Intermenstrual Postcoital (pedunculated submucous fibroid)
Pain	Mild (hyaline degeneration) Moderate (red degeneration in pregnancy) Severe (torsion of pedunculated subserous)

is rarely encountered and should be confirmed either by hysterosalpingogram or hysteroscopy. Fibroids cause low backache, especially if large and the uterus is retroverted. Torsion of pedunculated fibroids is rare and causes acute pain.

Fibroids feel firm, smooth and rounded and the uterus is distorted. The differential diagnosis is from ovarian tumours. It is difficult to distinguish between a subserous fibroid and an ovarian or other tumour mass by only abdominal palpation and bimanual vaginal examination. The advent of skilled diagnostic ultrasonography and measurement of the ovarian tumour marker CA 125 precludes the need to proceed to a blind laparotomy. Transvaginal ultrasound also measures endometrial thickness and distinguishes endometrial polyps from small submucosal fibroids. However, hysteroscopy is the most accurate method of diagnosing submucosal fibroids, particularly when associated with heavy bleeding and another diagnosis could be endometrial carcinoma. These techniques have greatly reduced the need for hysterectomy and myomectomy in recent years.

Medical Treatment

Fibroids tend to grow during pregnancy and regress after the menopause. Thus, it has always been assumed that oestrogen withdrawal in some form or another may be an effective treatment. The anti-oestrogen danazol induces an artificial menopause and some shrinkage of the fibroids but the androgenic side-effects of acne and weight increase makes it unpopular. Partial agonists of gonadotrophin (LHRH), such as goserelin, shrink fibroids by 40–50% during treatment, but prolonged use increases the risk of developing osteoporosis. This, in turn requires the occasional addition of a small amount of prophylactic "addback" oestrogen. It is also an expensive drug. Some surgeons prescribe LHRH agonists pre-operatively for 3 months before attempting hysterscopic resection of submucosal fibroids or to shrink large fibroids enough to attempt a vaginal hysterectomy. Abdominal myomectomy, was initially thought to be easier after a brief course of LHRH agonist but enuclation of mural fibroids at operation, paradoxically, can often be more bloody and difficult.

Leiomyomata contain both oestrogen and progesterone receptors, and as in the endometrium, the amount of progesterone receptors is oestrogen-dependent. Therefore progesterone too can influence fibroid size. This has therapeutic implications when considering oral contraception or hormone replacement therapy in women with fibroids. Oestrogens tend to 'feed' and maintain leiomyomata. This may also account for why progestogens are partially successful in controlling heavy abnormal vaginal bleeding in the presence of fibroids.

Fibroids generally do not cause pain so this symptom presenting as a new complaint in a patient with known fibroids requires further investigations to exclude other causes. These include ovarian carcinoma in the post-menopausal woman, endometriosis, pelvic inflammatory disease, adenomyosis and torsion of an ovarian cyst in the younger woman. Once fibroid pain is suspected, it may be caused by 'red degeneration', which can be relieved by a non-steroidal anti-inflammatory drug (NSAID) such as mefenamic acid. Infarction commonly occurs in pregnancy and NSAIDs are very effective in relieving this excruciating pain.

Surgical Treatment

Today the indications and indeed the need for major surgery to treat fibroids is reduced. Patients are better informed about the advantages and disadvantages of particular operations. Moreover, they are increasingly reluctant to undergo abdominal hysterectomy as the definitive treatment, as young women wish to conserve their uterae. Gynaecologists too, are reluctant to perform a myomectomy as it is technically difficult and often bloody. Small silent fibroid uterae are best left undisturbed. The patient should be seen regularly, to detect any possible increase in size. Serial ultrasound and diagnostic hysteroscopy should be performed. Exocervical fibroid polyps can be avulsed or twisted off. Hysteroscopic resection of small submucosal fibroids is an accepted form of treatment by an experienced minimal access surgeon. Endoscopic techniques to remove large subserous fibroids can be difficult. The old axiom 'Never touch or attempt to remove a fibroid in a pregnant uterus' remains true today. Blood loss can be massive and potentially life-threatening.

However, abdominal hysterectomy is the treatment of choice for the very large fibroid uterus. This can often be removed by intraoperative myomectomy with the help of a myomectomy metal screw which also serves as upward traction on the uterus. A cervical fibroid should be carefully removed through a vertical incision just above the fibroid. Care should be taken when removing a broad ligament fibroid because of proximity of the uterine vessels and ureters and the potential distortion of the normal anatomy. The use of the myomectomy screw, again, is helpful. It is often difficult to conserve the ovaries when removing a massive fibroid uterus, so patients should be advised and warned at the pre-operative consultation. It is no longer considered necessary to remove the cervix at every hysterectomy. A subtotal hysterectomy may therefore be considered for the very large fibroid uterus or if there is substantial preoperative haemorrhage.

Vaginal hysterectomy may be performed if there is sufficient utero vaginal descent and the uterus is not larger than a 12-week size pregnant uterus. This depends on the experience of the surgeon. More parametrial clamps and ties are necessary and it is often difficult to remove the fundus of the uterus. Vertical splitting of the uterus into two halves can help extraction. Furthermore, concurrent bilateral oophorectomy is difficult and is associated with haemorrhage. Morcellation or piecemeal removal of the uterus is daunting and fraught with difficulty — so is best avoided. Laparoscopic assisted vaginal hysterectomy (LAVH) for the small fibroid uterus can be considered by an experienced surgeon.

ADENOMYOSIS

This is an enigmatic benign condition, often clinically unsuspected by gynaecologists, as it is a histological diagnosis following post-hysterectomy examination of the uterus. It occurs when foci of active endometrium penetrate the myometrium. Eighteen per cent of hysterectomy specimens have adenomyosis. It is said to be self-limiting and does not affect fertility. It should be considered in the differential diagnosis of secondary spasmodic dysmenorrhoea in women with associated heavy periods. This means pain occurring with the onset of menstruation in a mature woman who previously had never experienced such a pain with her periods. This must be distinguished from congestive dysmenorrhoea, which means pelvic pain occurring just before the onset of menstruation. The uterus feels tender, mobile and slightly enlarged on gentle bimanual vaginal examination with no other adnexal mass or cervical excitation tenderness. Endometriosis and pelvic inflammatory disease should be considered and excluded by laparoscopy and other tests. However, if normal and there are no fibroids and there is a thickened myometrium relative to the endometrium (greater than 10 mm), as the sole finding on ultrasound, then adenomysis should be suspected.

Treatment

Non-steroidal anti-inflammatory drugs such as mefenamic acid may be ineffective. A trial of the intrauterine coil coated with the progesterone, levonorgestrel can alleviate both the spasmodic dysmenorrhoea and heavy periods. Patients must be warned that this device takes up to 3 months or more to be effective. Endometrial resection is contraindicated in the presence of menstrual pain. However, endometrial thermal ablation is not, and therefore, should be considered. A hysterectomy may be performed as a last resort if the above treatments fail.

Histology

Adenomyosis, unfortunately, is diagnosed after microscopic examination of the removed uterus. The endometrial stroma together with evidence of chronic haemorrhage, such as haemosiderin, is seen to lie within the myometrium. Endometrial glands may or may not be seen. There is usually continuity between the glandular tissue of adenomyosis and the endometrium of the uterine cavity.

ENDOMETRIAL POLYPS

These polyps usually, are benign and are the main cause of inter-menstrual bleeding. Hysteroscopy, particularly in women over 40 years, is mandatory to exclude the possibility of endometrial carcinoma. Hysteroscopy has revealed that endometrial polyps are more common than previously realised. An endometrial biopsy must be performed, and the polyps removed using hysteroscopic techniques.

23

Endometriosis

Endometriosis is a benign gynaecological condition in which endometrial glands and stroma are found invading tissue outside the endometrial cavity. The most common sites are the pelvic peritoneum and the ovary, but it may also be found in the recto-vaginal septum and on the bowel. Finally, it may also be found, rarely, in distant sites, e.g. the umbilicus, the lung and the eye.

The symptoms are characteristically dysmenorrhoea, pelvic pain and deep dyspareunia and it is these symptoms which may be manifestations of other pelvic conditions which make the diagnosis and management of patients with endometriosis complex.

DEFINITION

There is difficulty in defining exactly what constitutes the disease endometriosis. Recently it is agreed that occasional spots of endometrium, which temporarily are present on the pelvic peritoneum, do not constitute an abnormality and are better referred to as ectopic endometrial deposits. It is not believed that these isolated infrequent lesions are symptomatic. Endometriosis as an entity is characterised by invasive lesions which distort both the peritoneal surface and the underlying tissue, thereby giving rise to the symptom complex.

An endometrioma is a blood-filled cystic lesion of the ovary. This lesion contains old menstrual blood which is derived from endometrial deposits on the surface of the ovary.

Lesions that occur in the recto-vaginal septum are usually a mixture of muscle and endometrial deposits and are probably derived from Müllerian remnants and generally have an appearance which is more reminiscent of adenomyosis.

INCIDENCE

The precise incidence of endometriosis in the population is unknown. It is probable that around 10% of women have some degree of endometriosis, but some 20% have ectopic endometrium. However, recent studies have suggested that minor endometrial deposits may be seen in as many as 80% of laparoscopies for sterilisation or other unrelated reasons other than pelvic pain, so the phenomenon of ectopic endometrium is probably extremely common. The progression, however, to invasive endometriosis is much less frequent.

PATHOGENESIS

There are two main theories proposed to explain the occurrence of pelvic endometriosis.

Retrograde Menstruation Theory

It seems that almost all women retrogradely menstruate at the time of their period to some extent and this menstrual fluid, which flows down the fallopian tube, pools in the Pouch of Douglas. It contains menstrual blood, including endometrial cells, and a local immune mechanism normally eradicates these cells. A failure of this immune mechanism to work efficiently will leave endometrial cells attached to the peritoneal surface and they produce vascular epidermal growth factor (VEGF) which stimulates local neovascular growth, thereby sustaining the endometrial deposit, which then multiplies and sheds its endometrial lining cyclically, as does the endometrium within the endometrial cavity of the uterus. These endometrial deposits invade below the surface of the peritoneum in tissue planes that involve peritoneal nerves, and it is this mechanism that causes the pain associated with endometriosis. Endometrial deposits which attach to the ovarian surface seem to become involuted by the capsule of the ovary and begin to produce menstrual blood within the inclusion cyst which then grows monthly with increasing menstrual supply to form the endometrioma.

The Metaplasia Theory

In this hypothesis, endometriosis is supposed to result from metaplastic changes in the peritoneum of the pelvis under stimulation from undetermined stimuli (but dependant on the presence of oestrogen), and the resulting metaplasia gives rise to endometrial cells which then invade as described above.

Recto-vaginal endometriosis almost certainly is derived from Müllerian remnants that undergo hyperplasia over time with resultant myometrial cell and endometrial cell growth. These deposits lie within the recto-vaginal septum and cause cyclical pain as the endometrial cells shed their menstrual loss into the myometrial deposit.

Distant sites of endometriosis, such as lung etc. may arise by local metaplasia or as a result of haematogenous or lymphatic spread of endometrial cells which, on reaching a particular target, implant and cause symptoms.

SYMPTOMS AND SIGNS

Endometriosis of the pelvis produces three characteristic symptoms — dysmenorrhoea, deep dyspareunia and pain on defaecation.

The dysmenorrhoea usually begins from the onset of menstruation and most patients report that they have had painful periods throughout their life. This dysmenorrhoea in the teenage years is usually primary in nature, i.e. begins with the onset of menstruation. However, as the years progress they develop secondary dysmenorrhoea with pain beginning some three or four days prior to the onset of menstruation and extending into the early part of menstruation, but eventually the pain being relieved as menstruation proceeds.

Dyspareunia is usually deep and occurs when the deposits in the Pouch of Douglas distort the anatomy, including the utero-sacral ligaments and then during the act of intercourse, movement of the cervix results in severe pelvic pain as the utero-sacral ligaments are stretched and the peritoneum stimulated. Recto-vaginal disease causes severe pain during penetration which may lead to apareunia. The presence of endometriomas without disease in the Pouch of Douglas may be painless and the presenting symptoms may be related to ovarian enlargement. Superficial dyspareunia may (secondarily) occur due to fear and anticipation of deep dyspareunia.

Progressive endometriosis leads to adhesion formation between the bowel and the uterus, cervix and vagina posteriorly, and in these circumstances, defaecation may become extremely painful. If the endometriosis invades through the bowel wall, the patient may declare the symptoms of cyclical rectal bleeding.

Some patients will give a history of pre-menstrual and post-menstrual spotting, although the exact mechanism by which this occurs remains unknown. The presence of endometriomas may cause midcycle pain, although periovarian scarring will also cause pain in mid-month, as ovulation leads to ovarian enlargement and this may again stretch the peritoneum causing midcycle pain. Following ovulation, the ovarian volume decreases and the symptom disappears.

Finally, as the disease progresses and the architecture of the pelvis becomes distorted, infertility may be a presenting symptom. However, mild and minimal disease are not thought to contribute to infertility.

Examination of the patient may reveal tender nodules in the Pouch of Douglas or utero-sacral ligaments and/or adnexal swellings due to endometriomas. In severe disease the uterus may be tender and fixed, often in retroversion, due to pelvic adhesions. However, it is important to realise that clinical examination may reveal no signs whatsoever in patients who can have considerable disease.

DIFFERENTIAL DIAGNOSIS

The differential diagnosis for chronic pelvic pain includes irritable bowel syndrome, chronic pelvic inflammatory disease, benign or malignant ovarian cysts and chronic urinary tract infections. The most common diagnostic dilemma is irritable bowel syndrome. The nerve supply to the sigmoid colon and rectum are shared with the uterus and ovaries and therefore differentiation between the symptoms caused by these adjacent structures is difficult for the woman to differentiate.

INVESTIGATION

Patients with a history suggestive of endometriosis need to have a laparoscopy as this is currently the only definitive way of making the diagnosis. Imaging the pelvis with ultrasound may help to distinguish cystic structures in the ovary which may have an appearance consistent with endometriomas, as opposed to benign fluid-filled ovarian cysts. However, definitive laparoscopy will be required.

The appearances of peritoneal endometriosis range from red, flared lesions to clear, to yellow, to brown, to black, as the lesions undergo a series of changes which result in the deposits of haemosiderin and these deposits result in changes of colour. The most active form of endometriosis is a red lesion with altered peritoneal vasculature surrounding it. The peritoneum may be distorted and false pockets called lacuna may form. The utero-sacral ligaments are a favourite site for deposits, which invade and cause nodular swelling of the ligament itself (Fig. 23.1). The ovary, if it contains an endometrioma, is enlarged and the cystic structure, if aspirated, will reveal couplet-like material, hence the term chocolate cyst of the ovary (Fig. 23.2). In more severe disease, the ovaries tend to become adherent to the peritoneum of the lateral pelvic side wall or to the utero-sacral ligaments and if both ovaries are involved in this process, the Pouch of Douglas becomes completely obliterated to view. Adhesions thereafter may involve the rectum and sigmoid colon and in the most severe disease, small bowel may become adherent to the pelvic organs. Endometriosis between the anterior uterine wall and the bladder is less common but may occur, and occasionally, lesions may be seen invading through the bladder wall. These circumstances may give rise to cyclical haematuria and the diagnosis is made on cystoscopy. Patients who present a symptom of cyclical rectal bleeding should have a sigmoidoscopy or colonoscopy

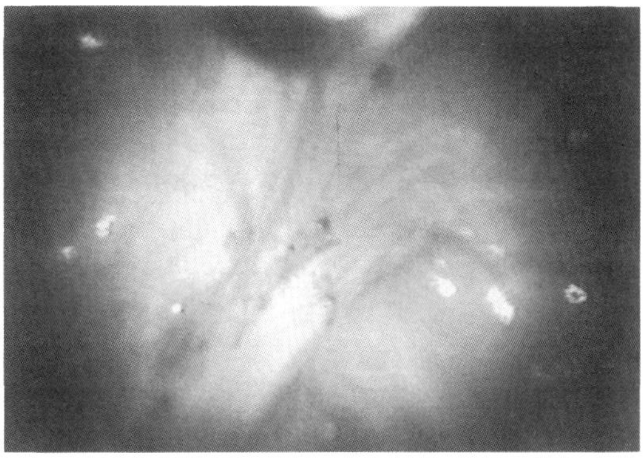

Fig. 23.1 *Peritoneal endometriosis.*

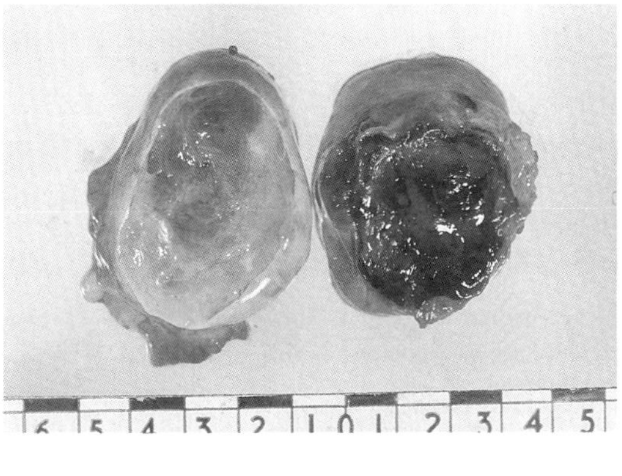

Fig. 23.2 *Endometrioma in an ovary.*

THE AMERICAN FERTILITY SOCIETY
REVISED CLASSIFICATION OF ENDOMETRIOSIS

Surname:..

First name:..

Date of birth:..

Hospital number:..

Date: .... Laparoscopy / Laparotomy

Stage I	(Minimal)	1 - 5
Stage II	(Mild)	6 - 15
Stage III	(Moderate)	16 - 40
Stage IV	(Severe)	>40

Total: ....

PERITONEUM	**Endometriosis**	**<1 cm**	**1 - 3 cm**	**>3 cm**
	Superficial	1	2	4
	Deep	2	4	6
OVARY	R Superficial	1	2	4
	Deep	4	16	20
	L Superficial	1	2	4
	Deep	4	16	20
	POSTERIOR CULDESAC OBLITERATION	**Partial** 4	**Complete** 40	
OVARY	**Adhesions**	**<1/3 enclosure**	**1/3 - 2/3 enclosure**	**>2/3 enclosure**
	R Filmy	1	2	4
	Dense	4	8	16
	L Filmy	1	2	4
	Dense	4	8	16
TUBE	R Filmy	1	2	4
	Dense	4*	8*	16
	L Filmy	1	2	4
	Dense	4*	8*	16

*If the fimbriated end of the fallopian tube is completely enclosed, change the point assignment to 16.

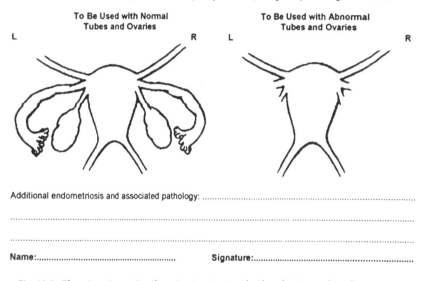

To Be Used with Normal Tubes and Ovaries

L R

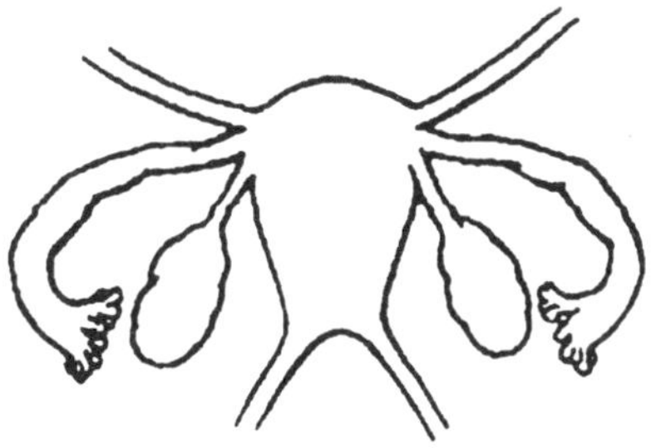

To Be Used with Abnormal Tubes and Ovaries

L R

Additional endometriosis and associated pathology: ....

....

....

Name:.. **Signature:**..

Fig. 23.3 *The American Fertility Society Revised Classification of Endometriosis.*

in order to establish whether or not lesions have perforated through the bowel wall. These investigations are best done when the patient is menstruating as bleeding points are clearly visible at this time. At other times, it is easy to miss the lesion and a false negative examination reported.

All patients who have a diagnostic laparoscopy in whom endometriosis is diagnosed should have their degree of severity of disease

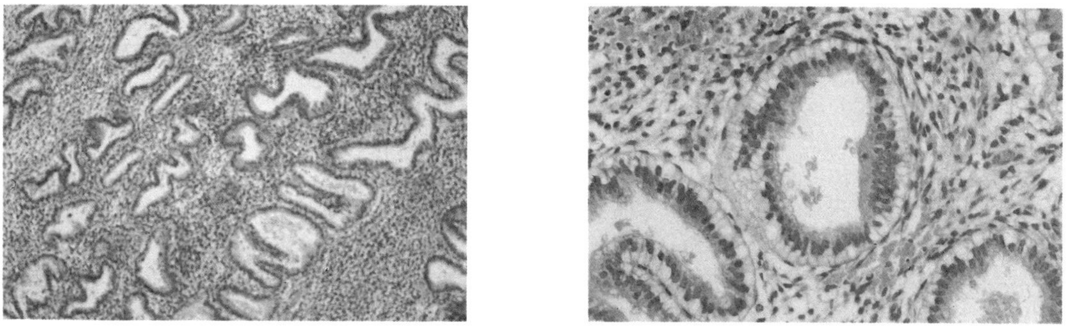

(a) (b)

Fig. 23.4 *Early secretory endometrium with subnuclear vacuolisation evident at high magnification. Stroma and glandular epithelium are readily apparent.*

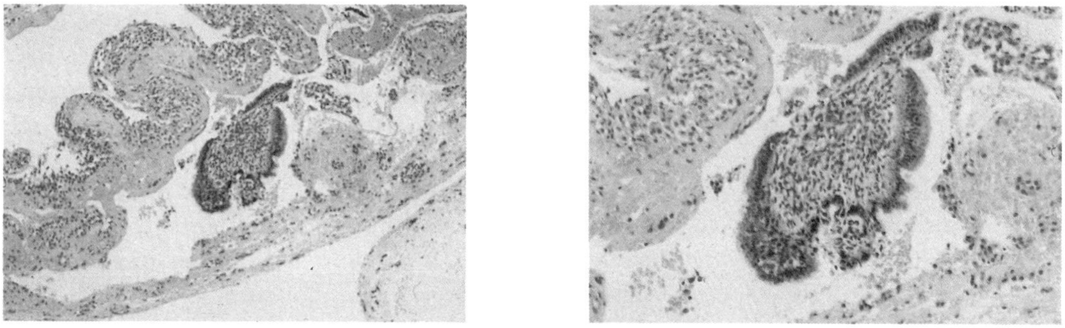

(a) (b)

Fig. 23.5 *Peritoneal endometriosis with surrounding reactive mesothelial hyperplasia. Stroma and glandular epithelium are demonstrated.*

recorded on the American Fertility Society scoring system chart (Fig. 23.3).

HISTOLOGY

Biopsy specimens from either peritoneal lesions or from endometriomas reveal characteristic histological findings of glands and stroma in the biopsy. These histological findings are similar to the architecture seen from an endometrial biopsy (Figs. 23.4 and 23.5).

TREATMENT

The treatment of a patient with endometriosis depends on a number of factors. Firstly, fertility may be an issue, either because the presenting symptom may be infertility, or secondly, the patient may be young and for whom fertility has not yet become an issue. Here, conservative management is essential in order to keep the options of fertility open. Secondly, the extent of the disease. Thirdly, the age of the patient. Fourthly, the wishes of the patient, and lastly, the involvement of other organs, in particular the bowel and renal tract and subsequent damage that may occur to them.

Treatment strategy may involve surgical approach, a medical approach or both.

Surgical Treatment

Patients with endometriomas require these to be removed. Medical treatment has no impact at all on endometriomas, and without surgical excision, the symptom complex will persist. Endometriomas of the ovary should be removed laparoscopically if safely possible and only in extremely large endometriomas, in excess of 10 cm in diameter, should an open approach be taken for this particular lesion. The cyst should be drained and then excised using either laser or cutting diathermy and any residual cyst wall ablated using the laser. Patients in whom fertility is an issue and in whom peritubal adhesions have developed, may have these divided at the same time to improve their prospects of fertility. All residual endometriosis on the peritoneum should be either lasered or diathermied in order to destroy the deposits.

The problem with the conservative approach is the risk of recurrence and all patients who have this type of conservative surgery and who need to conserve their fertility should consider maintenance therapy (see later).

In patients in whom recurrent surgery has failed, or in whom fertility is not an issue, hysterectomy and bilateral salpingo-oophorectomy is a curative procedure which tends to be reserved for women in their forties, for whom no other option exists. Subsequent oestrogen replacement therapy is required in pre-menopausal women.

Recto-vaginal endometriosis needs wide excision if it is to be successfully treated. This may be done with radical laparoscopic surgery or by open laparotomy and surgical excision, depending on the experience of the operator. It is imperative that in all surgical procedures, as much endometriosis as can be seen, must be ablated or removed to ensure that the prospects of long-term symptom relief are optimised.

Medical Treatment

A number of medical therapies are available for the management of endometriosis, but it is important to realise that none of them are anything other than palliative, and in some 70% of patients who receive medical treatment, recurrence will occur at some stage in the future. There are three mainstays of medical therapy.

GNRH agonists

This group of drugs work by eventually down-regulating the pituitary, thereby preventing FSH release. The removal of this stimulus to the ovary renders the ovary inactive and the patient becomes temporarily menopausal. As endometrial deposits are oestrogen-dependant, this brings about regression of endometrial deposits and with this the reduction or relief of pain. These drugs are usually used for a six-month course, but there are considerable side-effects of hypo-oestrogenism including hot flushes, vaginal dryness and the risk of bone loss from trabecular bone. These side-effects may be countered by using add-back oestrogen and progestogen therapy, without effecting the efficacy of the drug on the disease. Although the use of add-back therapy means that GNRH analogues could be used over prolonged periods of time, trial of this long-term type of approach are limited.

Medroxyprogesterone acetate

A synthetic progestogen, may also be used in the treatment of endometriosis. The principle behind its use is that the progestogen causes the ectopic endometrium to undergo decidualisation, which holds the cells from further division and eventually the cells undergo atrophy.

High doses of medroxyprogesterone acetate are required over a period of six to nine months to be therapeutic, but this may be continued over longer periods of time for maintenance therapy to avoid recurrence.

Danazol

This androgen derivative is used less frequently in the treatment of endometriosis nowadays because of its wide-ranging side-effect profile.

Androgens are known to have a direct effect on endometrial cell growth, reducing endometrial division and inducing atrophy. However, the androgenic side-effects of weight gain, hirsutism and acne due to increased circulating free testosterone, make its use less popular than in the past.

RECURRENT ENDOMETRIOSIS

Medical treatment of endometriosis has a recurrence rate of between 40% and 70% and therefore some attempt at maintenance therapy really must be considered in all patients who are maintaining their uterus and ovaries. There are two strategies involved in this. Firstly, the use of a monophasic oral contraceptive pill, which given continuously prevents menstruation. As the primary theory of endometriosis is based on retrograde menstruation, prevention of menstrual loss is logical. Many women find they get breakthrough bleeding after three or four months of continuous pill taking, and therefore menstruation may occur about three times per year. However, this may be very successful in reducing recurrence. It is also possible to use long-term progestogens, so long as the side-effects are tolerated and they too may be instrumental in preventing menstruation and endometrial recurrence.

SUMMARY

Endometriosis is a severe disease in some women and causes long-term pelvic pain. All patients with chronic pain find it debilitating and the psychological impact of this must be borne in mind. Clinicians need to be sympathetic to this particular group of patients who need to be handled sensitively, and preferably by a clinician who has an expertise in this disease process.

24

Endometrial Cancer

INCIDENCE

Endometrial cancer (EC) is more common in industrialised societies, and epidemiological studies have indicated its association with economic growth and dietary factors. Worldwide, there are 150,000 new cases per year and it is the fifth most common cancer in women. In England and Wales, EC is the second most common gynaecological cancer after the cancer of the ovary (approximately 4000 new cases per year). However, in the Unites States, it is the most common gynaecological cancer and the fourth most common female cancer, after the breast, lung and bowel cancer (approximately 34,000 new cases per year). Asian immigrants to the United States develop a risk similar to the local community, higher than their background risk in Asia.

The average age of patients who develop EC is 60 years (over 90% of cases occur over the age of 50) and it is very rare in women less than 40 years old.

AETIOLOGY

The exposure of the endometrium to oestrogens is the strongest risk factor; therefore early menarche, late menopause, nulliparity, infertility due to anovulation (especially due to polycystic ovaries), obesity (due to aromatisation of androgens in the fat issue) are all associated with an increased risk of EC.

Dietary factors (high fat intake) and diabetes (abnormal carbohydrate metabolism) have been shown to increase the risk of EC. Iatrogenic causes include the administration of unopposed oestrogen in the form of hormone replacement therapy (HRT) or tamoxifen. On the contrary, prolonged use of the combined oral contraceptive pill offers considerable protection (50% reduction of risk).

Tamoxifen is a non-steroidal oestrogen antagonist used in the treatment of breast cancer, but it has weak oestrogen agonist activity on the endometrium. Tamoxifen reduces the risk of breast cancer by 50%, but increases considerably the risk of EC. The National Surgical Adjuvant Breast and Bowel Project (B-14 trial) from the United States showed a corrected 2.5-fold increased risk of endometrial cancer in women with oestrogen receptor-positive breast cancer confined to the breast and with negative axillary nodes. As breast cancer is very common, it is expected that gynaecologists will see increasing numbers of women with abnormal bleeding due to tamoxifen. Ultrasound may show intrauterine lesions or increased endometrial thickness. All those women should undergo hysteroscopy and endometrial biopsy. Hysteroscopic findings include endometrial polyps, hyperplasia and cancer. However, endometrial cancers secondary to tamoxifen treatment tend to be well differentiated and carry a good prognosis. There is no agreement whether patients on tamoxifen should undergo screening for endometrial carcinoma, by ultrasound or endometrial biopsy, and for how long; nevertheless, early investigation of irregular vaginal bleeding is mandatory.

Rarely, EC can develop simultaneously with ovarian cancer or it can be caused by oestrogen-producing ovarian tumours, like granulosa-theca cell tumours.

A small proportion of endometrial cancers are not oestrogen-related and they tend to have a poorer prognosis. They are usually poorly differentiated and occur more often in Black and Asian women.

A very small proportion is related to genetic factors. Lynch II Syndrome (hereditary nonpolyposis colon cancer) presents as a combination of familial colon cancer (Lynch I syndrome) and other adenocarcinomas, including endometrial, ovarian, gastrointestinal, urinary and breast tumours. The responsible gene has been located on chromosome 2p.

PATHOLOGY

Endometrial Intraepithelial Neoplasia (EIN)

Contrary to the clearly defined premalignant histological categories of the cervix, vagina, vulva, prostate and gastrointestinal tract, the precancerous process in the uterus is not clearly defined The Endometrial Collaborative Group (an international affiliation of eminent gynaecological pathologists) has recently proposed a clear nomenclature, which is likely to be adopted in the future (Table 24.1). The advantage of the new proposed system is that there is clear distinction between endometrial hyperplasia (EH), endometrial intraepithelial neoplasia (EIN) and adenocarcinoma. This can offer better guidelines for treatment. EH, being a non-premalignant lesion, can be treated with progestagens; EIN can be treated by either progestagens or surgery; and frank adenocarcinoma by surgery. Close cooperation between the histopathologist and the gynaecologist is important, especially in young women who present with any of the above lesions and want to preserve their fertility. In all these cases, a thorough hysteroscopy, endometrial curettage and histological assessment are mandatory.

Simple, complex and atypical endometrial hyperplasia carry a risk of 1%, 3% and 29%, respectively of progressing to EC.

The most common histological type is endometrioid adenocarcinoma (85%). It carries a good prognosis because of its early presentation with irregular bleeding (usually postmenopausal). One in five of these tumours are associated with squamous differentiation and their prognosis is related to the degree of the squamous differentiation; the correct term is "endometrial adenocarcinoma with squamous differentiation" and not "adenoacanthoma" or "adenosquamous carcinoma", as they used to be called in the past, depending on the appearance of the squamous component.

Other unusual histological types are mucinous, serous papillary, clear cell and squamous carcinomas. They all carry a poor prognosis, except for the mucinous adenocarcinoma.

Endometrial adenocarcinoma can spread directly to adjacent structures (myometrium, fallopian tubes, ovaries, cervix and rarely to the pubic bones). Also, it metastasises to the pelvic, para-aortic and rarely inguinal lymph nodes. Haematogenous spread to the lungs is a rare event.

Table 24.1
Nomenclature

— Simple Non-Atypical Hyperplasia — Complex Non-Atypical Hyperplasia	— Endometrial Hyperplasia (EH)
— Simple Atypical Hyperplasia — Complex Atypical Hyperplasia	— Endometrial Intraepithelial Neoplasia (EIN)
— Adenocarcinoma	— Adenocarcinoma

PROGNOSTIC FACTORS

The identification of factors that influence the survival of cancer patients helps the clinician to individualise the treatment and minimise the morbidity related to various modalities.

Stage

The stage of EC at presentation is the most important factor of survival. Although most

Table 24.2
*Endometrial Cancer, Five-Year Survival According to Stage**

Stage I	72%
Stage II	56%
Stage III	31%
Stage IV	10%

*Based on the old clinical staging (1988 FIGO report). Incomplete staging in many cases and deaths from other causes may have influenced survival. Following the introduction of the new FIGO staging, the survival for Stage I is reported to be 83% and 71% for Stage II. The overall five-year survival in the England and Wales is 70%.

endometrial cancers present at Stage I, the survival according to stage is similar to that of cancer of the cervix (Table 24.2).

Except for a few patients who are not fit for surgery, complete surgical staging should be performed. The FIGO (International Federation of Gynaecology and Obstetrics) surgical staging is presented in Table 24.3.

Table 24.3
FIGO Staging of Endometrial Cancer

Stage	Ia	Tumour limited to the endometrium
	Ib	Invasion to less than one-half of the myometrium
	Ic	Invasion to more than one-half of the myometrium
Stage	IIa	Endocervical glandular involvement only
	IIb	Cervical stromal invasion
Stage	IIIa	Tumour invades serosa and/or adnexae and/or positive peritoneal
	IIIb	Cytology
	IIIc	Vaginal metastases Metastases to pelvic and/or para-aortic lymph nodes
Stage	IVa	Tumour invades bladder and/or bowel mucosa
	IVb	Distant metastases including intra-abdominal and/or inguinal nodes

Age

Older age at presentation is associated with increased risk of higher stage and poorer histological grade.

Histology

The depth of myometrial invasion correlates with the involvement of lymph nodes and the histological grade. Lymphovascular invasion is more likely to be found in the presence of high-grade tumours and advanced stage, and it is an independent factor of survival. Lymph node metastasis is a poor prognostic indicator but it is not routinely performed during surgery. The risk of lymph node metastasis increases in linear fashion with increasing histological grade and myometrial invasion. This may in part explain the surprisingly low survival rate in patients classified with Stage I disease, who have not undergone full staging.

Peritoneal Cytology

Although it is logical to assume that positive cytology is associated with decreased survival, this has not been confirmed from various studies. However, in general it should be regarded as an adverse prognostic sign, especially in the presence of other factors. It is unknown whether iatrogenic spread of malignant cells at the time of diagnostic hysteroscopy has any adverse effect.

Hormonal Factors

As in breast cancer, tumours with positive oestrogen and progesterone receptors have a better prognosis.

Genetic Factors

Recently, mutations in codons of the *Ki-ras* oncogene, the tumour suppressor gene *p53*, decreased amounts of epidermal growth factor (EGF) receptors and over-expression of *HER 2/neu* oncogene have been associated with advanced stage and poor prognosis. These developments offer new exciting prospects of possible identification of precancerous lesions and early treatment or even therapeutic strategies through gene therapy.

CLINICAL PRESENTATION AND INVESTIGATIONS

The average age at presentation is 60 years and 90% of patients present with post-menopausal bleeding. In pre-menopausal women, EC is always associated with irregularities of the menses (menorrhagia or intermenstrual bleeding). Occasionally, when the cervical canal is stenosed, patients may present with pelvic pain and discharge due to the enlarged uterus and the presence of haematometra or pyometra. In cases of advanced EC, ascites, or palpable masses may be felt on abdominal, vaginal or rectal examination. Rarely, endometrial cancerous cells may be found on a routine cervical smear or an asymptomatic pelvic mass on CT scan or ultrasound performed for unrelated reasons.

Post-Menopausal Bleeding (PMB)

This is a very common complaint and it counts for 5–10% of referrals in the UK outpatient departments. Its incidence is likely to increase in view of the improved life expectancy. It has to be investigated thoroughly because 12% in total of those women have a primary or secondary cancer and 8% have endometrial cancer.

The ideal investigation for PMB has not been defined. Transvaginal ultrasound is used to measure the endometrial thickness (ET), which should be no more than a few millimetres in post-menopausal women. The finding of an endometrial thickness of less than 5 mm at transvaginal ultrasound reduces the likelihood of endometrial carcinoma by a factor of 10. In women with PMB not using HRT, this reduces the risk from approximately 10% to 1%. Ultrasound has the advantage of being easy to perform and is not expensive or invasive.

A histological sample may be obtained in an outpatient setting using a pipelle sampler which relies on suction to approximate the curette to the endometrium and to draw the sample into the collection tube. Very good accuracy may be obtained with this very simple technique but false negative rates are between 5% and 15% and it may be uncomfortable, particularly if the endocervical canal is narrowed.

The endometrium may be visualised directly using a hysteroscope, either in the outpatient clinic without anaesthesia or under general anaesthetic. The lowest false negative rate is associated with D&C under general anaesthetic (2–6%).

Sonohysterography (instillation of fluid into the uterine cavity during ultrasound), 3-D scanning, Doppler and colour flow have also been investigated, but there is no evidence so far that they are superior to hysteroscopy. MRI of uterus and pelvis may show extension of the tumour in the cervix or myometrium, which may influence the extent of hysterectomy at surgery. However, this is not currently routine practice.

DIFFERENTIAL DIAGNOSIS

In most cases, post-menopausal bleeding is due to uterine atrophy. Less often, it is related to benign endometrial polyps or endometrial hyperplasia. Cervical and vaginal cancer can also present with PMB and no other symptoms.

Haematuria due to bladder cancer and blood loss due to colon cancer can also be mistaken for PMB. It goes without saying that a thorough clinical examination is the key to the successful diagnosis and to arranging the necessary investigations. This is especially important for women who do not belong to the main risk group of patients (post-menopausal with PMB). A breast examination and a cervical smear should always be part of the initial assessment.

SURGERY

Complete surgical staging requires ideally a midline incision, although a low transverse one can give adequate access to pelvis and may improve postoperative recovery in a great proportion of patients with EC, who are obese and have various medical problems.

Table 24.4
Surgical Staging for Endometrial Cancer

Cytology of peritoneal fluid
Inspection of the abdomen, pelvis and vagina
Biopsy of any suspicious lesions
TAH+BSO
Omentectomy in high-risk patients (with serous and clear cell tumours)
Suspicious pelvic and para-aortic lymph nodes should be removed
Sampling of pelvic and para-aortic lymph nodes*

*This is recommended for cases of unfavourable histological type and grade, evidence of more than half myometrial invasion, extension of the tumour to the cervix or outside the uterus and tumour size of more than 2 cm. A randomised prospective trial is taking place now and its results will be available in a few years (the ASTEC trial).

A total abdominal hysterectomy and bilateral oophorectomy (TAH+BSO) is routinely performed. However, in order to produce complete surgical staging, certain rules should apply (Table 24.4).

Radical Hysterectomy (RH)

There is no evidence that this improves survival in Stage I disease; however it can be considered when there is preoperative evidence of tumour extension into the cervix (Stage II).

Vaginal Hysterectomy (VH) and Laparoscopy

In many centres, patients have been treated with VH, laparoscopic oophorectomy and lymph node sampling in order to reduce the surgical morbidity and improve the postoperative recovery. We should be cautious with this approach until we know the long-term results of these operations and, especially the possible adverse effect that CO_2 pneumoperitoneum may have on tumour cells spread, as suggested in animal studies. However, VH, on its own, is a very valuable option in medically unfit patients and can be used as a palliative procedure in advanced cases.

RADIOTHERAPY

Radiation therapy can be given according to the following techniques:

- Interstitial vaginal brachytherapy (directly within the tumour)
- Intracavitary vaginal or intrauterine brachytherapy (adjacent to the tumour)
- Pelvic external beam therapy
- Combined external beam and brachytherapy.

Post-Operative Treatment

It is generally accepted that patients with Stage Ia and Grades 1, 2 tumours (no myometrial invasion, well and moderately differentiated) do not benefit from adjuvant radiotherapy. Patients with stage Ib, Grades 1 and 2 (extension to the inner half of the myometrium) are given vaginal brachytherapy. The rest of the patients are usually offered vaginal brachytherapy and external beam pelvic irradiation.

Whole abdomen irradiation can be used in the presence of intra-abdominal metastases outside the pelvis, although it is associated with increased morbidity.

Radiotherapy as Primary Treatment and for Palliation

Patients who are unfit to undergo surgery can be given primary intracavitary radiotherapy (patients with severe chronic illnesses, morbidly obese and very elderly). Radical radiotherapy in early stage disease has comparable effects on survival to surgery. Also, with advanced disease, palliative radiotherapy can produce satisfactory local control.

Intracavitary treatment with or without external beam radiotherapy can be given according to the clinical staging, the assessment of risk of extrauterine spread and the medical condition of the patient.

CHEMOTHERAPY

The role of chemotherapy is limited to treating recurrences and in patients with advanced disease. Although responses can be as high as 30%, they are short-lived. The most commonly used agents are cisplatin, doxorubicin, epirubicin and cyclophosphamide.

Recently, taxol, a highly effective taxane against ovarian cancer, has been included in randomised trials for EC.

HORMONAL TREATMENT

Oestrogen and progesterone receptors are present in 60% of cases of endometrial adenocarcinoma, and progesterone receptors have been shown to be a prognostic factor of survival. Progestogens are mainly given for recurrent disease, as there is no evidence that they are useful as part of the adjuvant therapy. Medroxyprogesterone acetate is the most commonly used agent with responses of up to 30%.

Tamoxifen shows both agonist and antagonist activity with oestrogen receptors. It is a first-line treatment in breast cancer with excellent responses in patients with oestrogen receptor-positive tumours. However, tamoxifen has not produced a better response than progestogens in EC.

GnRH Analogues

GnRH receptors are found in most endometrial cancers; however, no consistent responses have been reported and their use is limited in cases of recurrent tumours that have not responded to chemotherapy and progestogens.

There is no evidence that oestrogen-only hormone replacement therapy (HRT) in patients radically treated for early stage disease has an adverse effect. However, for patients who are considered at a high risk of recurrence, medroxyprogesterone acetate may be used to control vasomotor symptoms (hot flushes) at a dose 20–40 mg per day.

As in breast cancer, where responses of 30% for recurrent disease have been observed, a potentially useful group of drugs could be the aromatase inhibitors. They block the aromatase complex, and therefore, the peripheral conversion of androstendione and testosterone to oestrogens. Clinical data are lacking at the moment.

UTERINE SARCOMAS

They are rare, highly malignant tumours, accounting for 5% of uterine malignancies. Uterine sarcomas are more commonly encountered in Afro-Caribbean women and patients with a history of previous radiation therapy to the pelvis. The staging is similar to EC, although they have a far more aggressive behaviour and poorer prognosis. They metastasise by haematogenous (lungs), lymphatic spread or direct extension and are associated with previous irradiation of the uterus (for carcinoma of the cervix).

Leiomyosarcomas

They are the most common type of uterine sarcomas and occur more frequently in Afro-Caribbeans. Benign uterine leiomyomas (fibroids) rarely undergo malignant change (0.5%).

Leiomyosarcomas usually present as a rapidly growing pelvic mass or with irregular vaginal bleeding. In the latter case, curettings obtained at hysteroscopy may show a submucosal sarcomatous lesion.

The most important prognostic factor is the number of mitoses found per 10 high power fields (HPF). Tumours with more than 10 mitoses/10 HPF have a very poor prognosis, although the overall 5-year survival rate is 40%.

Other types of uterine sarcomas are mixed Müllerian sarcomas and endometrial stromal sarcomas. Again these are more common in Afro-Caribbean patients, present with post-menopausal bleeding and have a generally poor prognosis.

Treatment of Uterine Sarcomas

A staging laparotomy should always be performed in order to identify the extent of the tumour. A total abdominal hysterectomy and bilateral salpingo-oophorectomy should be performed. Inspection of the abdominal cavity, peritoneal cytology and sampling of pelvic and para-aortic lymph nodes is recommended. However, in most of the cases, the disease is incurable because of the presence of distant metastases at the time of surgery.

Mixed Müllerian tumours and endometrial stromal sarcomas are radiosensitive tumours, and radiotherapy can achieve local control and good palliation in a proportion of cases.

Several chemotherapeutic agents have been used with little success. Doxorubicin is active against leiomyosarcomas, and cisplatin and ifosfamide against MMMTs. However, their use has not significantly improved survival in clinical trials.

Medroxyprogesterone acetate is the only hormonal treatment used with sarcomas. It has produced long periods of remission in patients suffering from low-grade endometrial stromal sarcoma, a slow-growing tumour.

FURTHER READING

Lurain J.R. (1996). Uterine cancer. In *Novak's Gynecology*, 12th edn. Berek J.S. (ed). pp. 1057–1110. Baltimore: Williams & Wilkins.

Management of Gynaecological Cancers (1999). In Bulletin of the effectiveness of health service interventions for decision makers. *Effective Health Care* **5**(3) (ISSN: 0965-0288). London: The Royal Society of Medicine Press.

Quinn M.A., Anderson M.C., Coulter C.A.E. Soutter W.P. (1997). Malignant disease of the uterus. In *Gynaecology*. Shaw R.W., Soutter W.P., Stanton S.L. (eds). pp. 585–603. London: Churchill Livingstone.

Rogerson L., Jones S. (1998). The investigation of women with post-menopausal bleeding. *Review No. 98/07*. London: Royal College of Obstetricians and Gynaecologists.

25

Urinary Problems and Prolapse

URINARY PROBLEMS

Introduction

Urinary problems are common in women — particularly incontinence and urinary tract infections. This chapter briefly discusses urinary tract infection in gynaecology, but concentrates on urinary incontinence and urogenital prolapse.

Urinary Tract Infection

Lower urinary tract infection (UTI) is one of the most common conditions presenting to general practitioners, gynaecologists and urologists. Incidence increases with age occurring in 1–2% in schoolgirls to 5–10% in older women. Recurrent infections in middle age rarely cause upper renal tract damage, but single and recurrent bouts of infection cause much distress. Significant infection is regarded as a concentration of organisms $> 10^5$/ml in a clean catch or midstream specimen of urine. Others suggest that a bacterial concentration of 10^2/ml would be more useful. Eighty five per cent of lower urinary tract infections in general practice are caused by *Escherichia coli (E. coli)* count and other coliforms. The presence of pus (pyuria) plus a high bacterial count presents no diagnostic problem, but pyuria with few organisms requires further investigation. Cystitis may be acute or chronic, and not all are bacterial. Causes of abacterial cystitis include a large number of hypersensitive enigmatic conditions such as atrophic cystitis, interstitial cystitis, urethral syndrome and post-radiation cystitis. Apart from atrophic vaginitis, these conditions are often difficult to diagnose and treat. The symptoms of cystitis are increased frequency, voiding less than every hours and more than 7 times per day, and urgency of micturition. Nocturia is being awakened more than once a night with the desire to micturate. Dysuria or pain on micturition, in bacterial cystitis is a burning or scalding pain experienced during voiding. There may be associated bladder and loin pain if the infection extends to the upper renal tract. A dull supra-pubic ache experienced whilst the bladder fills, occurs with abacterial cystitis. Empirical treatment of an acute UTI should start immediately after a midstream specimen of urine has been collected with an appropriate antibiotic sensitive to *E. coli*. The course of treatment should be as short as possible to ensure patient compliance and to prevent a subsequent candidal vaginitis. This treatment may be suitable for the patient but is disliked by microbiologists because of the increased risk of drug-induced resistant strains of *E. coli*.

Urinary Incontinence

Urinary incontinence is defined as the involuntary loss of urine causing a social or hygienic problem. It is rarely life-threatening being either a nuisance, becoming embarrassing and distressing, or intolerable interfering with lifestyle requiring wearing of padded protection all the time. Urinary incontinence is estimated to affect around 2.6–3 million women in Britain. Recent studies suggest up to 30% of women may be affected. It affects women of all ages, but the incidence increases with age. Those who suffer from incontinence are often too embarrassed to admit that they have a problem. In over 90% of cases, urinary incontinence is caused by stress incontinence or detrusor instability. Overflow incontinence is relatively common, especially in elderly women.

Incontinence history

A detailed accurate history will yield clues as to the diagnosis. It is surprising the number of questions are required in a thorough incontinence history! The patient should be asked how often she micturates during the day and night, how long she can last between each micturition, how long she can delay micturition once she gets the urge? If frequency is the complaint, why does she void so often? Is it because of severe urgency, or convenience or an attempt to prevent a leak? The severity of her incontinence should be ascertained. Is it a nuisance, embarrassing, or intolerable? Does stress incontinence occur during coughing, sneezing or laughing, or only during heavy physical exercise, and what exercise? Does stress urinary incontinence occur during intercourse; if so, on entry or on deep penetration? Is her stress incontinence minimal or is it uncontrollable? Is her urgency constant and not relieved by micturition? Is her urgency because of pain or discomfort which is unrelieved by voiding? Is she aware of being incontinence or does she just find herself wet? Does she suffer from post-micturition dribble or enuresis? Does she have to wear protective pads, and if so, how often do they have to be changed? Does she have difficulty starting micturition? Does she have a weak constant stream? Does she have to strain or tilt forward to maintain stream? Has she ever been in urinary retention?

The patient should be asked about specific disorders, such as multiple sclerosis, spinal cord injury, lumbar disc injury, myelodysplasia, diabetes, stroke, or Parkinson's disease, which are known to affect bladder and sphincter function. Drugs can also affect bladder function — clonidine exacerbates stress incontinence and sympathomimetic drugs, such as ephedrine or tricyclic antidepressants (e.g. imipramine), may cause urinary retention and overflow incontinence. A bladder diary containing a frequency/volume chart and written details of her incontinence problems gives vital information about bladder function, provided it is properly completed by the patient.

Physical examination

Examination of the patient in the left lateral position, with a Simm's speculum, gives good information about the bladder. The mobility of the bladder neck can be seen, the presence of a cystocoele or a cystourethrocoele, vaginal prolapse, or rectocoele can be ascertained. Stress incontinence can be demonstrated on coughing, provided the patient has not politely emptied her bladder just before the consultation. Atrophic vaginitis can also be seen. Pelvic examination reveals uterine size and presence of any large pelvic masses. Pelvic floor strength can be roughly gauged by asking the patient to squeeze her levator ani muscle against the examiner's two fingers at the end of the vaginal examination. Contraction of the anal sphincter should be observed as a lax sphincter may a sign of neurological damage.

Stress incontinence

Stress incontinence denotes a symptom or a sign but not a diagnosis. Genuine stress incontinence (GSI) is a diagnosis made following urodynamics and is defined as the leakage of urine per urethra due to raised intraabdominal pressure, in the absence of detrusor activity. It commonly affects the middle-aged and elderly or the puerperal patient. Stress incontinence was previously thought to be caused by the loss of the posterior urethrovesicle angle as a result of increased intra-abdominal pressure such as coughing, or by a change in the angle of inclination of the urethral axis. Urinary continence depends upon a positive pressure gradient from the urethra to the bladder, thus ensuring that urethral pressure is always greater than the bladder pressure except during micturition. The urethral sphincter in women is weak and urethral closing pressure is maintained by the effects of collagen, elastic tissue and urethral smooth and striated muscle. Incontinence does not occur in normal women because the proximal urethra and bladder neck lie above the pelvic floor. Coughing increases the intraabdominal pressure, which is transmitted to this weak urethral sphincter increasing its closing power. Whenever the proximal urethra and bladder neck lie below the pelvic floor, as in a cystourethrocoele, the increased intra-abdominal pressure is not equally transmitted, so inefficient closure occurs, which cannot resist the increased intravesical pressure and incontinence results. The 'hammock' hypothesis is an alternative theory of female continence. Continence is maintained by compression of the urethrovesical junction against the hammock of the anterior vaginal wall during an increase in intraabdominal pressure. Any damage or weakening to the supports of the anterior vaginal wall contributes to both genital prolapse and stress incontinence. The aetiology is therefore multifactorial. It is associated with vaginal delivery (particularly prolonging bearing down in the second stage or, ironically a precipitant rapid delivery), the menopause and a congenital weakness in the pelvic floor (due perhaps to abnormal collagen composition), multiparity, constipation, obesity, chronic cough, and anything which causes increased pressure on, or damages the nerve supply to the pelvic floor. Patients complaining of stress incontinence may or may not have associated frequency, urgency and urge incontinence. Demonstrable stress incontinence proves that the patient is incontinent, but does not diagnose the underlying condition.

Unstable Bladder, or Detrusor Instability (Motor Urgency)

Detrusor instability or the unstable bladder presents with a history of frequency of micturition, sometimes as often as every 30–60 minutes, urgency of micturition, nocturia and urge and stress incontinence. It is a social problem, often perceived by the sufferer as possibly a serious organic problem. The detrusor muscle of the bladder contracts frequently and excessively, increasing the intravesical pressure markedly, and causing the frequent desire to micturate. Once urine reaches the proximal urethra, the micturition reflex is triggered and severe urgency and urge incontinence will follow. The International Continence Society (ICS) defines an unstable bladder as one that is shown to objectively contract, spontaneously or on provocation, during the filling phase while the patient is attempting to inhibit miturition. The precise cause of detrusor instability is unknown in many cases, but it can follow pelvic surgery. Once the process starts, it can rapidly worsen as the woman responds to all the desires to micturate and temporariliy loses the ability to suppress these, thereby establishing a vicious circle. Nocturia is a common symptom but also may reflect on the patient's excessive fluid intake or insomnia, or that she is taking diuretic drugs at the wrong time.

Overflow Incontinence

Overflow incontinence presents as constant dribbling, or voiding of small amounts of urine at frequent intervals, and stress incontinence. It can be caused by a lower motor neurone lesion, a pelvic mass, or inflammation of the urethra, vulva or vagina. Retention of urine can occur after pelvic surgery, epidural anaesthesia or following drugs such as ganglion blockers, anticholinergic drugs, β-adrenergic stimulants and tricyclic antidepressants. The diagnosis is based on a large residual volume after micturition found on ultrasound or by catheterisation. If the bladder is hypotonic, cholinergic agents particularly bethanechol chloride may be helpful. If there is outflow obstruction urethral dilatation, urethrotomy or intermittent self-catheterisation may be considered.

Diagnosis

Careful history-taking and careful examination and use of a detailed symptom questionnaire will differentiate up to 80% of cases of genuine stress incontinence from detrusor instability. However, there is too much overlap of symptoms between different causes to make a reliable diagnosis without resorting to objective tests such as urodynamics. Inspection of the patient's bladder diary is very helpful. Careful examination of fluid intake may reveal for example, an excessive addiction to tea, which happens to have a diuretic effect. A midstream specimen of urine must always be sent for culture to exclude a urinary tract infection. A random blood sugar measurement is also an essential preliminary investigation. Basic urodynamic investigations such as subtracted cystometry are then performed. This involves measuring the intraabdominal pressure and subtracting it from the measured vesical pressure to reveal the actual detrusor muscle pressure. This distinguishes genuine stress incontinence from detrusor instability in the majority of cases, but these are time-consuming and expensive. These should be confined to patients with: mixed symptoms, voiding difficulties before attempting surgery to confirm neurological disorder, and in patients with previous failed surgery. Videocystourethrography gives a visual display of the descent and rotation of the bladder neck, simultaneously combined with subtracted cystometry. It is reserved for complicated cases such as recurrent incontinence after previous surgery.

Treatment

An accurate diagnosis must be made before proceeding to treatment, as genuine stress incontinence can be cured by surgery, but detrusor instability is not remedial to surgery. Conservative treatment has few complications and should be offered to all women who have genuine stress incontinence before embarking on surgery. Pelvic floor exercises, encouraged by interested physiotherapists can be successful in young, highly motivated patients with mild genuine stress incontinence.

Surgical procedures for treatment of genuine stress incontinence

There are numerous types of operation to elevate the bladder neck and proximal urethra to an intraabdominal position to increase urethral sphincter closing pressure. Failure to cure genuine stress incontinence initially offers less chance of successful repair at successive operations, so choice of a suitable procedure is important. Suprapubic procedures such as the Marshall-Marchetti-Krantz operation, Burch colposuspension and various sling procedures give better results than the traditional anterior colporrhaphy. Needle bladder neck suspension procedures are reserved for the overweight, surgically difficult patient. Peri-urethral injection techniques with collagen, macroplastique or autolgolous fat, can be performed as day cases. They are suitable for the infirm but are effective only for 2–3 years. Laparoscopic colposuspension is another recently developed technique, but it remains unevaluated. Sub-urethral fascial sling procedures have been traditionally reserved for patients with recurrent stress incontinence and possible intrinsic sphincter deficiency. Another recent development is the tension-free vaginal tape procedure which is performed under local or spinal anaesthesia. An artificial prolene mesh tape is inserted loosely under the urethra to act as a hammock. The patient returns home after 24 hours and resumes normal activity within 2 weeks. Early follow-up studies suggest this tension-free tape to be effective.

Treatment of Detrusor instability

Detrusor instability is difficult to treat and patients are taught Frewen's regimen of bladder drill and exercises to improve the tone of the perineal muscles, so strengthening the pelvic floor. Frewen's regime involves: (1) re-emphasising and re-training the ability to resist urge incontinence and (2) simultaneously reducing frequency of micturition by deliberately increasing the time between voiding. This has to be done gradually. If successful, not only is frequency improved, but also urgency nocturia and even stress incontinence will be reduced. This gives the patient more understanding of her problems and the realisation that self-treatment is important and usually successful. Frequent follow-up and reassurance leads to improvement in symptoms. An unstable bladder can be converted to a stable one in 80% of patients by these measures. The ganglion blocker, emepronium bromide, produces temporary relief of symptoms, and the tricyclic antidepressant imipramine helps those with nocturia or enuresis as well as reducing urgency and urinary frequency. Oxybutynin hydrochloride acts in two ways on the detrusor muscle, possessing anticholinergic activity and a direct spasmolytic effect. It has unfortunate side-effects, common to all anticholinergic drugs. These include dry mouth, constipation, nausea, blurred vision, and facial flushing which accounts for poor patient compliance. It has been superceded by tolterodine, another anticholinergic with less side-effects. If sensory urgency is the main symptom and there is also moderate to severe atrophic vaginitis, concurrent local application of a small amount of oestrogen cream, for example 1 g nocte for a week, then once a week for a month, is beneficial. Systemic absorption of this small amount of oestrogen is minimal and has no detrimental effect on the endometrium.

Fistulae

Vesico-vaginal and utero-vaginal fistulae occur after pelvic surgery and irradiation therapy for pelvic malignancies, but in developed countries they are very uncommon. In developing countries, vesico-vaginal fistulae commonly occur after prolonged labour, causing pressure necrosis of the bladder. These fistulae cause continuous incontinence, and clinically, the patient awakens early in the morning with the bed soaked. There is no previous history of enuresis. These patients are, understandably aggrieved and angry and want this fistula repaired as soon as possible. A low vesico-vaginal fistulae, which is not adjacent to the ureteric orifice may be repaired by the vaginal approach but it is a delicate, awkward and prolonged operation. It has to be performed by an experienced vaginal surgeon. Today, most high vesico-vaginal and uretero-vaginal fistulae are repaired successfully by urologists through the abdominal approach.

GENITAL PROLAPSE

This can be defined as descent of adjacent organs through the fascial layers and into the vagina and sometimes beyond. Their definitions are shown in Table 25.1. Traditionally, uterine prolapse is classified — first, second or third degree. First degree prolapse is defined as the cervix descending to the lower third of the vagina on straining. Second degree prolapse means that the cervix is visible at the introitus on straining, whilst third degree or procidentia refers to passage of the entire uterus outside the vagina.

Most women who develop genital prolapse are multiparous. Only 2% of women with prolapse are nulliparous. Cows and sheep characterically have prolonged labours and develop prolapse, while horses and goats tend to have rapid labours do not develop prolapse.

Contributing factors towards development of genital prolapse are listed in Table 25.2. Bearing down in labour before full cervical dilatation subjects the uterine supports to undue strain, and undoubtedly, contributes to the development of prolapse later in life when lack of oestrogen causes changes in collagen which

Table 25.1

Descent of structure	Terminology used
Urethra	Urethrocele
Bladder	Cystocele
Small bowel	Enterocele
Rectum	Rectocele
Uterus	Uterovaginal prolapse

Table 25.2
Causes of Genital Prolapse

Weakened supports	Increased downward pressure
Congenital weakness (neuropathy, myopathy) e.g. spina bifida	Chronic cough
Multiparity	Constipation
Traumatic vaginal delivery	Abdominal masses
Large babies	Ascites
Inadequate perineal repairs	Uterine tumours
Failed postnatal exercises	
Poor nutrition	
Old age (hormone deficiency)	

weakens these uterovaginal supports. An understanding of the functional anatomy of the pelvic floor shows why genital prolapse can occur. The bony pelvis is like a bowl with no base except that provided by the platform of the levator ani and coccygeus muscles, and by the pelvic fascia. The coccygeus muscle consists of the ischio-, ilio- and pubococcygeus muscles which blend together on each side into a shelf that slopes medially downwards to produce a gutter effect in the midline pierced by the urethra, vagina and anal canal. These muscles arise from the ischial spines and pelvic bone to be inserted into the coccyx, and anococcygel raphe and perineal body. These pelvic floor muscles normally contract to counteract any raised intraabdominal pressure such as sneezing, laughing or coughing. A layer of fascia lies between these muscles and the peritoneal areolar tissue about the pelvic organs. Condensation of this fascia forms ligaments, such as the transverse cervical and uterosacral ligaments, which support the uterus, as well as the pubovesical fascia supporting the bladder and the rectovaginal fascia supporting the rectum.

Clinical Symptoms

Prolapse rarely starts during pregnancy, but symptoms may occur soon after delivery, stress incontinence being the most common. It is usually encountered in middle-aged and elderly women, who are often embarrassed and reluctant to visit the doctor until prolapse has been present for some time. Eighty per cent complain of a dragging sensation in the vagina or are aware of "something coming down". They may also complain of backache and urinary symptoms such as urgency, frequency, stress incontinence, or rarely, urinary retention. This occurs when there is a large cystocoele with good urethral support leading to occlusion of the urethrovesical angle. The sensation of the bowel being incompletely empty after defaecation or tenesmus, occurs when there is an associated low rectocoele. Sometimes, the patient has to apply digital pressure on the rectocoele from the vagina to promote complete defaecation. These women often reluctantly admit to the passage of inappropriate flatus per rectum which is socially embarrassing. Keratinisation and decubitus ulceration of the exposed cervix occurs in procidentia caused by persistent exposure and rubbing of the epithelium, which in turn, results in bleeding and discharge, especially when infected.

Diagnosis

Genital prolapse is confirmed by careful examination and categorised into the three degrees mentioned above. The patient is first examined lying supine with legs abducted and drawn up. Third degree uterovaginal prolapse will be obvious. The vulva and introitus should be examined and the patient asked to cough, so demonstrating any stress incontinence. Second degree prolapse may also be seen. A double bladed speculum is then inserted, a cervical smear taken and any ulceration or keratinisation of the cervix or vagina noted. When this speculum is withdrawn slowly, enterocoele and rectocoele may be seen. A bimanual examination is then performed to identify any enlargement of the uterus or pelvic masses. The woman is then examined in the left lateral position with the right knee raised above the left one, with a single blade Sims speculum. This exposes the anterior and posterior vaginal walls and clearly reveals any cystocoele and, when it is withdrawn, a rectocoele or enterocoele will be seen. Finally, a rectal examination will distinguish an enterocoele from a high rectocoele. The differential diagnosis includes any swelling at the introitus which, on superficial examination, may be mistaken for a true prolapse, but can consist of large cervical polyps, pedunculated fibroids, vaginal and Bartholin's cysts, and very rarely, chronic inversion of the uterus.

Prophylactic Treatment

Ninety five per cent of genital prolapse occurs in multiparous women, so prophylactic measures during and after labour are important. The second state of labour should not be too long and patients must be prevented from bearing down before full dilatation. Postnatal exercises to tighten the perineal muscles, and drawing the anus forward are vital and every patient should continue these throughout the puerperium.

Ring or shelf pessaries are inserted in elderly patients who are unfit for surgery. Ring pessaries are also used for temporary relief of symptoms in prolapse occurring immediately after childbirth while awaiting the effects of involution and pelvic floor exercises. They are also used for relief of symptoms in those women awaiting surgery. Pessaries should be changed every three months to prevent impaction and vaginal ulceration. Application of local oestrogen creams improves the post-menopausal vaginal skin. In cases of procidentia, the uterus should be gently re-inserted before proceeding to surgical repair at a later date. The use of local oestrogen cream will improve the condition of the vaginal mucosa before surgery.

Surgical Treatment

Today, fit patients with second or third degree uterovaginal prolapse, who are past childbearing age, undergo a vaginal hysterectomy with anterior and posterior colporrhaphy, if there is associated cystocoele and rectocoele. If there is associated genuine stress incontinence, then widely placed urethral buttress sutures should be inserted. Others advocate a concurrent Burch colposuspension to ensure permanent correction of the weak urethral sphincter, but the surgeon is then left with the dilemma of a combined vaginal and abdominal operation with increased operating time and resultant morbidity. Current opinion suggests a suspension procedure should be performed first, to correct the genuine stress incontinence, and subsequently perform a vaginal hysterectomy, as a separate operation, especially in younger women. The Manchester operation consists of amputation of the cervix, tightening of the uterosacral ligaments and anteversion of the uterus by tightening the transverse cervical ligaments in front of the cervix, as well as anterior colporrhaphy and posterior colpoperineorhaphy posterior vaginal wall repair. Most gynaecologists today perform a vaginal hysterectomy and colporrhaphies in preference to this procedure. However, it is sometimes performed in infirm patients who would not withstand a vaginal hysterectomy, or in younger women with a hypertrophied cervix without much uterine descent or in those wishing to keep the uterus. Vault prolapse can occur in up to 10% of patients following vaginal hysterectomy, if care is not taken to excise any enterocoele, or if a sufficiently high posterior colporrhaphy is not performed, or if the vaginal vault is not supported by suturing it to the transverse cervical ligaments. The middle-aged and elderly patient should be questioned about intercourse, and due care taken at operation to prevent removal of excessive vaginal skin leading to a narrowing of the introitus.

Post-Hysterectomy Vault Prolapse

Today, more vaginal hysterectomies are being performed, and so it seems the incidence of vault prolapse has increased. Traditional operations to correct this defect include closure of the enteocoele sac and plication of the uterosacral ligament, or closure of the vagina by colpoclesis. These narrow the vagina, making intercourse impossible and often fail so other techniques have been promoted. Sacrospinous fixation involves hitching the apex of the prolapsed vault onto the left sacrospinous ligament. This is performed 'blind' per vaginam, and is not for the occasional operator. The dome of the vault can also be hitched to the sacrum by the abdominal route — the abdominal sacrocolpopexy. Conservative treatment with various pessaries of different shapes and sizes usually fail, but may be the only remaining option in the old and infirm lady.

26

Diseases of the Vulva

The vulva is continuous with the distal vagina and is essentially a dermatological organ composed of skin, subcutaneous tissues and glands. It includes the mons pubis, labia majora and minora, clitoris, vestibule of vagina, bulb of the vestibule and the greater vestibular or Bartholin's glands.

SYMPTOMS OF VULVAL DISEASE

The vulva is subject not only to conditions affecting the skin over the rest of the body, but also to some diseases that occur here more frequently and to others that affect only the vulva. The dense nerve innervation to the vulval skin means that even mild conditions may result in severe symptoms of pain or pruritus.

Pruritus vulvae is the term used for chronic vulval itching where no cause is evident. In practice, it is often applied to any woman with a vulval itch regardless of aetiology. Occasionally, it can be due to systemic disease such as diabetes, uraemia or renal failure.

Vulvodynia describes vulval pain or vulval burning. Often it may be an isolated symptom but can be associated with dyspareunia. Examination of the vulva may not reveal any evidence of pathology. Biopsy may be required to exclude a pathological cause. Treatment is often difficult and often involves topical steroid creams. If thought to be neuralgic in origin, amitriptyline may be useful and has an anti-depressant effect in patients who may have an underlying affective disorder.

Vulval bleeding or the presence of a palpable lesion needs to be investigated early as it is important to exclude an invasive lesion.

DISORDERS OF THE GLANDS

The labia majora are covered with hair-bearing skin in contrast to the labia minora and thus may be involved by boils affecting the hair follicles which may be recurrent in the patients with diabetes. The vulval skin also has sweat glands which are subject to recurrent abscess formation in the condition hydradenitis suppurativa where the gland and duct which have different developmental origins do not link up.

Two larger constant glands called vestibular or Bartholin's glands are present in the vaginal entrance posteriorly and communicate via a short duct that is prone to blockage. The gland may swell and become infected causing acute discomfort. It may be possible to excise a diseased but uninfected gland, but marsupialisation or deroofing of the cyst cavity to create a permanent track is the preferred first option to minimise recurrence.

ULCERATION OF THE VULVA

Due to its relation to the lower genital tract, the vulva may become involved in sexually transmitted diseases either directly or as a result of irritation from the offensive discharge. Ulceration of the vulva may result from herpes genitalis. The primary attack can be very mild indeed with only focal areas of itching. Alternatively, it may present with systemic upset, marked swelling of the vulva with the presence of multiple diagnostic vesicles, enlarged inguinal lymph nodes and occasionally urinary retention. Treatment with antiviral agents is helpful if recognised in the early phase but management is otherwise supportive with catheterisation to alleviate urinary retention until the pain and swelling settle spontaneously. Secondary attacks are common but generally less severe and self-limiting. The differential diagnosis includes other causes of vulval ulceration such as syphilis, Crohn's disease and Behcet's disease. The last is a chronic ulcerative disease affecting the vulva, mouth and eye which may cause severe scarring. The underlying cause is not known but treatment with steroids is sometimes beneficial. Threadworm infestation can cause intense vulval itching and anal pruritus especially in children. Diagnosis depends on isolating the worms.

DERMATOLOGICAL DISORDERS OF THE VULVA

The vulva is subject to a variety of specific dermatological conditions. These have been classified by a number of systems and are generally called vulval dystrophies. Some believe that the clinical manifestations are a continuum of a single process but most divide these into a variety of subheadings.

Lichen Sclerosis

This condition is distinguished by the presence of amorphous changes in the epidermal layer. The patient often presents with severe pruritus which is made worse by excoriation caused by scratching. Although showing predominantly atrophic features usually distributed symmetrically on each side of the midline of the vulva, it may show hyperkeratosis in the form of raised white lesions termed leukoplakia which may be indistinguishable from precancerous changes. The condition may affect the vulva extensively with resorption of the labia minora and fusion of the labia anteriorly to bury the clitoris. The introitus may become scarred and stenosed causing superficial dyspareunia which can be distressing in younger patients. The clinical appearances is usually typical but biopsy may be required in those who do not respond to treatment. Potent topical steroid therapy is normally required to alleviate pruritus and the condition usually follows a relapsing course with maintenance therapy often indicated. A small number of these women develop vulval carcinoma and should be warned to seek advice if the symptoms change.

Squamous Cell Hyperplasia

This is a diagnosis of exclusion and applies to those cases where a biopsy has shown hyperplasia but without any demonstrable cause. This can result from persistent rubbing of previously normal skin, psoriasis and following chronic candidal infection.

Allergic Dermatitis

Due to the dense nerve innervation, the vulva is particularly prone to symptomatic allergic or irritant dermatitis. The patient may complain of vulval pruritus as a result of exposure to perfumed toiletries, hair shampoo, biological washing powders or synthetic materials. The skin may appear generally reddened with possible excoriation and secondary infection. Such symptoms may result from excessive washing or vaginal douching in patients who have worries over cleanliness or odour. After exclusion of likely sensitising agents and treatment of secondary infection, treatment with steroids is often required.

Lichen Planus

This is an uncommon condition of unknown aetiology. Vulval pruritus is the common presenting symptom and on examination white well demarcated plaques may be seen. Examination of the mouth may also reveal their presence on the buccal mucosa. The condition is normally self-limiting but steroid therapy may be required.

VULVAL INTRAEPITHELIAL NEOPLASIA (VIN)

Hyperplasia of the epidermal layer may be accompanied by dyskaryotic changes of the cells with mitotic figures and loss of maturation as the cells reach the surface. This is analogous to the development of precancerous cells in the cervix and is known as vulval intraepithelial neoplasia (VIN). The severity of VIN depends on the degree of dyskaryosis exhibited by the cells and in VIN 3, there is full thickness replacement of the epithelium with severely dyskaryotic cells and frequent mitosis of the basal cells. It is thought that human papillomavirus may be implicated but the association is not as strong as with CIN. Such patients often give a history of previous treatment for CIN. VIN may be asymptomatic and noticed incidentally as a leukoplakic lesion but patients mainly present with pruritus. The area may be isolated or be part of a field change affecting the vulva in a widespread fashion and extending to surround the anal canal.

The risk of malignancy for those with VIN I is small but is greater for women with high grade lesions. It can be difficult to differentiate clinically between the hypertrophic florid lesions sometimes seen with VIN III and an early invasive lesion. Multiple biopsies are required to exclude a malignancy. Opinion is divided as to whether excision of precancerous lesions or close surveillance should be undertaken. Recurrence is common after excision even when a vulvectomy has been undertaken. Thus conservative management of extensive recurrent lesions is often adopted unless symptoms are severe or there is a suspicion of invasion. Treatment with topical steroids often alleviate symptoms but does not affect the underlying pathology. Topical retinoids have also been used with limited success.

CARCINOMA OF THE VULVA

Carcinoma of the vulva is a rare condition with approximately 800 cases annually in the United Kingdom. Thus, a general practitioner may diagnose only one new case in his professional career. Squamous cell cancer accounts for 90% with the remainder composed of malignant melanoma, carcinoma of Bartholins gland and the very rare verrucous carcinomas.

Vulval carcinoma develops from a background of VIN in over two-thirds of cases. These invade locally initially but patients are often elderly and tend to present late when the disease may be more advanced. In countries where chronic inflammatory conditions such as lymphogranuloma inguinale and schistosomiasis may predispose to its development, it may affect younger women.

The tumour may appear as an ulcer but may also be exophytic or difficult to distinguish from extensive VIN III. A histological diagnosis is mandatory prior to planning the extent of surgical treatment as the appearances may be mimicked by condylomatous warts.

Local invasion predominates with relatively late spread to the regional lymph nodes situated in the groin. These comprise the nodes which lie on the inguinal ligament, the superficial femoral lymph nodes lying above the cribriform fascia and a deep group lying medial to the femoral artery and vein. For small laterally placed invasive cancers, the lymphatic drainage is likely to be confined to the regional nodes on the same side. For larger tumours and those that arise from midline structures such as the clitoris or perineum, bilateral spread is more common.

Staging of Vulval Cancer

The risk of spread to the regional lymph nodes is dependent on tumour grade, size of lesion, depth of invasion and presence of lymph-vascular space invasion. The risk of lymph node involvement is negligible if the depth of tumour invasion is less than 1 mm. Such tumours are termed microinvasive disease and radical, local excision with adequate margins is usually sufficient.

For frankly invasive lesions that fall outside this category, inguinal lymph node dissection is also required. A staging procedure under

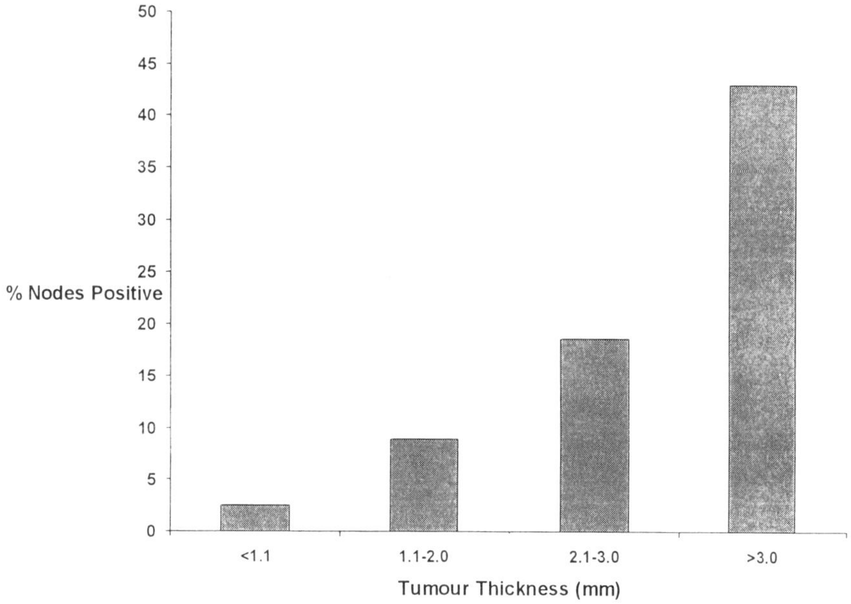

Fig. 26.1 *Effect of tumour thickness on risk of lymph node metastasis.*

Table 26.1
Staging of Carcinoma of the Vulva

Stage	Definition
I	Confined to vulva and/or perineum, 2 cm or less maximum diameter. Groin nodes are negative.
II	Confined to vulva and/or perineum, more than 2 cm maximum diameter. Groin nodes are negative.
III	Tumour of any size with any of the following: Adjacent spread to the lower urethra and/or vagina, or anus. Unilateral regional lymph node metastases.
IVa	Tumour invades any of the following: Upper urethra, bladder mucosa, rectal mucosa, pelvic bone. Bilateral regional lymph node metastases.
IVb	Any distant metastases including pelvic lymph nodes.

general anaesthetic is performed to assess the true extent of the disease and the involvement of surrounding structures. A full thickness biopsy is taken and the presence of any satellite lesions noted. A combined clinical and surgical staging system is now recommended by FIGO (1989) which includes histological information from regional lymph nodes and improves the prognostic value somewhat for such a system.

Treatment

The changing surgical treatment of vulval carcinoma demonstrates how with good case selection, treatment may be individualised to minimise complications and yet still adhere to the basic concepts of surgical treatment for malignant disease. Traditional management for vulval carcinoma was radical vulvectomy and bilateral en bloc dissection of the regional lymph nodes. This was accomplished via a butterfly type incision from the anterior superior iliac spine with radical wide excision of the vulva. Closure of the wide resection was difficult and often broke down completely. Long term psychological side effects were common from such a mutilating procedure although survival rates were good. The knowledge that regional lymph node metastases was by embolic spread rather than local invasion in the vast majority of cases meant that separate incisions to remove the groin nodes but leaving still a skin bridge in between would not compromise local control. In most patients with vulval carcinoma, the disease is unifocal and the remainder of the vulval skin is either unaffected or exhibits low grade VIN. Thus radical local excision of the lesion (ensuring good tumour margins even if this requires sacrifice of important structures such as the lower part of the urethra or clitoris) has largely replaced radical vulvectomy. For those patients with multifocal disease, radical vulvectomy is still appropriate however.

In those patients with small tumours that are laterally placed on the vulva, unilateral groin lymph dissection on the same side only is sufficient as long as these prove negative. With involvement of the ipsilateral nodes, the possibility of diversion of the lymph drainage to the contralateral side increases and these should be removed also.

The main complication from the operation remains, namely wound infection and breakdown, but this is less common and more easily managed with the modified technique. With the removal of the superficial and deep femoral lymph nodes that drain the leg and disruption of the lymph channels that return lymph to the pelvis, lymphocysts are common at the site of operation. These improve with conservative management but lymphoedema of the lower limbs may occur to varying degree and in rare cases can be very severe. This is particularly so in those patients that subsequently require radiotherapy. Selective lymph node dissection to minimise such side effects is currently under investigation by identification of a possible sentinel node to which the tumour cells spread preferentially and if this is negative, no further dissection is required. Until such studies are rigorously validated, systematic node dissection should be undertaken because recurrence in the groin nodes is almost invariably fatal.

Pelvic radiotherapy is indicated if more than two nodes are involved. Radiotherapy is sometimes used to shrink the tumour preoperatively so that surrounding essential structures may be spared and thus avoid the need for exenteration to achieve local control.

Outcome

When the disease is confined to the vulva with no regional lymph node metastases the 5-year survival is over 90%. With unilateral groin node metastases, this drops to 50–75% and this falls 30% when there is bilateral involvement.

With wide local excision preserving vulval issue, there is likely to be an increase in recurrent local disease. Further local excision gives approximately a 50% survival.

Groin recurrence is usually fatal. Such lesions are locally infiltrating causing severe distress and suffering to the patient over a protracted period prior to death. Thus although patients with vulval cancer are often elderly and frail, it is mandatory that such patients still receive full surgical treatment at the outset to gain local control and prevent such a disastrous situation arising.

Rare Forms of Vulval Cancers

Melanoma accounts for approximately 5% of vulval tumours and it occurs more frequently on the vulva than the skin area should suggest. For this reason and as exposure to sunlight is normally rare, excision of any pigmented lesion

Table 26.2
Results of Treatment

FIGO stage	Corrected 5-year survival (%)
I	98%
II	85%
III	46–74%
IV	31–50%

on the vulva should be considered. The usual appearance is often an enlarging mole although amelanotic forms may occur. Beyond the critical depth of 0.7 mm, the risk of spread to lymph nodes is considerable. Unfortunately, this has already occurred in almost one-third of patients at presentation. Treatment requires wide local excision with margins of 3–5 cm. By contrast, management of the regional lymph nodes is expectant with excision only when clinically involved. Outcome is poor with 5-year survival rates in those who are node negative of 50% falling to only 10–15% in those who are found to be node positive.

Verrucous carcinoma is a rare very slow growing neoplasm which resembles condilomata accuminata macroscopically and histologically. Basal cell carcinomas may also be found on the vulva. Wide local excision is usually sufficient in such cases as risk of lymph node metastases is low. Bartholins gland carcinomas are equally often adenocarcinomas and squamous cell carcinoma. Due to their location deep within the skin, they tend to arise more deeply with frequent local invasion and lymph node spread at diagnosis. These should be distinguished from adenoid cystic carcinomas (similar to salivary gland tumours) which are locally invasive but have a low risk of distant spread. Both have a poor prognosis.

27

Diseases of the Cervix

PHYSIOLOGY AND HISTOLOGY OF THE CERVIX

The cervix uteri is a cylindrical structure composed of fibromuscular tissue and is continuous with the corpus or body of the uterus. It is lined internally by delicate columnar epithelium and glandular tissue, which produces mucus dependent on the phase of the menstrual cycle. The external surface of the cervix or ectocervix is covered by squamous epithelium, which is relatively resistant to trauma and continuous with the vaginal epithelium. The external entrance to the cervix leading into the endocervical canal is termed the external os, which in those who are nulliparous, is circular but following childbirth remains as a horizontal slit. The site where the squamous and columnar cells meet is termed the squamocolumnar junction. This is variable in position and may lie on the external surface of the cervix or hidden from view in the endocervical canal. At menarche, the cervix grows and everts so that the endocervical epithelium is exposed on the ectocervix. The endocervical epithelium is 'transformed' gradually into squamous epithelium by a process of squamous metaplasia spreading inwards towards the cervical os from the squamocolumnar junction. This area is known as the transformation zone. When the process of squamous metaplasia is deranged, premalignant and malignant disease of the cervix develops.

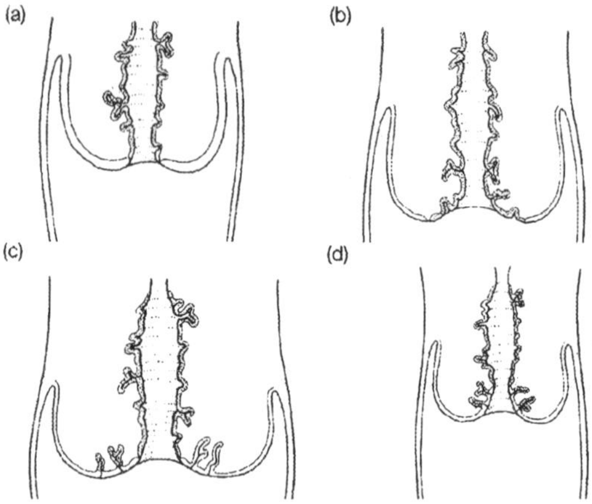

Fig. 27.1 *The changes that take place during a woman's life.* ***(a)*** *The small prepubertal ectocervix is covered by squamous epithelium and the squamocolumnar junction lies at the external os.* ***(b)*** *After menarche, during pregnancy or while taking the oral contraceptive pill, the cervix grows and everts, exposing columnar epithelium on the ectocervix.* ***(c)*** *The exposed columnar epithelium undergoes metaplasia to squamous epithelium until the squamocolumnar junction is at the external os again.* ***(d)*** *After the menopause or when oestrogen levels fall, the cervix shrinks and the squamocolumnar junction is drawn into the endocervical canal.*

BENIGN DISEASE

Cervical Ectopy

This condition is also called a cervical ectropion or erosion. The term erosion is particularly inappropriate because it implies wrongly that the condition is abnormal. Ectopy arises when the thin endocervical epithelium is exposed on the ectocervix as described above (Fig. 27.1(b)). The blood vessels beneath this thin epithelial covering can be seen easily so the cervix appears red and inflamed.

Ectopy is usually not responsible for any symptoms but some patients present with postcoital bleeding or excessive vaginal discharge. An ectopy may bleed when a cervical smear is taken. More often, the ectopy is wrongly blamed for symptoms. A cervical ectopy will regress eventually. The alarming appearance may give rise to concern about malignancy but a cervix with an erosion feels rubbery while one with a cancer feels hard. Colposcopy is appropriate only if malignancy is suspected. Explanation and reassurance should normally suffice. Treatment by cautery, cryotherapy or large loop excision of the transformation zone (LLETZ) may be undertaken but is often unsuccessful and should be avoided unless symptoms are very distressing. The cervix should not be treated without prior colposcopy.

Nabothian Cysts

These are cystic structures on the cervix formed from gland crypts that have been blocked off and have filled up with mucus. They vary greatly in size and may distort the cervix very substantially. They are often yellowish in colour, especially when near the surface. The only relevance of these retention cysts is that they may make the cervix look very abnormal as they distort the surface and often have quite large blood vessels running over their surface. The feature of these vessels that distinguishes them from vessels on a cancer is that they branch like the roots of a plant, each tributary being smaller than the vessel from which it arises.

Cervical Polyps

Cervical polyps are benign polypoid growths usually of endocervical epithelium. They may cause postcoital bleeding but are usually asymptomatic. They nearly always have a narrow stalk and can be removed in the clinic without anaesthesia simply by twisting the polyp gently through several complete revolutions on the stalk until it falls off. It used to be said that curettage of the endocervix and the endometrium was necessary to remove any polyps in these locations. That is no longer done because it turned out nearly always to have been a fruitless exercise. Occasionally a cervical polyp is a fibroid. If the stalk is thick, it is safer to remove this in theatre in case of bleeding.

Sometimes, a polyp which appears to be growing on the cervix is actually intrauterine in origin and has been extruded through the cervix. Most commonly, these are fibroids, but in older women a malignant mixed Mullerian tumour may present in this way.

Infection of the Cervix

The cervix is remarkably resistant to infection but both chlamydia and the gonococcus can infect the cervix. Such patients may present with pelvic pain, dyspareunia, offensive discharge and postcoital bleeding. However there may be no symptoms and the diagnosis may only be reached as a result of contact tracing, or investigations as a result of infertility. The diagnosis is made by a lower genital tract infection screen including endocervical swabs placed in special transport media to help isolate chlamydia. Chlamydia are difficult to identify and a positive result does not always indicate an active infection. Treatment should be given where there is any doubt because of the risk of chronic pelvic inflammatory disease developing.

Chronic cervicitis is a much overdiagnosed condition. Rarely, it may follow an incompletely treated acute infection but usually no organisms are isolated. The patient complains of dyspareunia and excessive discharge. The cervix appears red and is tender on palpation. Symptoms are seldom alleviated by cervical diathermy.

Cervical warts may result from infection with human papillomavirus, typically types 6 and 12, although high risk types are also found. Most warts normally regress spontaneously with time but may be spread by sexual contact and patients may opt for treatment with cryotherapy, local application of liquid nitrogen, laser or diathermy ablation. Recurrence after such a treatment is common. A cervical smear should be performed and a lower genital tract infection screen to exclude preinvasive changes and coexistent sexually transmitted infections.

The Epstein Barr virus also grows commonly in the cervix. It causes no symptoms and its only relevance is that it is often responsible for the viral changes reported in cervical smears.

PREMALIGNANT DISEASE OF THE CERVIX

Squamous cell carcinoma of the cervix develops through a series of premalignant stages termed cervical intraepithelial neoplasia (CIN). With the advent of sensitive molecular biological techniques, human papillomavirus (HPV) has been found in almost all cases of squamous cell carcinoma of the cervix and in most patients with CIN. To date, over 100 subtypes of HPV have been isolated but only certain subtypes notably 16,18, 31 and 33 are associated with cervical neoplasia. HPV infection is very common indeed, with at least 60% of young women becoming infected by the end of 3 years. The vast majority of infected women do not develop precancerous changes and most clear the virus from the cervical epithelium within a year. HPV tends to gain entry at the transformation zone and may initially escape immune surveillance by remaining above the basement membrane. HPV is a DNA virus and the nuclear sequences from high risk subtypes become integrated into the host cell genome and cause the cell to be immortalised. Malignant transformation results from exposure to other carcinogenic agents and the cumulative genetic mutations that would normally lead to programmed cell death.

The Cervical Screening Programme

Progression from CIN to an invasive cancer may take 10–15 years. To be suitable for screening, a disease should be relatively common, ideally with a known natural history including an identifiable precancerous stage and cause significant morbidity and mortality if unrecognised. In addition, a treatment should be available that will have an impact on outcome. The test used should be acceptable to women, cost-effective and of high specificity and sensitivity. Cervical cancer is therefore suitable for a screening programme. This forms the rationale for the development of the national comprehensive cervical cytological screening programme implemented in 1988.

Under the current national screening guidelines, a cervical smear is recommended for all women between the ages of 20 to 65 years at 3- to 5-yearly intervals. Although annual smear tests have been proposed, this would be very much more expensive and not much more effective.

A cervical smear test requires the use of a cell sampling device to transfer cells from the transformation zone of the cervix where most abnormalities are located onto a microscope slide. A Papanicolaou stain is used to highlight abnormal cells (hence the alternative name of 'Pap smear'). The sampling device traditionally used is an Ayre's or Aylesbury wooden spatula but brush devices have been introduced to sample the endocervical canal.

Limitations of such a programme include incomplete or inadequate sampling of the cervix, poor transfer or fixation of exfoliated cells and difficulty with the correct interpretation of cellular abnormalities presented. It is thought to take 10 to 15 years for CIN to become invasive. Therefore, although a cervical smear may correctly identify the presence of an abnormality in only 75% of cases, given the length of premalignant stage, it is likely that subsequent cervical smears would correctly identify CIN before it has progressed to invasive disease. The success of such programmes is now undoubted

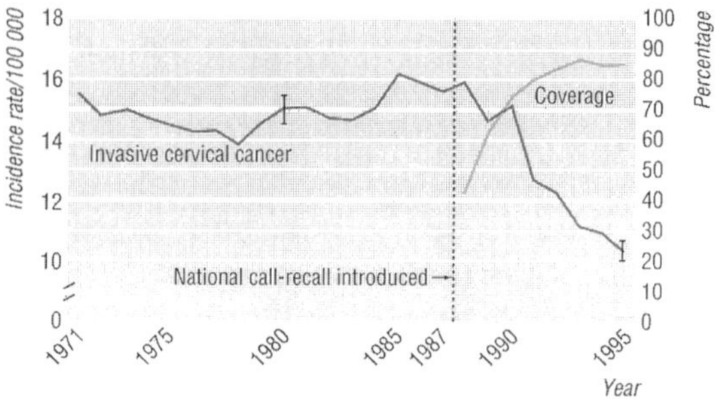

Fig. 27.2 *The incidence of invasive cancer has fallen as the coverage of the target population has increased (Quinn et al., 1999).*

and has resulted in the fall in the annual incidence of cervical cancer from approximately 16/100,000 women prior to the introduction of systematic a call and recall programme to currents rates of just over 10/100,000. Different primary screening methods are currently under evaluation including liquid based cytology and quantitative HPV testing.

CIN is normally asymptomatic and is usually identified following a cervical smear which demonstrates abnormalities of cervical cells. Normal cervical epithelium is characterised by an ordered maturation of plump parabasal cells near the basement membrane to superficial thin desquamated squamous cells with small inactive nuclei that are present throughout a normal cervical smear. Precancerous changes recognised on cervical smear include nuclear abnormalities, increased mitotic activity and disordered maturation such that cells with large nuclei that have failed to fully differentiate have reached the surface and are present on the cervical smear. As cervical smears report abnormalities in cells rather than histological tissue, the term dyskaryosis is used and are graded as mild, moderate or severe depending on the degree of abnormality present. Following the finding of dyskaryotic cervical cells, further investigation is recommended by colposcopy.

Colposcopy

A colposcope is a low power microscope typically of ×10–×40 magnification, which can be used to examine the surface of the cervix. Acetic acid (which highlights abnormalities as white) is used to aid identification of precancerous changes. A biopsy of this area is then commonly taken to provide a histological diagnosis.

As stated earlier, a cervical smear is a cytological specimen and therefore reported in terms of dyskaryosis, whereas a biopsy is a histological specimen and is normally reported as grades of cervical intraepithelial neoplasia. Such a term is slightly misleading in that the cells may have features of a malignancy, but the presence of an intact basement membrane means that the lesion is confined to the epithelial layers and therefore not truly invasive. CIN is normally graded as I (low grade), II and III (high or severe grade). There is some correlation between cytological findings and those of the histological biopsy but the terminology should not be regarded as interchangeable.

Natural History of CIN

There is a peak incidence of CIN between the ages of 25 to 35 and subsequently an increase in the numbers of invasive cancer 10 to 15 years later. The vast majority of patients who develop CIN however do not progress to cervical carcinoma, and many patients who have CIN I do not develop higher grades of CIN. Spontaneous resolution of low grade abnormalities may occur in as many as 50% of women over 2 years. Nonetheless, there is at least a 30% chance of CIN III progressing to invasive disease over a 20-year period.

Treatment

A colposcopic assessment must always be performed prior to treatment to confirm the diagnosis of CIN and to exclude a frankly invasive lesion. Opinion is divided regarding the need to treat CIN I at the outset or whether observation in the hope of spontaneous resolution over a number of years should be favoured.

There are a variety of treatment options available for the treatment of CIN which can be divided into excisional or ablative methods. The choice of treatment is largely governed by extent of disease and personal preference, but the aim is to remove the extent of CIN and the transformation zone to a depth of at least 7 mm (as CIN may occur in crypts and glands to this level). Over recent years, there has been a change in policy from the widespread use of a knife cone biopsy under general anaesthetic to cone biopsies which may be accomplished under local anaesthetic using electrodiathermy such as LLETZ (large loop excision of the transformation zone), NETZ (needle excision of the transformation zone) or laser. Ablative methods whereby the cells are destroyed by heat ('cold coagulation' at temperatures of

120°C, radical diathermy at much higher temperatures), cold (cryotherapy), or laser are now less popular and have the disadvantage of not providing a histological specimen to confirm grade of abnormality and completeness of excision margins.

Glandular Abnormalities of the Cervix

Glandular cells in the cervix can show dyskaryotic changes in the same way as squamous cells. These are described as cervical glandular neoplasia (CGIN) and high grade changes are also known as adenocarcinoma *in situ* (AIS). Pure glandular abnormalities are rare and often coexistent with squamous abnormalities. Much less is known about the natural history of glandular lesions and although such lesions are sometimes picked up by the national cervical smear programme, this is often fortuitous. The screening programme has far less effect on adenocarcinoma than on squamous cell carcinoma.

Glandular abnormalities cannot be detected reliably by colposcopy. Glandular lesions may occur throughout the endocervical canal but are usually close to the transformation zone. Treatment by the cone biopsy techniques used for treatment of squamous lesions often results in incomplete excision, and further surgery is often required, especially in older women. Careful long term follow-up with endocervical smears is essential even when the lesion appears to have been removed completely.

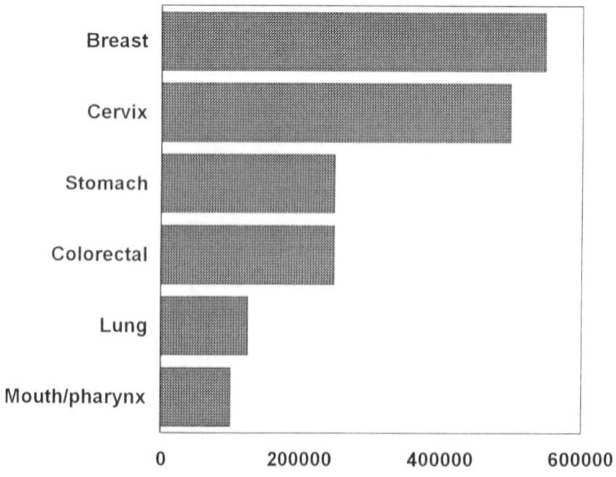

Fig. 27.3 *Estimated numbers of cases worldwide in 1975.*

CARCINOMA OF THE CERVIX

Cervical cancer is the second most common gynaecological cancer in the United Kingdom with almost 4000 cases annually. Thus it remains uncommon in comparison to breast, lung and colon cancer. However, it is more common than breast cancer in many developing countries and is still a major health problem worldwide with 500,000 cases annually. A large proportion of women with cervical cancer are young women.

Most cervical cancers arise near the transformation zone with 80% occurring on the ectocervix and the remainder in the endocervical canal. They may be exophytic, appearing as a cauliflower-type lesion or endophytic, causing an ulcer. If present in the endocervix, they may be invisible but expand the mid cervix to form a characteristically, hard, barrel-shaped cervix.

Eighty-five per cent of tumours are of squamous origin with the remainder adenocarcinoma or adenosquamous carcinoma. Adenocarcinomas are relatively more common in patients who are 35 to 45 years old where they may account for 30% of cases. In this age group, a marked relative rise in incidence has been seen over the past 20 years, probably because of more effective prevention of squamous cell lesions.

Aetiological Factors

Human papillomavirus has been implicated in the development of cervical intraepithelial neoplasia and cervical carcinoma. Other factors that have been shown to be associated with cervical cancer include behavioural factors such as smoking, number of sexual partners and age of first sexual intercourse. Such factors are often interrelated and can be correlated with social class. It should not be forgotten that these factors increase the risk only relatively. Most women who develop cervical cancer do not have any of these characteristics. Unfortunately many of the women who are at high risk of cervix cancer are those who default from the national screening programme and only present when symptomatic with advanced disease. Patients who are immunosuppressed, either by disease such as AIDS or pharmacologically such as after renal transplantation, are more at risk of CIN and progression to invasion.

Spread

Cervical cancer invades locally initially into the body of the uterus or to the vagina. Lateral spread is into the parametrium that in advanced disease may obstruct the ureter and become fixed to the pelvic side wall. In such cases, patients can present with obstructive renal failure. Occasionally, direct infiltration of the bladder and rectum can lead to fistula formation.

Spread may also occur via the lymphatic system to the pelvic lymph nodes that lie along the iliac blood vessels and then to the paraaortic nodes. Intractable leg and buttock pain may result from involvement of pelvic side wall nodes and infiltration of the sacral plexus. Scalene node metastases may be present in the neck. Blood borne metastases also occur to the lungs or brain.

Symptoms

Almost 50% of patients with cervical carcinoma are detected as a result of the cervical screening programme and therefore are asymptomatic. Although this represents a relative failure of the screening system to detect preinvasive disease, such cancers are often very early and have a good prognosis with the possibility of treatment by cone biopsy only. Although the cervical cancer screening programme is not designed to diagnose glandular lesions, the majority of screen detected adenocarcinomas are confined to the cervix.

Patients who present symptomatically have a worse prognosis as the tumour is often more advanced. The most common presenting symptom is irregular vaginal bleeding often with intermenstrual and postcoital bleeding.

Detection and Assessment

On examination of the cervix, a cancer may be obvious but sometimes the cancer is very small, hidden from view in the endocervical canal or is confused with inflammatory changes. Occasionally, the diagnosis is only apparent after histological examination of a cone biopsy performed for presumed CIN.

In the UK, the most common presentation is that of a macroscopic tumour apparently confined to the cervix. The most likely location of metastatic disease is in the pelvic lymph nodes, although early parametrial spread is often undetected. Tumour size is of prognostic significance but the grade of tumour is also important. Poorly differentiated tumours that invade the lymphvascular spaces are more likely to involve the pelvic lymph nodes. Therefore even apparent small primary cancers may have distant spread at the time of diagnosis.

The current staging system adopted by FIGO (International Federation of Obstetrics and Gynecology) is based on clinical findings typically performed by formal examination under anaesthesia (EUA) and cystoscopy. Standard investigations such as chest X-ray and IVP (to diagnose ureteric obstruction) that are routinely available may influence stage, but in order to allow uniformity of staging procedures for all health care systems, CT or MRI findings should not be incorporated. Many patients are treated by radiotherapy and therefore findings from surgical treatment should not change the stage.

Recent modifications to include tumour size in the classification for stage I disease were introduced in 1995 but lymph node involvement which remains the major prognostic indicator is not included. The current FIGO system is shown in Table 27.1.

Treatment

The treatment of carcinoma of the cervix is governed to a large extent by the stage of

Table 27.1
FIGO Staging System for Cervical Cancer 1999

FIGO stage	Definition
I	Carcinoma confined to the cervix/corpus.
IA	Invasive carcinoma diagnosed microscopically with maximal stromal invasion of less than 5 mm and maximum transverse diameter of less than 7 mm.
IA1	Microscopic invasive carcinoma with a depth of invasion of less than 3 mm and transverse diameter less than 7 mm.
IA2	Microscopic invasive carcinoma with a depth of invasion between 3 and 5 mm and maximum transverse diameter less than 7 mm.
IB	Clinically evident lesions confined to the cervix and microscopically diagnosed lesions falling outside the above criteria.
IB1	Carcinoma less than 4 cm in size.
IB2	Carcinomas greater than 4 cm.
II	Extension beyond the uterus but not to the pelvic side wall or to the lower third of the vagina.
IIA	Vaginal involvement but no obvious parametrial invasion.
IIB	Obvious parametrial invasion.
III	Extend to the pelvic wall and/or involves lower third of the vagina and/or causes hydronephrosis or non-functioning kidney.
IIIA	Extension to lower third of vagina; no extension to the pelvic wall.
IIIB	Extension to pelvic wall and/or causes hydroneprosis or non-functioning kidney.
IV	Extension beyond the true pelvis or has clinically involved the mucosa of the bladder or rectum.
IVA	Involvement of the mucosa of the bladder or rectum.
IVB	Distant metastases.

disease at presentation. For early stage disease (Ia), surgery is the preferred option whereas for those with locally advanced disease (IIb or greater), chemoradiotherapy is the treatment of choice. For patients with stage Ib carcinoma, either treatment may be used, and therefore the patients age, medical health and personal preferences may govern treatment method.

Surgery

For very early disease (Ia1), a large cervical cone biopsy with clear margins is adequate treatment. In those with stage Ia2 to Ib2 disease, a radical hysterectomy and pelvic lymph node dissection is required. This is also known as a Wertheim hysterectomy after the description by E. Wertheim from Vienna in 1905. The addition of pelvic lymphadenectomy to this procedure was advocated later by J. Meigs from Boston who gives his name to the operation in the US.

The operation involves removal of the cervix and body of the uterus together with the parametrium, upper third of vagina and part of the supporting cardinal and uterosacral supporting ligaments of the uterus. The pelvic lymph node tissue lying along the external, internal and common iliac vessels and in the obturator fossa is removed. Rarely, paraaortic node dissection is indicated. To achieve a radical central dissection, it is necessary to mobilise the ureters which run close to the cervix in the parametrial tissue.

Complications may rarely include ureteric obstruction or fistulae between ureters or bladder and the vagina. More commonly, because of disruption of the autonomic nerve supply to the bladder and rectum that occurs when the uterosacral ligaments are divided widely, loss of bladder and rectal sensation lead to incomplete emptying of bladder and bowel. This is the main reason for leaving an indwelling catheter in the bladder after the operation for several days. In most women, bladder function returns sufficiently to normal for the catheter to be removed after 7 to 10 days but some will require to empty the bladder with a catheter for several weeks or, in rare cases, several months. Even among those who are not dependant upon a catheter, many will remain aware of reduced bladder sensation for several years. In some, this is permanent. Analagous problems with the rectum and constipation occur with similar frequency.

The advantages of surgery include preservation of ovarian function and a much lower rate of dyspareunia than is seen following radiotherapy. Surgery also provides additional prognostic information from lymph node dissection, and retains the option of radiotherapy for the treatment of recurrent disease.

With carcinoma of the cervix becoming relatively more common in younger women and the increasing age of childbearing for social reasons in modern societies, it is not unusual for nulliparous women to present with invasive disease. If the tumour is small and apparently confined to the ectocervix, a radical excision of the cervix including the parametria and uterosacral ligaments termed a radical trachelectomy may be appropriate. A cervical suture is placed at the level of the internal cervical os to ensure cervical competence. This preserves the body of the uterus and patients have undergone successful pregnancies with delivery by caesarean section. The pelvic lymph nodes are also removed either by transperitoneal laparoscopic or an extraperitoneal approach. Only a limited number of such cases has been reported with relatively short follow-up so the efficacy of this new operation remains unknown. Radical hysterectomy remains the gold standard treatment for such cases.

Cancer of the cervix can sometimes present during pregnancy. If the pregnancy is early, then termination prior to curative treatment or prompt delivery of the baby if near term is recommended. However, if the diagnosis is reached at a time when the fetus is approaching viability or still at severe risk from the complications of extreme prematurity, then the patient needs to be carefully counselled with regards to her options of continuing with the pregnancy. There is no evidence that stage for stage cervical cancer in pregnancy has a worse prognosis, but delay may allow progression of the disease which doubles in volume every 7 weeks on average.

Radiotherapy

Traditionally this has been the treatment of choice for disease beyond the cervix and uterus, and in those who are elderly where the complications of vaginal stenosis and ovarian irradiation may be less relevant.

There are a number of different methods of utilising radiotherapy but the standard principles of delivering a lethal central and sidewall dose remain similar. The treatment is usually begun with external beam radiotherapy (teletherapy) to the whole pelvis. This is then followed by a high local dose of radiation given by intracavitary therapy (brachytherapy).

The whole pelvis is treated by external beam radiotherapy which is given in a number of small doses to reduce damage to surrounding normal tissues. The total dose is usually 50 to 60 Gy given in 30 to 35 daily fractions. The volume to be treated is defined by CT and tiny tattoo marks are placed on the patient's abdomen to align each treatment precisely with laser beams. Each treatment is usually given to 3 or 4 fields with radiation being delivered from front and back and from each side in order to achieve the highest possible dose in the tumour with the least amount of radiation to normal tissues. Each field is irradiated for only 1 to 2 minutes but the whole process takes 15 to 20 minutes as the linear accelerator delivering the treatment is positioned carefully for each field.

Brachytherapy involves the placement of a hollow delivery rod system into the lateral vaginal fornices and cervical canal. Radioactive sources are then driven up the hollow tubes into the cervix and vagina where they are left for a calculated time period to deliver a carefully calculated radioactive dose to the cervical tumour. In the Manchester and other similar techniques, treatment is planned to administer a set dose to point A, which lies 2 cm lateral to the midline and 2 cm above the vaginal fornix. Radioactive dose falls rapidly as the distance from the source increases. The radioactive sources are placed inside the tubes in a way that creates a treatment field that minimises the radioactive dose to the surrounding normal tissues such as the bladder and rectum. Thus an inverted pear-shaped field is used to cover the cervix, the upper vagina, parametria and uterosacral ligaments for the majority of cases. Formerly, implants were inserted in sealed applicators at the time of placement of the rods. This exposed staff to radioactivity and, when caesium or radium were used, treatment took 48 to 60 hours. With remote afterloading instruments and use of radiocobalt, radioactive material is kept in a shielded store until the patient is isolated and then loaded into the applicator. With high intensity radioactive sources, treatment may be limited to less than 1 hour. Medium intensity sources require longer treatment times.

After the first week of radiotherapy, most women begin to feel nauseated. Diarrhoea and fatigue are common. There is considerable variation between individuals in their sensitivity to radiotherapy. If an individual's maximum tolerable dose to normal tissues is exceeded, severe cystitis, colitis or proctitis may develop. These usually do not become apparent for 12 to 18 months. Radiation damage to the small bowel is less common but more serious. The risk of these complications is increased by previous surgery which may previously have resulted in adhesions. In some cases, fistulae develop.

Chemoradiotherapy

Recent research has shown that survival is improved when chemotherapy is given concomitantly with radiotherapy. The usual agent is cisplatin which probably acts as a sensitising agent making the cancer cells more susceptible to radiation. The chemotherapy regimens vary but the simplest is a weekly dose of cisplatin throughout conventional radiotherapy treatment. The side effects are more severe than with radiotherapy alone and may not be suitable for all patients especially those who are elderly or very frail.

Prognostic Factors

The stage at presentation affects outcome with those patients presenting with early stage Ia disease having a 95% 5-year survival, compared with 60% for stage II disease, 30% for stage III and 10% for stage IV. The largest group of patients present with stage Ib disease. Overall they have a 5-year survival of 80%, but this is a diverse group varying from those with small tumours of less than 1 cm diameter confined to the cervix to those with very large tumours of 8 cm or more that may invade throughout the body of the uterus. Other factors that influence outcome are the grade of tumour and the presence of lymph-vascular space invasion, both of which are related to the presence of lymph node metastases. Thus although the overall survival for stage Ib cervical cancer is 80%, this ranges from 95% in those who are node negative with small central tumours, to 50% in those with high risk central disease and positive lymph nodes.

In those patients who are found to have widespread metastatic cancer in the pelvic lymph nodes or incomplete excision of the central cancer, adjuvant radiotherapy may be advised. This may improve local control of the cancer, but the side effects are much increased following radical surgery, as bowel and bladder may be adherent to the pelvic side wall and the survival is probably not improved.

Recurrence of cervical cancer is most common within the pelvis but lung, brain or extrapelvic lymph nodes may be involved. Approximately 50% of recurrences occur within the first year with 80% by 2 years. Once recurrence is detected, the outlook is poor with subsequent 5-year survival rates of only 10%. If radiotherapy had not been used previously, then this may be a treatment option but normal structures are not able to withstand a second curative dose of radiotherapy. Recurrences on the pelvic side wall are generally thought to be inoperable but if an isolated mobile central recurrence occurs or patients have persistent central disease following chemoradiotherapy, surgical treatment by pelvic exenteration is potentially curative in 30% of carefully selected patients. Such an operation typically involves the en-bloc removal of the bladder, vagina, uterus and rectum with the formation of a colostomy and a urostomy to divert the urine. Occasionally, an anterior exenteration preserving the rectum or posterior exenteration preserving the bladder may be possible depending on the site of recurrence. Exenterative procedures are significant surgical undertakings with major changes in body image and sexuality, and are only appropriate after counselling, psychological assessment and as a potentially curative procedure.

Palliative Treatment

Patients may present with incurable disease or following recurrence are found not to be suitable for further curative treatment. Such patients may still benefit from supportive treatment to minimise symptoms as the cancer progresses. One of the aims of treatment for cervical cancer is to achieve local control of the cancer in the pelvis. Untreated cervical cancer is locally invasive and distressing symptoms may result from vesicovaginal and rectovaginal fistulae. Pain from vertebral bone metastases and involvement of the sacral nerves may be difficult to control by analgesic drugs and sometimes require surgical or chemical nerve ablation using phenol.

Death often results from renal failure as a result of ureteric obstruction. The temptation to alleviate this by nephrostomy or stenting of the ureters should be avoided in women with recurrent disease as it is only delaying the inevitable for a short time and substitutes an unpleasant, painful death for what would otherwise be a peaceful demise.

Patients should be managed by a multidisciplinary team which should include a palliative care consultant, and pain management team liaising with the primary care services and general practitioner. This should ensure that their physical symptoms and psychological needs are addressed and controlled to help maintain quality of life for as long as possible despite relatively advanced local disease.

28

Ovarian Pathology — Benign and Malignant

BENIGN OVARIAN TUMOURS

The ovary is composed of epithelial cells derived from coelomic epithelium, oocytes, which have differentiated from primitive germ cells and medullary and mesenchymal elements. With such embryological cell lines being represented in the ovary, it is hardly surprising that no other organ in the body produces such a number and diversity of tumours. Classification is therefore difficult.

Functional Cysts

Atretic cysts

When the graffian follicle or corpus luteum are undergoing natural degeneration they may become cystic. The cysts are small, often multiple and lined by granulosa cells, granulos lutein cells, theca lutein cells or connective and hyaline tissue. Such cysts are invariably symptomless.

Distention or retention cysts

Cystic enlargement of a normal ovarian component is so common as to be considered physiological. It is of no pathological significance, although if complicated by intracystic haemorrhage, the resultant tarry contents may be confused with endometriosis.

Follicular and theca lutein cysts

These cysts represent enlargements of unruptured graffian follicles. The ovum degenerates, but the granulose and thecal cells continue to secrete fluid. They rarely exceed 5 cm in size, are occasionally multiple and usually symptomless. Where granulose cells predominate, enough oestrogen may be produced to cause menorrhagia. When oestrogen or progesterone production is continuous, short periods of amenorrhoea occur. Repeated cyst formation may cause iliac fossa pain. Treatment is rarely required. The cysts often rupture spontaneously. Recurrent follicular cystic development can be suppressed by inhibiting ovulation with an oral contraceptive.

Corpus luteal cysts

A normal corpus luteum may become cystic, especially after haemorrhage into its cavity. Quite a large cyst can arise in the corpus luteum of pregnancy. Occasionally, the corpus luteum becomes cystic and continues to produce progesterone. This causes short spells of amenorrhoea followed by heavier than usual menstruation, thus mimicking early spontaneous abortion or ectopic pregnancy.

Compound lutein cysts

In the presence of trophoblastic disease, large multiple lutein cysts may arise in both ovaries. The excessive luteinisation is directly due to the production of human chorionic gonadotrophin (HCG) by the trophoblastic tissue. Once this tissue is removed, the hormonal stimulus disappears and the ovaries return to normal.

Solid luteoma of pregnancy

Solid foci, usually multiple, of luteal tissue may be found in the ovaries during pregnancy. They are caused by HCG stimulating theca or stromal cells. They are separatc from the corpus luteum and may be up to 10 cm in diameter. Usually symptomless they are found incidentally at caesarean section or laparotomy.

Benign Ovarian Pathology

Surface papilloma

This is a small, often multiple pedunculated surface growth with a marked connective tissue core. It is usually an incidental finding at laparotomy.

Mucinous or pseudomucinous cystadenoma

This is the most common primary tumour of the ovary, accounting for 30–40% of ovarian tumours (Fig. 28.1). It is unilateral in 90% of cases. Although its growth is slow, it may attain huge proportions. It is a multilocular cyst usually with a smooth, thick, fibrous wall. The lining membrane of the loculi is composed of tall, columnar, mucin secreting cells with darkly staining nuclei situated near their base. Rarely, papillary ingrowths are present within the cyst and may reflect malignant degeneration to an adenocarcinoma, which occurs in 5–10% of cases. The fluid within the cyst is mucinous, usually colourless and of variable consistency, containing a glycoprotein related to mucin. Although large in size, the cyst generally remains without adhesions and so can be removed without difficulty. A rare complication of a cyst which ruptures and leaks its contents into the peritoneal cavity is pseudomyxoma peritonei. Cells from within the cyst implant in the parietal and visceral peritoneum and omentum and continue to secrete mucin. Multiple adhesions form enclosing large masses of gelatinous material in all parts of the abdominal cavity. Even after removal at laparotomy, these gelatinous loculi tend to reform and the patient usually dies from cachexia after several operations. The condition may also occur after mucocoele of the appendix.

Serous cystadenoma (Fig. 28.2)

This cyst accounts for approximately 10% of ovarian tumours. It is usually smaller than the mucinous tumours and is bilateral in 30–50% of cases. The outer surface is commonly smooth and thin-walled and the entire cyst is unilocular. The contents are watery, and colourless, unless contaminated by blood pigments. The inner surface of the cyst wall nearly always contains papilliferous projections, often warty or cauliflower-like in appearance. These papillae range in number, being few and localised to one area, or fill the entire cyst, giving it a solid appearance, with all the gradations in between. These papillae may occur on the outer surface and cause ascites. Although such a cyst may

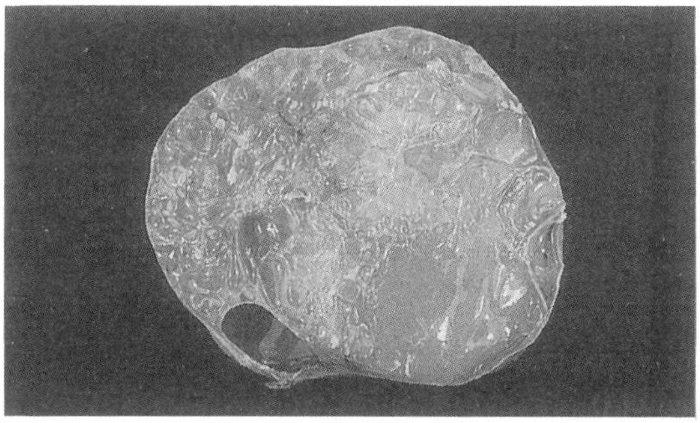

Fig. 28.1 *Benign mucinous multilocular cystadenoma. Small cystic spaces are present and some contain thick, glairy mucus.*

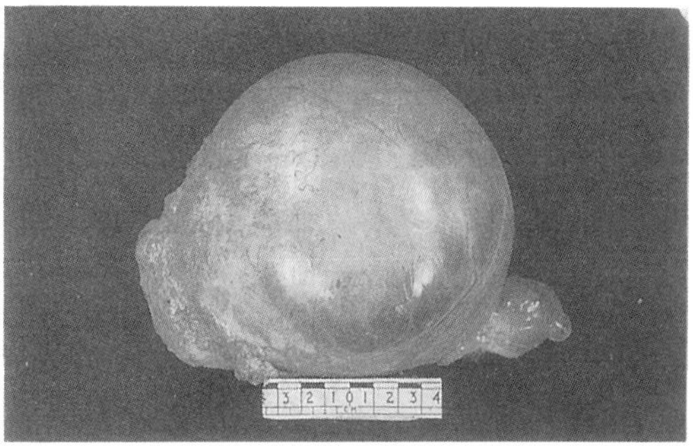

Fig. 28.2 *Benign serous cystadenoma of moderate size. Smooth outer surface with thin walls. The fallopian tube is stretched over the cyst.*

look malignant, the majority are histologically benign.

The lining cells are cuboidal or columnar and may be ciliated resembling the epithelium of the fallopian tube. Often small deposits of calcium are present in the stroma and are known as psammoma bodies. The epithelium may range from a well differentiated benign pattern to the marked atypia and anaplasia of malignancy. In those cysts where the epithelium adopts a more intermediate pattern, it can be difficult to allot the tumour into a benign or malignant category.

Fibroma

This tumour accounts for up to 5% of ovarian neoplasms. It is slow growing and rarely exceeds 12 cm in diameter. Usually spherical or ovoid in shape, it can be lobulated and is mobile. It is solid and hard, and its cut surface is white and whorled. It is bilateral in up to 10% of cases. It may replace the entire ovary or exist as a small surface nodule.

Histologically, it is composed of spindle cells of fibroblastic character. Plain muscle cells may or may not be present, but the tumour behaves in a similar fashion to a uterine fibroid. Hyaline change is common and most large fibromas show cystic changes caused by central necrosis due to inadequate blood supply. A fibroma of the ovary may cause ascites in 20% of cases. Often associated is hydrothorax which is usually right-sided. Meig's syndrome is the triad of ovarian fibroma, ascites and hydrothorax. The origin of the fluid is ariously ascribed to exudates resulting from irritation of the peritoneum by the tumour or an active secretion by the tumour.

Removal of the fibroma results in the spontaneous cure of the ascites and the hydrothorax. The findings always cause concern as they impart a clinical impression of malignancy.

Adenofibroma

This is often a small fibropapillary nodule occurring on the surface of the ovary. It is solid and behaves similarly to the fibroma. Histologically, it contains both fibromatous and glandular tissues.

Benign cystic teratoma or dermoid cyst

These tumours are unique in that all three embryological layers — ectoderm, mesoderm and endoderm — may be represented. They probably arise from varied differentiation of totipotent cells within the ovary. Some suggest that they may arise from parthenogenesis, where an ovum is stimulated to make a disorderly attempt to produce an embryo without first being fertilised.

Dermoid cysts account for 10–15% of ovarian tumours. They tend to occur at a relatively early age (18–30 years), and are usually symptomless. They are bilateral in 10% of cases. They rarely grow bigger than 12 cm in diameter and are usually unilocular with a thick, smooth capsule. They contain a thick, yellow, greasy, sebaceous fluid secreted by the glands within the tumour wall.

Histologically, the lining epithelium is a typically stratified squamous-like skin and contains the normal integuments of hair, sebaceous and sweat glands. Teeth and central nervous system components are not unusual and cartilage and gastrointestinal epithelium may be present. There is generally a nodal point in the cyst wall around which these tissues are distributed.

Although cystic teratomata are predominantly ectodermal in character, this is not always so, especially in the more solid variety. For example, when thyroid tissue predominates the cyst is called struma ovarii, and the glandular epithelium may be functional, capable of causing clinical hyperthyroidism. When other specialised tissues predominate, the cyst may be suffixed lipoma, myoma, chondroma or osteoma. Once a teratoma is suspected clinically, the diagnosis is easily confirmed by the typical multiple echogenecity found at ultrasound scan, or the presence of teeth within the pelvis on X-ray. In most cases, benign cysts can be enucleated intact, but the contralateral ovary should be carefully inspected to exclude the presence of small cysts.

Other benign connective tissue tumours

Other solid benign tumours that may arise from the connective tissue of the ovary include myoma, lipoma, chondroma, osteoma, haemangioma and lymphangioma. All are very rare with no distinguishing clinical pattern. Some of these may arise from a benign teratoma.

Clinical Features of Benign Ovarian Tumours

Benign primary ovarian tumours are most commonly found in women aged 40–60 years, the benign cystic teratoma being the exception.

Small tumours may be asymptomatic and found incidentally. When large, the patient may notice abdominal distension and the pressure effects of dyspepsia and frequency of micturition. Utero-vaginal prolapse may be exacerbated by an ovarian cyst.

The physical signs are not difficult to elicit. When pelvic, the ovarian tumour is distinguishable from the uterus as a smooth, mobile adnexal swelling. Endometriomata may be irregular and fixed, suggesting malignancy. As the tumour rises into the abdomen it may take up a central position, displacing the intestines above and to the sides. The tumour is dull to percussion centrally with areas of resonance in the flanks. The differential diagnosis and further investigations are considered later in this chapter.

Complications of Ovarian Cysts

These include:

1. Torsion of the pedicle
2. Rupture of the cyst
3. Haemorrhage into or from the cyst
4. Infection.

All present with pain, swelling and tenderness over the cyst. Laparotomy is indicated as soon as possible.

Treatment

The management of benign ovarian tumours is to a large extent dictated by the age of the patient. In young women, it is important to preserve ovarian function and future fertility, and so ovarian cystectomy is indicated. Where the adnexal tissues are necrotic from ischaemic damage due to torsion of the ovarian pedicle, salpingo-oophorectomy may be the only option. Total abdominal hysterectomy and bilateral salpingo-oophorectomy is generally accepted as the treatment of choice in those over 40, as the family is usually complete and there is the possibility of early malignant change within the cyst for which this operation would be the appropriate treatment. Whichever procedure is performed, meticulous histological examination of the tumour is imperative to confirm the nature of the tumour. If totally benign, no further treatment will be required.

MALIGNANT TUMOURS OF THE OVARY

The majority of them are serous tumours (75%) and are characterised by endosalpingeal type of cells, producing serous fluid and the formation of psammoma bodies, which are laminated calcospherites and may represent a response to local irritant agents causing adhesions and entrapment of the surface epithelium. Mucinous tumours (10%) are characterised by endocervical type of large cells producing mucin, but they are also similar to intestinal cells, resembling a metastatic gastrointestinal tumour. Endometriotic tumours (10%) are characterised by endometrial type of cells and may be associated with endometriotic deposits in the ovary, although the malignant potential of endometriosis is believed to be low. Clear cell tumours (2%) are characterised by tall cells with clear cytoplasm and hobnail type of cells. They resemble histologically cancerous uterine or vaginal cells associated with exposure to diethylstilbestrol (DES) *in utero*. Brenner tumours

Table 28.1
Types of Ovarian Malignancy

Epithelial tumours
Serous cystadenoma
Mucinous cystadenoma
Endometrioid adenoma
Clear cell adenoma
Brenner tumour
Mixed epithelial tumour
Undifferentiated
Unclassified
Germ cell tumours
Dysgerminoma
Endodermal sinus (yolk sac) tumour
Embryonal carcinoma
Immature teratoma
Choriocarcinoma
Gonadoblastoma
Mixed germ cell tumours
Stromal tumours
Fibrosarcoma
Granulosa and theca cell tumours
Sertoli-Leydig tumour
Gynandroblastoma, arrenoblastoma
Lipid cell tumour
Hilar cell tumour

are rare and characterised by transitional type of malignant epithelium, as seen in the bladder, and usually of very favourable prognosis as they present at an early stage. The types of ovarian malignancy determined histologically are shown in Table 28.1.

Incidence and Aetiology

Ovarian cancer rates show considerable variation among different parts of the globe, but it appears to be more common in industrialised societies, with high rates in Northern Europe and America. It is the fourth most common cancer in women in England and Wales, with an incidence rate of 20 per 100,000 women (6000 new cases per year), and lifetime risk of 1.5%. In the United States, 26,800 new cases are diagnosed per year with 14,200 women dying of the disease.

Ovarian epithelial cancer occurs more frequently in post-menopausal women and very rarely in women before the age of 35 years; it carries the worst prognosis among all gynaecological cancers because of its late presentation, 75% of patients at diagnosis have disease outside the gynaecological organs. Hence, the overall 5-year survival is only 25%. Unfortunately, despite the development of new potent chemotherapeutic agents and very aggressive cytoreductive surgery, the prognosis has not improved drastically in the last 50 years.

Table 28.2
Epithelial Ovarian Cancer, Five-Year Survival

Stage	%	Alive at 5 years (%)
I	26	73
II	15	46
III	41	19
IV	18	5

Epithelial ovarian cancers, the most common type, present usually in the post-menopausal period, whereas germ cell tumours, occur more often in young women and children. Suppression of ovulation appears to protect against ovarian cancer. Early menarche, late menopause, nulliparity, low parity, and possibly, late age at first birth are all associated with an increased risk of ovarian cancer. The use of the contraceptive pill has been recently associated with a decreased risk of ovarian cancer. Dietary factors may also have a role to play — suggested by the international variation of the disease.

Familial ovarian cancers account for approximately 5% of all cases and occur at a younger age.

Familial ovarian cancer. The vast majority of cases of ovarian cancer are sporadic although a small number of cases, up to 5%, occur in ovarian cancer families, usually in association with familial breast cancer. These cases tend to occur at a younger age and most of them are serous adenocarcinomas. Mutations of the *BRCA1* gene (located in chromosome 17q) and *BRCA2* gene (located in chromosome 13q) are the most common genetic associations. The lifelong risk of ovarian cancer in a carrier of a mutant BRCA1 gene is thought to be 30–40%

and of breast cancer 80–85% but varies with the particular mutation. The cloning of the BRCA genes offers the possibility of genetic screening of a high-risk population, however serious ethical dilemmas have to be considered.

Population genetic studies suggest an autosomal dominant pattern of inheritance with variable penentrance. A woman with two first-degree affected relatives has a risk of 50% of inheriting a mutant gene.

Lynch II syndrome (hereditary nonpolyposis colon cancer) presents as a combination of familial colon cancer (Lynch I syndrome) and other adenocarcinomas, including endometrial, ovarian, gastrointestinal, urinary and breast tumours.

Prophylactic mastectomy in affected individuals can reduce the lifelong risk of breast cancer by 90% but it is a mutilating operation, and hormonal manipulation, like tamoxifen, may be a reasonable alternative. Similarly, prophylactic oophorectomy could be considered in these women and offers very good reduction in risk, although primary peritoneal carcinoma may occasionally still occur.

Ovarian cancer and fertility treatment. Recent suggestions that infertile women have a higher chance of developing both ovarian and breast cancer have been linked to the potent ovulation agents used to induce ovulation. This assertion has not been substantiated by prospective studies and further epidemiological controlled studies are awaited in the future.

Screening

Ovarian cancer develops silently and presents very late. A screening test to detect the disease at an early stage could potentially save many lives but the ideal screening test for ovarian cancer remains elusive.

CA-125 (a serum antigen recognised by a murin monoclonal antibody produced by ovarian cancer cells) has been extensively studied in the UK. This blood test is an attractive option for screening because of low cost, simplicity and reproducibility. Unfortunately, CA-125 can be normal in as many as 50% of stage I cases and is raised in many other conditions (pregnancy, pelvic inflammatory disease, endometriosis, menstruation, pancreatitis and liver cirrhosis). It is more useful in the post-menopausal population where fewer false positives occur and if followed by ultrasound scanning as a secondary screen has a very low false positive rate. Whether the use of this screening strategy leads to reduced mortality from the disease is the subject of a current very large randomised trial.

Ultrasound has also been used in smaller studies with a high sensitivity to detect ovarian cancers. Unfortunately the false positive rate is high, leading to unnecessary surgery when asymptomatic adnexal masses are detected. Doppler ultrasound measurements of blood flow have been used to reduce the false positive rate but it still remains much higher than the sequential combination discussed above.

At the moment, it is justified to offer screening tests only to women with a familial predisposition to develop ovarian cancer defined usually as two or more first degree relatives (mother or sister) with ovarian cancer. Women with only one first-degree relative have a relative risk of 3 compared with the general population, and screening is not usually recommended except in the context of trials.

Pathology

Epithelial cancer is the most common (85%) and it arises from the germinal epithelium, which derives from the Müllerian duct. Consequently, the different histological types of epithelial ovarian cancer resemble other adenocarcinomas of the urogenital system.

Metastatic ovarian tumours (5%) can occur in relation other gynaecological primary tumours (fallopian tube, uterine and cervical adenocarcinoma). Also, they may be secondary to intra-abdominal tumours (Krukenberg tumours arising in the stomach) or extra-abdominal primaries (breast).

Ovarian cancers metastasise typically via the transcoloemic route by exfoliation and implantation of cells in the abdominal cavity. They are transported with the peritoneal fluid along the paracolic gutters and the mesentery. Malignant deposits can be found on the surface of any abdominal organ but they rarely invade the muscularis of the bowel.

Early lymphatic spread can occur to the pelvic, para-aortic or extra-abdominal lymph nodes. There is evidence that positive para-aortic lymph nodes can be found in as many as 15% of stage I cancers. Haematogenous spread can occur anywhere in the body and it is usually associated with advanced disease.

Prognostic factors

The stage at presentation is undisputedly the most influential prognostic factor. Various studies have shown that the age of the patient, the amount of residual disease after surgery and the volume of ascites influence survival. The spillage of tumour at the time of operation is a controversial parameter, which has not been clearly shown to influence survival. Clear cell histological type, poor histological differentiation and aneuploid tumours are all associated with poor prognosis. Many proto-oncogenes have also been studied and found to be associated with poor outcome (HER-2/neu which is found in 30% of ovarian cancers, the macrophage colony stimulating factor — MCSF, the epidermal growth factor — EGF). A common tumour suppressor mutated gene, the *p53* is found in 50% of cases and it is associated with a later stage of disease at presentation and rapid progression.

Clinical presentation

The peak incidence of ovarian cancer is about 62 years and one-third of ovarian tumours are malignant in post-menopausal women. Patients may complain of vague symptoms like abdominal discomfort, dyspepsia, urinary frequency, diarrhoea, irregular periods or post-menopausal bleeding. However, when the disease is in an advanced stage, they may present with weight loss, pelvic pain, loss of appetite and more characteristically with abdominal distension due to malignant ascites.

Typically, a hard solid fixed mass can be easily felt on abdominal palpation or bimanual pelvic examination. A rectal examination could also reveal a small tumour in a woman with a deep pelvis and give valuable information on its consistency.

It cannot be over-emphasised that persistent vague symptoms should not be easily attributed to ill-defined benign conditions, like irritable bowel syndrome. A simple gynaecological examination and a pelvic ultrasound may save a woman's life if a malignant tumour is discovered at an early stage. In a post-menopausal woman, the rule is that an ovarian cyst should be considered malignant until it is proven benign.

Differential diagnosis

Benign ovarian cysts, endometriomata, ovarian abscesses due to pelvic inflammatory disease (PID) and uterine fibroids may be confused with a malignant ovarian mass. Pelvic bowel tumours (both inflammatory and malignant), and very rarely, an ectopic pelvic kidney may also mimic an ovarian cancer.

Serum CA 125, a non-specific antigen, is a useful marker of ovarian malignancy although it can be raised in a variety of normal, inflammatory conditions. In post-menopausal women, a combination of raised CA 125 and the presence of a complex ovarian cyst has a 96% positive predictive value, but it is raised in only 50% of cancer cases confined to the ovaries.

Transvaginal ultrasound is easy to perform and it can easily identify the characteristic appearance of an ovarian cancer (multiloculated, irregular cysts with solid components). Computerised tomography (CT) and MRI do not improve the diagnostic accuracy, however CT has been shown to correctly identify the extent of metastatic disease and therefore may alter the management in a patient with advanced disease (administration of neo-adjuvant chemotherapy before debulking surgery). A CT scan, MRI, colonoscopy, barium enema or gastroscopy may be indicated when there is a suspicion of a gastric or bowel tumour in the absence of the characteristic findings of ovarian cancer. A plain chest X-ray should be routinely performed to detect solid metastases and more importantly pleural effusions. However, only thoracocentesis can give a definite cytological diagnosis. Paracentesis may be useful in the case of ascites and the absence of characteristic appearances on ultrasound.

There is no evidence that further routine radiological investigations improve the pre-operative diagnostic accuracy and should only be performed when there is suspicion of extrapelvic metastatic disease. An abdominal and kidney ultrasound and an intravenous pyelography may be indicated in the presence of related symptoms or abnormal liver and kidney biochemical investigations. If patients present with irregular bleeding, a cervical smear and an endometrial biopsy should be taken to exclude a metastatic growth or a second primary tumour. A breast examination should always be performed.

It is important to emphasise that ovarian cancer is a histological diagnosis; therefore a laparotomy should be undertaken without delay in doubtful cases. This is not very straightforward in pre-menopausal women who want to retain their fertility. If they present with a small, mostly cystic simple cyst on ultrasound, it may be worth waiting for two to three months and repeating the investigations before subjecting the patient to the risk of an unnecessary laparotomy.

Staging

This is a very important aspect of the treatment because it gives information on the biological behaviour of the tumour and influences the treatment strategy. It is a surgical staging and ideally should be undertaken by a gynaecological oncologist.

Table 28.3

The International Federation of Gynecology and Obstetrics (FIGO) Classification for Staging of Ovarian Cancer

I	Growth limited to the ovaries
Ia	Growth limited to one ovary; no ascites No tumour on the external surfaces; capsule intact
Ib	Growth limited to both ovaries; no ascites No tumour on the external surface; capsule intact
Ic	Tumour either stage Ia or Ib, but with tumour on the surface or one or both ovaries; or with capsule ruptured; or with ascites present containing malignant cells or with positive peritoneal washings
II	Growth involving one or both ovaries with pelvic extension
IIa	Extension and/or metastases to the uterus and/or the tubes
IIb	Extension to other pelvic tissues
IIc	Tumour either stage IIa or IIb, but with tumour on the surface of one or both ovaries; or with capsule(s) ruptured; or with ascites present containing malignant cells or with positive peritoneal washings
III	Tumour involving one or both ovaries with peritoneal implants outside the pelvis and/or positive retroperitoneal or inguinal nodes. Superficial liver metastasis equals stage III. Tumour is limited to the true pelvis but with histologically proven malignant extension to small bowel or omentum
IIIa	Tumour grossly limited to the true pelvis with negative nodes but with histologically confirmed microscopic seeding of the peritoneal surface
IIIb	Tumour involving one or two ovaries with histologically confirmed implants on abdominal peritoneal surface, none > 2 cm in diameter. Nodes are negative
IIIc	Abdominal implants > 2 cm in diameter and/or positive retroperitoneal or inguinal nodes
IV	Growth involving one or both ovaries with distant metastases. If pleural effusion is present there must be cytology to allot a case to stage IV

The latest 23rd edition of the International Federation of Gynecology and Obstetrics "Annual Report" shows that the 5-year survival for stage Ia is 87%. In the exceptional circumstances of a young woman with stage Ia, grade 1 cancer (well differentiated tumour, limited to one ovary with its capsule intact) who wants to preserve her fertility, a decision may be taken to perform an ipsilateral salpingo-oophorectomy and preserve the uterus and the other adnexum. The remaining ovary should be biopsied and an endometrial biopsy obtained. However, she should share the responsibility of this decision and have a pelvic clearance as soon as she completes her family. Alternatively, she could have healthy ovarian tissue preserved and use it in a surrogate pregnancy in the future. The latter is in its embryonic stage of development and further advances are awaited.

Surgery

The aim of surgery is to remove all visible disease as ovarian cancer is one of the few solid tumours that seem to respond to a combination of cytoreductive surgery and chemotherapy. Considering that maximum cytoreductive surgery carries a high morbidity in advanced disease and that the above statement has never been tested in a randomised prospective trial, the answer of improving survival could lie with developing more potent chemotherapeutic agents. However, removal of the bulk of the tumour affecting other organs, like the bladder and the bowel, is likely to improve the progression-free interval and, more importantly, the quality of life of the patient. These operations should be only undertaken by specialist gynaecological oncologists and in centres that can provide comprehensive pre- and post-operative care.

Cell kinetics, surgery and chemotherapy

Animal and molecular biology studies suggest that the extent of surgical debulking influences survival in patients with cancer. It has been shown that hamsters suffering from a solid tumour had a better response to chemotherapy if significant surgical reduction of the tumour is achieved. Reduction of 1 k of tumour to 1 g produced a better response to adjuvant cyclophosphamide, even if the total number of cells was only reduced from 10^{12} to 10^{9}. Therefore, the success of treatment depends on both the dose of the drug and the amount of tumour. As the tumour size decreases, cytotoxic drugs are more likely to eradicate minimal residual disease, as they are more active with rapidly growing cell populations. The less residual disease that is left, the more likely the cytotoxic treatment will be successful as less cycles of chemotherapy will be required. Therefore, the more aggressive the surgery and the earlier the administration of chemotherapeutic agents, the better is the treatment response.

Laparoscopic surgery

The vast majority of patients with ovarian cancer will have to undergo an open laparotomy through a midline incision in order to have an adequate debulking and staging procedure. However, it has been argued that cases of stage I cancers can be successfully managed laparoscopically.

The benefits of laparoscopic surgery are considerable; in experts' hands, the operative morbidity, the post-operative recovery and hospital stay are reduced. However, there is an increased risk of rupture of an ovarian cyst, especially big in diameter, during laparoscopic manipulation.

We believe that the introduction of laparoscopic surgery in everyday gynaecological practice is one of the major advances of the last fifty years. However, in the field of gynaecological oncology, it has to be introduced with great caution and only after proper evaluation in clinical trials. We believe that the standard treatment of patients with a pre-operative working diagnosis of ovarian cancer should always be by open laparotomy, unless the patients participate in clinical studies.

Chemotherapy

This is a combination of six courses of carboplatin and taxol. It has produced in patients with advanced stage disease a clinical response of 77%, median progression-free interval of 18 months and median survival of 37.5 months. All these parameters compare very favourably to previously used regimes.

Carboplatin is a second-generation platinum compound with less renal and neurological toxicity than cisplatin and it can be administered on an outpatient basis. It is however myelotoxic and is given at a dose of 75–100 mg/m^2.

Taxol (paclitaxel) is a taxane developed in the 1980s, which comes from the bark of the Pacific yew. It stabilises by polymerising the cell microtubules and blocks their division and growth. It is neuro- and myelotoxic and can cause severe anaphylactic reactions. It usually causes total hair loss and mild nausea and vomiting. It is given at a dose of 135–175 mg/m^2/24 hours.

Platinum-based treatment (neo-adjuvant chemotherapy) can be used prior to surgery in order to reduce the bulk of tumour and improve the chance of optimal debulking surgery.

In combination with surgery, the development of a plethora of new agents and efficient, not very toxic regimes is likely to have a sizeable impact on improving the survival of patients suffering from ovarian cancer.

Follow-up

CA 125 has a sensitivity of nearly 100% as a marker of residual disease or relapse. A literature review has shown that it can predict persistent disease in 97% of patients who undergo a second-look operation. It is mainly for this reason and its operative morbidity that diagnostic second-look laparoscopy has not become routine practice in the UK. However, it should be kept in mind that the negative predictive value of CA 125 is low (56%).

Unfortunately, the long-term survival of patients suffering of ovarian cancer has not improved dramatically over the last decade despite the development of new drugs.

Relapse of ovarian cancer

The outlook for patients is poor and treatment is only palliative. Other cytoreductive surgery, or chemotherapy or radiotherapy have all been used but with only a short increase in survival time.

Hormonal treatment (tamoxifen and GnRH analogues) has also been shown to stabilise the disease for short periods and give a partial response in a small proportion of patients.

Mifepristone, a potent abortificient because of its antagonistic activity on progesterone receptors, is a potentially useful agent against tumours with positive progesterone receptors. Its role has not been fully evaluated in clinical studies.

More recently, cytokines (-interferon, -interferon and interleukin-2) have been used as salvage treatment.

BORDERLINE EPITHELIAL TUMOURS

Also called tumours of low malignant potential, they constitute 10% of epithelial tumours and are characterised by epithelial proliferation, nuclear atypia and increased mitotic activity in the absence of stromal invasion.

Pre-menopausal women are mostly affected and these tumours carry a very good prognosis. The majority are serous or mucinous tumours and present at an early stage. Invasive and non-invasive deposits develop in up to 40% of patients causing intestinal adhesions. Intestinal obstruction is the cause of death in most patients who succumb to the disease.

There is no evidence that chemotherapy or radiotherapy has any role to play in the management of these tumours, but complete excision is associated with excellent chances of survival.

GERM CELL TUMOURS

They arise from primordial germ cells in the ovaries, although a few can be found in extra-ovarian sites along the migratory line of germ cells from the caudal yolk sac to the dorsal mesentery, which occurs during embryogenesis. They account for 10% of all ovarian cancers and 75% of them until the age of 20, although only one-third are malignant.

Germ cell tumours grow very fast and usually present with abdominal distension and pain. Occasionally, they may present as an acute abdomen because of torsion of the ovarian malignant cyst, causing pain because of cyst distension, haemorrhage and necrosis. They often cause irregular uterine bleeding and urinary frequency.

The differential diagnosis includes pregnancy, benign ovarian cysts, appendicitis and inflammatory conditions of the bowel.

Ultrasound is highly sensitive in demonstrating irregular ovarian cysts with solid components. Any adnexal masses over 2 cm in pre-pubertal girls and 8 cm in girls after the menarche, which do not regress after two months, should be treated with a great degree of suspicion for malignancy.

Germ cell tumours are hormone-producing tumours; therefore, tumour markers are very useful in the differential diagnosis and follow-up of these patients.

The definite diagnosis is provided by histology after laparotomy.

Dysgerminomas

They constitute one-third of germ cell tumours and up to 10% of all ovarian cancers in women below the age of 20. Histologically, they are characterised by anarchic growth of germ cells, which normally are found in primordial follicles. These large cells have irregular shape, clear cytoplasm and large nuclei with prolific mitotic activity. Extensive lymphocytic and plasma cell infiltration is usually seen and granulomatous formation is common. Macroscopically, they are usually large, smooth tumours organised in lobules. In a young nulliparous patient, surgery should be limited to removal of the affected ovary only because, even in the presence of disease elsewhere, these tumours are extremely chemo-radiosensitive. Dysgerminomas carry an excellent prognosis as most of them (80%) present at stage Ia, in which case the 5-year survival is 95%.

SEX CORD STROMAL TUMOURS

Granulosa stromal tumours constitute 1.5% of all ovarian malignant tumours and are rarely bilateral. They occur more frequently in post-menopausal women, when they characteristically present with abnormal uterine bleeding.

Commonly, they present as a smooth abdominal swelling as they can grow to 40 cm in diameter.

Histologically, they are characterised by the "Call-Exner bodies", which are clusters of ovoid cells, and their smooth, yellow appearance because of luteinisation.

Granulosa tumours have an excellent prognosis (90% 10-year survival rate), but tend to recur after many years. They are not particularly chemo-radiosensitive tumours; therefore complete surgical clearance is of paramount importance.

Androgen producing tumours (Sertoli-Leydig tumours, gonadoblastomas and hilar tumours) are very rare and usually present with signs of virilisation.

FURTHER READING

Anderson M.C., Lambert H.E., Rustin G.F., Soutter W.P. (1997). Carcinoma of the ovary and the fallopian tube. In *Gynaecology*. Shaw R.W., Soutter W.P., Stanton S.L. (eds). pp. 627–49. London: Churchill Livingstone.

Berek J.S., Fu Y.S., Hacker N.F. (1996). Ovarian cancer. In *Novak's Gynecology*, 12th edn. Berek J.S. (ed). pp. 1155–230. Baltimore: Williams & Wilkins.

Management of Gynaecological Cancers (1999). In Bulletin of the effectiveness of health service interventions for decision makers. *Effective Health Care* 5(3) (ISSN: 0965-0288). London: The Royal Society of Medicine Press.

McGuire W.P., Harris W.B. (1999). Chemotherapy of epithelial ovarian cancer. In *Gynecologic Oncology. Principals and Practice of Chemotherapy.* Deppe D., Baker V.V. (eds). pp. 212–40. London: Arnold.

McGuire W.P., Hoskins W.J., Brady M.F., *et al.* (1996). Cyclophosphamide and cisplatin compared with paclitaxel and cisplatin in patients with stage III and stage IV ovarian cancer. *New Engl. J. Med.* **334**: 1–6.

29

Cessation of Reproduction

THE MENOPAUSE

Definition

The menopause is the final cessation of menstruation, i.e. the last menstrual bleed. The menopause is diagnosed retrospectively after one year of ammenorhoea. The average age of the menopause is 50 to 51, and this does not appear to be influenced by factors such as race, height, weight, age of menarche, parity or other socio-economic factors, though smokers may experience an earlier menopause. Prior to the menopause, a woman's reproductive ability declines over a period of 3–4 years and this period of time is called the climacteric — 'a period of life specially liable to a change in health' (*Shorter Oxford English Dictionary*). This transitional phase of decreasing fertility is associated with menstrual disturbance associated with anovular cycles, vasomotor, psychological and other typical symptoms of the 'menopause'.

Premature Ovarian Failure

Ovarian failure before the age of 40 (premature ovarian failure) occurs in about 1% of the female population. Causes include:

- genetic factors (e.g. Turners syndrome XO)
- autoimmune disorders
- infection (mumps oophritis)
- iatrogenic factors (e.g. irradiation, cytotoxic drugs or surgery — bilateral salpingo-oophrectomy is performed for ovarian and endometrial carcinoma and may be performed for severe endometriosis or chronic pelvic pain
- idiopathic

Physiology

The menopause represents the endpoint of a series of physiological changes that begin during fetal life.

The ovary develops from primordial germ cells, which have migrated to the genital (gonadal) ridge from the endoderm of the yolk sac. At birth, the ovary contains all the potential germ cells that are likely to mature during the woman's reproductive life (about 1–2 million), but by the time the girl reaches puberty only 40,000 primary oocytes remain.

Each primary oocyte is found within an ovarian primordial follicle surrounded by follicular cells. After puberty, during each menstrual cycle follicles attempt to mature, but only one succeeds and ovulates leaving the corpus luteum to form in the ovary which then degenerates to form the corpus albicans (fibrous tissue). The follicles which fail to mature, degenerate to form atretic follicles. Follicle stimulating hormone (FSH) and luteinising hormone (LH) secreted by the pituitary serve to drive this ovarian cycle. The number of follicles that grow each day is a function of the total number of follicles remaining within the ovary and hence declines with age.

Menopause is reached when there are no more recruitable follicles within either ovary. The mean weight of the ovary begins to decrease at the age of 30 and with the passing of time, the ovaries become increasingly small until they mainly consist of fibrous tissue devoid of follicles.

As a consequence of ovarian failure at the menopause, there is a fall in the level of ovarian oestrogen production and hence circulating oestrogen levels. In response, by means of a

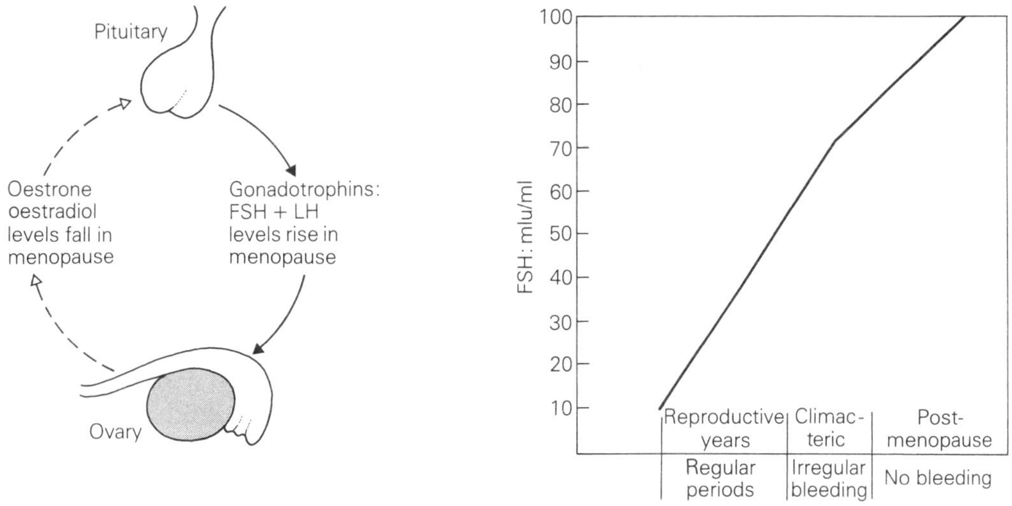

Fig. 29.1 *The pituitary ovarian axis at the menopause.*

feedback mechanism with the anterior pituitary, large amounts of FSH are produced (up to 10 times the level in pre-menopausal women) in an attempt to drive the ovaries to produce oestrogen. LH levels also rise up to threefold (Fig. 29.1). Plasma gonadotrophins and oestrogen concentration assessment, form the basis of the biochemical test to confirm the onset of the climacteric/menopause. However, it must be stressed that levels of oestrogen and gonadotrophins fluctuate widely during the climacteric and detailed biochemical investigations may be of little value in diagnosis.

Oestrogen continues to be produced in smaller amounts by theca cells in the ovary, and in a patient with post-menopausal bleeding secondary to endometrial hyperplasia or endometrial carcinoma, a theca cell tumour (thecoma) should be considered.

Symptoms

The great fall in oestrogen production, which accompanies the menopause, produces the local and systemic symptoms of the menopause as so many target organs are hormone deprived.

Vasomotor symptoms

Hot flushes are the characteristic symptom which occur during the climacteric and after the menopause. Fifty to seventy per cent of women experience hot flushes and up to 25% of women suffer for more than 5 years. A woman's ability to cope with these symptoms depends on the duration, frequency and severity of the attacks. When night sweats occur frequently they can produce insomnia, lethargy and loss of concentration during the day.

Though known to be mediated by the autonomic nervous system, the cause of these vasomotor symptoms is not known. The influence of the fall in oestrogen after the menopause on these symptoms is not yet understood, though it seems that all major sex steroids, oestrogens, androgens and progestogens may play a part.

Emotional and psychological problems

Anxiety, irritability, depression, forgetfulness, mood swings, loss of confidence and loss of libido are all common complaints around the menopause, especially in the 1–2 years prior to cessation of periods. Over 50% of women are reported to suffer such symptoms. Although many studies show beneficial effects of oestrogen therapy on psychological disturbances, it must be remembered that emotional problems do occur around middle age and can be wrongly attributed to the menopause. There are other domestic and emotional causes for psychological symptoms such as children leaving home, elderly parents, social or work circumstances where a sympathetic doctor, partner or family can be of significant benefit. Although there is no conclusive evidence for a relationship between the climacteric/menopause and affective anxiety disorders, both oestrogens and progestogens have neuroactive and psychoactive properties by modulating many aspects of brain function.

End-organ atrophy

The target organs of the genital tract are the vulva, vagina, cervix, uterus, bladder, urethra and supporting ligaments.

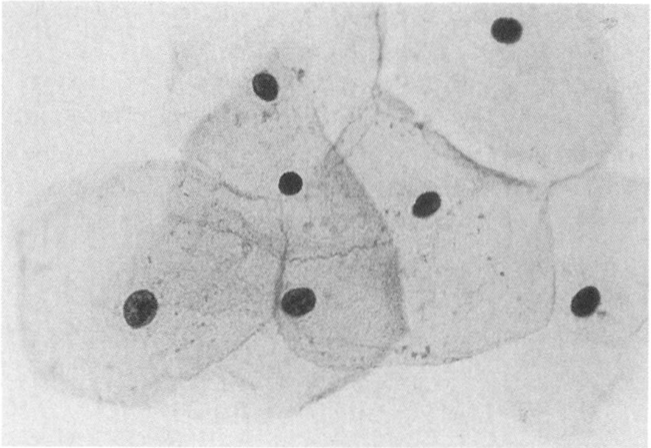

Fig. 29.2 *Mature squamous epithelial cells from normal vaginal epithelium (x125). (Courtesy of Dr E. Hudson, Northwick Park Hospital, London.)*

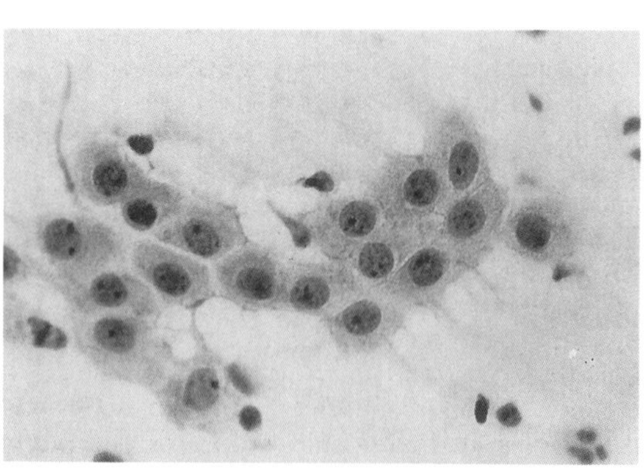

Fig. 29.3 *Squamous cells from atrophic vaginal epithelium (x125). (Courtesy of Dr E. Hudson, Northwick Park Hospital, London.)*

Oestrogen deficiency of the menopause causes the uterus to shrink as the myometrium converts to fibrous tissue. Atrophic changes in the epithelium of the cervix and vagina result in thinning and dryness. The vaginal pH rises to about 7.2, compared with 4.5 in the reproductive years, as there is no longer glycogen present for Doderleins bacilli to convert to lactic acid. This produces a susceptibility to infection plus atrophic vaginitis Figs. 29.2 and 29.3. Atrophic vaginitis may cause dyspareunia and may also be the cause of post-menopausal bleeding, a symptom requiring urgent investigation and treatment.

Histological point. Atrophic vaginal skin has a reduced number of superficial cells and an increased number of basal cells. These changes can be demonstrated cytologically on a lateral vaginal wall smear. The karyopyknotic index (KI), which is the proportion of superficial cells to basal cells provides useful and reliable information about oestrogen effects as oestrogen increases the number of superficial cells.

The external genitalia decrease in size and there is a loss of pubic hair. The transitional epithelium of the bladder trigone undergoes atrophy, and at cystoscopy, it is not uncommon to see atrophic changes resembling those in the vagina over the whole bladder epithelium. The urethra, which arises from the same ectoderm as the vaginal vestibule also appears to be under the influence of oestrogen. Atrophic changes in the bladder may cause dysuria, frequency and urgency, i.e. urethral syndrome or even detrusor instability.

Skeleton

Bone is constantly being remodelled throughout life, and at a cellular level this consists of bone resorption and bone formation. Osteoclasts are multinucleated giant cells found at the surface of bones undergoing resorption. They increase in number and activity in response to parathyroid hormone (PTH) and vitamin D and decrease in number and activity in response to calcitonin. Osteoblasts form bone tissue and are found at surfaces where bone is remodelling. They secrete collagen to form a non-mineralised bone called osteoid which in time matures into mineralised calcified bone. It requires 100–150 osteoblasts to form the amount of bone which can be broken down by a single osteoclast. Bone resorption is followed by bone formation, a phenomenon called coupling.

Once peak bone mass is achieved in the 3rd–4th decade of life, the amount of bone resorbed becomes greater than the amount of bone replaced (from age 40–50 years in both sexes), thus explaining the decline in bone mass with age. In women, bone loss prior to the menopause is approximately 3–5% per decade, paralleling that in men. However, at the menopause, with the fall in oestrogen levels, bone loss accelerates averaging 2% per year for the next 5–10 years, though this rate of bone loss varies from one woman to another.

Bone is considered osteoporotic if its density is more than 2.5 SD below the mean value for that of a young adult and a decrease in bone density of only 1 SD is associated with a three-fold increase in fracture risk. The vast majority of osteoporotic fractures are reported in post-menopausal women which can lead to deformity, pain and disability. The most common sites for these fractures are vertebral resulting in a reduction in height and in severe cases, a kyphosis, the distal radius and the neck of femur. All are associated with significant morbidity and even mortality.

Starting with a high peak bone density (a genetic factor), a later age of menopause, taking regular exercise, a healthy diet, non-smoking and the avoidance of excess alcohol will all help to reduce a rapid decline in bone density and help prevent osteoporosis. However, as previously described the oestrogen deficient state of the menopause significantly increases the risk of osteoporosis. Oestrogens have complex effects of skeletal homeostasis and effectively inhibit the rapid phase of bone loss associated with the post-menopausal period. Calcitonin and the bisphosphonates also effectively inhibit osteoclastic bone resorption in the post-menopausal period and may be appropriate alternatives for the treatment of osteoporosis in those women in whom Hormone Replacement Therapy (HRT) is contraindicated.

HRT almost halves the risk of osteoporotic fractures if used for 5–10 years beginning at the menopause and has also been reported to increase bone density by 5% in women with established osteoporosis.

Skin

Skin thickness declines after the menopause due to a decrease in skin collagen. This is potentially reversible with the use of oestrogen replacement.

Cardiovascular system

Men are 5 times more likely to suffer from heart disease than pre-menopausal women. In fact, prior to the menopause ischaemic heart disease (IHD) is rare in women who do not smoke, or suffer from hypertension or diabetes mellitus. However, after the menopause the difference in incidence of IHD between the sexes declines and it is therefore suggested that oestrogen deficiency contributes to the post-menopausal increase in IHD.

Results of many basic science and epidemiological investigations show that oestradiol replacement conveys a protective effect on the cardiovascular system in post-menopausal women, decreasing the risk of myocardial infarction or stroke by 50%. Twenty five to fifty per cent of the cardio-protective effect of oestrogen is afforded by its alteration of lipid and lipoprotein concentrations. This effect on lipids and lipoproteins depends on the sex steroid given, its dose and its route of administration. These oestrogen effects are also modified if a progestogen is added. Oestrogens generally decrease the overall cholesterol concentration specifically decreasing low density lipoproteins (LDLs) but increasing high density lipoproteins (HDLs). Progestogens have differing effects on the lipoprotein and lipid concentrations depending on their androgenicity, the more androgenic the properties of the progestogen, the more it will reverse the HDL raising effect of oestrogens.

Central nervous system

There is evidence now accumulating that oestrogens may help protect against Alzheimers disease or at least delay its occurrence. Alzheimers disease may have an oestrogen-dependent component, though the mechanism by which oestrogen may effect Alzheimers disease has not yet been clarified. Clearly this is an area where more research is needed.

Diagnosis

The diagnosis of the menopause is retrospective — the last period after 12 months of amenorrhoea. However, women may present complaining of climacteric/menopausal symptoms which are diagnosed by history, examination and if necessary investigation. Women may also present requesting hormone replacement therapy (HRT), not only for control of symptoms but as prophylaxis against the long-term consequences of the menopause, e.g. osteoporosis, coronary heart disease and Alzheimers disease.

History

Symptoms of the menopause are detailed above, and listed usefully below.

- Hot flushes/night sweats
- Sleep disturbance/fatigue
- Mood change, anxiety, irritability and loss of concentration
- Vaginal discomfort — from atrophic vaginitis and/or infection and vaginal dryness
- Dyspareunia
- Urinary incontinence — associated with detrussor instability
- Atrophic urethritis producing symptoms of urethral syndrome
- Ischaemic heart disease
- Fractures associated with osteoporosis
- Skin laxity associated with collagen depletion.

Any woman presenting with the above symptoms should have a brief exclusion of other conditions producing similar symptoms. It is also important to ensure that psychological symptoms are not being caused by other life events.

Examination

A sensitive but thorough physical examination should be performed, i.e. the blood pressure taken, the urine tested, the breasts examined and a pelvic examination performed. A high vaginal swab should be taken if there is evidence of infection. As in all examinations the woman must be put at ease and constantly reassured.

Investigations

Increased FSH and LH levels and decreased oestrogen levels will help to confirm the diagnosis.

Treatment

Climacteric/menopausal women should be treated sympathetically and with understanding. Explanation that there is a physiological basis for their symptoms is important, and a brief, basic description of the menopause assisted by written literature can help women understand. The mainstay of treatment of this oestrogen-deficient state is oestrogen replacement therapy combined with (where indicated in women with a uterus) additional progestogen supplementation.

For women in whom HRT is contra-indicated, not tolerated or not wanted, treatment options are aimed at specific symptomatic relief.

Non-HRT treatments

Evening primrose oil may offer some relief of vasomotor symptoms and clonidine can be used to reduce hot flushes and night sweats. For psychological symptoms, counselling and supportive measures are important non-medical options which can be employed to help cope.

Lifestyle changes such as stopping smoking, decreasing heavy alcohol intake and increasing exercise should be encouraged around the time of the menopause to help prevent osteoporosis if additional treatment is used or not. The bisphosphonates e.g. etidronate or alendronate have anti-bone resorptive properties and are used for the treatment of osteoporosis where HRT is contra-indicated. Calcium and vitamin D supplementation are useful for frail institutionalised women at high risk of osteoporosis where adequate dietary intake may be inadequate.

Again, advice on lifestyle adaptation is essential for women to reduce likelihood of coronary heart disease, e.g. cessation of smoking, adequate exercise and a healthy well balanced diet.

Women keen to avoid pharmaceutical HRT can gain some natural oestrogen replacement from soy produce and yam root.

Hormone Replacement Therapy

Oestrogen replacement therapy is the medication of choice for treatment and prevention of menopausal symptoms. The symptoms of the menopause which can be alleviated by treatment have been listed earlier in this chapter, however the potential side-effects and risks of oestrogen replacement will now be considered.

Side-effects and risks

Endometrial hyperplasia and carcinoma. The continual administration of unopposed oestrogen causes endometrial hyperplasia and an increase in the incidence of adenocarcinoma of the endometrium (an incidence about 8 times greater than that of the population norm). It is therefore essential that women with a uterus have a progestogen added to oestrogen replacement for at least 10–14 days per cycle to negate this excess risk.

Endometrial carcinoma is an oestrogen-dependent tumour. The treatment of choice for this malignancy is to perform a total abdominal hysterectomy and bilateral salpingo-oophrectomy. In the past, HRT use has been contra-indicated in these women. However, it is now understood that women with early stage, well-differentiated disease do not have decreased survival rates or increased recurrence rates when given oestrogen replacement. In fact, their quality of life is much improved when disabling menopausal symptoms are relieved. These women need to be fully counselled prior to prescribing HRT and be closely followed up.

Breast Cancer. Breast cancer is an important common female cancer with a lifetime incidence of 1:12. The potential influence of HRT on breast cancer must be considered as how it effects this background incidence. Meta-analysis of data has shown that there is a small but significant increase risk of breast cancer after 5 years of HRT use.

In women aged 50 years not using HRT, about 45 in every 1000 will be diagnosed with breast cancer over their next 20 years. If HRT is used for 5 years, 2 extra women per 1000 will be diagnosed, if used for 10 years, 6 extra women per 1000 will be diagnosed and if used for 15 years, 12 extra women per 1000 will be diagnosed. This increased risk persists for 5 years after therapy ends, but there is no increased risk of death from breast cancer in HRT users. In fact breast carcinoma diagnosed in HRT users is less likely to have spread beyond the breast than non-users. All women prescribed HRT should have these risks explained so they can make a balanced and informed choice about its use. All women using HRT must be encouraged to self-examine their breasts and have regular mammograms.

Many breast cancers are known to be oestrogen-dependent tumours, and exposure to exogenous oestrogens as in HRT could stimulate tumour cell growth, accelerate the disease, or promote relapse. Most post-menopausal women with breast carcinoma will be offered tamoxifen (see SERMS later) which may improve vaginal atrophy and have positive effects on bone and lipid profile. Tamoxifen will not relieve vasomotor symptoms and may stimulate the endometrium. Women who are disease free for 10 years after breast cancer can be considered cured and potentially offered oestrogen replacement therapy, though combination with high dose progestogens is recommended and full counselling is mandatory.

Venous thromboembolism (VTE). The administration of exogenous oestrogens in HRT has been shown to produce a modest increase in the relative risk of VTE. Epidemiological studies show the background risk of VTE in 45 to 64-year-olds to be 1:10000 women per year, whereas in those on HRT the risk is 3:10000 women per year. Therefore, the use of post-menopausal oestrogen is associated with one extra case of VTE in every 5000 users per year. This increased risk is highest in the first 12 months of use. The absolute risk of VTE with HRT is low and the benefits from therapy such as osteoporosis or coronary heart disease prevention outweigh the risk of VTE.

The mechanism by which HRT produces this increased risk is unclear. There are changes in the haemostatic system induced by oestrogen replacement, but it could be that an underlying thrombotic trait is unmasked (e.g. antithrombin 3, protein S or C deficiency, Factor V Leiden, antiphospholipid syndrome or hyperhomocysteinaemia).

Women who are to be commenced on HRT should have a personal and family history of VTE taken. Although a routine thrombophilia screen is not necessary in all women about to start HRT, it is recommended in women who have a positive personal or family history of VTE. If no thrombophilia is detected and the VTE was greater than one year ago and non-life threatening, the patient can be prescribed HRT. If a thrombophilia is detected, it is advised that HRT not be prescribed unless reviewed in a specialist centre with expertise in thrombphilias.

There is no indication for women to stop HRT prior to surgery as long as appropriate thromboprophylaxis is employed.

Liver disease. It has been recognised that women who use HRT are at greater risk of cholecystectomy compared with women who have never used HRT. Oestrogen-related cholestasis and jaundice are thought to be mediated by oestrogen-induced changes in hepatocyte membrane fluidity and are dose-dependent. These changes are more pronounced with synthetic oestrogens, e.g. ethinyloestradiol than the natural oestrogens commonly used in HRT. In fact, transdermal oestradiol which avoids high levels of oestrogen in the portal blood can be considered in all women with chronic liver disease who are post-menopausal as long as liver biochemistry is monitored.

Side effects of HRT. Post-menopausal women with a uterus using cyclical progestogens to protect the endometrium will have monthly withdrawal bleeds or 3-monthly bleeds if using tridestra (any irregular bleeding on HRT warrants further investigation of the endometrium). This can be avoided in an appropriately selected sub-group of women with continuous combined HRT. Other side-effects include breast enlargement, mastalgia, headaches, nausea and vomiting and depression. Women using progestogens may also experience fluid retention, bloating, increased appetite and irritability of mood.

Contraception. HRT does not have contraceptive properties and women are considered potentially fertile for 2 years after her LMP if less than 50 years of age and 1 year if greater than 50 years of age. Any potentially fertile woman using HRT should employ non-hormonal contraceptive measures.

HRT Regimens

The range and choice of HRT preparations is ever-increasing. As the variety grows, the best treatment option for each individual woman depends on the indication and convenience of use balanced against the potential associated risks. The decision to prescribe HRT should be taken only after fully explaining the benefits and risks to the patient, even providing her with accurate written literature so she can take on board and fully understand the information. Women are well known to comply poorly with HRT use and the more knowledge they have about the menopause and the benefits of HRT the more likely they are to comply.

Local oestrogens

Oestrogen-deficient vaginitis (even in women with a uterus) may be treated in the short-term with local oestrogen creams to improve the quality of the vaginal epithelium. Topical oestrogens should be used in the minimum effective amount thereby minimising systemic oestrogen absorbtion. If local oestrogens are used long term in a woman with a uterus, a progestogen needs to be added for 10–14 days per cycle to protect against endometrial hyperplasia. Commonly used local products include:

- Dienoestrol cream (contains dienoestrol)
- Vagifem tablets (contain oestradiol)
- Estring (releases 7.5 microgram oestradiol in 24 hours therefore producing minimal systemic absorption. It lasts 3 months.)

Systemic oestrogens

Natural oestrogens such as oestradiol, oestrone and oestriol offer a more appropriate profile for HRT than synthetic oestrogens such as ethinyloestradiol or mestranol.

Oral Preparations

Oral preparations contain naturally occurring human oestrogens such as oestadiol, oestrone and oestriol or conjugated equine oestrogens prepared from the urine of pregnant mares (which is 50% oestrone sulphate and other equine oestrogens, also considered to be natural). There is no evidence that one type of natural oestrogen is more effective than the rest in relieving climacteric symptoms or preventing osteoporosis or ischaemic heart disease.

Following oral ingestion, the administered oestrogen absorbed from the gut enters the hepatic portal vein to the liver where it undergoes modification by the liver, thereby reducing its bio-availability to under 10%. This is known as the 'first pass' effect. Therefore larger doses of oestrogen need to be used orally to ensure therapeutic levels of the active hormone are delivered systemically. Furthermore, the high levels of oestrogen in the hepatic system potentially exacerbate problems with VTE or liver disease.

Transdermal Preparations

Oestrogen is well absorbed through the skin and by doing so enters directly into the systemic circulation thereby avoiding the 'first pass' effect through the liver. Transdermal oestrogen administration produces a more natural oestrogen concentration. Patches either consist of oestradiol dissolved into a gel pressed against the skin by an adhesive backing (needing replacement twice weekly), or consist of a matrix where the hormone is embedded in the adhesive layer, making these patches thinner and lees irritant on the skin which may be replaced once or twice weekly.

Gels

Oestradiol gels which are administered in 0.75 microgram doses can be rubbed into the skin of the arms or legs twice daily to produce rapid absorption and good symptomatic relief again avoiding the 'first pass' effect.

Implants

Pellets of crystalline oestradiol can be implanted into the subcutaneous fat of the lower abdominal wall (doses of 25 or 50 mg) to release a small amount of oestradiol daily for 6 months after insertion. Tachyphylaxis has been demonstrated with implants where women request insertion of a new implant to relieve symptoms at shorter and shorter intervals. There may be recurrence of vasomotor symptoms at supraphysiological plasma concentrations of oestrogen, a problem to be watched for in women using this form of HRT. There is also evidence that after discontinuation of implants, endometrial stimulation may continue for up to 2 years and therefore prolonged progestogen protection may be required.

Testosterone (100 mg) implants can be used in conjunction with oestradiol implants to treat symptoms of loss of energy and loss of libido.

Additional progestogens

Women with a uterus need progestogens for at least 10–14 days of the cycle to abolish the effect oestrogen has on increasing the incidence of endometrial carcinoma.

Commonly used progestogens in HRT are the C-19 progesterones — norethisterone (0.7 mg–1 mg) and levonorgestrel (150 micrograms), and the C-21 progesterones — dydrogesterone (10–20 mg) and medroxyprogesterone acetate (5–10 mg), which are less androgenic. There is concern that the more androgenic progestogens may counteract the beneficial effects of oestrogen on lipid metabolism.

Sequential progestogen therapy is where progestogens are only provided for 10–14 days of the cycle, commonly via the oral or transdermal route. This use of progestogen is associated with regular predictable withdrawal bleeds, a side-effect considered a drawback by many women. To try to reduce withdrawal bleeds, continuous combined HRT (CCHRT) has been developed.

CCHRT was developed because most women prefer not to bleed while taking HRT. By administering a continuous dose of both oestrogen and progestogen, no withdrawal bleeds occur (and compliance improves) and the endometrium remains protected. CCHRT is available in oral or transdermal preparations but it is not recommended for all women. It should not be used in women who are perimenopausal as they have a high incidence of breakthrough bleeding and tends to be recommended for women 1–2 years ammenorrhoiec post-menopausally or those aged 54 years or more if on cyclical HRT through the menopause. There may be erratic spotting or bleeding vaginally in the first 3 months of administration of CCHRT. However, if this persists for longer, investigation of the endometrium is mandatory.

The progesterone releasing intrauterine system (Mirena) may be beneficial to administer progestogens directly to the endometrium when side-effects of systemic progestogens are intolerable. The Mirena intrauterine system (Schering Healthcare) which releases 150 micrograms of levonorgestrel daily is not currently licensed for this use, but its combination with oral or transdermal oestrogen may be an alternative to CCHRT.

Tibolone

Tibolone is a steroid hormone that has oestrogenic, progestogenic and androgenic properties. It effectively reduces vasomotor symptoms of the menopause, improves libido and sexual enjoyment and prevents osteoporosis without bleeding. It is safe for the endometrium and cardiovascular system, however, as yet its influence on the incidence of carcinoma of the breast has not been fully assessed. Again livial is advised for use in women 1 year after their last menstrual period especially those who had an adverse effect on conventional HRT.

Selective oestrogen receptor modulators (SERMS)

It is now understood that the oestrogen receptor is not a single entity and to date, two receptor types have been identified (ER alpha and ER beta). These receptors differ in distribution and affinity for oestrogens and by using this knowledge, molecules can be modified to develop drugs which are highly targeted to specific receptors. SERMS are molecules which have mixed oestrogen agonism and antagonism depending on the receptor they bind to. A first generation SERM, e.g. tamoxifen is known to impede bone loss, favourably modify the lipid profile, but stimulate the endometrium. Raloxifene is a second generation SERM which acts as an oestrogen antagonist on the endometrium and in the breast, but is an oestrogen agonist in bone and on the cardiovascular system. Early investigations show that raloxifene may prevent osteoporotic fractures and produce a favourable lipid profile, though it is unknown if this translates into a decrease in myocardial infarction. Raloxifene (60 mg daily oral dose) does not induce vaginal bleeding and nor will it help vasomotor symptoms. In fact the side-effect profile of raloxifene includes vasomotor symptoms, and a similar increase in relative risk for VTE as for oestrogen HRT.

POST-MENOPAUSAL BLEEDING (PMB)

Definition

Any bleeding after the menopause, but in practice any bleeding 6 months or more after the last period. PMB may originate from anywhere in the genital tract and the cause may be benign or malignant. It is important to realise that sometimes the woman may not know where the bleeding has come from, and it is assumed the bleeding is vaginal.

Aetiology of Post-Menopausal Bleeding

Benign causes

Uterine

- Atrophic endometritis — a totally atrophic endometrium may bleed
- Endometrial polyp
- Endometrial hyperplasia
- Fibroid
- HRT
- Tuberculosis (rare).

Cervical

- Atrophic cervicitis — large friable blood vessels on the atrophic cervix may bleed
- Cervical polyp.

Vaginal

- Atrophic vaginitis
- Infection
- Urethral caruncle — small red fleshy outgrowth at the urethral meatus, commonly a localised prolapse of urethral epithelium.

Malignant causes

Massive PMB rarely occurs unless it is due to malignancy.

- Cervical carcinoma
- Endometrial carcinoma/sarcoma — after the age of 60, endometrial carcinoma is 4 times more common than cervical carcinoma
- Vulval carcinoma — PMB on wiping or drying is a common presenting history
- Ovarian malignancy — when the endometrium is stimulated as a result
- Vaginal carcinoma — very rare
- Fallopian tube carcinoma — very rare.

Management

The management of any woman presenting with PMB includes taking an accurate history, examination and performing necessary investigations.

History

The clerking of any woman with PMB should involve a full past medical and drug history and the specific detailed history should include:

- When did the bleeding occur?
- How long did it last?
- Was there a precipitating factor (e.g. postcoital bleeding)?
- How much bleeding was there?
- Was the bleeding fresh or old blood?
- Is there a history of HRT or SERM use?
- Was it related to micturition or deafecation? — a clear bowel and urinary history is essential.
- Is there any weight loss?
- Are there any other symptoms?
- Age of menarche?
- Age at menopause?
- Obstetric history? (endometrial carcinoma is 3 times more common in nulliparous women)
- Any gynae surgery?
- Date of last smear test?
- Any family history of note?

Examination

A general examination is performed with attention paid to detecting lymphadenopathy, masses in the breast or abdomen. A careful speculum and bimanual examination should be performed, allowing the lower genital tract and cervix to be inspected for possible causes.

Investigations

Any woman presenting with PMB should have formal investigation of the uterine cavity without delay. The methods of investigating the uterine cavity are as follows.

Hysteroscopy

The visualisation of the uterine cavity using a narrow, flexible or rigid telescope inserted through the cervix. Abnormal endometrium is visualised through the cervix and confirmed by directed biopsy. This can be performed as an outpatient procedure though some women may require a general anaesthetic for adequate assessment. This is presently the investigation of choice for PMB.

Ultrasound

Transvaginal ultrasound can assess not only the ovaries in a woman presenting with PMB, but also the endometrial thickness. By measuring the symmetrical double layer thickness of the endometrium, an assessment of the endometrium and uterine cavity can be gained. Women with a cut-off endometrial thickness of 4 mm or less can be reassured that they have a negligible chance of endometrial malignancy though other endometrial pathology may be missed.

Endometrial sampling

Dilatation and Curettage (D&C)

D&C involves dilatation of the cervical canal and curettage of the endometrial cavity. The curettings obtained can be examined histologically. Less than 75% of the endometrium is sampled during this procedure and as such endometrial cancer can be missed. It is a less effective way of diagnosing endometrial cancer than hysteroscopy and directed biopsy.

Pipelle

This endometrial sampler has the advantage that it can be inserted through the cervix without prior dilatation and therefore can be used in an outpatient clinic to sample the endometrium. However, the pipelle has been shown to only sample 4–5% of the endometrium, and should only be used as an adjunct to other methods of visualising the endometrial cavity.

Treatment

Treatment depends on the diagnosis. Lesions of the bowel or bladder will require referral to the appropriate specialist. Carcinoma of the uterus and cervix will be discussed in the appropriate chapters.

FURTHER READING

Br. J. Obs. Gynae. (1996). **103**(13): 1–108.

Kearney C., Purdie D. (2000). Selective Oestrogen Receptor Modulators (SERMS). *Obs. Gynae.* **1**: 6–10.

Hormone replacement therapy and venous thromboembolism (1999). *RCOG Greentop Guideline No. 19.*

Collaborative Group on Hormonal Factors in Breast Cancer (1997). Breast cancer and hormone replacement therapy: Collaborative re-analysis of data from 51 epidemiological studies of 52,705 women with breast cancer and 108,411 women without breast cancer. *Lancet* **350**: 1047–59.

30

Contraception

In comparison with economic trends or national crises, specific contraceptive measures have probably contributed little to population trends. Events such as the Depression of the 1920s and 1930s, followed by World War II in the 1940s have had much more profound effects on populations than the advent of the oral contraceptive pill or intrauterine devices. However, for the individual couple, the ability to control and space their family using one or several current methods as appropriate is very important to the well-being and happiness of parents and other children.

TRADITIONAL METHODS

Safe Period

This method depends on the avoidance of intercourse at a time when conception might take place. Despite an apparently regular 28-day cycle, the timing of ovulation is not precise and the duration of survival of ovum and sperm is variable. The ovum is likely to be capable of fertilisation for 24–26 hours after ovulation, but sperm may survive in the female genital tract for up to 3 days. The pre-ovulatory infertile period is difficult to recognise and is calculated on the basis of previous cycles and the date of the last menstrual period. If the cycles are irregular and short, then the pre-ovulatory safe period is correspondingly short and unpredictable. Ovulation can be recognised in some women by a change in their cervical mucus, which becomes clear and copious, and/or mild midcycle lower abdominal pain (mittelschmerz). A significant rise (0.5°C) in the basal body temperature occurs shortly after ovulation, but this is an imprecise method of detecting ovulation on a regular basis. The post-ovulatory safe period will commence 2 days after it is thought that ovulation has occurred. The failure rate of this method is of the order of 30 per 100 woman years because of the difficulty of predicting the time of ovulation accurately. Attempts are being made to detect ovulation more precisely by means of recording temperature or pH changes in the vagina or by improving the ability of the woman to assess her own cervical mucus. It is not possible to say whether these techniques will be reliable in practice or whether they will reduce the failure rate significantly.

Coitus Interruptus (Male Withdrawal)

This has been an important method of limiting family size throughout the world for many centuries. Its use in developed countries has been, and still is, declining. There are no apparent side-effects of the method. However, if the female partner is to achieve orgasm and the male is to withdraw before any seminal fluid is expelled, he must exercise concentration and self-control. The frequency with which the method is used is difficult to assess, but it may be that the method is practised regularly or occasionally by 20% of social groups 3, 4 and 5, and somewhat less frequently by social classes 1 and 2. The failure rate is equally difficult to determine, but is probably of the order of 22 per 100 woman years. The main advantages of both these methods are that there are no health hazards and they do not require intervention from outside personnel, while the main disadvantage is a high pregnancy rate.

BARRIER METHODS

Condoms

These are latex rubber sheaths usually 0.04 mm in thickness. They are sometimes lubricated with spermicide, usually teat-ended to collect the ejaculate and are sold in a variety of colours and styles. To be successful, they must be rolled onto the full length of the erect penis before penetration and after ejaculation the penis should be withdrawn before the erection is lost, lest the condom slip off or there is leakage of the seminal fluid from around its base. Care should be taken not to tear the condom during its application. Condoms are extremely strong and they are unlikely to burst during intercourse. Most claims of 'burst sheaths' probably reflect improper use or failure of use. Popularity of the condom varies considerably from country to country, its use being high in male dominated societies such as Japan, to being low in some South American countries and Australia. Use in Western Europe is about one-third of contraceptive users.

Advantages of the method are that it is good for people having casual relationships or couples having infrequent intercourse. The condom provides protection for either partner against acquiring gonorrhoea. The risks of acquiring AIDS (Autoimmune Deficiency Syndrome) through sexual intercourse is markedly reduced by the use of condoms. Their use in all casual sexual encounters is strongly advocated. Especially thick and stronger condoms are needed for use in anal intercourse.

The quoted failure rates vary greatly. Obviously, there is considerable scope for user failure, particularly if a condom is not used at every act of intercourse. In studies involving regular, well motivated users, the failure rate is about 4 per 100 woman years.

There is now a female condom which is made from thin latex. It lines the vagina and covers the cervix. It is held in place by a rim which fits over the vulva. It is not widely used yet as it is difficult to fit and use easily. There is reduced sensation for the male. It has not been used widely enough to have reliable figures for use effectiveness, but it is likely to be similar to the male condom.

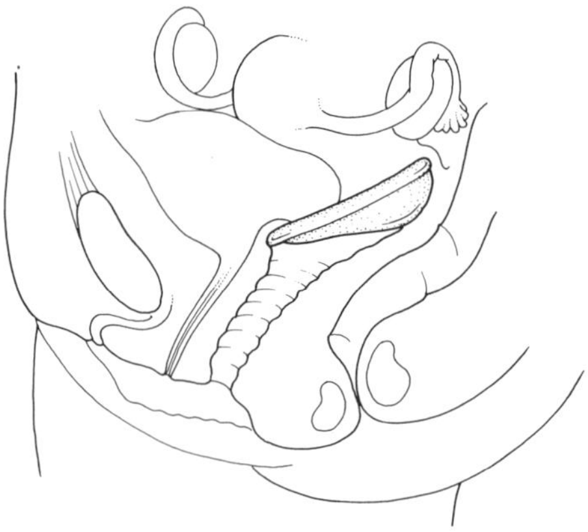

Fig. 30.1 *Diaphragm in position.*

Diaphragms

These are made of latex and have a flat, circular spring edge or a coiled arcing spring which is more flexible and possibly more comfortable to wear. They are of variable size (45–100 mm) and have to be individually fitted. The diaphragm lies in the posterior fornix behind the cervix posterosuperiorly and behind the pubic symphysis anteroinferiorly (Fig. 30.1). The cervix is thus covered by the dome of the diaphragm. Before insertion, the diaphragm must have spermicide applied to both of its surfaces, so that there is a layer of spermicide retained by the diaphragm over the external cervical os. This is as important as the actual barrier in the mode of action of the diaphragm. Spermicidal pessaries should not be used as the fats contained in them can damage the rubber. The diaphragm can be left *in situ* for 6–8 hours after first intercourse and will be effective for that time unless dislodged. It must then be removed, washed, dried and stored in a cool, dark place to prevent deterioration of the rubber. Use of the diaphragm is small, being about 4–5% of contraceptive users. It is more popular among higher social classes and in developed countries.

Again, there is considerable scope for user failure, but if used regularly by well motivated women, the failure rate in some large scale studies in the UK is between 2 and 3 per 100 woman years. The advantages of this method are that it is free of health hazards and is suitable for occasional intercourse. Used regularly it can be reliable. The disadvantage is that the user must be happy with the idea and technique of insertion and this may not be aesthetically acceptable to many women.

Spermicides

The use of spermicide cream with the diaphragm is essential, while some condoms incorporate a spermicidal lubricant. Spermicidal pessaries, tablets or pastes used alone are not very effective. Results reported in the literature quote failure rates of from 2 to 25 per 100 woman years. Clinical impressions suggest that the higher figure is more likely. The most commonly used agent in spermicides is nonoxynol-9 (nonylphenoxypolyethoxyethanol). Other compounds are being investigated together with the use of devices such as vaginal rings which may slowly release the spermicide.

Contraceptive sponges containing spermicide are available, but their efficacy has never been tested in large studies, and it is doubtful if they can provide anything other than some protection for occasional intercourse.

A variety of new spermicides are being studied in trials.

Intrauterine Device (IUD)

Intrauterine devices can be either inert silastic or be medicated. These have copper wire wound round the stem or contain a progestogen. The presence of the device in the uterine cavity does not alter endocrine function and ovulation takes place normally. A number of hypotheses have been put forward concerning their mode of action. The IUD leads to a leukocytic infiltration of the endometrium, the so-called sterile inflammatory response, and the devices themselves have many macrophages adhering to them. These can phagocytose spermatozoa and this may be why there are very few sperm which reach the fallopian tube in the presence of an intrauterine device. There is increased prostaglandin production from the endometrium with an IUD *in situ*, and this, in turn, may lead to enhanced myometral activity, particularly during the late luteal phase of the cycle. Uterine contractions of up to 100 mmHg in strength may interfere with implantation of the blastocyst. Subtle and, as yet, undocumented biochemical changes in the endometrium probably also occur which may affect implantation. The larger the inert device, the lower the pregnancy rate, but there will be higher rates of removal for pain and bleeding.

Copper in the form of wire has been added to the vertical stem of devices to reduce their size and to maintain a low pregnancy rate. The surface area of copper is 200–300 mm^2 and this allows copper at the rate of 50 μg per day to be released for up to 3 years. More recently, copper has been added to the horizontal arm of a T device to give 380 mm^2 of copper. This device has a pregnancy rate of 2 per 100 woman years and a life of 6 years. Copper enhances the endometrial 'inflammatory' response already described and allows the smaller device to give a lower pregnancy rate. Copper interferes with endometrial biochemistry, depressing oestrogen binding and thymidine uptake into DNA, impairs glycogen storage and inhibits metabolic enzymes such as lactate dehydrogenase. Despite this, if pregnancy does take place, there is no evidence that either the inert or copper-containing device causes congenital abnormalities. The use effectiveness of IUDs varies from almost zero to about 8 per 100 woman years. Factors that affect the pregnancy rate are the ability of the fitter (a device placed improperly in the uterus will be more likely to drop out unnoticed), the loss to follow-up rate and the duration of the study (long-term users tend to have a lower pregnancy rate than short-term users). In general, the pregnancy rate is accepted as being about 3 per 100 woman years and does not vary significantly from one device to another.

Recently a T-shaped device releasing levonorgestrel has been developed (Minerva). This device is an effective contraceptive but also reduces menstrual blood loss. It lasts for 5 years but is expensive at £89. It is now being used in an unlicensed way for the treatment of menorrhagia.

The advantages of the intrauterine device are that it is not coitally related, it is simple, lasts for 3 or more years and has no effect on endocrine function, with few serious side-effects. Its disadvantages are that it may cause heavier periods or occasionally intermenstrual spotting. Its main disadvantage is a small increased tendency to pelvic inflammatory disease. The method is not the best for young, nulliparous, sexually very active women. Development of pelvic pain and dyspareunia in someone wearing an IUD requires immediate attention to diagnose, and if necessary, treat pelvic inflammatory disease. Usually, the device would be removed during treatment and its replacement carefully considered afterwards. A history of recurrent pelvic inflammatory disease would be a contraindication to the use of an IUD. Valvular heart disease, because of the risks of bacteraemia and endocarditis, is a very stong contraindication to the use of an intrauterine device.

ORAL CONTRACEPTION

Oestrogen/Progestogen Containing Pills

These are taken daily for 21 days followed by 7 'pill free' days. Some brand packets (ED) contain 28 pills, the last 7 of which are inert, the reason for this being that pill-taking can be continuous. The dose of steroids used in the combined pill has continued to decline. Few preparations contain 50 μg of ethinyloestradiol, most containing between 20 and 35 μg. Doses of progestogens have also declined and many preparations include 0.5 or 1.0 mg of norethisterone or 250 μg of levonorgestrel. A second generation of progestogens has been introduced recently with fewer androgenic properties and so with supposedly fewer thrombotic side-effects. These are gestodene, desogestrel and norgestimate (current combined preparations are listed in Table 30.1). The concept of varying progestogenicity clearly applies to dose, but the relationship of one compound to another is more complex, as each compound affects different tissues in different ways.

Whether there are differences in intracellular biochemistry caused by different progestogens remains to be evaluated. Until we know more about the intracellular changes caused

Table 30.1
Hormone Content of Combined Oral Contraceptives

Preparation	*Progestogen*	*Preparation*	*Progestogen*
Ethinyloestradiol 20 μg		Ovranette	levonorgestrel 150 μg
Femodette	gestodene 75 μg	Ovran 30	levonorgestrel 250 μg
Loestrin 20	norethisterone 1 mg		
Mercilon	desogestrel 150 μg	**Ethinyloestradiol 35 μg**	
		Binovum	norethisterone 0.5&1 mg
Ethinyloestradiol 30 μg		Brevinor	norethisterone 0.5 mg
Eugynon 30	levonorgestrel 250 μg	Cilest	norgestimate 0.25 μg
Femodene	gestodene 75 μg	Norimin	norethisterone 1 mg
Femodene ED	gestodene 75 μg	Ovysmen	norethisterone 0.5 mg
Loestrin 30	norethisterone 1.5 mg		
Marvelon	desogestrel 150 μg	**Ethinyloestradiol 50 μg**	
Microgynon 30	levonorgestrel 150 μg	Norinyl 1	norethisterone 1 mg
Microgynon 30ED	levonorgestrel 150 μg	Ovrin	levonorgestrel 250 μg
Minulet	gestodene 75 μg	Schering PC4	levonorgestrel 250 μg

Triphasic pills not listed.

by progestogens, it is prudent to use the smallest effective dose in the circumstances.

Mode of action

The combined pill acts by inhibiting the release of Gonadotrophin Releasing Hormone (GnRH) and so of gonadotrophins, which in turn, causes inactive ovaries and anovulation. This is the combined effect of both the oestrogen and progestogen components. The progestogen alters the cervical mucus so that it becomes thick and difficult for sperm to penetrate. There are alterations of endometrial biochemistry which could impair implantation, but these have not yet been fully determined. These three actions make the combined pill a highly effective contraceptive.

The method failure is less than 0.5 per 100 woman years and the overall failure rate is about 1.5 per 100 woman years. The ability to take tablets regularly is important in maintaining the efficacy, as forgetting even one or two tablets can allow ovulation to take place. Interaction with other drugs, such as some antibiotics, or failure of absorption due to gastroenteritis are also common reasons for failure of the method. The drugs listed in Table 30.2 may cause interaction with the pill's steroids.

Advantages of the method are its efficacy and that it is not coitally related, but there may be others, such as reduced menstrual loss or diminished dysmenorrhoea. Disadvantages are the need to take tablets daily, an increased vaginal discharge due either to increased cervical mucus or a tendency to candida infections, weight gain and headaches in some users. There are also wide-ranging metabolic effects which have been extensively investigated during the past 20 years. The oestrogen component acting via hepatic oestrogen receptors alters protein synthesis. This manifests through the changes in enzymes, binding and transport proteins, and proteins involved in the coagulation mechanism. The pill causes increased risk of thrombosis, possibly through raised coagulation factors and fibrinogen and increased platelet adhesiveness. This may cause venous thromboembolism in susceptible individuals, namely those with a previous history of deep venous thrombosis or those with varicose veins and thrombophlebitis. In women with a family history of venous thromboembolic disease, antithrombin III deficiency in plasma should be excluded.

There are alterations in lipids, such as increased triglyceride levels as well as a reduction in the high (HDL) and an increase in the low density (LDL) lipoprotein fractions of

Table 30.2

Drugs Causing Interaction with Steroids in Oestrogen/Progestogen Pill

The following drugs may possibly reduce contraceptive efficacy, as measured by an increased incidence of breakthrough bleeding or pregnancy:

1. amidopyrine; anti-inflammatory agents such as oxyphenbutazone and phenazone;
2. phenacetin;
3. anticonvulsants such as phenytoin, primidone and ethosuximide;
4. antibiotics such as ampicillin, chloramphenicol, rifampicin, sulphamethoxypyridazine and nitrofurantoin;
5. barbiturates such as hexobarbitone, phenobarbitone and methylphemobarbitone;
6. sedatives such as chlordiazepoxide, chlorpromazine and meprobromate and chloral hydrate derivaives used as hypnotics;
7. vasoconstrictors; such as dihydroergotamine.

Oral contraceptives may alter the dose required of the following groups of drugs:

1. anticoagulants;
2. tricyclic antidepressants such as imipramine;
3. corticosteroids;
4. insulin or oral hypoglycaemic agents.

cholesterol, the latter being caused by the progestogen component. Arterial thrombosis may result in susceptible women — those who already have abnormal lipids, obese women, and those who smoke heavily, particularly over the age of 35. It is debatable as to whether or not pill steroids cause impairment of glucose tolerance. Many of the studies were carried out on the higher dose pills used 10 to 20 years ago. The current pills probably have no significant effect on carbohydrate metabolism, except in susceptible women such as latent diabetics, i.e. those with a history of abnormal carbohydrate metabolism in a previous pregnancy.

Carcinogenesis and the pill is a controversial issue. Pill use early in the reproductive era has been associated with a higher incidence of breast cancer in some studies, but not in others. This has been attributed to the progestogen component. An association between the pill use and carcinoma of the cervix has also been suggested. While the former may be a genuine anxiety, the latter is more likely to be due to the acquisition of sexually transmitted carcinogens, although the effect of the sex steroids on the cervical epithelial cells cannot be entirely disregarded. Multicentre case control studies involving several countries have not shown any positive association between oral contraceptive use and either breast or cervical cancer, but have suggested a protective effect against endometrial cancer.

Hypertension may be caused or exacerbated by the combined pill in about 1% of users. Biochemical mechanisms are not clear, but may involve altered rennin-angiotensin or aldosterone production. Regular checks of blood pressure in pill users is mandatory. The combined pill may reduce milk volume and is not the contraceptive of first choice for lactating mothers.

Triphasic Pills

These contain oestrogen and progestogen in varying amounts rather than constant amounts. The active tablets are taken for 21 days followed by 7 placebo pills. The dose of oestrogen is usually 30 μg but rising to 40 μg in mid cycle The dose of progestogen is less during the first 10 days of the 21-day tablet cycle, and more during the second 10 days, thereby reducing the total dose of steroid ingested. Their efficacy and side-effects are similar to those of the combined pill. The names of these preparations are Logynon, Synphase, Tri-Minulet, Triadene, Trinordiol and Trinovum.

Progestogen Only Pills

These contain small doses of norethisterone (0.35 mg), levonorgestrel (30 or 75 μg) or ethynodiol diacetate (0.5 mg) and are taken daily on a continuous basis. They alter ovarian function, but do not inhibit ovulation in more than 50% of cycles. Persistent follicular cysts with relatively high circulating oestrogen levels may occur in a proportion of users. The mode of action is on the ovary, on the endometrium and on cervical mucus. Failure rates have varied widely from one trial to another. It is generally accepted that the true failure rate is about 4–6 per 100 woman years. The main advantage of the method is the relative absence of metabolic side-effects due to the low dose of progestogen used and the absence of oestrogen. There is no effect on milk volume or composition and so this is a method of choice for the lactating woman. The disadvantages are: (1) that the tablets must be taken daily and preferably at a constant time of day to maintain adequate blood levels, and (2) irregular menstrual bleeding, caused by all progestogen only contraceptives.

The brands available in the UK are Femulen, Micronor, Microval, Neogest, Norgeston and Noriday.

POST-COITAL CONTRACEPTION

Prevention of pregnancy up to 48 hours, or even longer, after unprotected intercourse can be effective. The methods used are 2 high dose combined oral contraceptive tablets 12 hours apart or the insertion of an intrauterine device as soon as possible after coitus. Both methods alter the endometrium to prevent implantation or they interrupt this process in its early stages. The failure rates vary between 2 and 6 per 100 woman years in trials, the lower pregnancy rate being when the method was initiated within 48 hours and preferably within 24 hours. The method is not widely used presumably because of lack of information among the people who most need it. Schering PC4 is marketed as such a preparation while Levonelle-2 is a progestogen only post-coital pill to avoid the nausea induced by the oestrogen component.

INJECTABLE HORMONAL CONTRACEPTIVES

These consist of intramuscular injections of either medroxyprogesterone acetate 150 mg given every 12 weeks or norethisterone oenanthate 200 mg given either every 8 or 10 weeks. Their use has been surrounded by much unwarranted controversy, but gradually scientific facts are being accepted and these two injectables are now licensed for use in a large and increasing number of countries including the UK. They act by inhibiting ovulation as well as by exerting the other progestogenic contraceptive effects on the endometrium and cervical mucus already described. Consequently, they are very effective contraceptives with failure rates of about 0.5 per 100 woman years and it is easy to differentiate user from method failure. The advantages of the method are: (1) its efficacy; (2) it is a non-coitally related method; (3) despite irregular bleeding, there may be increased haemoglobin levels and increased weight gain, both of which may be of value in developing countries. A disadvantage of the method is the irregular bleeding similar to that seen with other progestogen only methods, the cause of which is still uncertain. The high plasma levels of progestogen, particularly during the first 4–6 weeks of the injection interval, lead to suppression of the hypothalamic-pituitary-ovarian axis and endometrial atrophy causing variable periods of amenorrhoea in a number of users. Compared with the combined pill, there is a relative absence of metabolic changes. Synthetic progestogens do not significantly alter the coagulation factors, and while there is an increase in plasma insulin, this is compensated for by insulin antagonism in the tissues, so that carbohydrate tolerance is not altered. Liver function tests are not altered. Milk volume and composition are not altered by injectable progestogens and so the method is a suitable one for lactating women, provided it is started 6 weeks after delivery. Transfer to the infant of tiny amounts of progestogen in breast milk should be avoided during the first 6 weeks of life.

Plasma lipids are altered by progestogens, particularly by the 19 nortestosterone derivatives. High density lipoprotein cholesterol is reduced by about 25% in users of norethisterone oenanthate. There is a slight, but inconsistent and insignificant elevation of low density lipoprotein cholesterol. High density lipoprotein cholesterol (HDLC) is a transport form of lipid and so its reduction will increase the deposition of cholesterol and atheroma formation. However, there is no epidemiological evidence to suggest that injectable progestogens increase the risks of myocardial infarction.

Existing compounds in smaller doses, with or without oestrogens, are being tried as monthly injectables, as are new compounds such as esters of levonorgestrel.

Vasectomy

The identification of the vas deferens, excision of a 2 cm segment of it and the separation of the cut ends by doubling them back on each other, is usually a simple operation performed under local anaesthetic. It prevents access of sperm from the testes into the ejaculate, but about 30 ejaculations are required to empty the seminal vesicles of live sperm. At least one sample with azoospermia is necessary before the method can be deemed to be effective.

The failure rate is low. The incidence of circulating antibodies to sperm increases from 2% to over 50% after vasectomy. Even though reversibility can be accomplished anatomically, fertility is markedly reduced because of these antibodies.

NEW METHODS

Four approaches to alternative methods of contraception are currently being investigated. These are (1) release of existing steroids or variations of them from different vehicles; (2) alteration of the hypothalamic-pituitary axis inhibiting spermatogenesis; (3) chemical methods of inhibiting spermatogenesis; and (4) immunological interference with implantation.

The method of releasing existing steroids, in this case levonorgestrel, is from 6 subcutaneous implants releasing 40–45 μg per day (Norplant).

Implant

Norplant consists of six silastic tubes, each 2.5 cm long and 3 mm in diameter, containing levonorgestrel crystals. They are inserted subcutaneously in the upper arm using a trochar and cannula after a small skin incision is made under local anaesthetic. The failure rate is about 1 per 100 woman years and protection can be given for up to 6 years (Norplant 6). Removal can be difficult. Single devices of the same dimensions releasing levonorgestrel from sesame oil, contained within a polymer shell, and double devices releasing levonorgestrel from crystals within a silastic tube (Norplant 2) are being tried.

A single implant releasing etonorgestrel (Implanon) and which lasts for 3 years has recently become available.

The advantages are the provision of an effective method of contraception for a long time without patient involvement. The disadvantages are irregularity of the menstrual cycle, which diminishes with duration of use, and those of an invasive procedure for insertion and removal.

Alterations of the Hypothalamic Pituitary Axis

This has been carried out using synthetic peptides which are analogues of GnRH and which act either as antagonists or as agonists of this compound. The antagonistic analogues act by competitive binding to pituitary receptor sites, abolishing the LH surge and so inhibiting ovulation. Administration is intranasally or by injection and only small scale studies have been carried out. Long-term effects and contraceptive efficacy have not been investigated. GnRH agonists, such as buserelin or nafarelin, given intranasally, have been investigated more fully and found to inhibit ovulation regularly. These compounds act by desensitising the pituitary so that it fails to respond to oestradiol, thereby abolishing the LH surge required for ovulation. Oestradiol levels are reduced as a result of ovarian suppression, the endometrium becomes inactive and there are bleeding irregularities.

Alternative routes of administration, such as implants or injectables, will be tried in the future, as well as the possibility of combined therapy with an agonist given intermittently together with a progestogen to improve cycle control.

Chemical Methods of Inhibiting Spermatogenesis

A number of compounds are being investigated that may inhibit spermatogenesis. The most widely known of these is gossypol, found as a trace contaminant of cotton seed oil in China. Its efficacy in preventing sperm maturation and reducing motility and capacity for fertilisation is being assessed. Certain side-effects have been reported after large doses, including hyperkalaemia and subsequent cardiac arrthymias.

Immunological Methods

The concept of inducing antibodies to HCG by vaccination, thereby preventing implantation, is an attractive one. However, the difficulties must not be underestimated. These are (1) variability of antibody titre induced, and (2) the variability from person to person of its duration of action. Successful animal studies have led to preliminary studies in humans. However at this stage, the approach must be considered as very much an experimental one.

FURTHER READING

Fraser I.S., Wiesberg E.A. (1981). A comprehensive review of injectable contraception with special emphasis on depomed-toxyprogesterone acetate. *Med. J. Aust.* **1**(1): 1–19.

Hafez E.S.E., ed. (1979). *Human Reproduction, Conception and Contraception,* 2nd edn. Hagerstown, Maryland: Harper and Row.

Harper M.J.K. (1983). *Birth Control Technologies.* London: Heinemann Medical.

Hawkins D.F., Elder M.G. (1979). *Human fertility control.* London: Butterworth.

Snowdon R., Williams M.Z., Hawkins D. *The IUD. A Practical Guide.* London: Croom Helm.

31

Sterilisation and its Reversal

The verb 'to sterilise' is defined as to wash, to cleanse, to clean or to purify. In the gynaecological context, it is defined as being barren or not fertile. It is the process where an otherwise fertile person is rendered infertile. It is important to remember that this is applied equally to the male as well as the female.

HISTORY

Safe effective sterilisation has only been around for as long as there has been safe and effective anaesthetic agents. Prior to safe anaesthesia, ways of attempted sterilisation normally centred around causing some form of inflammatory or infective process within the uterine cavity of the female. These were usually with caustic agents which "burnt" the lining of the uterus and hence set up a severe inflammatory reaction which caused an Asherman's type syndrome. Unfortunately, these were performed in a very uncontrolled way and quite often resulted in horrendous injuries and even death to the female. It is of interest that no comparable methods were employed in the male!

After the introduction of safe anaesthesia, this allowed multiple methods of sterilisation to be performed both on the male and female.

REASONS FOR STERILISATION AND PATIENT DISCUSSION POINTS

The vast majority of patients are sterilised because as a couple they feel that they have completed their family. These patients tend to be over 30 years old and already have two or more children. The decision in this case is relatively straightforward as long as the doctor concerned is happy that both partners consent to the procedure and they realise the consequences of the operation, the risks of the procedure, as well as the failure rate involved. These days, it is essential medicolegally that the failure rate is not only carefully explained to both partners, but that a note is made in the patient records that this has been discussed.

The risks of the procedure vary from the male to the female. The female sterilisation is generally performed under general anaesthetic, although in some countries it is routinely done under local anaesthetic. There are the usual risks of the laparoscopy itself which must be fully explained. Male sterilisation on the other hand is generally done under local anaesthetic and the post-operative complication rate small. When discussing sterilisation, it is important that both partners are present and both forms of sterilisation are discussed. It should be noted though that in some societies, it is very unlikely that the male will agree to be sterilised as they feel this is restricting their masculinity.

In some situations, sterilisation is not so straightforward and the two main areas of concern here are single women who have not had any children and the mentally handicapped. The gynaecologist will occasionally get women who are in their twenties who are adamant that they do not want, or ever want, children and do not want to use other forms of contraception such as the pill. These patients have to be considered with a great deal of tact as well as understanding. Although it is up to the individual practitioner, it would be unusual to sterilise someone under the age of 30 who has not had any children or completed their family. There are circumstances though where the patient repeatedly visits the gynaecologist over a period of years requesting the procedure. If the gynaecologist is completely sure that the patient fully understands the implications of the procedure, then this can be performed. It must be said that a lot of young women in their early twenties do not have a strong maternal instinct, but several years later, the maternal instinct grows and they would regret it if they had been sterilised at that early age.

The gynaecologist will also get requests from parents or guardians of mentally handicapped children who are sexually active and where the parents or guardians are concerned about the possible results of this sexual activity resulting in a pregnancy. The gynaecologist is not allowed to act on the consent from the parent or guardian but has to seek legal approval for this to be carried out. With any patient where the gynaecologist is not sure about the medical competence of the patient, then further opinion should be sought.

A lot of women will ask about the possible increase in menstrual blood loss after sterilisation. It should be explained to them that there is *not* an increase, only a *perceived* increase. On the other hand, sterilisation is often carried out in the mid to late thirties, when menstrual loss may be increasing for other reasons. Large trials have shown that sterilisation itself is not a factor.

FEMALE STERILISATION

The vast majority of sterilisation procedures performed on the female involve some form of occlusion of the fallopian tubes. Initially this was simply by taking the entire tube away on both sides (bilateral salpingectomy) or even a portion of the tube on both sides (partial salpingectomy). This would therefore stop the sperm getting to the egg, fertilising it and then allowing it back into the uterine cavity. Indeed, total and partial salpingectomies are still commonly used and are still one of the most effective ways of sterilising the female.

Salpingectomies and partial salpingectomies were generally performed at open operation or laparotomy. As long as the fallopian tubes are not badly damaged or encased in adhesions then this is generally a straightforward procedure but does still require the abdomen to be opened.

To try and make the sterilisation procedure easier, other ways to damage and occlude the tube were found. The tube can be burnt or diathermised, which again will occlude it along the length that the diathermy is applied to. This was initially carried out with monopolar diathermy which was applied with forceps similar to those used to cauterised bleeding points that are found during any major operation. Unfortunately, this burning had an unacceptably high rate of adverse affects most commonly resulting in burns to other organs such as the bowel. This ultimately causes perforation and unless diagnosed and treated can lead to death. It was in view of these unacceptable side-effects of diathermy that other, not only simpler, but safer methods were designed.

In the 1970s, laparoscopy was introduced on a widespread basis. Laparoscopy was not only very useful for diagnostic reasons in gynaecology, but it was realised that less invasive ways of sterilisation could be performed. This coincided with improvements in techniques to occlude the tube using specially designed clips or rings.

Clips

One of the first clips that was used was the Hulka Clemens. This was very successful and was used for many years. Indeed in some parts of the world it is still used. It was applied with a special applicator and was placed on the isthmic portion of the tube. The clip itself went right across the tube and was fixed there by a permanent catch within the clip itself. Occasionally, these clips would fall off or not occlude the total lumen of the tube. They were also rather fiddly to apply and hence generally had a higher complication and subsequent failure rate than was desired. This led to the introduction of the Filshie clip. This was a special silicon and titanium clip that was much easier to apply, had a lower complication rate and hence a lower failure rate. This is now the most commonly used clip throughout the world.

Rings

A special distensible ring, the Fallope or Yoon ring, was developed that could also be applied laparoscopically. A small loop of the fallopian tube was pulled through a special instrument and then the ring, rather like an elastic band, was applied to the base of this loop. This loop then became necrotic, creating a significant obstruction between two portions of the tubal lumen. Unfortunately the ring was difficult to use, difficult to apply over a satisfactory loop of tube and had a much higher failure rate than the Hulka Clemens clip. However, it was very cheap and predominantly took off in the Third World.

Both the clips and the rings were applied through a second laparoscopic port of between 5 and 8 mm under direct vision.

CURRENT TECHNIQUES

Both open and keyhole, or laparoscopic, techniques are still currently used in female sterilisation.

Open Techniques

It is still appropriate under certain circumstances to do a partial or total salpingectomy. The most common indication for an open procedure these days is at the same time as the caesarean section. This is most commonly performed if the patient has already had three or more caesarean sections and wishes to be sterilised at the same time as the delivery of the baby. Generally, a partial or total salpingectomy is performed, although a clip or diathermy can also be applied to the tube.

Laparoscopic Techniques

The Filshie clip is by far the most commonly used form of laparoscopic sterilisation at present. It is applied under direct vision and ideally should be applied under video control so more than one person can ensure that it is applied in the correct place on the fallopian tube. In the present medicolegal climate, it is also useful to have a colour printout after the application of both clips.

With the growing use of laparoscopic surgery, some centres now perform bipolar coagulation which is inherently far safer than the monopolar that was previously used and caused a lot of the burns. Bipolar forceps are extremely exact and can be applied across the tube and burnt in a safe manner. The main benefit to this is that it is a cheaper way as the instruments are re-usable and clips do not have to be purchased.

In some circumstances, a partial or total salpingectomy can also be performed laparoscopically as long as there is correct instrumentation and correct skills available. This is generally performed if there has been some other disease to the tube, such as infection, which is giving the patient symptoms such as recurring infection or pelvic pain. In these situations, both the tubes can be removed to try and alleviate the symptoms as well as to sterilise the patient.

The benefits and problems of the various methods are shown in Table 31.1.

Future Techniques

Most of these centre around less invasive techniques to occlude the fallopian tube. Various hysteroscopic techniques have been studied including injection forms of "super glue" into the proximal portion of the tube hysteroscopically. Unfortunately though this is relatively easy, the tubes can re-canalise and the failure rates were unacceptable. In view of this, various types of plastic and titanium coils have been developed where these are inserted, again hysteroscopically, but have a lower failure rate. Unfortunately, these are still very expensive and require a general anaesthetic, but would have the additional benefit that reversing them would be even easier as they should be able to be removed hysteroscopically. At present, there are several ongoing studies into these sort of hysteroscopic occlusive techniques, and it might

Table 31.1
Benefits and Problems of Different Sterilisation Techniques

Methods	Pros	Cons
Salpingectomy	Very low failure rate. Good if tube diseased	Irreversible and interventional
Partial salpingectomy	Very low failure rate	It can be reversed but the initial operation is a lot more tricky and prone to bleeding. It can only be reversed if the fimbria were left.
Diathermy	Very cheap and can be used laparoscopically. Can be reversed if not too much burnt	Has to be used by an experienced operator but is safe as long as bipolar is used
Clips	Very low failure rate and easy to learn	Clips are expensive and must be applied correctly.
Yoon rings	Cheap and can be applied laparoscopically	More difficult to reverse as a greater amount of tube has been damaged. Difficult to apply

be that in the future, these are even safer and more preferred by the patient.

MALE STERILISATION

Sterilising the male, vasectomy, is where a portion of the vas deferens is removed or occluded surgically. This is a relatively straightforward procedure that involves one or two small (less than 1 cm) incisions in the scrotum, the vas identified, the associated neurovascular bundle stripped off it, and then the vas divided. It can be just cauterised but the re-canalisation rates are too high. Most practitioners would remove a small portion of the vas and send this for histology to confirm that it was indeed the vas. The ends of the vas can then either be folded back and tied, or cauterised and tied. The resultant gap then significantly reduces the chance of any re-canalisation occurring. The operation is generally carried out under local anaesthetic and should take approximately 20 minutes.

The possible post-operative complications with vasectomy are infection, haematoma and post-operative pain. All of these should have a low incidence and the procedure can be covered with prophylactic antibiotics.

The most important point to remember with a vasectomy is that the male is not immediately sterile. Indeed, the patient should be advised that until he has had two semen samples that have shown total azoospermia, he should still be considered as fertile. These samples are produced by masturbation and generally produced between 4 and 8 weeks after the initial procedure. As soon as he has two confirmed azoospermic samples, then he can be considered sterile.

Long-Term Effects

One of the worries that most men have regarding vasectomy is: what happens to all the sperm that are produced, and if there are any long-term detrimental consequences. They need to be re-assured that the sperm is just re-absorbed from within the testis itself and this does not cause a problem. The main long-term consequences of vasectomy are mild scrotal pain and this has a low incidence in most patients.

STERILISATION REVERSAL

Female

The main questions that need to be considered with reversal of sterilisation are: whether it should be done, the way the initial sterilisation was performed, and the subsequent success rates of the reversal procedure.

Should it be done?

A lot of clinicians feel that with the limited resources of the NHS that unless there are exceptional reasons, a routine reversal should not be performed at all. If the patient is still with her current partner and the children are all alive, then most people would feel this is an inappropriate use of NHS resources. If the patient wants to pursue this privately, then this would be an option.

However, there are always tragic circumstances where reversals are appropriate on the NHS, and these range from the deaths of any children through fires or car crashes, or more commonly, separation of the parents. It is an unfortunate fact that nowadays many get divorced and may want to have children with their new partner. Although the children tend to stay with the female partner in any divorce, if her future partner has no children, then again she may wish to procreate with him.

Method of reversal and success rates

The less damage that has been done to the tube, the easier it is to reverse. If the patient had a salpingectomy or the entire tube burnt with diathermy, then these are not reversible. If a partial salpingectomy or a clip sterilisation has been performed, then these can be reversed. This should be done by a surgeon skilled in microsurgery and an operating microscope used. It is important the tubes are repaired in a very accurate fashion and then re-anstomosed under the operating microscope. The tubes should be repaired in two layers with some very fine non-absorbable sutures inserted to the tubal mucosa, and then the tubal serosa closed over this. It is possible for reversal to be done laparoscopically, although not only does this take considerably longer, but also the success rates are significantly lower. In expert hands, a laparoscopic reversal will give pregnancy rates of 65%, whereas in expert hands by open microsurgery it is possible to get over 85% pregnancy rates with a single clip sterilisation. As a general rule, the more the tube has been removed or damaged, the lower the success rates.

It is also possible to bypass the entire tubes altogether with techniques such as *in vitro* fertilisation, but when comparing the two techniques if a reversal is possible, it should always be performed in the first instance as the success rates are significantly higher. The only exception to this is if there is a concurrent severe sperm problem as well.

Although the duration of time from the initial sterilisation to the reversal is not significant, the age of the female plays a very important part in obtaining subsequent successful pregnancies.

Male

It is generally easier to reverse a vasectomy than a female sterilisation, but this again should be performed in a microsurgical way to get the best results. The longer the amount of vas removed again, the more difficult the re-anastamosis will be and the more likely that a stricture will have occurred post-operatively. The success rates of getting sperm into the ejaculate after reversal of vasectomy should be around 90%. As with any operation on the testis or vas, it is an unfortunate fact that anti-sperm antibodies can be produced by the patients own immune system as a result. These antisperm antibodies then cause the sperm to clump together and can significantly reduce the effectiveness of the reversal. The amount of anti-sperm antibodies produced increases with time, and it is because of this fact that it is generally not worthwhile reversing vasectomies if there is greater than 5 years from the time of the original operation to the reversal. Although the man's age is not as important as the females, the duration between these two operations is of importance.

If a man does undergo reversal of vasectomy, this should be performed in a centre not only with the appropriate microsurgical skills, but in a centre than can freeze a piece of testicular tissue taken at the same time as the reversal is performed. This is important in situations where the reversal fails and no sperm are ejaculated. Sperm can then be extracted from this testicular tissue and be used for an IVF/ICSI cycle. This would prevent him from having to have a further operation to obtain the tissue.

SUMMARY

There are now many safe forms of sterilisation both on the male and female side. It is important that all methods and all possible reasons to do one or the other are fully discussed with both partners. The patient should *always* be warned about failure rates and should generally be advised that sterilisation is not a reversible procedure. However, for whatever circumstances a reversal is necessary, then this should be performed in appropriately skilled hands where success rates can be very high.

32

The Role of Minimum Access Surgery

INTRODUCTION

Minimum access surgery (MAS) utilises telescopes with TV attachments as well as other small instruments that can fit down through 5–10 mm incisions to perform certain procedures that would otherwise require much more invasive and open surgery. These techniques are commonly called "keyhole" surgery and have been around for the last 20 years. They have only been in common usage though over the last 5 to 10 years. The two main areas of MAS (sometimes called minimum invasive surgery) are laparoscopic and hysteroscopic. Laparoscopic surgery is where a telescope is inserted through a 10 mm incision in the umbiiicus after the abdomen has been insufflated with carbon dioxide gas to examine the abdominal and pelvic contents. Extra ports (normally 5 mm), are then inserted into other locations in the abdomen through which instruments such as graspers, scissors and lasers are inserted. Laparoscopies themselves are divided into diagnostic and therapeutic. Diagnostic laparoscopies are where the surgeon only looks inside the pelvis to diagnose gynaecological diseases such as endometriosis, fibroids or any pelvic scarring. Therapeutic laparoscopy is where treatment is performed inside the pelvis to try and ressolve some of the pathology seen. It is the therapeutic options that would be further discussed in this chapter.

Hysteroscopy is where a small telescope, normally around 3–4 mm, is inserted through the cervix to examine the uterine cavity. Diagnostic hysteroscopy examines the uterine cavity to see whether there are any abnormal areas, contributing for instance to menorrhagia, or any abnormal structure such as fibroids or adhesions contributing towards pain or infertility. Therapeutic hysteroscopy is where other micro instruments are then inserted along an operating channel in the hysteroscope to try and resolve these problems.

Reasons for Minimal Access Surgery

The main reasons for minimal access surgery are:

- Cosmetic
- Faster recovery time
- Fewer post-operative complications
- Cost benefits.

As the patient is having several small incisions, these are generally more cosmetic than a large Pfannensteil or sub-umbilical midline scar.

The incisions are between 5 and 10 mm, and as a general rule, patients are in hospital only as a day case or perhaps one night. Patients not only spend a far shorter time in hospital than for an open procedure, but are also back to normal day-to-day living and working in a significantly shorter period of time. They also experience less post-operative pain due to the smaller incisional sites.

Minimal tissue trauma occurs, strict haemostasis should also be performed and the tissues are not allowed to dessicate. This results in less post-operative adhesion formation and fewer post-operative complications such as haemorrhage, infection and even pneumonia. (The patient who is at high risk of post-operative pneumonia is more likely to be able to cough adequately following minimal access procedures than they are after having a large incisional wound).

Taking all the above points into account, there is also an overwhelming cost benefit to the Health Service with these procedures — even taking into account the cost of the equipment.

Training and Equipment

Anybody utilising this equipment should be fully trained in its use and there are several excellent courses available, taking the surgeon from the most basic level to the most advanced. The most advanced courses are often carried out abroad where the live pig model can be utilised to give increased realism during the training. There is no place for untrained surgeons to be using this sort of equipment and there have been several patient deaths in the past when insufficiently trained surgeons have attempted these procedures.

Equipment must be of high quality so that there are good views of the operation site and instruments for incision making and haemostasis in good working order. Due to the complexity of the equipment, the capital costs of setting up a theatre for a range of such procedures is about £70,000.

LAPAROSCOPIC PROCEDURES

Endometriosis

Endometriosis is one of the conditions which is best suited for laparoscopic treatment, most commonly with some form of laser energy. A carbon dioxide or fibre laser can be used to safely and adequately ablate any peritoneal endometriotic deposits. This is an extremely effective way of improving the symptoms from this debilitating disease and very good results can be obtained from it. If endometriotic cysts have been found in the ovary, then lasers can also be used to open the ovary and, after drainage, to ablate the cyst wall within the ovary itself. Treatment of endometriosis in this way cannot only significantly improve the pain, but also improve the subsequent fertility of patients who have previously been infertile. Indeed, today all forms of minimal and moderate grades of endometriosis that require surgery should be treated laparoscopically. The only place for open surgical treatment would be if there is a frozen pelvis where laparoscopic techniques could not be safely used.

Pelvic Adhesions

Pelvic adhesions can contribute towards pelvic pain and infertility. Laparoscopic adhesiolysis is carried out utilising very small scissors, laser energy, or if the adhesions are vascular they can be coagulated and then cut with the scissors. Most adhesions can be divided with the above methods to get exceptionally good results to alleviate the majority of symptoms. Similar to endometriosis, the only cases where this cannot be performed laparoscopically is where the pelvis is completely obliterated with dense adhesions and the various structures cannot be safely elucidated.

Laparoscopic adhesiolysis has also the added benefit that the adhesions are less likely to re-form as less trauma has been performed to the peritoneal structures and the tissues are not dessicated as they would be at open procedure. Drying out of tissues leads to further fibrosis.

Ectopic Pregnancy

Ectopic pregnancy is one of the few areas in MAS that has been studied, both for cost effectiveness as well as outcome. The general conclusions and recommendations from the Royal College of Obstetricians & Gynaecologists is that the vast majority of ectopic pregnancies should be treated laparoscopically. All modes of treatment can be used from linear salpingotomies, partial salpingectomies up to and including total salpingectomies. This does depend on the severity of the ectopic and the skill of the surgeon.

Tubal Surgery

There is very little place for laparoscopic surgery in the area of tubal microsurgery. Though most forms of tubal surgery *can* be done laparoscopically, they can often take up to 7 or 8 hours for a cornual resection and re-anastomosis, but most importantly the results are seldom as good as for open microsurgical procedures. The only crossover in this area is that of distal tubal disease. If the tube has only mild distal disease, then some surgeons will get as good results by performing a laparoscopic salpingostomy as others will by an open salpingostomy.

Adnexal Surgery

The vast majority of ovarian cysts, salpingectomies and oophorectomies can now be performed by laparoscopic procedures. The main concern with this tends to be if the underlying pathology is malignant and the worry that you may therefore not perform such an adequate staging procedure, or that you might seed the malignancy further. Most surgeons will therefore not perform these techniques laparoscopically if there is a high index of suspicion that the underlying pathology is malignant. On the other hand, some gynaecological cancer specialists will still do it laparoscopically but take great care to put the tissue in specially designed bags which would prevent dissemination of any fluids or tissue throughout the pelvis.

Polycystic Ovarian Syndrome

Ever since Stein and Leventhal treated this condition by wedge resection of the ovary, the therapeutic treatment of the above condition by damaging the ovary has continued. The previous wedge resections performed at laparotomy were very invasive and the post-operative complication rate in the form of adhesions was very high. It has now been found that patients who are resistant to Clomid can be made to spontaneously ovulate, or be made sensitive to Clomid, by drilling several holes in each ovary. It does not seem to matter how these ovaries are drilled, whether it is with a diathermy point or with a laser. It appears that the mere fact of damaging the ovarian cortex gives the therapeutic result which improves the hormonal millieu and corrects some of the abnormalities noted with the syndrome. Unfortunately, the effect is not permanent and only lasts between 12 and 24 months.

Myomectomy

The only limiting factor here is the size of the uterine corpus. Obviously, if the fibroids extend up to the umbilicus then a laparoscopy cannot be safely performed and this treatment is not possible. If though the fibroids are smaller and it does allow safe laparoscopy, then the fibroids can be removed laparoscopically. The fibroids are morcellated by an electric 'liquidiser' type of machine so that it can then be removed through a 10 mm port. The resultant defect is then sutured very carefully. It is important though to realise this is *not* an optimal technique for the patient who is still desirous of fertility. Most reproductive surgeons feel that it is a technique that should only be used in a patient who has completed her family but still wants to retain her uterus for psychological reasons.

Hysterectomies

Hysterectomies are possible laparoscopically, either by doing a laparoscopic assisted vaginal hysterectomy (LAVH) where the first two pedicles are taken laparoscopically and the third vaginally. The uterus is removed vaginally. It is also possible to do a subtotal hysterectomy where again the first two pedicles are taken laparoscopically, the cervix is then left behind and the uterus morcellated and removed through a 10 mm port. A total laparoscopic hysterectomy where all the pedicles are taken and the vaginal vault closed is also possible but is time-consuming, and in most situations does not offer any further benefit to the patient. Indeed even though all these techniques are possible, the rate for laparoscopic hysterectomies performed has decreased greatly over the last

5 years as more people realise the value of a traditional vaginal hysterectomy in suitably experienced hands. The major benefit of the laparoscopic approach is that if there are adhesions around the uterus from previous infection or surgery, then these can be divided prior to a vaginal hysterectomy being performed, and if the ovaries need to be removed, then by dividing their pedicles laparoscopically it can make the vaginal approach easier.

Laparoscopic Colposuspension

It is now possible to do a laparoscopic colposuspensions, and indeed the laparoscope gives possibly the better view of the extraperitoneal space where the sutures are applied. It does though require a high level of surgical skill in placing and tying the appropriate suture. Although there are several surgeons around the country that have done more than 20 of these procedures, the long-term results have yet to be validated against the open procedure.

HYSTEROSCOPY

Menorrhoagia

This is without doubt one of the most useful techniques in the investigation of the menorrhagic patient is hysteroscopy. It can not only be used to diagnose any pathology that may be contributing to the menorrhagia, but also allows a biopsy to be taken under direct vision. This is very useful if abnormal areas are seen in the uterine cavity which can sometimes be missed by blind curretage ('D & C'). If medical treatment options have been used and the patient still complains of menorrhagia, then the endometrium can either be resected with a loop resectoscope or ablated with a laser. This is a very successful option in most patients, and even though only approximately 30 to 40% of patients will be amenorrhoeic afterwards, a further 30 to 40% of patients will have a significant decrease in their menstrual loss, and be satisfied with this. There are also other techniques available hysteroscopically which destroy the endometrium through the use of hot water, microwave energy or direct contact with electrically conductive plates placed within the uterine cavity itself. Whereas the normal diagnostic hysteroscope has a diameter of 3 to 4 mm, the transcervical instrument that either ablates or resects the endometrium has a diameter of approximately 7 mm.

Sub-Mucus Fibroids

Fibroids that predominantly protrude into the uterine cavity (submucous), can be very elegantly removed transcervically. This is done with a transcervical instrument identical to that used to resect the endometrium. The fibroid is resected in multiple chips until it is flushed with the uterine surface. The surgeon then waits 5 to 10 minutes to see if any more of the fibroids will be pushed from the uterine corpus itself, if this happens, further fibroids are then resected. The results from transcervical resection are extremely good with relief from pain, menorrhagia and infertility.

Intrauterine Adhesions

Intrauterine adhesions (Asherman's Syndrome) can be formed from over enthusiastic curettage of the pregnant uterus or from other infective or inflammatory processes. They can be diagnosed either by hysterosalpingography or by diagnostic hysteroscopy. After they have been diagnosed, a hysteroscope with an operating bridge over it can be inserted under direct vision, and then a small pair of scissors inserted down the operating bridge. The adhesions between the posterior and anterior surface of the uterine cavity can be very carefully divided under direct vision and an intrauterine contraceptive device inserted for 3 months to prevent them reforming.

Congenital Abnormalities

Patients who have had a septate uterus diagnosed previously (normally by a combination of laparoscopy and hysteroscopy) can have the septum divided hysteroscopically. This is a far better way than having it performed by open procedure as it is much less invasive and is much less likely to cause any post-operative problems such as formation of adhesions. It is essential that a laparoscopy is performed before the division is performed to ensure you are dividing a septum and not a bicornuate uterus. A similar hysteroscope and operating bridge to that used for intrauterine adhesiolysis is inserted and the septum is very carefully divided longitudinally until small blood vessels are seen in it. This would be a sign that you have reached normal myometrium. As the septum is scar tissue, the septum itself does not bleed on cutting. Electrosurgery and laser can also be used to divide the septum but there is more likely to be thermal damage to the endometrium which could possibly cause problems in future cycles if the patient is still desirous of fertility.

SUMMARY

Minimal access surgery is now an accepted and widely used modality in gynaecological surgery. Over half of all gynaecological surgery can be performed safely and effectively laparoscopically, but it is most important to still realise that just because you *can* perform it, does not mean you *should*. The surgeon should be adequately trained with correct equipment and always take into account the patients best interest before deciding to do any minimal access procedure.

33

Female Infertility

FEMALE INFERTILITY

Whether termed infertility or sterility, the inability to reproduce is a problem which can become all-consuming for the couple concerned. Both partners *should* be seen together in the clinic throughout their management. Often the man is unable to attend, but at some stage in the management it should be insisted that he be involved. The physician must be constantly aware of the psychological well-being of the couple, sensitive to the stresses and strains of the situation and sympathetic to any fear or anxieties that arise. Subfertility is an emotionally charged situation and, even before the couple enters the consulting room on their first visit, all sorts of psychological pressures, fears and other anxieties will have arisen. Most people will feel a mixture of embarrassment at their problem, and a fear and anxiety that something serious is wrong. As investigations and treatment proceed, these feelings may give way to frustration or even hopelessness at the lack of results. Emotional rapport with the physician is of extreme importance from the very start, so that fears can be allayed, the stress of the situation partly defused and confidence built up between both partners and the physician.

The rates of normal conception (Fig. 33.1) show that 10% of 'normal couples' i.e. couples who conceive without medical help, will not conceive during the first year of attempting to get pregnant. When should investigations start? The fact that a couple seek medical help means that they perceive that there is a problem. Thus it is important to take the request for help seriously from the start, although the vigour of investigation may be modified somewhat if the duration of exposure to pregnancy has been short.

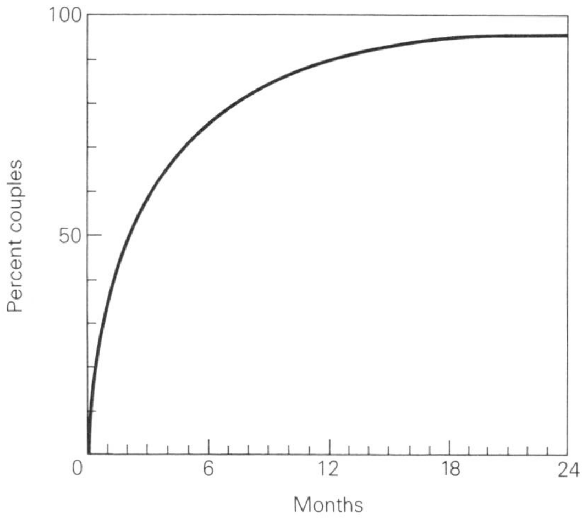

Fig. 33.1 *Normal conception rates.*

Potential areas leading to inability to reproduce will be considered under the headings of (1) defects in ovulation, (2) cervical problems preventing the entry of spermatozoa into the uterus, (3) structural problems interfering with ovum transport, and (4) failure of implantation.

OVULATION

In the average infertility clinic, 30% of couples seen will have some defect concerning maturation of the ovarian follicle. Any variation in the subtle interplay of hormonal balance, whether at hypothalamic, pituitary or ovarian level, may lead to a defect in follicular development, ovum release or maintenance of corpus luteal function. There are many signs suggestive of ovulation, but perhaps the only definite proof is pregnancy.

Menstrual History

Regular menstrual bleeding does not necessarily indicate ovulation, but scanty irregular menses is more suggestive of anovulation. Primary amenorrhoea, which means no spontaneous bleeding before 18 years of age, unusually presents as infertility, and the underlying cause, for instance Turner's syndrome or gynaetresia, can usually be diagnosed by an accurate clinical history and examination. Secondary amenorrhoea — cessation of menstruation after the regular occurrence of normal menstrual periods — and oligomenorrhoea, defined as scanty, irregular bleeding, may be due to many defects (Table 33.1) and treatment is by the induction of regular ovulation. Special investigations may include hysterosalpingography to exclude intrauterine pathology and measurement of follicle stimulating hormone (FSH), luteinising hormone (LH) and prolactin. If the ovary has failed prematurely (all ovaries fail at the menopause), serum FSH and, to a lesser extent, LH levels will be raised, and the diagnosis is confirmed by ovarian biopsy, when no primordial follicles will be seen. Other, less common, causes of secondary amenorrhoea are due to abnormal thyroid function (hyper- or hypo-) and pituitary tumours. Thyroid function tests (T4:TSH) and X-ray examination of the sella turcica of the pituitary fossa will aid diagnosis.

Table 33.1
Causes of Secondary Amenorrhoea and Oligomenorrhoes

Hypothalamic	Weight change
	Drugs (oral contraceptives, tranquilisers)
	Psychological disturbances
Pituitary	Adenoma
Ovarian	Premature ovarian failure
	Polycystic ovarian syndrome
Uterine	Synechiae
	Asherman's syndrome
	Cervical stenosis

Cervical Mucus

Because of the high levels of circulating oestrogen, the pre-ovulatory mucus is clear and of low viscosity allowing the free passage of spermatozoa. It has the property of forming into threads when stretched between two points (Spinnbarkeit) and, when spread on a microscope slide, it dries in the form of 'fern-like' structures (ferning). At the time of maximum mucus production, the cervical os is open to its greatest extent, but after ovulation, it closes and the mucus abruptly becomes scant, sticky, viscous and impenetrable to sperms. Women can be taught to recognise these changes in the cervical mucus both in quantity and consistency, and this is one of the most useful symptomatic markers of ovulation.

Mastalgia, which is pain or tingling in the breasts, reflecting distension or fluid retention secondary to the pre-ovulatory oestrogen rise, and Mittelschmerz, which is unilateral, midcycle pain of ovulation felt in the iliac fossa are inconstant markers.

Basal Temperature

During an ovulatory cycle, the body temperature shows a biphasic pattern with a rise of about 0.5°C following ovulation. Classically, there is a slight temperature fall (approximately 0.3°C) immediately pre-ovulation, followed by a rise in response to the thermogenic effect of progesterone or its metabolites. The resting basal body temperature is taken daily, usually orally in the morning before getting out of bed and recorded on a temperature graph: the basal temperature chart (BTC). This biphasic chart may indicate ovulation and, occasionally, the pre-ovulatory fall in temperature may be a useful predictor of ovulation. However, this pre-ovulatory fall is often recognised only in retrospect and hence its clinical predictive value is limited. The BTC is cheap and simple to complete and hence is a popular aid in the investigation of the infertile couple. Its usefulness, however, is extended beyond that of recording basal temperature by enlarging the data recorded to include the pattern of menstruation (duration, periodicity and degree), symptoms of mastalgia and cervical mucus changes. Hence, a well completed BTC will give a comprehensive summary of all the symptomatic changes already discussed. The frequency of intercourse should also be recorded, information which is often quite revealing and important.

Endometrial Biopsy

The endometrial lining is one of the end organs of hormonal effect, and histological changes, mainly reflecting progesterone effect, are well documented. Pre-menstrual endometrial biopsy is rarely justified except when genital tuberculosis is to be excluded. Endometrial biopsy increases the risk of uterine infection, necessitates dilatation of the cervix with risk of damage and, if over vigorous, may lead to intrauterine adhesions and hence compound the infertility problem.

Hormones

Radioimmunoassay has enabled the measurement of most hormones involved in the ovulation mechanism. For the detection of ovulation in a menstruating woman, it is usually sufficient to measure the raised plasma progesterone levels in the potentially luteal phase of the cycle (usually Days 19–25). Values of 30 nmol/l or more are highly suggestive of ovulation and adequate luteal function. Various relatively cheap, easy to use kits are available over the counter which many couples find helpful. They usually measure the LH surge. The detection of hyperprolactinaemia may also be important.

Visualisation

Perhaps the best method of detecting ovulation is actually to visualise the ovary. This may be done by direct visualisation at time of laparotomy or conveniently at laparoscopy or by means of ultrasound scanning. The dominant pre-ovulatory follicle measures about 25 mm in diameter, and rupture and ovum release results in the formation of the characteristic punctate 'stigma'. The remaining granuloma cells then appear haemorrhagic (corpus haemorrhagica) and later have a yellow appearance (corpus luteum). These characteristic changes on the ovarian surface may be visualised directly at laparoscopy. Using ultrasound, either transabdominal (with a full bladder) or a vaginal probe, the developing fluid-filled follicles can be observed easily, and the subsequent disappearance of the dominant follicle may indicate ovum release.

In practice, a combination of these investigations and signs — usually BTC, cervical mucus observation, serum progesterone assays and possibly laparoscopy — are used to arrive at a diagnosis of anovulation or ovulation.

Treatment

First, general measures should be considered. A sudden increase in weight, or more commonly, loss of weight as seen typically in anorexia nervosa may act at the hypothalamic level to interfere with hormonal release. Simple advice on diet or perhaps psychiatric aid may be sufficient to regain hormonal balance. Other, more nebulous factors, such as stress or a great desire for pregnancy, may influence the higher centres of the brain and treatment by reassurance and the alleviation of stress may often lead to conception. Derangement of other endocrine systems, e.g. thyroid, may need to be investigated and treatment instigated. The main treatment, however, of anovulation is by ovulation induction using either:

1. Clomiphene citrate or tamoxifen, or
2. Gonadotrophins, or
3. Gonadotrophin releasing hormone, or
4. Bromocriptine.

Clomiphene citrate, which is a weak oestrogen with anti-oestrogenic actions, is the treatment of choice for patients with anovulatory cycles and oligomennorhoea and should always be tried first in patients with secondary amenorrhoea with normal FSH, LH and prolactin levels. Clomiphene's main action is at the hypothalamic level where, by virtue of its anti-oestrogenic action, it causes an increased output of pituitary gonadotrophins. It is usually prescribed for 5 consecutive days, starting at a dose of 50 mg daily and increasing to 100 mg, but rarely to a maximum of 200 mg, until ovulation, as monitored by ultrasound progesterone levels, is occurring. The mild anti-oestrogenic effect of clomiphene on the cervical mucus may be minimised by commencing it early in the cycle, e.g. Days 2–6. Occasionally, this effect may need to be counteracted by taking oral oestrogen in midcycle. In the absence of spontaneous menstruation, a withdrawal bleed may be stimulated by prescribing norethisterone 5 mg twice daily for 5 days, and clomiphene is then added on the day after bleeding starts. There is about a 10% incidence of twin pregnancy following clomiphene therapy. Human chorionic gonadotrophin may sometimes be added in the middle of clomiphene stimulated cycles to enhance ovulation and improve luteal function.

Gonadotrophin therapy, a mixture of FSH and LH or FSH alone, acts directly on the ovaries, and hence dosage and response must be carefully monitored by oestrogen assays and ultrasound to avoid over-stimulation, multiple follicle development and multiple pregnancies. Gonadotrophins should only be used in centres where good hormonal and ultrasonic monitoring of ovarian function is readily available.

Gonadotrophin releasing hormone (GnRH), when given in pulsatile doses, by portable infusion pumps, is extremely effective in treating defective hypothalamic function. Its use must be confined to specialised centers.

Dopamine agonists such as bromocriptine or cubergoline inhibit secretion of prolactin by the anterior pituitary and are the specific treatment of anovulation due to hyperprolactinaemia. The response is monitored by serum prolactin assay. Hyperprolactinaemia will also be suspected if clinically galactorrhoea is demonstrated and, in this circumstance, serum prolactin assays are mandatory. Serum prolactin levels may also be raised by stress, certain drugs (e.g. phenothiazides, methyldopa, and benzamines) or by a pituitary microadenoma. If hyperprolactinaemia is demonstrated, the possibility of pituitary enlargement must be investigated by X-ray, using tomograms if necessary, before treatment by bromocriptine is started. If a pituitary tumour is demonstrated, this may be treated by surgery, radiotherapy or pharmacologically.

In such circumstances, the patient must be closely watched during a subsequent pregnancy for signs of pituitary enlargement by assessment of visual fields and if necessary by X-rays.

CERVICAL FACTORS

The postcoital test (PCT) involves the examination of cervical mucus on a slide under the microscope within 24 hours after intercourse. This should ideally be performed when the cervical mucus is most receptive to sperm penetration, i.e. at ovulation, with maximum oestrogen effect. At the time of this examination, the following are noted: (1) whether there is evidence of oestrogenisation as seen by dilatation of the cervix; (2) the quantity and quality of the mucus (the ability to stretch being the Spinnbarkeit); (3) the numbers of sperm per high power field; and (4) whether the sperm are moving in a linear direction.

Thus the presence of many motile spermatozoa in thin clear mucus should indicate that:

1. The act of coitus occurs satisfactorily.
2. Good plentiful mucus is circumstantial evidence of ovulation.
3. There is no cervical barrier to the progress of healthy spermatozoa.

The most common reason for poor mucus or lack of spermatozoa is that the examination is performed at the wrong time in the cycle, or that the woman is not ovulating. Hence, a negative test must be repeated and ovulation confirmed.

If no spermatozoa are seen, this may be due to failure in coital technique, and persistently absent sperm in the presence of good mucus should raise the possibility of either a male factor, or stress and a psychological problem. The repeated finding of lack of progressive sperm movement raises the infrequent possibility of immunological factors, e.g. sperm antibodies, which have an inhibiting effect on normal sperm. This may be clarified by demonstrating cervical hostility *in vitro*.

Cervical problems may be difficult to treat. Mucus production may be stimulated by exogenous oestrogen, e.g. ethinyl oestrodiol 0.01 mg daily, and a local lesion, e.g. infection or an erosion, should be treated. However, when sperm fail to penetrate the mucus, therapy is very disappointing. Intrauterine artificial insemination with husband's sperm (AIH) may be used in these circumstances with benefit.

STRUCTURAL PROBLEMS

Interference with ovum release, failure of its capture by the fimbrial portion of the tube (the so-called ovarian unit) and subsequent transport of the fertilised ovum into the uterine cavity, caused by structural distortion, accounts for perhaps 20–25% of couples attending the infertility clinic. This distortion may be major, such as complete occlusion of the fallopian tube or more subtle, such as minor peritubal adhesions interfering with the tubo-ovarian mechanism. The most common causes of such problems are infection or post-operative adhesion formation. Resolution of infection causes an inflammatory response and subsequent fibrosis, which may lead to adhesions covering the ovaries or distorting the fallopian tubes. Complete occlusion of the tube may occur and, most commonly, the most sensitive and vulnerable portions of the tube are affected, i.e. the narrow cornual isthmic portion of the tube, a cornual block, or conglutination of the fimbriae causing a hydrosalpinx. Even if tubal patency is not disturbed, the mechanism of function may be disrupted by destroying the fine sensitive cilial lining of the fallopian tube and interfering with ovum transport. Post-infective distortion is commonly symmetrically bilateral. A similar mechanism causes pelvic adhesions and distortion following any traumatic operative procedure such as ovarian cystectomy. This damage may be aggravated by post-operative infection but post-operative adhesions may disrupt the pelvic anatomy and function.

The history may be suggestive of anatomical abnormalities contributing to the infertility problem, but confirmation of this diagnosis will be by hysterosalpingogram (HSG) and laparoscopic assessment. The X-ray demonstration by HSG allows the diagnosis of intrauterine pathology, e.g. adhesions or synaechiae and tubal occlusion (Figs. 33.2–33.5).

Introduction of a laparoscope subumbilically into a pre-formed pneumoperitoneum of CO_2 allows direct visualisation of the uterus, fallopian tubes, their motility and their relationship with the ovaries as well as the ovarian surface for signs of ovulation and adhesions. Laparoscopy is a safe procedure with experience and is best performed under general anaesthesia, because manipulation of the pelvic organs necessary for adequate visualisation of the surfaces is painful. Dye may be introduced through the cervix and tubal patency demonstrated. Increased vascular markings on the

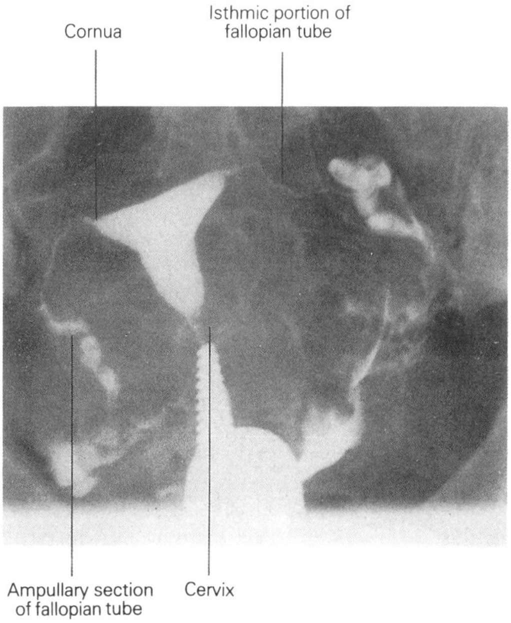

Fig. 33.2 *Normal pelvis.*

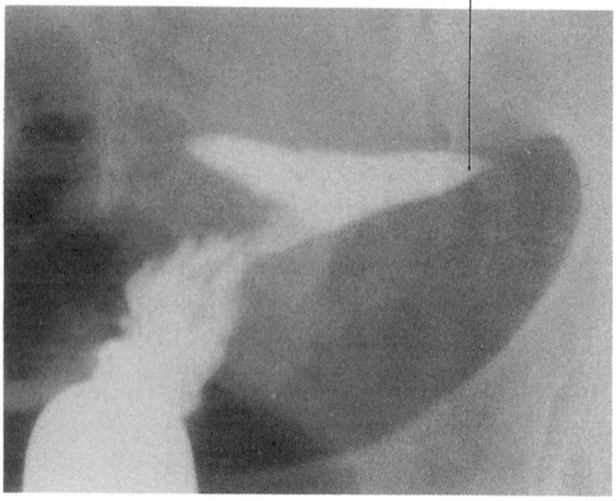

Fig. 33.3 *Bilateral cornual block.*

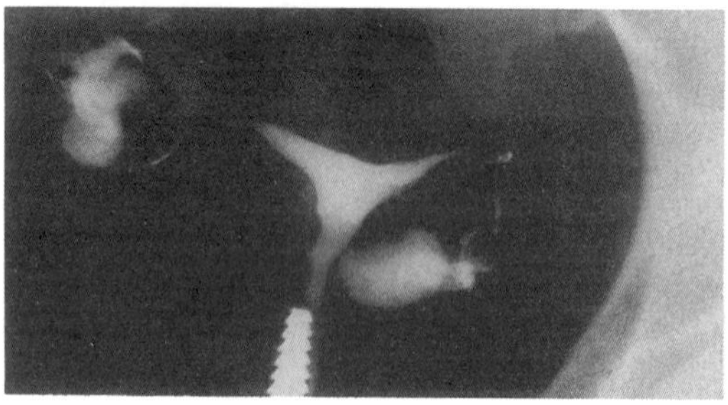

Fig. 33.4 *Bilateral hydrosalpinges.*

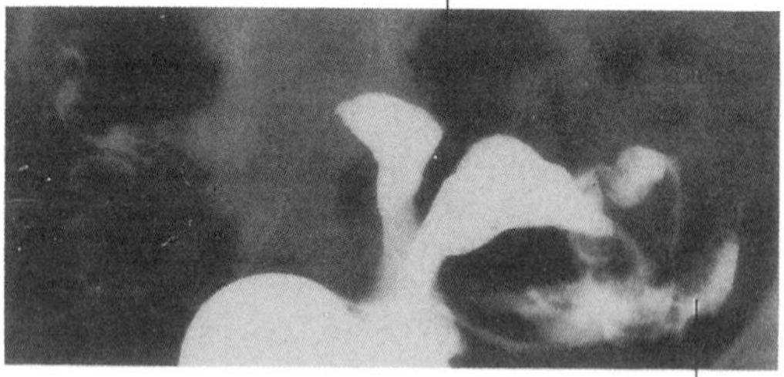

Fig. 33.5 *Septate uterus.*

external tubal serosa may indicate underlying intraluminal pathology.

Treatment of structural problems is by surgical correction, division of adhesions, and restoration of anatomy. However, even if tubal patency results, there will always be some residual scarring and damage, especially to the sensitive cilial lining of the tube. Thus results as judged by subsequent intrauterine pregnancy rates are disappointingly poor. The use of magnification allows for greater attention to detail, better conservation of healthy tissue, better restoration of anatomy and decreased post-operative adhesion formation. The correct use of the operating microscope requires special training and experience. However, its major contribution to infertility surgery has been not only to give better results, but also to teach all gynaecologists involved in fertility surgery a respect for sensitive tissues, and a better attitude towards conservation of healthy tissue, preservation of anatomy and a decrease in post-operative adhesion formation.

Endometriosis may also affect fertility by distortion of pelvic anatomy, prevention of ovum release or complete tubal blockage. The diagnosis is made by laparoscopy. Treatment may be by surgery — removing or cauterising the endometriotic deposits and restoring the pelvic anatomy — or medically. Medical treatment is danazol, a gonadotrophin inhibitor, or one of the GnRH analogues. They inhibit ovulation and cause endometrial atrophy. Danazol is used in doses of 200–800 mg daily for 3–6 months.

Danazol is usually used in the milder forms of endometriosis, surgery being indicated when there is gross distortion. Another situation is the finding of minor endometriotic deposits on structures such as the uterosacral ligaments in infertile patients. Although not obviously interfering with the pelvic function or anatomy, it is postulated that the release of prostaglandins (mainly Pg $F_{2\alpha}$) by this ectopic endometrium interferes with tubal transport. The evidence for this is not conclusive.

Uterine leiomyomata may, by their size, cause anatomical distortion or tubal occlusion. Treatment by surgical removal, myomectomy, may be attempted but great care must be taken at the time of operation to avoid post-operative adhesion formation or haematoma in the uterus that subsequently becomes infected. GnRH analogues also have a place in reducing the size of fibroids, thus reducing symptoms or making surgery easier.

UNEXPLAINED INFERTILITY

Even with the increase in knowledge of the normal physiology of conception and also the many advances in the treatment of abnormalities which can occur, it has become apparent that there is a small group of couples who, at the end of investigation, appear 'normal' but remain infertile. These couples with 'unexplained infertility' form a difficult and demanding group for the clinician. Sometimes, on closer screening, it is apparent that the results of some of the tests are, in fact, inadequate or 'border-line', or alternatively that some areas have been overlooked, such as minor endometriosis or intrauterine pathology. Before making the diagnosis, it is important to be sure that:

1. The infertility evaluation was complete in terms of most modern standards
2. The results of studies and observations were appropriately interpreted
3. Factors, which were considered within normal limits during investigation, have not changed during the period of evaluation.

Making this diagnosis has some benefits. First, it ensures that the couple has been properly investigated and that no diagnosable abnormality has been missed. Secondly, it may allow a positive approach to counselling the couple by offering alternative treatments, for example various drugs and hormonal combinations or techniques such as *in vitro* fertilisation (IVF) and gamete intrafallopian transfer (GIFT). *In vitro* fertilisation is an expensive treatment suitable for women who have irreparable tubal disease or absent tubes, but who are otherwise fertile. The technique is described in Chapter 34. It is a stressful procedure involving detailed monitoring of the stimulated ovarian cycle, collection of eggs, preparing of fresh sperm, fertilisation and embryo culture, and finally re-implantation of the embryo should it fertilise satisfactorily. Thirty per cent of embryo replacements continue to viable pregnancies.

Gamete intrafallopian transfer is a simpler procedure than IVF. Induced ovulation and egg and sperm collection are the same. The egg and sperm are then inserted into the distal end of the fallopian tube at laparoscopy. Hopefully, fertilisation will then occur in its natural environment, namely in the ampulla of the fallopian tube. This means that a culture laboratory is not necessary but, of course, the woman must have normal tubes. The method is not suitable for those with tubal disease, but may be of some value in cases of unexplained inferility.

It is important to explain to both partners that not only has no abnormality been detected, but that there is always a possibility of spontaneous pregnancy occurring. However, it is not enough to offer open-ended psychological support, and the time usually comes when it is important for both partners and the physician to face the facts and acknowledge that, given our present state of knowledge, nothing more can be done and that persistent infertility is a definite possibility. The acceptance of the fact and the psychological adjustment required are important, if the couple are to maintain a balanced healthy attitude. At this time, it may be appropriate to raise the possibility of adoption, if this has not already been considered. Accepting the fact of probable childlessness requires social and psychological adjustment with re-arrangement of emphasis on to other things such as career interests or hobbies. An open, honest, three-way discussion by the couple and their physician should set the foundation for this, often difficult, realisation.

SCHEDULE FOR INVESTIGATION

The aim is to collect as much information as quickly as possible, so that therapy can be started without delay. Each return visit should have a number of objectives, so that investigations are completed in a minimum of time and inconvenience to the woman.

First Visit

1. History

Take details of:
   a. Duration and type of infertility;
   b. Previous gynaecological and surgical history, and previous infertility history and treatment;
   c. Menstrual, sexual, contraceptive and medical history.
2. General and gynaecological examination
3. Investigation
   a. General
      Basal temperature chart (BTC)
      Prolactin assay
      Arrange progesterone and second pro lactin assay about Day 21 of cycle (midluteal phase)
      Bring seminal analysis (SA)
   b. Specific
      If history indicates, arrange hysterosalpingogram (HSG) and/or laparoscopy.

Second Visit

1. Timed midcycle for postcoital test.
2. Review hormones, BTC and SA.
3. Arrange HSG (if done too early, this may be traumatic and discourage patient) or book laparoscopy.
4. Arrange repeat of any abnormal tests.

Third Visit

1. Review all data.
2. If HSG normal, then arrange laparoscopy.
3. If SA X 2 abnormal, arrange examination of male.
4. If PCT abnormal, repeat and review ovulation/mucus.
5. If anovulation, commence treatment, clomiphene citrate.

Fourth Visit

Definite abnormality should by now be identified and appropriate treatment instigated. Review findings and outline subsequent management. If no abnormalities are detected, and laparoscopy has not yet been performed, it should be done at this stage.

FURTHER READING

Chamberlain G.V.P., Winston R.M.L., eds. (1981). *Tubal Infertility*. London: Blackwell Scientific Publications.

Insler V., Lunenfeld B., eds. (1986). *Infertility: Male and Female*. Edinburgh: Churchill Livingstone.

Muse K.N., Wilson E.A. (1982). How does endometriosis cause infertility? *Fertil. Steril* **38**: 145–152.

Pepperell R.J., Hudson B., Wood C., eds. (1981). *The Infertile Couple*. Edinburgh: Churchill Livingstone.

Royal College of Obstetricians Guidelines. 1997 — The Initial Investigation and Management of the Infertile Couple; 1998 — The Management of Infertility in Secondary Care; 2000 — The Management of Infertility in Tertiary Care.

34

Assisted Conception

We can define assisted conception methods as infertility treatments in which fertility drugs are used in order to enhance ovulation or superovulation with timed coitus, intrauterine insemination of washed sperm from the partner or from a donor, or *in vitro* fertilisation (IVF-ET), or gamete intrafallopian transfer (GIFT).

Probably, IVF is the most widely used and is also known as "test tube baby " technique. It is based on collection of eggs, fertilisation with sperm outside the body, and then transfer to the woman's uterus. This treatment was pioneered in humans by Steptoe and Edwards in 1978. The first IVF baby born in the world was Louise Brown, in England, over 20 years ago.

Indication for *In Vitro* Fertilisation

A — Probably the most common indication for this approach is the tubal factor. Infertility due to tubal damage is responsible for more than 30% of cases of female infertility. Some of these can be repaired by surgery, but in the most severe cases IVF is the most realistic option.

B — Ovarian dysfunction, when induction of ovulation using clomiphene citrate (Clomid, Serophene) or gonadotrophins has failed to produce a pregnancy inspite of good ovarian response. The largest group of patients are those with polycystic ovarian syndrome.

C — Patients with no response to fertility drugs. Prognosis in these cases is very poor, probably because there is a more important underlying problem of ovarian function such as poor ovarian reserve or failure.

D — Patients suffering from endometriosis of different degrees can be good candidates for this type of treatment.

E — Cervical factor: when the cervix of the uterus has been severely damaged by a surgical procedure such as a cone biopsy or a very traumtic forceps delivery.

F — Couples with multifactorial reasons for their infertility, male and female combined.

G — Couples with a high risk of producing offspring with severe malformation; the use of IVF with pre-implantation diagnosis can be a solution.

H — Patients whose uterus has been removed with conservation of the ovaries or have a severely scarred uterus as a result of infection such as tuberculosis, or traumatic damage after curettage or myomectomy causing intrauterine adhesions and Asherman's Syndrome. Egg collection is possible and once eggs have been fertilised, embryos can be transferred to a surrogate mother.

I — Couples with severe male factor. IVF and intracytoplasmatic sperm injection (ICSI) offer a good prognosis. In men with azoopermia due to a mechanical cause such as sterilisation, congenital absence of the vas, obstruction after surgery or infection, sperm can be extracted surgically, by puncture or open surgery.

J — It is possible that in males with some degree of testicular failure, when no sperm are ejaculated or sperm are immotile, sperm that are capable of fertilising *in vitro* can be obtained by testicular biopsy.

Assessment of the Couple

It is most important that couples are fully investigated before assisted conception takes place. This involves a hysterosalpingogram, to assess the uterine cavity and tubal lumen. Vaginal ultrasound is used to assess ovarian volume, morphology and accessibility for egg retrieval. Hormone levels such as FSH, LH, and prolactin at the beginning of the cycle (preferably days 2–3) and progesterone level in the middle of the luteal phase are needed to assess patterns of ovulation.

The male factor should be assessed with a sperm count and examination of washed sperm. In males with severe oligospermia or azoospermia, FSH/LH and testosterone levels should be measured. High FSH levels are an indicator of testicular failure. Some of these men (3–5%) can have an associated chromosomal abnormality such as a balanced translocation, that may pass to their offspring or become unbalanced and produce an abnormal child. For these reasons, their karyotype should be examined.

Laparoscopy and hysteroscopy are very important investigations and are generally carried out in most infertile patients. They offer an unique opportunity of assessing fully the state of the tubes, ovaries and the uterus. This will help to decide if the cause of the infertility is a mechanical one, and whether or not it can be treated by surgery or if IVF is the only way forward.

Is a laparoscopy always necessary before IVF? The answer is no, for patients with a history of multiple laparotomies, previous salpingectomy/previous tubal surgery or a severe male factor, ICSI is the only option possible. A laparoscopy will be unnecessary, because it will be most unlikely that it will change the patient's management, and in the cases of previous laparotomy the morbidity due to adhesions can be serious.

Regimens for Superovulation

The number of mature oocytes collected in an IVF cycle is of crucial importance for the success of the treatment. The patients must go through a process of ovarian stimulation known as a superovulation. Assuming that ovarian funcion is within normal limits, the normal process of selection of a single follicle and ovulation must be overriden in order that the ovary can produce more than one mature egg.

The strategy of superovulation is based on an increase in the number of follicles with complete maturation, using clomiphene citrate or more frequently with gonadotrophins in the human or recombinant form.

Whichever drugs are used, the idea is to overcome the gonadotrophin threshold necessary for multiple precursor follicles and then to support follicular development, overriding the process of natural selection of a single follicle. One of the problems that all these regimens of superovulation have is the asynchrony between the follicles. Sometimes only a very few are ripe (20 mm in diameter) by the time that the LH surge starts. Smaller follicles (less than 15 mm in diameter) are unsuitable for collecting eggs for fertilisation.

Since analogues of luteinising hormone releasing hormone (LHRH) were introduced in regimens of superovulation, important improvements on the outcome of IVF have been achieved. The spontaneous release of gonadotrophins by the pituitary gland can be abolished, using LHRH analogues, protecting oocytes from inappropriate exposure to luteinising hormone (LH), which is detrimental to maturation of eggs. These analogues produce temporary hypogonadotrophic hypogonadism, reducing the production of follicle stimulating hormone (FSH), allowing the stimulation of follicles in an early stage of recruitment with exogenous gonadotrophins. This accounts for the increased production of oocytes using this method of superovulation. Due to the fact that analogues abolish the spontaneous LH surge, ovarian stimulation is much more controlled, with logistic advantages of timing the hCG and egg collection. Egg collections are generally done on weekdays in the morning and the cancellation rate is due to incorrect ovarian response and abnormal

LH surges which are very low, compared with the unsuppressed cycles.

Monitoring

Good monitoring is essential for a successful egg harvest. It is based on a series of ultrasound scans in order to measure the size and number of follicles produced and on blood samples to measure oestrogen levels. Using both parameters, we can ascertain the degree of maturity of the oocytes and time of the injection of the hCG in suppressed cycles and when to go ahead with the egg retrieval.

When is a patient ready for egg collection? In general, it is accepted when at least three follicles with a diameter of 18 mm or more are present and oestrogen levels on the day reach 3000 nmol or more. According to the number of follicles, hCG (10,000 units) should be given and 32–34 hours later, egg collection is carried out (Fig. 34.1).

Once sperm are produced, they are prepared by a process called swim up and wash. Sperm are put in a test tube with culture medium for a period of two hours and the most active ones swim to the surface. Among these, the most active are selected and are used for insemination. Approximately 150,000 are required per egg in order to achieve 75–85% fertilisation rate. In ICSI procedures, sperm are injected directly into the oocyte.

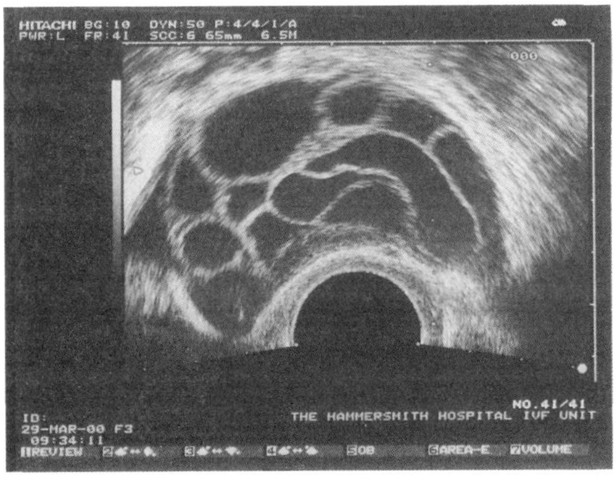

Fig. 34.1 *Multiple follicles prior to egg collection.*

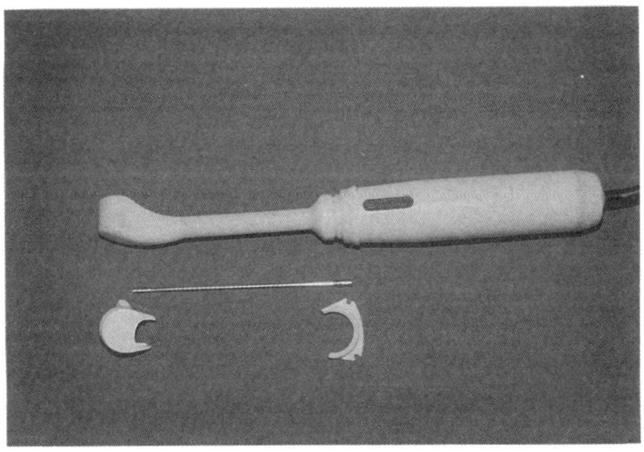

Fig. 34.2 *Vaginal ultrasound probe.*

Egg Retrieval

Historically, egg retrievals were performed by laparoscopy. Since the development of sophisticated ultrasound machines, the approach has changed radically.

The introduction and development of vaginal transducers made the vaginal approach easy to perform and very well accepted by the patients and staff. It is true that this approach is not suitable for all patients but it is for the the great majority, leaving other routes for specific cases (Fig. 34.2). The procedure is done as a day case, under sedation and local anaesthesia. In patients with difficult ovaries situated in a high position in the pelvis, or in patients with very low pain thresholds, general anaesthesia is necessary.

Gamete Intrafallopian Transfer (GIFT)

Pregnancies obtained as a result of this approach were first published as an alternative method to IVF. This method was based on the fact that if the sperm and egg were placed in the natural site of fertilisation, the ampulla of the fallopian tube, pregnancy rates will be much higher than those with IVF.

Egg collection is done by laparoscopy or ultrasonically guided via the vagina. Two or three eggs are mixed with sperm which have been previously prepared and transferred into the ampulla of the fallopian tubes with a very fine catheter through a second abdominal puncture.

This is possible only in patients with macroscopically normal tubes, in couples with unexplained infertility or some degree of male factor.

Today, this procedure is hardly used in Europe, but in some parts of the USA, it is still popular especially among the older group of patients, because it allows for the transfer of a larger number of oocytes. There is no hard evidence that the use of this method has improved the pregnancy rate in either young or old patients.

Embryo Transfer

Embryo transfers are done two or three days after egg retrieval, but in exceptional circumstances can be delayed up to 5 days. In general, it is a very simple but very important procedure. A fine catheter loaded with the embryos is placed through the cervix into the uterine cavity. In most units this is done with ultrasound guidance (abdominal) to ensure that the catheter is in the right place and has not bent on itself and remains in the cervix. This reassures the patient and the doctor about the place where the embryos have been lodged. In a small number of patients when the cervix has been severely damaged and scarred by previous surgery, general anaesthesia or sedation is required.

All patients must have a cervical assessment before they start the cycle to see if there is going to be any difficulty with the procedure. A small group of patients require a cervical dilatation, which is done under general

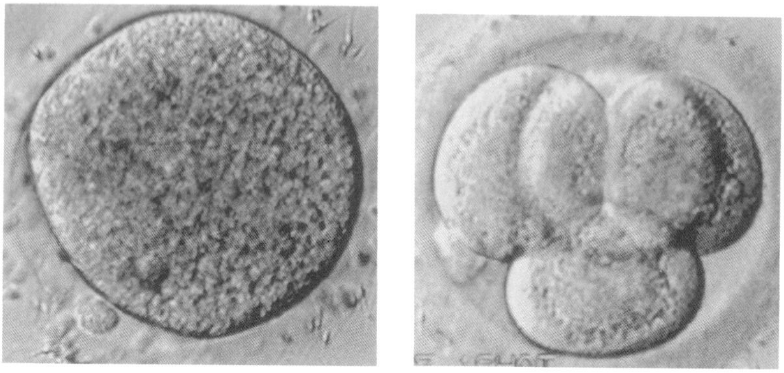

(a)

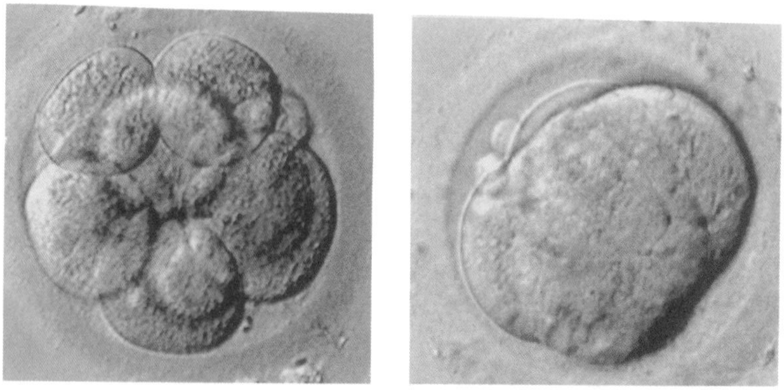

(b)

Fig. 34.3 *Human embryos at 4–8 cell stage.*

anaesthesia before the start of ovarian stimulation.

There is not yet a method that is able to select the best embryos.

At the moment, the morphological criteria are used to select the embryos and are based on the number of cells (blastomeres), fragments or degenerated cells which are present. These are scored and the ones with the best morphology transferred.

Most embryos transfers are done at the cleavage stage of 4–8 cells. [Figs. 34.3(a) and (b)]. Blastocyst transfers on day 5 after egg collection are done sometimes (Fig. 34.4). The reason for this is is to try to select the best embryos, with the idea that if they survive and cleave up to the blastocyst stage *in vitro* the chance of producing a pregnancy is much higher. Some authors have published a 50% pregnancy rate. Unfortunately, not every patient has enough embryos which survive that period of time *in vitro*. More than 35% of the patients may not have embryos to transfer if this approach is used.

In the same way that sperm and egg are transferred through the fimbrial end of the fallopian tube with GIFT, embryos can be transferred but there is no evidence so far that the use of this method offers higher chances of conception than transcervical transfer.

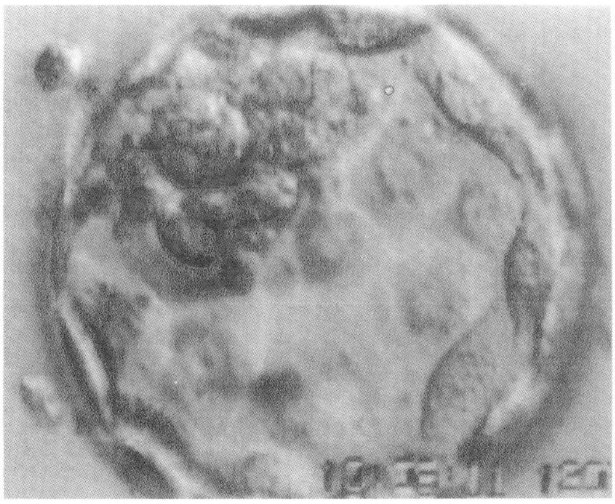

Fig. 34.4 *Human blastocyst.*

Intracytoplasmatic Sperm Injection

At the begining of the IVF era, fertilisation *in vitro* was only achieved by placing a reasonably large number of sperm (>150,000) with each egg in a Petri dish. In couples with severe male factors, fertilisation rates were very low or nil.

In recent years, treatment of the male factor has changed with the use of different methods of microsurgical fertilisation. Opening the zona pellucida to facilitate the entry of the sperm so that it will be able to penetrate the cytoplasm were followed by ICSI, when the sperm is injected directly into the cytoplasm.

ICSI is undoubtedly one of the greatest achievements in the treatment of male infertility. Males with very low sperm counts or even a single sperm were given the possibility of fathering children, when before, the only alternative was the use of donor sperm.

With the development of this technique and further experience, sperm obtained surgically by testicular biopsy could be used to fertilise oocytes, producing embryos and consequently pregnancies with normal children. Men with obstructive azoospermia or with some degree of testicular failure are able to be treated successfully.

The prevalence of chromosome abnormalies in males varies from 2.15% up to 8.6% in males with subfertility compared with the normal fertile population of 0.7% to 1%. In 4.3% of the couples in which ICSI is required, there is a chromosomal abnormality present, the most common being the classic Klinefelter syndrome (47XXY). Patients with obstructive primary azoospermia must be investigated if they are carriers of cystic fibrosis or one of the mutations in the CFTR gene.

Does ICSI *per se* increase abnormalities? Probably not, but at the moment there is not enough evidence to draw any conclusion. *De novo* chromosome abnormalites are very rare, but still possible. This type of abnormality is probably more common in cases in which the male has a chromosomal abnormality or balanced translocation which may be transmitted to the offspring or become unbalanced and produce a malformation.

Pre-Implantation Diagnosis

The possibility of being able to produce embryos *in vitro*, and consequently pregnancies, has provided the possibility of diagnosing some of the large numbers of genetic defects and prevent transmission, using pre-implantation diagnosis (PGD).

Genetic diseases are common and most of these problems are chromosome related. It is known that, for example, breast cancer, diabetes and heart disease are genetically transmitted. Single gene defects are as a result of a mutation. More than 10,000 are known but fortunately the majority are very rare. Around 20 mutations are responsible for 80% of the major genetic disorders in the United Kingdom. The prevalence of a chromosome syndrome and a single gene disorder is 2%.

Single Gene Defects are:

a — Recessive genetic defects: when both parents carry the misprint of the gene and pass it to the childrens' chromosomes. They are the most common of genetic diseases. In the UK, cystic fibrosis is the most frequently found among this type of defect.

b — Dominant gene defects: when a copy of such a gene is inherited fron one of the parents and causes the disease. Huntington's chorea is one of them.

c — Sex-linked defects: only affects boys. The mother carries the gene defect in one of the X chromosomes. The child inherits the affected X-chromosome and suffers the disease, for example Duchenne muscular dystrophy and haemophilia. Other reasons for using this approach is when one of the parents has a high risk of transmitting a chromosome abnormality, such as a translocation. The majority of these couples have repeated miscarriages and/or are infertile.

Like any other technique PGD has its failures:

A — The possibility of misdiagnosis, due to the technique itself, or that the material obtained from the embryo is not representative, or contamination from other genetic material in the laboratory.

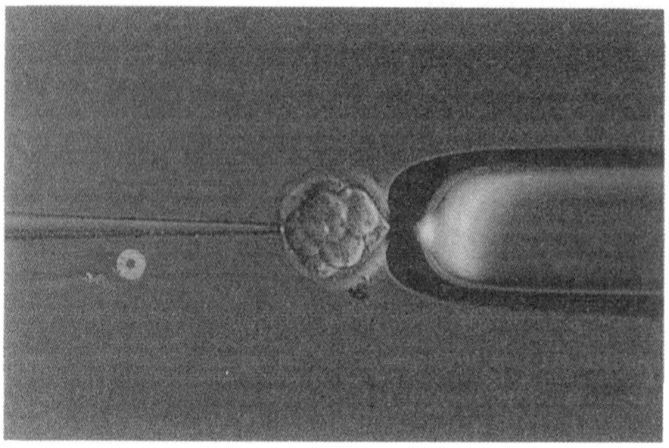

(a)

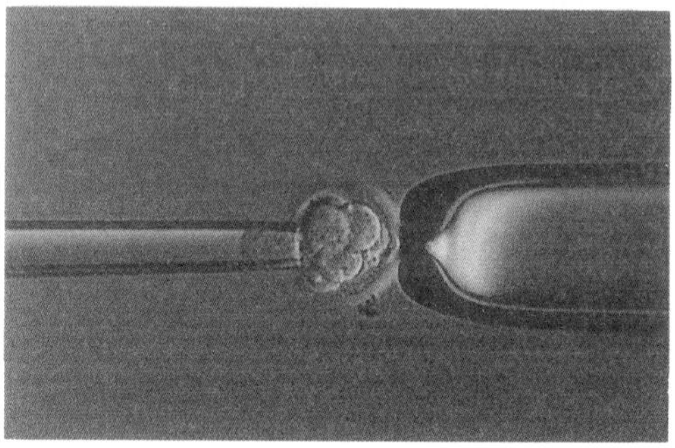

(b)

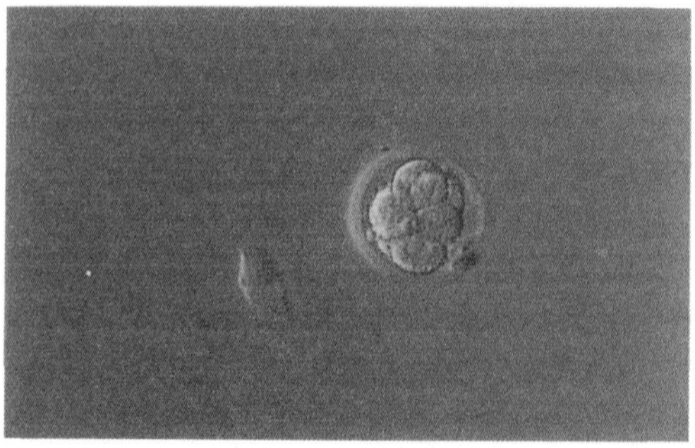

(c)

Fig. 34.5 *Removal of a cell from human embryo for pre-implantation diagnosis.*

B — Embryos can occasionally be subject to mosaicism. It is not known how frequently this occurs. PGD is very dependent on the IVF technique, so failure of fertilisation or cleavage of embryos may render the attempt to a failure.

C — It is very important to remember that there is no guarantee that a pregnancy will be achieved and go to full term, and that the child will be normal. These techniques are very specific to one disease or problem. The fetus can still be affected by other problems and be abnormal.

Pre-implantation diagnosis is based on a two-stage process. *In vitro* fertilisation is used in order to produce embryos, which are screened for specific disorders or to established their sex (sex-linked disorders), and unaffected embryos transferred. After fertilisation, the embryos are cultured for 2 to 3 days (6–10 cell stage). One or two cells are then removed for embryo biopsy [Figs. 34.5(a)–(c)]. This is performed by making a hole in the zona by enzymatic digestion. With micromanipulation, the cells (blastomeres) are removed, with no detrimental effect on development of the embryo. These cells are then broken up to obtain the DNA for analysis. There are two basic methods used currently:

a — Analysis of the DNA for a specific single gene defect using PCR (polymerase chain reaction).

b — Analysing the chromosome with the special staining technique FISH (flourescent *in situ* hybridisation).

Pregnancy Outcome

Chances of conception after a single IVF cycle are, in general, low (Table 34.1). Age is the most important factor in the outcome of IVF. In a study conducted by our IVF unit, one of the largest series published so far using one standard treatment protocol, more than 9000 cycles were reviewed. Women of 20 to 25 years old had a pregnancy rate of 48% compared with 8% over the age of 41. The overall miscarriage rate was 3% in the 20 to 25 years age group compared with 20% in 40-year-old women. This figure can go up to 50%.

Biochemical pregnancy, when beta-hCG rises transiently, is a positive indicator for subsequent success. In normal fertile women, there is good evidence that early pregnancy loss is a very common event. In our series, 36.4% of the patients conceived in the second cycle following a biochemical pregnancy in their first. The chances of a pregnancy after the first cycle of IVF is 26% which is similar or better than in a month of normal intercourse. In the UK, the cumulative pregnancy rate is 32% after 3 months of intercourse, and 55% after 6 months in a fertile population. We found 54% of cumulative pregnancy rate after the third cycle, reaching 72% after the 6th IVF cycle, in our own unit.

Cryopreservation

With the use of superovulation regimes, multiple embryos are created but not all of these can be transferred. This surplus of embryos can be frozen and the advantages of this

Table 34.1

Clinical Pregnancies and Live Birth Rate. Female Cause of Infertility (HFEA Annual Report 1999)

Factor	Number of cycles	% of all cycles	Clinical pregnancy rate (%)	Live birth rate (%)
Tubal disease	11,254	32.5	18.2	14.9
Endometriosis	3005	8.7	20.2	16.3
Unexplained	16,414	47.4	20.3	17.2
Others	7116	20.5	21.0	16.8

procedure have been recognised from the early stages of the evolution of IVF.

One of the most important factors in cryopreservation is the quality of the embryos which are to be frozen. A survival rate of 78% in morphologically regular embryos compared with 20% when embryos have uneven blastomeres or fragmentation has been reported.

Embryos can be frozen at different stages of development, but in general it is accepted that freezing at the blastocyst stage is less efficient than at the pro-nuclear or early cleavage stages.

COMPLICATIONS

Ovarian Hyperstimulation

Probably one of the most common complications of assisted conception is ovarian hyperstimulation. It is the direct consequence of excessive multiple follicular responses to ovarian stimulation. The patient presents in general 7 to 10 days after embryo transfer with nausea or vomiting, abdominal pain and distension, ascites, enlarged ovaries, and sometimes oedema, pleural effusions and some degree of oliguria. There are different degrees to hyperstimulation — from the most mild to severe.

Mild ovarian hyperstimulation is probably more frequent than reported. Severe cases occur in between 1% and 3% of the stimulated cycles. Some of these patients required admission to intensive care due to the severity of respiratory symptoms, oliguria or anuria. Treatment consists of restoring fluid balance with intravenous fluid administration, paracentesis and drainage of a pleural effusion if there are respiratory symptoms. Due to the high levels of estradiol, subcutaneous low molecular weight heparin is necessary to prevent deep venous thrombosis. Antibiotics are not in general required, unless there are signs of specific infection.

Probably the most important predisposing factor is polycystic ovaries. These patients have the tendency to produce multiple follicles when using very low doses of gonadotrophin.

None of the strategies considered for prevention of ovarian hyperstimulation, such as follicular aspiration before administration of hCG and administration of human albumin at the time of oocyte retrieval, are effective. Probably the only way of preventing the problem is remembering the possibility of its occurrence and the use of low doses of gonadotrophins in patients with predisposing factors.

Ectopic Pregnancy

Although embryos are transferred into the uterine cavity, ectopic implantations in the tubes or the cervix and most unusually in the ovary are still possible. Ectopic pregnancies occur in 5% of the pregnancies achieved though IVF, compared with 1% from natural conception, and no relationship has been found between ectopic pregnancies and number of embryos transferred).

Combined intra- and extrauterine pregnancy (heterotopic pregnancy) is estimated to occur naturally in between 1:15,000 and 1:3,0000. With IVF, it occurred in 2.9% of clinical pregnancies.

Multiple Pregnancy

Multiple pregnancy can be considered as a side-effect of assisted conception technologies. Pregnancy rates are very strongly related to the number of embryos transferred. A large number of embryos are still transferred in unregulated countries with high multiple pregnancy rates. In the UK, as in the majority of European countries, no more than three embryos are transferred in a single cycle. In our unit, more than 80% of patients have only two embryos tranferred (Table 34.2).

In the older group of patients (>38 years of age) who required a very high dose of gonadotrophins, or who had had previous failed attempts, the transfer of three embryos is reasonably safe, because statistically the chance of producing a multiple pregnancy is very low.

Intrauterine insemination or timed coitus is not an exception. For that reason, the insemination or coitus should take place only

Table 34.2

Pregnancy Rates for 2 and 3 Embryo Transfers (HFEA Annual Report 1999)

Number of embryos transfered	Number of cycles	Live birth (% of number of cycles)	Multiple birth rate (% of number of live births)
2	5435	26.0	24.9
3	7760	254.7	34.3

*There were 58 cycles where only one embryo was transferred.

when no more than two follicles, within the criteria (18–19 mm diameter) are present, and the couple must be advised of the risks and refrain fron having unprotected sexual intercourse during that cycle if these criteria are not met.

Ovarian Cancer

The suggestion that there is an association between the use of fertility drugs and ovarian cancer has been one of the most worrying problems in reproductive medicine as a long-term side-effect or complication of assisted conception technology. Analysis of the most recent data does not support a direct relationship between ovarian stimulation and ovarian cancer. It is possible that "fertility drugs" may have a role in increasing the number in some special categories of tumours, but only large randomised prospective epidemiological studies will be able to answer this difficult question.

Regulations

England was the first country in the world with an authority to regulate assisted conception and embryo research — Was first organised through a consultation committee chaired by Lady Warnock and after a long period of discussions with researchers, clinicians and members of the public, their recommendations were issued. As a result of these recommendations and heated debates in Westminster, Parliament created the Human Fertilisation Embryology Authority (HFEA) in 1990.

The function of this authority is to license and monitor clinics where *in vitro* fertilisation (IVF), donor insemination (DI) and human embryo research are carried out. It also regulates the storage of gametes and embryos.

Other functions are: to produce a code of practice, to keep a register of donors, to keep under review research on embryos and to advise the Secretary of State.

There is a standard fee charged to the patient for each cycle. All cycles are recorded and consent forms must be signed by both partners for each individual procedure and every time these procedures are carried out. Units that carry out research on embryos must be licensed for that particular project.

35

Reproduction and the Male

ANATOMY

The male reproductive system consists of the testes, epididymes, vasa deferentia, seminal vesicles, prostate, the penis (including its erectile tissue), urethra and accessory structures including the bulbo-urethral glands.

Testes

The testis lies supported in the scrotum by the scrotal tissue and spermatic cord. Its dimensions are approximately $4 \times 3 \times 2$ cm and is ovoid in shape. It is covered in a dense fibrous fascia, the tunica albuginea, which is invaginated posteriorly as the mediastinum. Internally, it is divided by fascial septa into some 200 lobules, these septa radiating from the mediastinum. Each lobule contains some three or more seminiferous tubules supported by stroma containing the interstitial cells of Leydig. The seminiferous tubules are lined by cells that produce spermatozoa and are of two types, the supporting cells of Sertoli and the spermatogenic cells themselves. The efferent ducts converge as the rete testes in the mediastinum, efferent ducts from the rete pass superiorly to the apex of the testis and into the head of the epididymis (Fig. 35.1).

The blood supply of the testis is from the testicular artery which arises from the abdominal aorta just below the renal arteries and courses downwards and laterally behind the peritoneum to enter the deep inguinal ring and thence the spermatic cord. This wayward course is due to the embryological origin and descent of the testis *in utero*. The venous drainage enters the pampiniform plexus in the spermatic cord and then into the testicular vein which empties into the inferior vena cava on the right and into the left renal vein on the left. Lymph drains to the lumbar lymph nodes and thence to the mediastinum.

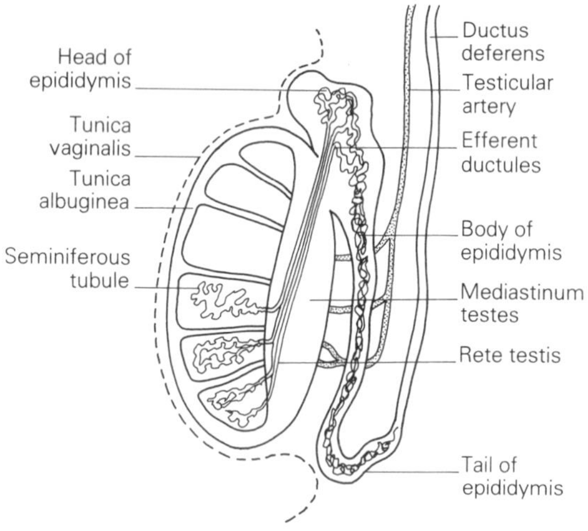

Fig. 35.1 *Cross-section though the testis.*

Epididymis

The epididymis is essentially a long (6 cm) convoluted tube lined by pseudostratified columnar epithelium and is usually described as having a head, body and tail. The head is closely apposed to the upper pole of the testis where the efferent ducts of the rete testis perforate the tunica albuginea. The body lies posterior and lateral to the testis and descends to its lower pole, where the tail is attached by dense fibrous tissue and the reflection of the tunica vaginalis. The tail drains into the ductus deferens.

Blood supply is from the testicular artery and venous drainage is similar to the testis.

Ductus Deferens (Vas Deferens)

The ductus deferens is a thick-walled muscular tube consisting of an internal mucosa and submucosa with three well-defined layers of smooth muscle — an internal longitudinal layer, which fades out proximally, and an inner circular and external longitudinal layer. It courses from the tail of the epididymis superiorly into the posterior part of the spermatic cord, through the superficial inguinal ring and along the inguinal canal to enter the pelvis, separating from the other structures in the cord to pass, initially, superiorly, anterior to the external iliac artery and then, posteriorly, into the pelvis on its lateral wall, crossing the ureter on the posterior surface of the bladder to join the duct of the seminal vesicle as the common ejaculatory duct. This duct pierces the prostate to open into the prostatic urethra through the veru (verumontanum) on its posterior wall (Fig. 35.2 and Fig. 35.3).

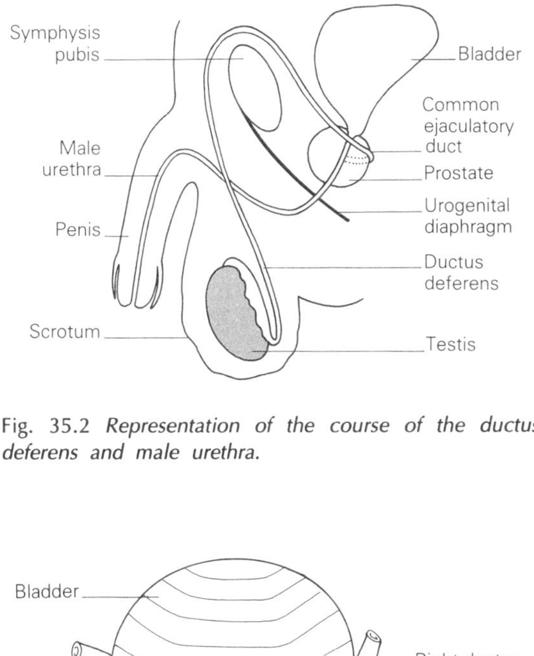

Fig. 35.2 *Representation of the course of the ductus deferens and male urethra.*

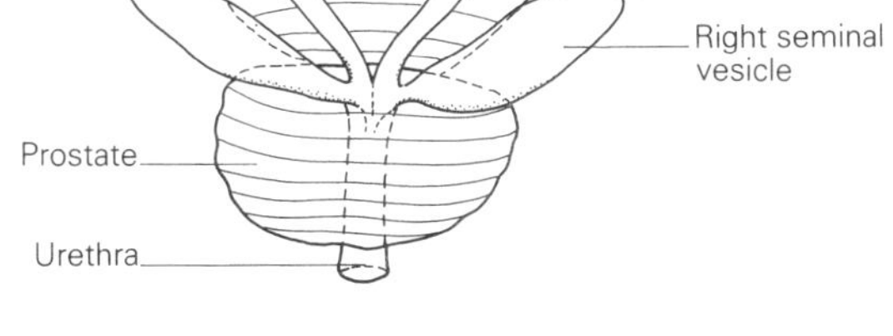

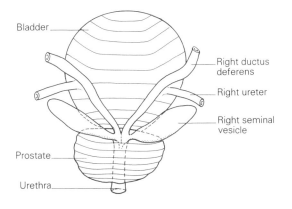

Fig. 35.3 *Posterior representation of bladder and prostate.*

Seminal Vesicles

The left and right seminal vesicles lie attached to the posterior wall of the bladder, just superiorly and posteriorly to the prostate (Fig. 35.3). Each vesicle, approximately 6 cm long, joins the ductus deferens as the ejaculatory duct. The ureters lie somewhat superiorly and medially to each vesicle with the ductus deferens crossing the ureter from above.

Each vesicle is lined with pseudostratified columnar epithelium with diverticulae containing goblet cells that secrete a large part of the seminal fluid. They do not form a reservoir for spermatozoa. Surrounding the mucosa is a muscular layer, thinner and less well-defined than that of the ductus, but nevertheless, with a discernible inner circular and outer longitudinal coat. Sympathetic nervous stimulation leads to contraction of the prostate, seminal vesicles and vasa deferentia with partial bladder neck closure which produces ejaculation. The blood supply comes from the inferior vesical and middle rectal arteries and the venous drainage is via the prostatic and pelvic plexuses. Lymph vessels backtrack along the arteries.

Prostate

The prostate is a walnut-sized gland, weighing approximately 8 g in the young adult male and has a tendency to enlarge with age. It is inferior to the bladder surrounding the prostatic part of the male urethra. It is supported, anteriorly, by the puboprostatic ligaments and, inferiorly, by the urogenital diaphragm and lies directly behind the symphysis pubis. Posteriorly, it is separated from the rectum by the rectovesical fascia of Denonvilliers (Figs. 35.2 and 35.3).

It can be easily palpated through the rectal wall and feels, to the examining finger, to have a median sulcus separating the gland into right and left lobes. Structurally, the prostate is enveloped in a thin capsule which is firmly adherent and continuous with the stroma of the gland. It contains smooth muscle fibres, which necessarily surround the urethra and can be seen to be continuous with fibres from the neck of the bladder, thus forming the involuntary sphincter of the urethra. The stroma of the gland itself consists of much elastic tissue and smooth muscle fibres, in which are embedded many epithelial glands that drain, via 25 or so ducts, into the urethra in the sulcus lateral to the verumontanum.

Blood supply comes from the inferior vesical and middle rectal arteries and some from the internal pudendal. Venous drainage is via the prostatic plexus and veins to the internal iliac veins. A rich nervous innervation of both sympathetic and parasympathetic origin is found. Lymph drains to the hypogastric, sacral, vesical and external iliac nodes.

Penis and Male Urethra

The penis is the male organ of copulation. It contains erectile tissue that brings about an increase in length and rigidity to enable vaginal penetration to occur.

It consists of two parts — the root, attached to the urogenital diaphragm, and the body, which hangs limply and is completely covered in loose fitting skin. Internally, the penis consists of three main parts — the left and right corpora cavernosa, and the median corpus spongiosum. The corpora cavernosa take origin from the base of the pubic arch and the lateral aspect of the urogenital diaphragm, here called the crura. Passing forward, these two corpora meet in the midline and continue into the body of the penis. The corpus spongiosum contains the bulb and spongy parts of the male urethra and arises in the midline from the urogenital diaphragm. Here the urethra pierces the urogenital diaphragm to enter the corpus. The corpus continues forward into the pendulous portion and expands

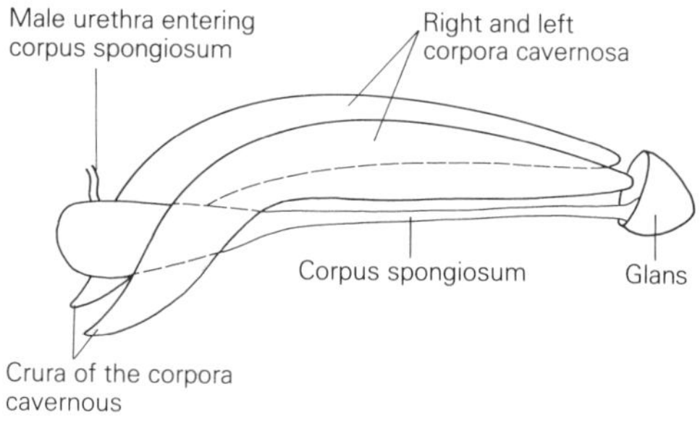

Fig. 35.4 *Diagrammatic representation of the corpora.*

distally as the glans penis. It lies on the ventral aspect of the two corpora cavernosa (Fig. 35.4).

Each corpora is surrounded by a strong fibrous membrane called the tunica albuginea. The tunica of the two corpora cavernosa are fused in the midline as the septum penis. Surrounding the three corpora is a loose fitting layer of fascia (Buck's fascia) that is continuous with fascia from the anterior abdominal wall and, covering the whole, is a loose layer of skin that distally extends as a hoodlike structure, the prepuce, which covers the glans penis. The body of the penis is supported by the suspensory ligament attached to the front of the pubic symphysis and blending with the tunica albuginea of the corpora cavernosa.

The blood supply is derived from the internal pudendal artery via three main branches. The bulbar artery pierces the urogenital diaphragm to enter the corpus spongiosum. Just distal to this artery, a second branch, the urethral artery, also pierces the diaphragm to follow the course of the urethra. Lastly, the penile artery divides into two branches — the deep artery, which pierces the urogenital diaphragm to supply each crura and corpus cavernosum, and the dorsal artery, which passes forward, under the arcuate ligament, into the dorsal aspect of the penis deep to the fascia. The dorsal artery sends some 5 or 6 circumflex branches around the shaft, forming a rich anastomosis, branches of which perforate the tunica albuginea and supply the corpus cavernosum as well.

Many arteriovenous anastomoses exist in the corpora and these play an important part in the mechanism of erection.

The venous drainage can be divided into three components.

1. *The superficial veins:* a rich network that merges as the superficial dorsal vein and empties usually into the left saphenous vein, but variants are common, e.g. the right saphenous vein, the epigastric and even the femoral veins.
2. *The intermediate veins* deep to Buck's fascia that drain into the deep dorsal vein which passes under the suspensory ligament and anterior to the anterior free edge of the urogenital diaphragm into the prostatic plexus.
3. *The deep veins* which drain the corpora directly into the pudendal prostatic plexus.

Emissary veins exist that communicate between the corpora and the deep dorsal vein and, also anastomoses exist between the superficial and deep dorsal veins. There are also veins communicating between the corpora spongiosum and the corpora cavernosa.

The nerve supply of the penis is composed of autonomic and somatic nerves. Tumescence occurs following stimulation of the parasympathetic nerve fibres from sacral segments 2, 3 and 4, while detumescence occurs following stimulation of sympathetic nerve fibres originating from the 10th and 11th thoracic to the second lumbar spinal segments. The pudendal nerve is primarily responsible for penile sensation and for contraction of the bulbar spongiosus and ischiocavernosus muscles which contribute to increased rigidity during erection and expulsion of ejaculatory fluids.

Lymph drains from the skin to the superficial inguinal nodes, from the glans to the deep inguinal and external iliac nodes, and from the urethra to the hypogastric and common iliac nodes.

Male urethra

The male urethra is divided into several parts — the prostatic part, within the prostate, 3 cm long, connects the bladder with the membranous part; the spongy urethra lies within the corpus spongiosum and terminates at the external urethral orifice. The urethra is lined with transitional epithelium throughout, except distally, where it becomes squamous.

PHYSIOLOGY

Normal male potency requires all the intrinsic parts of the reproductive system to function correctly and in conjunction. The various stages involved are spermatogenesis, transport of active spermatozoa, production of semen, erection and ejaculation.

Spermatogenesis

Spermatogenesis occurs in cycles, each consisting of three stages of approximately 23 days. Successive phases of the cycle occur at consecutive intervals along the length of the tubule. In the first place, the primitive germ cells replicate by mitotic division and produce several generations of spermatogonia. Each spermatogonium divides into two diploid primary spermatocytes, which undergo a meiotic or reduction division with the formation of two haploid spermatocytes. A second maturation division then occurs, resulting in four haploid spermatids arising from every primary spermatocyte. After a number of nuclear and cytoplasmic changes, the spermatids become spermatozoa. The mature spermatozoa is an actively motile cell consisting of two main parts. The head is covered in its anterior two-thirds by the acrosomal cap, and the tail provides motility and correct orientation at the time of fertilisation.

Steroidogenesis

Leydig cells of the testes produce 90% of circulating testosterone. The remainder comes from the adrenals and peripheral conversion of precursor steroids. Androgens are important for the development of the fetal genitalia and for the development and maintenance of secondary sexual characteristics and normal sexual activity. The very high intratesticular concentration of testosterone may be necessary for germ cell maturation.

Endocrine control of spermatogenesis

The testes are affected by the gonadotrophins, luteinising hormone (LH) and follicle stimulating hormone (FSH) (Fig. 35.5). Testicular hormones exert a negative feedback on LH production and, to a small extent, that of FSH. However, the failure of androgens to suppress FSH to normal levels after castration suggests an additional feedback mechanism. Inhibin, a peptide produced by the Sertoli cells, may be responsible for this. The Sertoli cells are probably the sole target for FSH within the testes. In response to both testosterone and FSH, they produce a high affinity androgen binding protein which maintains the high androgen content within the seminiferous tubules. Significantly elevated levels of LH and FSH are found in infertile men with severe degrees of germ cell damage. Normal levels of reproductive hormones in males are shown in Table 35.1.

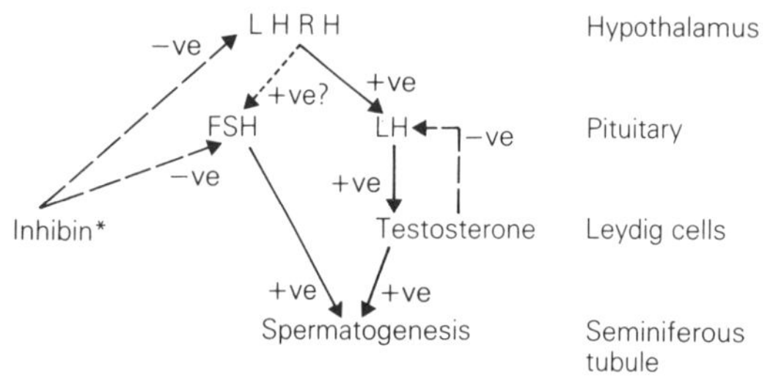

Fig. 35.5 *Hormonal control of spermatogenesis. Inhibin is a polypeptide hormone found in high levels in the seminiferous tubules. It has been shown to decrease FSH secretion. It is thus postulated that this hormone is the feedback required to control FSH secretion. It may prove to be useful as a male contraceptive.*

Table 35.1
Normal Levels of Reproductive Hormones in Males

Testosterone	10–28 nmol/l
Luteinising hormone	4–14 iu/l
Follicle stimulating hormone	1.5–8 iu/l
Prolactin	75–375 mu/l

Table 35.2
Chemical Content of Seminal Fluid

Seminal vesicle	50–80% (alkaline)	Fructose Phosphotidylcholine Vitamin C Prostaglandins Flavins
Prostate	15–30% (acid)	Spermine Citric acid Cholesterol and phospholipids Zinc Acid phosphatase Phosphatase and bicarbonate buffers
Cowpers glands		Enzymes Plasminogen activator

Semen

The bulk of the ejaculated fluid consists of secretions from the seminal vesicles and the prostate gland, 60% being produced from the seminal vesicles. Normal semen has a pH of 7.3–7.5 and a reasonable ejaculate volume would be 2.5–5 ml containing approximately 100×10^6 spermatozoa per ml (less than 20×10^6 normal spermatozoa per ml is likely to render the individual subfertile).

The chemical content of semen is summarised in Table 35.2. For semen to be impregnated, a two-part mechanism occurs — erection and ejaculation.

Erection

Erection involves the lengthening and increased rigidity of the penis and is essentially a vascular phenomenon. There has been much debate in the medical literature as to the relative importance of various events that occur. It would appear, however, that there are three components to erection.

1. Increased arterial flow.
2. Active relaxation of sinusoidal spaces within the corpora cavernosa.
3. Active and passive venous constriction.

Stimulation of the nerve supply to the corpora cavernosa produces a three-phase response.

1. *Latent phase:* the shaft increases in length with an increase in arterial flow (both systolic and diastolic) with no change in intracorporeal pressure, suggesting decrease in resistance to flow.
2. *Tumescence:* the corpora harden and there is an increase in intracorporeal pressure and, at the same time, arterial flow remains increased.
3. *Full erection:* the intracorporeal pressure reaches 5–10 mmHg below that of systolic aortic pressure and the flow decreases, but does stay higher than the pre-stimulation level.

Three pathways regulate penile smooth muscle relaxation — cGMP, cAMP and hyperpolarisation. Vasoactive intestinal polypeptide produced in the non-adrenergic non-cholinergic nerves, prostaglandins E1 and E2 in smooth muscle and neural or circulating catecholamines result in the stimulation of specific receptors coupled to G proteins. This activates adenylate cyclase and catalyses the formation of cyclic adenosine monophosphate cAMP. The increased concentration of cAMP stimulates cyclic AMP dependent protein kinase which results in a decrease in intracellular calcium and other ions and causes relaxation of the smooth muscle. Noradrenaline and adrenaline work by increasing intracellular calcium mobilisation resulting in smooth muscle contraction.

Nitric oxide causes relaxation by activating synthesis of an intracellular second messenger cyclic guanosine monophosphate (cGMP). The accumulation of cyclic GMP sets in motion a cascade of events at the intracellular level including hyperpolarisation, closure of voltage activated calcium channels, sequestration of calcium by intracellular organelles and a decrease in intracellular calcium. The result of these combined events is relaxation of the smooth muscle.

Venous leakage does cause some cases of human erectile dysfunction and this suggests that active venous constriction is a required mechanism. Venous leakage can be demonstrated by such techniques as dynamic cavernosography.

Ejaculation

Ejaculation is essentially a spinal reflex, but higher centres are also intricately involved. There are three phases:

1. Seminal emission
2. Formation of a pressure chamber
3. Expulsion of fluid from the urethra.

Seminal emission is controlled via the sympathetic nervous system and noradrenaline can be found in large quantities within the vas and ejaculatory ducts. Sympathetic stimulation results in contraction of the smooth muscle within the seminal vesicles, ejaculatory duct and prostate to express secretions into the prostatic urethra. As emission occurs, pressure increases within the urethra, between the vesicle neck and the urogenital diaphragm. It is this increase in pressure that forces fluid into the bulbar urethra. An intact and functioning bladder neck is required to prevent retrograde ejaculation into the bladder. Rhythmic contractions of the bladder neck under alpha-adrenergic stimulation have been demonstrated during ejaculation and, at the same time, relaxation of the external sphincter under somatic control via pudendal nerves allows semen to pass through the urogenital diaphragm into the bulbar urethra. Finally, expulsion of semen from the urethra is brought about by rhythmic contractions of the bulbospongiosus and bulbocavernosus muscles also under somatic control by the pudendal nerves.

Premature ejaculation is generally ascribed to anxiety. However there is evidence that hypersensitivity of the penile skin is present. There are many drugs which delay ejaculation and these can be used with effect to treat this condition. Alternatively counselling by a sex therapist may help.

Orgasm

Orgasm is the sensation of pleasure that normally accompanies the sequence of events already described. Part of the pleasure of orgasm is the feeling of tension and inevitability associated, temporarily with contraction of smooth muscle in the seminal vesicles and prostate, with the development of the pressure chamber and, finally, the release of ejaculation. Whether the contraction of smooth muscle is appreciated at a cortical level is unknown as, in other parts of the body, smooth muscle contraction is rarely associated with conscious appreciation.

The nervous pathways are obviously complicated and probably involve sensory information in both autonomic and somatic systems. Sensation, via the pudendal nerves, probably starts the sequence and a positive feedback circuit can be envisaged. As each phase begins, further sensory afferents are stimulated and the sensations summate as orgasm on ejaculation.

Orgasms can occur without sensory stimulation of the genitalia, as seen in the phantom orgasmic imagery of paraplegics and stimulation of the septal area of the brain can lead to the experience. It would appear, therefore, that there is a cortical association area that, when stimulated, leads to orgasm, either via sensory afferents or by some other mechanism.

Orgasm can occur without emission and ejaculation in this way and, similarly, emission and ejaculation can be brought about without local stimulation (the nocturnal emissions of adolescence).

Orgasm is, as yet, a subjective phenomenon, the neurophysiology involved being complicated and ill-understood.

Absence of orgasm

Congenital anorgasmia is a rare, but well defined, cause of total absence of ejaculation. Repression of the normal sexual responses, possibly brought about by an over-strict upbringing prevents the individual from achieving climax and ejaculation. Ejaculation can often be provoked by vibration but may require transanal electrical stimulation.

INFERTILITY

In the past, male dominated societies have been unable and unwilling to accept the fact that the male partner of an infertile marriage could be responsible. This is exemplified by many of the ancient gods such as Osiris of Egypt, Frey of Sweden and Priapus of the Romans being depicted with an erect or enlarged phallus. In India, 'sterile' women would visit temples of Siva, where they would press their naked bodies against the massive phallus of the god's statue.

Between 8% and 15% of marriages are childless, though not all of these are involuntary. Male disorders are responsible in 30% of couples and contributory in a further 20%. It is now accepted that the investigation and treatment of infertility involves both partners, and most centres now run clinics where the husband and wife are seen and investigated together. In younger couples, this is normally after two years of unprotected intercourse, though in couples where one partner is over the age of thirty, this period should be considerably less.

Treatment of the Male Problem

Until recently, the aim was to give the couple a prognosis based on the length of time of trying, testicular size, hormone levels, sperm count (Table 35.3) and testicular biopsy.

A very small proportion would be offered treatment of a varicocoele, an epididymovasostomy or deroofing of a Müllerian duct cyst or obstructed ejaculatory ducts.

Table 35.3
Abnormalities of Sperm Count

Azoospermia	Absence of sperm in the ejaculate
Severe oligospermia	$< 5 \times 10^6$ spermatozoa/ml
Oligospermia	$< 20 \times 10^6$ spermatozoa/ml
Asthenospermia	< 60% motile at 3 hours

The question that now needs to be asked is whether assisted reproduction technology should supersede attempts at surgical repair. The investigation of the infertile male now goes well beyond the conventional semen analysis. An increasing number of sperm function tests have now been described, including sperm capacitation, sperm morphology, sperm viability, measurement of reactive oxygen radicals, assessment of sperm ATP, acrosome reaction, etc.

The clinical history and physical examination are aimed at determining the likely cause, so that appropriate investigations for the individual patient, rather than a full battery of tests for all, can be carried out.

History and Examination

It is essential to see both partners together and individually. A history of a previous child does not exclude either partner from further investigation.

Fertility status is often a good reflection of general fitness, particularly in relation to smoking, alcohol intake and obesity, all of which impair spermatogenesis. The frequency and timing of intercourse is important, but knowledge of the fertile period is not essential. In cases where sexual intercourse is infrequent, due to absence of one or other partner, this knowledge becomes more important.

Occupational history

Exposure to pesticides, cadmium, lead, arsenic and zinc, and a variety of organic chemicals impairs spermatogenesis. Occupations which result in an increase in scrotal temperature, for example boiler workers, long-distance lorry drivers and fighter pilots, may impair fertility.

Drug history

Drugs used in the treatment of nematodes and many drugs used in the treatment of malignancy significantly affect spermatogenesis sometimes permanently. These include most alkylating agents, e.g. chlorambucil, cyclophosphamide, nitrogen mustard and melphelan. Other drugs such as sulphasalazine used in the treatment of ulcerative colitis results in oligospermia. Cimetidine and spironolactone inhibit androgen action, and ethanol, marijuana and opiates, through a variety of different mechanisms, may affect spermatogenesis (Table 35.4).

Medical history

Impaired spermatogenesis may occur in men with a history of undescended testes or previous scrotal or inguinal surgery. Many infections, including mumps, syphilis, gonorrhoea, tuberculosis and typhoid may result in an orchitis.

Table 35.4
Drugs Commonly Affecting Fertility

Chemotherapeutic agents	Effect	Recovery
Mustine Vincristine Prednisolone and Procarbazine	Invariable profound oliogospermia	Rare
Doxorubicin bleomycin Vinblastine docarbazine	Occasional azoospermia	Occasional
Chlorambucil	Azoospermia	Usual
Anabolic steroids	Oliogospermia	Usual
Sulphasalasine	Oliogospermia	Usual
Cimetidine Spironolactone	Androgen inhibition	Usual
Propranolol	Decreases motility	Usual

Epididymitis may result from infections due to *Chlamydia, Escherichia coli, Haemophilus, Klebsiella, Schistosoma haematobium, Histoplasma capsulatum, Toxoplasma* and *Blastomyces.* Some congenital chromosomal disorders also affect fertility, e.g. prune belly syndrome, cystic fibrosis, Kartagener's syndrome and Klinefelter's syndrome. Damage to the pituitary or hypothalmus may result in secondary infertility.

Physical examination

This is aimed at identifying syndromes associated with infertility and local abnormalities, which may impair sperm production or transport. The male partner should be examined in both the erect and supine positions with all clothes removed to assess build and any other general abnormalities suggestive of endocrine or chromosomal abnormality. In Klinefelter's syndrome (XXY), the limbs are disproportionately long in proportion to the trunk and gynaecomastia may be present. Gynaecomastia is also found in men with hyperprolactinaemia, though most men with this condition usually present with impotence or lack of libido rather than infertility. It is unusual for men with pituitary failure to present primarily with infertility.

Local examination

The penis. Meatal stenosis, phimosis or hypospadias may result in ineffective ejaculation and require correction. If erectile dysfunction is a problem it is more likely to be of psychogenic origin, if it was of rapid onset, occurs with one partner but not another, and with the maintenance of early morning or nocturnal erections. Such men and their partners should be seen by a psychosexual counsellor. Men with organic erectile dysfunction who are trying to produce a pregnancy should not be treated with intraurethral prostaglandins.

Scrotal contents. The testes should be examined for their position, consistency and size, the latter being measured by using an orchiometer for a more accurate assessment of volume. The epididymes are more often affected by infection than the testes. A hard irregular epididymis is often associated with a past history of venereal disease, bacterial epididymitis or tuberculosis. A swelling in the head of the epididymis may be associated with an obstruction. Both vasa deferentia should be palpated, as bilateral absence accounts for up to 2% of men attending an infertility clinic. The presence of a varicocoele should be sought with the patient standing, breathing quietly and also during a Valsalva manoeuvre. The use of Doppler or thermography increases the diagnostic accuracy. Ninety per cent of varicocoeles occur on the left, but they can occur solely on the right, or rarely bilaterally.

Abdomen. Both groins should be examined for scars from previous herniorrhaphies or attempts to locate or bring down an undescended testis. The prostate should always be examined and the expressed prostatic secretion collected and examined for the presence of white blood cells and bacteria.

Investigations

Seminology

Seminal analysis should be carried out after 3 days' abstinence from sexual intercourse and at least two samples, 3 weeks apart, should be examined. No more than 2 hours should pass from the time of ejaculation to the time of examination. The seminal fluid should be produced by masturbation and collected into a glass container with a screw cap. If coitus interruptus is used, the sperm-rich first part of the ejaculate is often lost. Condoms containing spermicides should not be used. Routine analysis (Table 35.5) will report volume, liquefaction, viscosity, motility, the presence of sperm agglutination, bacteria and leucocytes. The sperm density, i.e. numbers of sperm per ml, must always be related to the total sperm count. The percentage of abnormal forms is also

Table 35.5
Seminal Analysis — Normal Values and Common Causes of Abnormalities

Normal range	Abnormality	Common causes
Volume (2–6 ml)	Low	Inadequate collection, absent prostate and seminal vesicles, retrograde ejaculation
	High	Prolonged abstinence
Concentration (> 60 × 10^6 spermatozoa/ml)	Low	Chronic systemic disorders, acute febrile illness. Toxic agents or drugs, accessory gland infection, varicocoele, cryptorchidism
	High	Low seminal volume
	Absent	Epidydimal obstruction, absent vasa, absent spermatogonia. Drugs, toxic agents, pituitary failure, retrograde ejaculation
Motility (> 60% showing forward progressive at 3 hours)	Low	High scrotal temperature, occupations, varicocoele
Liquefaction complete in < 20 minutes	Failure	Prostatic infection
Agglutination > 10%	> 10%	Infection, antibodies
Bacteria None	Present	Prostatic infection, contamination, non-sterile container
Fructose	Absent	Absent prostate and seminal vesicles

reported. Unless the patient is azoospermic, it is difficult, using the above measurements, to provide an accurate prognosis for the individual patient.

Endocrine studies

It is not necessary to carry out endocrine studies in all patients. The majority of patients presenting with infertility have hormone changes secondary to seminiferous tubule damage rather than any primary endocrine abnormality. Acquired lesions of the pituitary may give rise to hypogonadotrophic hypogonadism, but this is usually associated with other pituitary defects, which require more urgent treatment.

Hyperprolactinaemia is usually associated with loss of libido and its significance in men presenting with infertility is doubtful on present evidence. A high FSH level in the presence of small testes signifies significant testicular damage, but not necessarily complete absence of sperm production, which can only be identified by carrying out a testicular biopsy.

Antibody studies

Autoantibodies to certain spermatozoal antigens can exert pathological effects causing infertility. Antibodies to sperm surface antigens are usually detected by agglutination or complement-mediated cytotoxic reactions. Approximately 10% of men from couples with unexplained infertility have antisperm antibodies. It is usual to examine their serum first and to test seminal plasma in all those with serum antibodies. Antibodies are more likely to be found in couples with a poor postcoital test, i.e. < 5 motile sperms per high power field present in normal pre-ovulatory cervical mucus. Antibodies are also likely to be present when there is massive agglutination of fresh semen.

A useful test for screening spermatozoa for antisperm antibodies is the mixed erythroctye spermatozoa antiglobulin reaction (MAR) test, which can detect both IgG and IgA antibodies. Using an indirect version of the technique, serum antibodies can be determined while a direct technique determines antibodies bound to the surface of spermatozoa in the ejaculate.

The clinical significance of serum titres of antibodies is determined using the sperm cervical mucus contact test. Using fertile donor sperm and normal cervical mucus as controls with sperm and cervical mucus from the infertile couple, positive evidence as to which partner is likely to have significant antibodies can be obtained. A positive reaction is shown by a change in sperm motility when in contact with cervical mucus. The spermatozoa change from a progressive movement to a characteristic non-progressive shaking or jerking movement.

Testicular biopsy

Testicular biopsy may be indicated in the following situations:

1. Azoospermia with a mild elevation of FSH to distinguish between obstruction, germinal cell damage, maturation arrest of the developing spermatozoa or the Sertoli cell only syndrome, where the patient is born without spermatogonia.
2. Severe oligospermia with normal FSH.
3. In fertility of long duration with non-contributory tests on both husband and wife. Certain rare disorders of meiosis may be detected by meiotic analysis.
4. Where chemicals or cytotoxic agents might be implicated as a cause of fertility.
5. Extraction of sperm from the testis or epididymis for assisted reproduction techniques.

Treatment of Specific Clinical Situations

Varicocoele

The mechanisms by which a varicocoele affects testicular function and how often this occurs in the male population is not known. Many patients with varicocoeles have normal fertility. One suggested mechanism is the bilateral elevation of testicular temperature. Reflux of adrenal metabolites, changes in prostaglandin levels and alteration in testosterone levels have also been reported in association with a varicocoele. There are many reports of improvement in semen quality and an increased rate of pregnancy after varicocoele ligation. However, there are also reports questioning the efficacy of varicocoelectomy in subfertile men. In one controlled study, no changes were seen in motility and motile sperm count following varicocoelectomy compared with preoperative sperm counts when there were less than 10 million per ml. Treatment of a varicocoele by embolisation of the testicular veins is the treatment of choice. The treatment of varicocoeles is still controversial and before infertility is ascribed to the presence of a varicocoele, it is important to ensure that the female partner is normal.

Azoospermia

The complete absence of sperm on seminal analysis is usually due to a blockage of sperm transport or spermatogenic arrest, i.e. a failure at some stage during sperm production, in which case the plasma FSH will be normal. Other causes such as anorchism, germinal aplasia (Sertoli cell only syndrome) or previous cytotoxic therapy will usually be associated with an elevated FSH level. The presence of small testes and grossly elevated FSH levels requires counselling of the couple with regard to the almost hopeless prognosis. However, the absence of sperm production can only be shown by performing a testicular biopsy. If the FSH and testicular size are normal, operation should be advised. This enables the testes and epididymes to be inspected, to perform vasography, to biopsy the testicles and carry out any reconstructive procedure that may be indicated. The results of surgery for obstruction in the epididymis, however, are not good.

If mature spermatozoa are present, these may be used in assisted conception techniques.

Antisperm antibodies

If it has been decided that antisperm antibodies are significantly interfering with fertility and that the wife has patent tubes and ovulation is occurring regularly, then treatment of the male partner should be initiated. Treatments include artificial insemination after sperm washing, prednisolone, given either as a long-term low dose regimen or in a high dose given to the male on days 21–28 of his wife's menstrual cycle. Side-effects such as dyspepsia, haematemesis, diabetes, acne or avascular necrosis of bone may occur and the patient must be advised accordingly. The degree of response to treatment can be checked using the MAR and postcoital tests.

Erectile and ejaculatory disorders

Organic impotence due to previous trauma, operations, priapism, neuropathy or vascular insufficiency are probably best treated, provided there is no contraindication, by the phosphodiasterase inhibitor sildenafil or by autoinjection of vasoactive drugs. The results of microsurgical revascularisation of the penile arteries have so far been disappointing. Patients with psychogenic impotence should be seen by a therapist with a particular interest in this type of disorder. Ejaculatory disorders, such as premature ejaculation or failure to ejaculate, usually require psychosexual counselling. Premature ejaculation sometimes responds to treatment with Clomipramine taken an hour before intercourse. A complete inability to ejaculate may be treated using a vibrating device or electrical stimulation. Retrograde ejaculation is the most common cause of an absent ejaculate. The semen passes backwards through the bladder neck into the bladder. This is usually due to congenital dysfunction of the bladder neck, previous surgery to the bladder neck such as bladder neck incision, or surgical injury causing damage to the sympathetic supply to the bladder neck. It is common in diabetics with autonomic neuropathy. It is sometimes helped by ejaculating with the bladder full or taking a sympathomimetic agent such as ephedrine an hour before intercourse. Occasionally, surgery may be required, or retrieval from the bladder of semen by post-ejaculatory catheterisation and artificial insemination.

Other Treatments

The Human Fertilisation of Embryology Authority (HFEA) licenses and monitors clinics which carry out IVF. Successful treatment occurs in approximately 20% of couples.

Artificial insemination

This may be used in men with premature ejaculation, erectile dysfunction or anatomical abnormalities.

In vitro fertilisation

This may be used in men with a low sperm count. After hormone stimulation eggs are collected from the female and mixed with sperm. Fertilisation occurs in a culture dish.

Intracytoplasmic sperm injection

Eggs are again collected after hormone stimulation, a single sperm being injected directly into each egg. A maximum of three fertilised eggs can be transferred back into the uterus.

Surgical sperm recovery

Sperm can be collected from either the testis or the epididymis by open surgery or microaspiration.

Donor insemination

Sperm from an anonymous donor is utilised. The anonymity of the donor may not be protected in the future.

FURTHER READING

Royal College of Obstetricians and Gynaecologists Guidelines, Internet www.rcog.org.uk/guidelines/infertile.html

Whitfield H.N., Hendry W.F., Kirby R.S., Duckett J.W., eds. (1997). *Textbook of Genitourinary Surgery*, 2nd ed., Vol. 2, pp. 111–23. Oxford: Blackwells Science, Publishers.

Index